Handbook
of
Neurorehabilitation

NEUROLOGICAL DISEASE AND THERAPY

Series Editor

WILLIAM C. KOLLER

Department of Neurology
University of Kansas Medical Center
Kansas City, Kansas

Handbook

of

Neurorehabilitation

edited by

David C. Good
Bowman Gray School of Medicine
Wake Forest University
Winston-Salem, North Carolina

James R. Couch, Jr.
The University of Oklahoma Health Science Center
Oklahoma City, Oklahoma

Marcel Dekker, Inc.   **New York•Basel•Hong Kong**

Library of Congress Cataloging-in-Publication Data

Handbook of neurorehabilitation / edited by David C. Good, James R.
  Couch, Jr.
      p.   cm. – (Neurological disease and therapy ; v. 24)
      Includes bibliographical references and index.
      ISBN 0-8247-8822-2 (alk. paper)
      1. Nervous system–Diseases–Patients–Rehabilitation.   I. Good,
  David C. II. Couch, James R. III. Series.
      [DNLM: 1. Nervous System Diseases–rehabilitation.   W1 NE33LD
  v.24 1994 / WL 100 H2368 1994]
  RC350.4.H36 1994
  616.8'043–dc20
  DNLM/DLC
  for Library of Congress   93-42706
                                                                              CIP

The publisher offers discounts on this book when ordered in bulk quantities.
For more information, write to Special Sales/Professional Marketing at the
address below.

This book is printed on acid-free paper.

Marcel Dekker, Inc.
270 Madison Avenue, New York, New York 10016

Current printing (last digit):
10 9 8 7 6 5 4 3 2 1

PRINTED IN THE UNITED STATES OF AMERICA

Series Introduction

An increasingly important area of neurology deals with rehabilitation after neuronal injury. The basic knowledge of neuronal recovery and plasticity has increased greatly in the recent past. It has become apparent that with the appropriate intervention we can increase the prospects of recovery for a variety of neurological conditions. Nonetheless, in many neurological residency training programs there is little emphasis on neurological rehabilitation. The *Handbook of Neurorehabilitation* attempts to fill this void in knowledge for all physicians who care for neurologically impaired patients. General concepts of neurorehabilitation are discussed first, followed by an in-depth discussion of outcome measures that are important in the rehabilitation process. The authors next discuss a variety of treatments, both medical and nonmedical. The use of these strategies to improve the quality of life for patients with neurological deficits is undoubtedly an important one and one that is sometimes overlooked. Specific medical problems such as bladder dysfunction and pain management are also discussed. Lastly, The *Handbook of Neurorehabilitation* discusses specific disease entities and problems in rehabilitation that are unique to these conditions, including such important entities as stroke, traumatic brain injury, spinal cord injury, multiple sclerosis, and neurodegenerative diseases.

The *Handbook of Neurorehabilitation* by Drs. Good and Couch and their contributors provides current, up-to-date information on the important area of rehabilitation. The book is comprehensive, yet practical in its approach in keeping with this series. The information presented in this book, if properly applied to the patient with nervous system injury, will undoubtedly result in better care of patients with these neurological problems.

William C. Koller

Preface

During recent years, there has been a growing interest in the rehabilitation of neurological disease for a number of reasons. Research has suggested that the nervous system possesses greater degrees of plasticity than once thought. The aging population will result in more patients with neurological deficits and chronic neurological disease. With the "graying of the population," there is also increased financial and social pressure to ensure that elderly persons remain independent and active for as long as possible. There is new inquisitiveness about traditional rehabilitation concepts as well as an interest in determining which are effective and the neurophysiological basis for this effectiveness. Finally, there is a growing interest in rehabilitation on the part of physicians who care for patients with acute neurological conditions.

Despite the increased interest in neurological rehabilitation, most neurological training programs have lagged behind in providing an adequate experience in this area. Furthermore, while many rehabilitation textbooks have been written, very few have been dedicated solely to neurological conditions or written from the perspective of neurological clinicians.

Obviously, not every topic can be discussed. However, the topics have been chosen to meet the needs of clinicians who care for common neurological conditions. Important aspects of the scientific basis for rehabilitation are examined. Much of the book is intended to provide a practical source of information.

The first portion of this book deals with the underlying scientific evidence and theory that provide the basis for clinical neurorehabilitation. In the second portion, important organizational and social factors that are important to the rehabilitation process are introduced. The available methods for assessing current functional status and predicting outcome are also reviewed. The third section of the book discusses specific treatments available to clinicians interested in neurorehabilitation, including traditional approaches, as well as new concepts and ideas, some of which are in their infancy. The next section is devoted to the practical management of specific medical problems common to many patients undergoing rehabilitation, regardless of diagnosis. The final section is devoted to the rehabilitation of specific types of neurological illness or injury.

We would like to thank the many contributors to this volume for their dedication in producing a unique text. We hope the reader captures some of the excitement that the new interest in neurorehabilitation has engendered, is motivated to learn more about this area and, most importantly, is inspired to apply what is learned to the betterment of patient care.

David C. Good
James R. Couch, Jr.

Contents

Contributors

Mindy L. Aisen, M.D.   Chief of Spinal Cord Injury, Department of Neurology, Cornell University Medical College, The Winifred Masterson Burke Rehabilitation Hospital, Inc., White Plains, New York

David N. Alexander, M.D.   Director of Stroke Rehabilitation, Center for Diagnostic and Rehabilitation Medicine, Daniel Freeman Hospital, Inglewood, and Assistant Clinical Professor, Department of Neurology, UCLA School of Medicine, Los Angeles, California

Michael P. Alexander, M.D.   Director, Stroke Programs, Braintree Hospital, Braintree, and Associate Professor, Department of Neurology, Boston University School of Medicine, Boston, Massachusetts

Hugues Barbeau, Ph.D.   Professor, School of Physical and Occupational Therapy, McGill University, Montreal, Quebec, Canada

Michael J. Brennan, M.D.   Medical Director, The Rehabilitation Center of Fairfield County, Bridgeport, Connecticut

James R. Couch, Jr., M.D., Ph.D.   Professor and Chairman, Department of Neurology, The University of Oklahoma Health Sciences Center, Oklahoma City, Oklahoma

Mary L. Dombovy, M.D.   Assistant Professor, Department of Neurology and Orthopedics, University of Rochester, and Chairperson, Department of Physical Medicine and Rehabilitation, St. Mary's Hospital, Rochester, New York

Rodger J. Elble, M.D., Ph.D.   Director, Center for Alzheimer Disease and Related Disorders, and Interim Chairman, Department of Neurology, Southern Illinois University School of Medicine, Springfield, Illinois

Joyce Fung, P.T., Ph.D.   Research Associate, R. S. Dow Neurological Sciences Institute, Portland, Oregon

David A. Gelber, M.D.   Assistant Professor, Department of Neurology, Southern Illinois University School of Medicine, and Medical Director of Rehabilitation, Memorial Medical Center, Springfield, Illinois

Larry B. Goldstein, M.D.   Assistant Professor of Medicine, Division of Neurology, and Assistant Research Professor, Center for Health Policy Research and Education, Duke University, and Durham Department of Veterans Affairs Medical Center, Durham, North Carolina

David C. Good, M.D.   Associate Professor of Neurology, Director of Rehabilitation, Bowman Gray School of Medicine, Wake Forest University, Winston-Salem, North Carolina

Susan T. Iannaccone, M.D.   Associate Professor, Department of Neurology, University of Texas Southwestern Medical Center, Dallas, Texas

Patricia B. Jozefczyk, M.D.   Associate Professor, Department of Neurology, University of Pittsburgh School of Medicine, Pittsburgh, Pennsylvania

Douglas I. Katz, M.D.   Clinical Director, Traumatic Brain Injury Program, Braintree Hospital, Braintree, and Assistant Professor, Department of Neurology, Boston University School of Medicine, Boston, Massachusetts

Laurie Laven, M.D.   National Rehabilitation Hospital, Washington, D.C.

Richard B. Lazar, M.D.   Assistant Clinical Professor, Schwab Rehabilitation Hospital and Care Network, and Departments of Physical Medicine and Rehabilitation, and Neurology, Northwestern University Medical School, Chicago, Illinois

Laura Lennihan, M.D. Assistant Professor, Department of Clinical Neurology, College of Physicians and Surgeons of Columbia University, New York, and Director, Department of Stroke Rehabilitation, Helen Hayes Hospital, West Haverstraw, New York

Bala V. Manyam, M.D. Professor, Department of Neurology, and Director, Parkinson's Disease and Movement Disorders Clinic, Southern Illinois University School of Medicine, Springfield, Illinois

Catherine A. Mateer, Ph.D. Director, Good Samaritan Neuropsychological Services, Good Samaritan Hospital, Puyallup, Washington

John W. Michael, M.Ed., C.P.O. Director, Professional and Technical Services, Otto Bock U.S.A., Minneapolis, Minnesota

Norman S. Namerow, M.D. Medical Director, Center for Diagnostic and Rehabilitation Medicine, Daniel Freeman Memorial Hospital, Inglewood, and Clinical Professor, Department of Neurology, UCLA School of Medicine, Los Angeles, California

Ronald Pak, M.D. Department of Physical Medicine and Rehabilitation, University of Rochester and St. Mary's Hospital, Rochester, New York

Russell K. Portenoy, M.D. Director of Analgesic Studies, Pain Service, Department of Neurology, Memorial Sloan-Kettering Cancer Center, New York, and Associate Professor of Neurology, Cornell University Medical College, White Plains, New York

Steven J. Price, M.D. Attending Neurologist, Department of Medicine, Appleton Medical Center, Novus Health Group, Appleton, Wisconsin

Sarah A. Raskin, Ph.D. Neuropsychologist, Good Samaritan Neuropsychological Services, Good Samaritan Hospital, Puyallup, Washington

Michael J. Reding, M.D. Associate Professor of Neurology, Department of Neurorehabilitation, Cornell University Medical College, The Winifred Masterson Burke Rehabilitation Hospital, Inc., White Plains, New York

Peter W. Rossi, M.D. Medical Director, Rehabilitation Hospital of South Texas, Corpus Christi, and Clinical Assistant Professor, University of Texas at San Antonio Health Science Center, San Antonio, Texas

Susan M. Rubin, M.D. Neurologist and Fellow in Neurophysiology, Department of Neurology, Northwestern University Medical School, Chicago, Illinois

Randall T. Schapiro, M.D. Director, Fairview Multiple Sclerosis Center, and Clinical Professor, Department of Neurology, University of Minnesota, Minneapolis, Minnesota

I
GENERAL CONCEPTS

1

History and Physical Examination in Neurorehabilitation

Norman S. Namerow

Daniel Freeman Memorial Hospital
Inglewood, and
UCLA School of Medicine
Los Angeles, California

INTRODUCTION

Assessment of the patient undergoing neurorehabilitation will vary considerably depending on the nature of the underlying neurological illness, the patient's deficits, and, to a certain extent, the setting in which the examination is performed. For example, the evaluation of the hospitalized severely brain injured patient with cognitive and corticospinal tract impairment will differ from the inpatient recovering from Guillain-Barré syndrome or the outpatient with spinal cord injury. The physician will therefore need a repertoire of clinical tests from which to draw in order to perform a comprehensive examination, yet must be capable of performing a more selective and detailed examination, as the situation warrants.

Because of its general nature this chapter will be broadly descriptive, but each portion of the chapter can be found in greater depth in a variety of articles and texts [1–5]. A special effort, however, will be made to relate the traditional history and physical examination to the needs of patients participating in rehabilitation.

The assessment of the patient undergoing neurorehabilitation requires a basic neurological examination coupled with a detailed musculoskeletal examination and a general physical examination. In addition, the examination must also include the vital aspect of function. This consideration of function makes the neurorehabilitation examination unique. That is, beyond the concept of impairment, which is the focus of most examinations, there must also be a consideration of how the patient functions, and whether and to what extent he or she has a disability. This disability, in turn, may result in a social or vocational handicap. The difference between impairment, disability, and handicap must be clearly understood for the effective communication of a patient's status. Reference is made to the World Health Organization Definition of Disease Outcome for further discussion on this important issue [6] (also see Chapter 7).

THE HISTORY

As with all examinations, the clinician should begin with careful history taking. This has the dual purpose of elucidating what has occurred medically prior to the patient coming to the physician's attention and is the first step in assessing behavioral, cognitive, and language functioning. During the process of taking a history, the physician can quickly gauge the patient's attention span, distractibility, memory, impulsiveness, perseveration, confusion, language disturbance, and other cognitive functions. Behaviors are also important to note, especially in patients referred for such rehabilitation programs as pain management and brain injury.

As indicated previously, the functional aspect of both the history and physical examination sets the neurorehabilitation evaluation apart from other specialty examinations. It is particularly important to have a good sense of the patient's functional abilities just before the injury or illness that necessitated referral to the neurorehabilitation service. Goal setting and discharge planning will be highly dependent upon the patient's previous level of function, as well as the patient's desired functional level after illness. It is not unusual to find the acute hospitalization history and physical examination, as well as consultations, to be inadequate for rehabilitation purposes. These may refer to an injury or the onset of symptoms, but often do not spell out how the patient was functioning before the injury or illness, if assistive aids were utilized, or if the illness had an impact on work performance, mobility, or independence. It is therefore particularly important that a family member or significant other be available to provide these important aspects of the history, especially if the patient has cognitive or language deficits.

The chief complaint is typically the medical condition or symptom that brought about the patient's functional impairment, and for rehabilitation purposes this is usually self-evident. However, less obvious problems may also affect rehabilitation. For example, disuse myopathy in a patient who has had a protracted and disabling illness must be clearly identified in addition to the primary illness and its main symptoms. Whatever the underlying diagnosis, there must be physical impairments resulting in functional disabilities that warrant rehabilitation therapy. The typical example would be a patient with stroke (diagnosis) with a right hemiparesis, hemisensory loss, hemianopsia, and aphasia (physical impairments), producing an inability to transfer, walk, or communicate (disabilities).

The past medical history and system review are crucial to determining a patient's rehabilitation program and establishing goals and objectives. Functional limitations as a consequence of various diseases, in addition to the chief complaint and primary diagnosis, must also be identified. In occasional cases, comorbidity and a superseding illness may prevent optimal rehabilitation. For example, angina may be a limiting factor in the rehabilitation of an individual who had a recent cerebrovascular accident (CVA) and an associated hemiparesis. A thorough system review is therefore mandatory, focusing on conditions that have the potential to impede rehabilitation efforts. Also of concern are bladder and bowel symptoms associated with the presenting problem.

The personal and social history must be reviewed in some detail. The availability of a strong family structure may be more important in determining the patient's discharge destination than any therapeutic effort. The neurorehabilitation history would not be complete without a detailed vocational or school history. Both clinician and patient must have a target activity and functional level to aim for, and, depending upon the desired scope and level of postillness activity, objectives and therapeutic options may widely vary.

THE PHYSICAL EXAMINATION

The physical examination is basically that which most general medical clinicians perform on their patients, but with three additions. Beside the general physical examination, detailed neurological and musculoskeletal evaluations must be performed. Also, the patient's physical functional abilities must be documented as thoroughly as the location of the examination will allow. More detailed functional performance can be supplied by individual therapists (e.g., occupational therapists) who can typically provide a real-life situation in which to gauge the patient's abilities.

The order of examination is not as important as the concept of developing a system of approach so that no aspect of the patient's clinical condition is overlooked. I prefer to evaluate the patient by performing the neurological examination first, perhaps from long familiarity with this procedure. During the motor portion of the neurological examination, a more expansive musculoskeletal examination can be done. Following the neurological aspects, a more general examination including an evaluation of the neck, heart, lungs, abdomen, skin, genitalia, bladder, and bowel can be completed. Many details of the neurological and muscle examination will not be discussed in depth here; such examinations have been well described in many texts that are readily available. De Jong's *The Neurological Examination*, for example, is an excellent reference that describes many examination techniques [1]. Additional useful references are texts by Chusid [4] and Haymaker [2].

A careful physical examination of a patient referred for neurorehabilitation will occasionally uncover unsuspected abnormalities resulting in a change in diagnosis. The rehabilitation physician should examine the patient with the intent of determining how abnormalities demonstrated on examination may result in functional disabilities or affect the rehabilitation program. This requires a shift in mental paradigm away from the traditional use of the physical examination for the diagnosis of illness. In the following description of the neurological and musculoskeletal examinations, areas of special relevance to rehabilitation will be highlighted in order to facilitate this subtle but important shift in focus.

The neurological examination begins with an assessment of the patient's mental functioning and cognitive status. First, orientation is assessed by seeking recognition of person, place, time, and events. Comment should be made on the patient's attention span, ease of distraction, the presence and level of confusion, perseveration, and the ability to recall specific information. The patient should be tested for ability to follow one-, two-, or three-step commands. Attention can be tested by offering a series of digits and asking the patient to repeat the digits in sequence. A normal response would be to remember six digits forward and at least five digits backward. Short-term memory for new information can be tested by asking the patient to remember three words, then requesting the patient to repeat these words after 3 min. Recent memory and attention are both critical for the acquisition of the new skills important for a successful rehabilitation outcome. Although of less importance to rehabilitation, remote memory may be assessed by asking for historical information such as place of birth, schools attended, telephone numbers and names of family and friends, and names of actors or characters on favorite television shows. Additional information to be obtained concerns the patient's fund of knowledge (current events, geography) and his or her ability to calculate. The ability to abstract can be assessed by offering the patient proverbs or a brief story and asking for an interpretation. An inadequate or concrete response would be an indication of frontal lobe dysfunction. During the interview, appropriateness of thought and action should also be noted. Evidence of inappropriateness or poor judgment suggests that the patient may have poor insight into his or her deficits, may be uncooperative during therapy, and may be at risk for injury during physical tasks.

The mental status examination should also include the patient's mood and affect. A determination of euphoria or whether the patient's affect is blunted or flattened should be made. A flattened affect may be due to depression, but may also be related to medication or reflect a poverty of animation and initiation secondary to frontal lobe dysfunction. Depression and frontal lobe dysfunction may both affect rehabilitation outcome but should be differentiated, since each is managed differently. Inappropriate laughter or crying, both a sign of frontal lobe disease or injury, should also be identified. These symptoms are very distressing to patients and families and can be disruptive to the rehabilitation process. For a more formal but still brief cognitive evaluation, the Mini-Mental State Examination can be used (Table 1). This instrument is reliable and its utility has been demonstrated

Table 1 Mini Mental State Examination

Maximum Score	Score	
		Orientation
5	( )	What is the (year) (season) (date) (day) (month)?
5	( )	Where are we: (state) (country) (town) (hospital) (floor)?
		Registration
3	( )	Name three objects, 1 sec to say each, then ask the patient to repeat all three after you have said them. Give one point for each correct answer. Continue repeating all three objects until the patient learns all three. Count trials and record.
		Attention and Calculation
5	( )	Serial 7s. One point for each correct response. Stop after five answers. As an alternative, spell "world" backward.
		Recall
3	( )	Ask for the three objects named in Registration. Give one point for each correct answer.
		Language
2	( )	Name a pencil and watch.
1	( )	Repeat the following "No ifs, ands, or buts."
3	( )	Follow a 3-stage command: "Take paper in your right hand, fold it in half, and put it on the floor."
1	( )	Read and obey the following: CLOSE YOUR EYES.
1	( )	Write a sentence.
1	( )	Copy a design
30		
		Assess level of consciousness along a continuum
Alert	Drowsy	Stupor Coma

Source: From ref. [7].

over the past 18 years [7]. The Mini-Mental State is especially valuable as a screen for dementia, which may impair rehabilitation efforts.

Next, the cranial nerves should be tested (nerves I–XII). Olfaction (I) can be tested by opening a small container of coffee or cloves beneath one of the patient's nostrils, then the other. Occasional patients undergoing rehabilitation may have an impaired sense of smell, especially patients with inferior frontal brain injury or basilar skull fractures disrupting the olfactory nerves. It is important to document visual acuity (II). At the bedside this is typically recorded with a handheld vision chart, and with ocular correction (the use of eyeglasses). In an office setting, a 20-foot visual acuity testing lane is a better means of measurement. Visual fields should be tested to gross confrontation, and the fundi should be visualized. Poor visual acuity or the presence of a visual field defect is common in patients undergoing rehabilitation and may require compensatory strategies. Pupillary responses and extraocular movements should be documented. Abnormal movements such as a gaze palsy (dysconjugate eye movements), nystagmus, or paresis of ocular muscles (III, IV, VI) should be noted. When ocular paresis results in diplopia, subjective dizziness and altered depth perception may affect the patient's ability to participate in rehabilitation. Facial sensation (V) should be tested next. All three divisions (ophthalmic, mandibular and maxillary) of the 5th cranial nerve should be evaluated for both light touch and pain. It is important to test the corneal reflex and the nasociliary response, since these may be the only ways to determine if sensory loss is present in a patient who is unable to communicate. Motor function of nerve V can be tested by palpating the masseter muscles during jaw clenching. Facial strength (VII) should be assessed by observation (facial asymmetry), and by testing strength of the frontalis, orbicularis oculi, and orbicularis oris muscles. Peripheral VII nerve lesions will weaken the entire face, while central lesions will primarily affect the lower facial muscles. In addition to altered cosmesis, facial weakness may affect labial articulation and result in pocketing of food inside the cheek, requiring compensatory techniques. Sensory VII nerve function (taste) can be tested by using salt or sugar solutions placed on the anterior and lateral portions of the tongue. Test one side and then the other, with the patient's tongue protruded. Hearing (VIII) can be adequately tested with a tuning fork or by whispering in one or the other ear and eliciting an appropriate response from the patient. In an elderly population hearing loss is very common, and may be of such severity that communication with family and professional staff is impaired.

The position of the uvula and the direction of retraction of the uvula on stimulating the pharynx should be observed (IX, X), along with the size of the tongue and the direction the tongue points on forced protrusion (XII). The protruded tongue will deviate toward the side of weakness. Dysfunction of cranial nerves IX, X, and XII results in a variety of disturbances of articulation and phonation, as well as oropharyngeal dysphagia. Testing the strength of the sternocleidomastoid muscles (XI) and trapezius muscles (XI) bilaterally completes the formal cranial nerve examination.

At this point, it is often convenient to perform some brief functional testing related to the cranial nerves. First the patient's swallowing competency should be tested. The patient's ability to cough and swallow his or her own saliva should therefore be checked. If both are weak, offer a small amount of pureed food. If the patient chokes or otherwise does not swallow appropriately, more accurate testing should include videofluoroscopy, which is now available in most major medical centers.

The rate and rhythm of speech should be noted next, as well as the clarity of enunciation. Dysarthria is a common neurological observation in patients with both central (brain stem and brain) and peripheral (brain stem and nerve) lesions. At this time, the patient's language and ability to communicate should be further evaluated by assessing the ability to understand and follow simple one- and two-step commands. The patient's ability to express him- or herself and name objects and their use should also be noted. Look for word finding problems, circumlocutory speech, and fluent expression. One may offer the patient a magazine or newspaper and document the ability to read and understand what is being read. Writing is tested next. It is important during all these activities to document whether there is unilateral neglect, particularly following right parietal lesions. Neglect may affect vision or body organization and in some patients can be one of the most frustrating impairments limiting rehabilitation.

The next major neurological system to examine is the motor system. Strength and tone of all muscle groups in the upper and lower extremities should be documented. The most prevalent means of documenting strength is to utilize the British scheme of 5 as normal strength, 4 for mild weakness but with active movement against resistance, 3 as the ability to move a joint against gravity, 2 when there is movement only if gravity is eliminated, 1 when a flicker of motion is present, and 0 when no motion or muscle contraction whatsoever is observed [8]. In the specific case of a patient with a spinal cord injury, a frequently used classification scheme for residual function is shown in Table 2 [9]. Muscle innervation and resultant joint movement are briefly summarized in Table 3 [3]. It should be stressed that muscles must be observed for atrophy and fasciculations, as well as tested for strength. As the motor system is tested, the examiner should consider the functional implications of the pattern of weakness detected. As part of the motor examination, it is also important to test the patient's ability to stand and walk. The gait is described as to speed, fluidity, stiffness, unilaterality of deficit, associated arm movements, and the ability to turn and pivot without diffi-

Table 2 Frankel Classification of Residual Function

Grade	Description of Deficit
A	Complete loss of function: no motor or sensory function below level of lesion
B	Paralysis below lesion level; sensation preserved
C	Some motor activity preserved below lesion level
D	Functional motor strength preserved below lesion level
E	Recovery with no neurological deficits

Source: From ref. [9].

Table 3 Muscle Innervation

Joint	Movement	Main Muscles	Nerve	Main Roots
Shoulder	Adduction	Latissimus dorsi	Thoracodorsal	C(6)–7–8
		Pectoralis major	Pectoral	C6–T1
	Abduction	Supraspinatus	Suprascapular	C5 (6)
		Deltoid	Axillary	C5 (6)
	Flexion	Deltoid		
	Extension	Deltoid		
		Latissimus dorsi		
	Internal	Latissimus dorsi		
	Rotation	Subscapularis	Subscapular	C5–6
	External	Teres minor	Axillary	C4–5
	Rotation	Supraspinatus		
		Infraspinatus	Suprascapular	C5 (6)
Elbow	Flexion	Brachialis	Musculocutaneous	C5–6
		Biceps	Musculocutaneous	C5–6
		Brachioradialis	Radial	C5–6
	Extension	Triceps	Radial	C6–7–8
	Supination	Biceps		
		Supinator	Radial	C(5)6(7)
	Pronation	Pronator teres	Median	C6–7
Wrist	Flexion	Fl. carpi radialis	Median	C6–7
		Fl. carpi ulnaris	Ulnar	C7–8
	Extension	Ext. carpi radialis longus and brevis	Radial	C6–7(8)
		Ext. carpi ulnaris	P. interosseous	C7–8
Metacarpo-phalangeal	Flexion	Lumbricales	Median and ulnar	C8–T1
		Interossei	Ulnar	C8–T1
	Extension	Ext. digitorum	Radial	C7–8
Interpha-langeal	Flexion	Fl. digitorum sublimis	Median	C(7)–8–T1
		Fl. digitorum profundus	Median and ulnar	C7–8–T1

Table 3 Continued

Joint	Movement	Main Muscles	Nerve	Main Roots
	Extensor	Ext. digitorum		
		Lumbricals		
	Adduction	Interossei		
	Abduction	Interossei		
Thumb	Flexion	Fl. pollicis longus	Median	C7–8–T1
		Fl. pollicis brevis	Median	C8–T1
	Extension	Ext. pollicis longus	P. interosseous	C7–8–T1
		Ext. pollicis brevis	P. interosseous	C8–T1
	Adduction	Add. pollicis	Ulnar	C8–T1
	Abduction	Abd. pollicis longus	P. interosseous	C7–8
		Abd. pollicis brevis	Median	C8–T1
	Opposition	Opp. pollicis	Median	C6–7–8
Trunk		Diaphragm	Phrenic	C3–4–5
		Rhomboids	Dorsal scapular	C5
		Serratus ant.	Long thoracic	C5–6–7
		Sacrospinalis gp.	Segmental at all levels	
		Intercostals	Segmental	T1–12
		Rectus abdominis	Segmental	T5–12
		Levator ani	Pudendal	S3–4–5
Hip	Flexion	Iliopsoas	Femoral	L2–3
		Tensor fascia lata	Sup. gluteal	L4–5
	Extension	Gluteus max.	Inf. gluteal	L5–S1–2
		Hamstrings	Sciatic	L5–S1–2
	Adduction	Adductor gp.	Obturator	L2–3–4
	Abduction	Gluteus med.	Sup. gluteal	L4–5–S1
		Gluteus min.		
Knee	Flexion	Hamstrings		
	Extension	Quadriceps	Femoral	L2–3–4
Ankle	Plantar flexion	Gastrocnemius	Tibial	S1–2
		Soleus	Tibial	L(5)–S1–2
		Tibialis post.	Tibial	L5–S1
	Dorsiflexion	Tibialis ant.	Peroneal	L4–5
	Inversion	Tibialis post.		
	Eversion	Peronei	Peroneal	L4–5–S1
Toe	Plantar flexion	Fl. digitorum long.	Tibial	L5–S1(2)
		Fl. digitorum brev.	Tibial	L5–S1(2)
	Dorsiflexion	Ext. digitorum long.	Peroneal	L4–5–S1
		Ext. hallucis long.	Peroneal	L5–S1–2

Source: From ref. [3].

culty. In particular, look for symmetry of movement. A slight delay in thigh flexion during the swing phase of gait may be the only sign of mild spasticity. Toe and heel walking are also used to stress the plantar flexors and dorsiflexors of the foot, and thereby identify minimal weakness. At this time, one should also measure the patient's ability to perform tandem gait, which is a test for balance and coordination.

Spasticity is measured by passively moving the major joints and noting resistance or a "catch" of increased tone. This can be documented utilizing the Ashworth Scale [10] (see Table 4). Excessive spasticity may predispose to contractures and difficulty with bed and chair positioning, which in turn may result in skin breakdown and decubitus ulcers. Spasticity is often associated with other features of the "upper motor neuron" syndrome, including hyper-reflexia, mass spasms, and abnormal "synergy patterns" of motor movement.

The possibility of a movement disorder is considered next. First, observe the patient for a resting tremor or other involuntary movements. Walking rapidly may also illuminate an underlying movement abnormality. Coordination testing is performed next. This is done by asking the patient to perform a patting maneuver with each hand on the palm of the opposite hand. While alternating movements are performed, the patient is observed for dys-diadochokinesis. Next performed are maneuvers, such as the finger-to-nose test, that can demonstrate an intention tremor typical of cerebellar disease. Past pointing and rebound, which reflect inability to check a movement, can also be looked for at this time. In the lower extremities, the heel-to-knee-to-shin test demonstrates ataxia when there is cerebellar incoordination or severe proprioceptive loss. Limb incoordination, whether clumsiness or true ataxia, results in functional disability, and will need to be addressed in the patient's plan of rehabilitation.

The deep tendon reflexes are examined next. It is important to note that reflexes will vary in a given patient depending upon the patient's level of anxiety and muscle tension. Reflexes are rated 0–4, with 0 denoting an absent

Table 4   Ashworth Scale

Score	Muscle Tone
1	No increase in tone
2	Slight increase in tone; catch felt when affected limb (joint) extended/flexed
3	Tone increased, but affected part easily extended/flexed
4	Tone considerably increased; passive movement difficult
5	Affected limb rigid in extension or flexion

Source: From ref. [10].

(abnormal) reflex and 4 a pathologically brisk reflex. Two is considered normal, with 1 diminished and 3 brisk, but within the normal range. Reflex responses should be symmetrical. Reflexes should at the least be tested at the biceps, triceps, and brachioradialis tendons in the upper extremities, along with finger jerks. If necessary, pectoral reflexes can be elicited. Knee jerks and ankle jerks should be obtained in the lower extremities. The patient should be tested for clonus, especially at the ankle and patella. Clonus can occasionally impair function, the best example being sustained ankle clonus, which may be triggered by standing or merely by placing the sole of the foot on a wheelchair foot rest. Babinski's sign (great toe extension and fanning of the remaining toes) should be looked for. The presence of Babinski's sign is pathognomonic of an upper motor neuron disturbance, and the clinician should expect associated impairments, such as spasticity, which may affect the patient's rehabilitation. Babinski's sign can be elicited by stimulating the reflexogenic zone on the lateral sole of the foot. If there is too much withdrawal, other tests to identify an extensor toe sign should be performed, such as the Chaddock or Oppenheimer [1]. It is also important to test the jaw jerk. A pathologically brisk jaw jerk can localize pathological involvement to an intracranial or upper pontine level, and may be the only way of determining such a level. The examiner should be familiar with the superficial reflexes, including the abdominal, cremasteric, and anal reflexes. These are primarily useful in localizing spinal lesions. The pattern of sensory and motor impairments commonly associated with lesions at a given level leads to a better overall picture of the disability the patient will experience. The glabella, palmomental, and snout reflexes can be elicited as well. The inability to suppress the glabella response (Meyerson's sign) is seen in patients with extrapyramidal syndromes, while the palmomental and snout reflexes are seen in patients with organic diseases of the frontal lobes. The segmental spinal levels that mediate the various reflexes are shown in Table 5 [3]. For completeness, superficial and visceral reflexes are included.

The sensory examination is the least reliable method of evaluation but nonetheless should be performed. Loss of sensation can cause a lack of important feedback resulting in "sensory ataxia," and may compound functional loss due to motor weakness. In addition, sensory loss is a major predisposing factor for pressure sores. The four basic modalities of pain, light touch, vibration, and position sense should be tested. In addition, the examiner should have in his or her repertoire tests to evaluate temperature and higher integrative sensory functions, such as two-point discrimination, tactile localization, graphesthesia, and stereognosis. Extinction on double simultaneous stimulation may be a manifestation of unilateral neglect, and should be assessed. The segmental dermatomal distribution of superficial sensation and peripheral nerve sensory patterns is shown in Figure 1 [4]. The

Table 5 Spinal Levels Mediating

Reflexes	Afferent Nerve	Center	Efferent Nerve
Superficial Reflexes			
Corneal	Cranial V	Pons	Cranial VII
Nasal (sneeze)	Cranial V	Brainstem and upper cord	Cranials V, VII, IX, X and spinal nerves of expiration
Pharyngeal and uvular	Cranial IX	Medulla	Cranial X
Upper abdominal	T7, 8, 9, 10	T7, 8, 9, 10	T7, 8, 9, 10
Lower abdominal	T10, 11, 12	T10, 11, 12	T10, 11, 12
Cremasteric	Femoral	LI	Genitofemoral
Plantar	Tibial	S1, 2	Tibial
Anal	Pudendal	S4, 5	Pudendal
Deep reflexes			
Jaw	Cranial V	Pons	Cranial V
Biceps	Musculocutaneous	C5, 6	Musculocutaneous
Triceps	Radial	C6, 7	Radial
Periosteoradial	Radial	C6, 7, 8	Radial
Wrist (flexion)	Median	C6, 7, 8	Median
Wrist (extension)	Radial	C7, 8	Radial
Patellar	Femoral	L2, 3, 4	Femoral
Achilles	Tibial	S1, 2	Tibial
Visceral reflexes			
Light	Cranial II	Midbrain	Cranial III
Accommodation	Cranial II	Occipital cortex	Cranial III
Ciliospinal	A sensory nerve	T1, 2	Cervical sympathetics
Oculocardiac	Cranial V	Medulla	Cranial X
Carotid sinus	Cranial IX	Medulla	Cranial X
Bulbocavernosus	Pudendal	S2, 3, 4	Pelvic autonomic
Bladder and rectal	Pudendal	S2, 3, 4	Pudendal and autonomics

Source: Adapted from ref. [4].

patient should also be asked to stand upright with feet together and eyes opened and then closed to assess balance. Loss of balance only with eyes closed (a positive Romberg maneuver) indicates proprioceptive loss in the lower extremities.

Following the neurological examination, the patient should be examined from a musculoskeletal perspective. This portion of the examination is often neglected by clinicians trained in the neurosciences. Range of motion of all joints of the upper and lower extremities should be documented. Clinicians practicing neurorehabilitation should have a basic understanding of the normal degree of motion allowed by all joints. The presence of contractures and painful joints must be noted. Full joint motion is critical for optimal biomechanical function, and any limitation can compound problems caused by neurological impairment. For example, a weakened quadriceps muscle may be unable to stabilize a knee with a fixed flexion contracture during ambulation. For patients with primary complaints of cervical or low back pain, a careful examination of spine range of motion must be made (flexion, extension, lateral rotation, and tilt to left and right). In addition, palpation can reveal paraspinal muscle spasm or tenderness. Posterior spinal process tenderness should be determined. Sciatic notch tenderness, straight leg raising, and Lasegue's maneuver are physical methods of assessing the low back and a possible radiculopathy, and the neurorehabilitation specialist should be familiar with their use. Patrick's maneuver (hip flexion and lateral rotation) is positive in patients with hip disease. Gaenslen's maneuver can be useful in determining sacroiliac joint disease as a cause of low back pain.

After the above has been completed, the examiner can assess the patient's overall medical status. The ears, nose, and throat should be examined. Auscultation of the neck may reveal the presence of a bruit, which can be critical for a patient with ischemic stroke. Auscultation of the heart and lungs should be performed and, if necessary, percussion and palpation of the chest follows. The abdomen should be palpated for tenderness, abdominal organs, and masses, and auscultated for bowel sounds and bruits. The suprapubic area should be gently palpated for possible urinary retention and a distended bladder. The extremities should be examined for coloration, temperature, and the presence of other pathological signs such as clubbing or edema. Special attention should be directed toward evidence of deep venous thrombosis in patients with leg weakness, or those who have been subject to prolonged bed rest. One of the most common serious medical complications in an inpatient rehabilitation population is deep venous thrombosis and subsequent pulmonary embolus.

The patient's skin must be carefully examined. This should include not only the skin of the face, anterior trunk, and extremities but also skin over the posterior surfaces. In particular, especially if the patient is thin, the status of

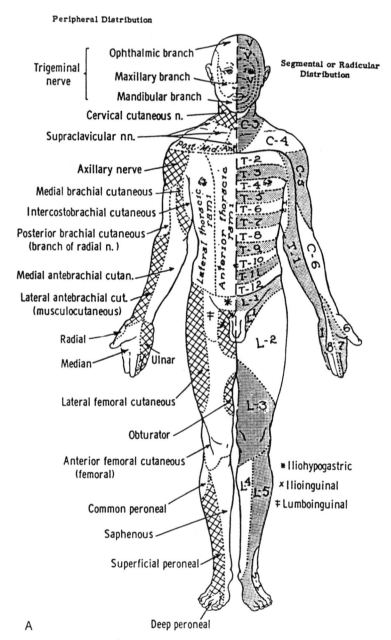

Figure 1   Cutaneous innervation (from ref. [4]).

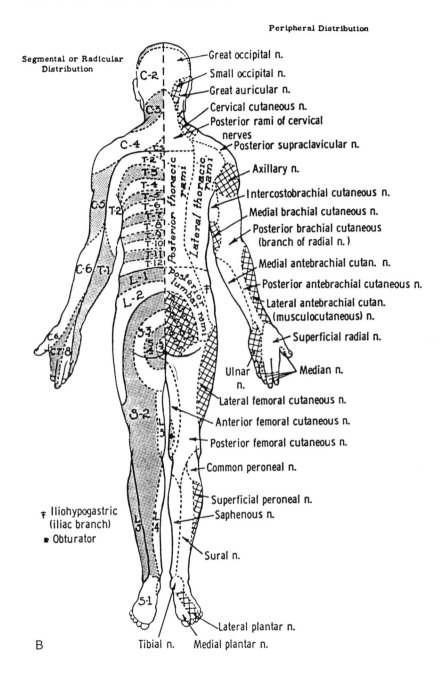

Peripheral Distribution

Segmental or Radicular Distribution

Great occipital n.
Small occipital n.
Great auricular n.
Cervical cutaneous n.
Posterior rami of cervical nerves
Posterior supraclavicular n.
Axillary n.
Intercostobrachial cutaneous n.
Medial brachial cutaneous n.
Posterior brachial cutaneous (branch of radial n.)
Medial antebrachial cutan. n.
Posterior antebrachial cutaneous n.
Lateral antebrachial cutan. (musculocutaneous) n.
Superficial radial n.
Ulnar n.
Median n.
Lateral femoral cutaneous n.
Anterior femoral cutaneous n.
Posterior femoral cutaneous n.
Common peroneal n.
Superficial peroneal n.
Saphenous n.
Sural n.
Lateral plantar n.
Tibial n.   Medial plantar n.

† Iliohypogastric (iliac branch)
* Obturator

B

Table 6   Classification of Pressure Sores

Grade 1	Skin reddened and inflamed, especially over a bony prominence
Grade 2	An ulcer that is superficial and involves just the dermis
Grade 3	An ulcer that extends into the subcutaneous tissue
Grade 4	An ulcer that involves subcutaneous tissue and muscle, and may extend to the bone
Grade 5	An ulcer that also involves a joint or a visceral cavity

Source: From ref. [11].

the skin over bony prominances such as the sacrum, buttocks (ischia), hips, and heels is an essential part of the examination. Decubitus ulcers or pressure sores, if present, are typically classified as grade 1–4, as explained in Table 6 [11]. Skin folds should also be examined for the presence of fungal infection or other abnormalities.

The external genitalia should also be assessed, especially if a Foley catheter is in place. If the patient is wet, voiding may be occurring around an obstructed catheter. In patients who self-catheterize, look for urethral discharge or ulcerations. A rectal examination should also be performed. This is essential for not only determining rectal sphincter tone but also to palpate the prostate and feel for polyps, masses, and the presence of stool within the rectum. Fecal impactions are not infrequent in patients with chronic neurological conditions.

FUNCTIONAL ASSESSMENT

The functional assessment is a unique feature of the neurorehabilitation examination. The rehabilitation specialist must see how well the patient performs functional tasks that require the integration of multiple physical and mental skills. At the bedside it is important to check mobility by asking the patient to roll from side to side, perform prop ups, and attempt to get out of bed. Next, the patient should be asked to sit at the edge of the bed. The clinician should note whether the patient needs assistance or not and, if so, how much assistance is necessary. Once the patient is seated, sitting balance is determined. Head and truncal control are documented and, if necessary, the patient's ability to adjust while seated can be tested by slightly pushing the patient from the front or from the side. Poor sitting balance generally precludes safe standing and ambulation. If capable, the patient should next be asked to stand and observation made of the patient's posture and balance.

The physician may employ a mock bathroom and ask the patient to perform such simple tasks as combing hair, brushing teeth, and washing hands. The ability to utilize simple hospital/household equipment such as the telephone can also be assessed. One may go a step further and ask the patient to put on and take off clothing of the upper and lower body. The ability to cut food and to chew/swallow are additional functional activities that are relatively easy to evaluate at the bedside. Functional assessment beyond this level usually requires the assistance of an occupational therapist and utilization of such facilities as a model kitchen and bathroom.

Evaluation of gait has already been discussed as a part of the neurological examination. However, gait is a functional motor activity and must also be considered in this context. Casual gait should be tested first. If this is performed well, heel, toe, and tandem walking must be assessed next. If the patient is unable to walk unaided, the examiner should determine how much physical assistance is required or if an assistive device (walker or cane) is indicated. These should be provided and the patient's abilities noted. The ability to shift weight to each extremity, the ability to advance each leg, and the pattern of motor movement during ambulation are especially important. The presence of weakness or relative imbalance of muscle tone may result in gait deviations that could be improved with an orthosis. If the patient is in a wheelchair, the physician should monitor the patient's ability to transfer to and from the chair, and also his or her ability to propel a wheelchair.

A more global measure of functional abilities may be obtained by using functional assessment scales that include a variety of functional activities, including mobility and the ability to perform activities of daily living. These are discussed in Chapter 7. In the past, two functional assessment scales were commonly used to monitor patient progress: the PULSES profile [12] and the Barthel Index [13]. More recently, there have been efforts to establish a uniform national data set, which has led to the Functional Independence Measure (FIM) [14], which is more comprehensive and sensitive to change.

SPECIAL EXAMINATIONS

The Comatose Patient

Not infrequently, the rehabilitation physician may be asked to evaluate a patient at a low cognitive or functional level (Rancho scale I or II) (see Table 7) [15]. Most commonly, the patient has had a head injury and evaluation is requested for prognosis and rehabilitation potential. The patient's level of consciousness should first be identified. A typical hierarchy would go from awake and alert to somnolent, obtunded, stuporous, and finally, coma. To this list must be added the persistent vegetative state (PVS): patients have stable vital functions, may have their eyes open, and may demonstrate primitive reflexes, but remain oblivious to verbal and other stimuli and remain mute

Table 7   Ranchos Los Amigos
Cognitive Recovery Levels

Level	Response/Description
I	Unresponsive to all stimuli
II	Generalized response
III	Localized response
IV	Confused–agitated
V	Confused–inappropriate
VI	Confused–appropriate
VII	Automatic–appropriate
VIII	Purposeful–appropriate

Source: From ref. [15].

and otherwise unresponsive. The patient demonstrates no awareness of self or the environment [16]. For patients with impaired consciousness, special examination techniques must be employed, but the most important consideration is to first make good passive observations. A few extra minutes simply watching the patient may be very rewarding in understanding the scope and extent of the patient's injuries. The examiner should look for spontaneous eye opening. If the eyes open and tonically deviate to one side or the other, or if there is skew deviation, it should be documented. Deviation of the eyes to one side may be seen with a frontal lobe lesion on the side to which the eyes gaze. An irritative frontal lesion may tonically deviate the eyes to the opposite side. It should also be noted if the patient scans the room or tracks people in the environment. If the eyes are kept closed, the lids may be held up and the position and movements of the eyes can then be observed. Further passive observations include watching for spontaneous movement of the limbs and listening for vocalizations or attempts at speaking. Restless movements of the limbs are to be differentiated from repetitive, jerking movements that might signal focal seizure activity. In this regard, particular attention should be paid to the orbicularis oris, orbicularis oculi, and mentalis muscles in the face and the intrinsic muscles of the hand, since twitches in these areas may be the only indication of focal seizure activity.

Spontaneous speech or vocalizations should be documented. When there is no spontaneous activity, it is appropriate to try to stimulate the patient to observe a response. Calling out to the patient may elicit a response when no spontaneous attempts at speech are made. Speech is usually a late event in the sequence of recovery following a moderate or severe traumatic brain injury (TBI). One should first speak or call out to the patient in a firm and nonthreatening voice. Simple one-step commands should be used (e.g.,

"Open your eyes" or "Move your hand"). The examiner must wait an adequate length of time, since there may be a considerable time delay before the patient responds to any given command. If there is no response to verbal stimulation, it is appropriate next to attempt tactile stimulation. This should first take the form of gently shaking the patient's shoulder or a limb while calling out his or her name. If this is unsuccessful, a more painful stimulation can be tried. This must be done with the greatest of sensitivity and concern for the patient. Unrestrained deep painful stimulation is never warranted. Squeezing the heel cord or applying pressure over the sternum, nail bed, or the supraorbital nerve are common methods to apply a painful stimulus. This type of stimulation can elicit various reactions, including semipurposeful attempts to brush away the noxious stimulus or abnormal limb flexion or extension (decorticate and decerebrate) responses.

In cases of traumatic brain injury, documentation of the patient's responses can be formalized by utilizing the Glasgow Coma Scale. This scale has been used to categorize the severity of a brain injury and is based on the patient's best eye opening (E), motor (M), and verbal (V) responses (Table 8) [17]. The scale is graded from 3 to 15 by summing the E, M, and V responses. A score of 13–15 would indicate mild impairment, 8–12 represents moderate impairment of function (i.e., a moderate head injury), while any score below 8

Table 8   Glasgow Coma Scale

Observe	Patient's Best Response	Score
Eye opening	Opens eyes spontaneously	E4
	Opens eyes to command	3
	Opens eyes to pain stimulus	2
	Eyes will not open to any stimulus	1
Motor response	Obeys simple commands	M6
	Localizes painful stimulus	5
	Withdraws from painful stimulus	4
	Flexion response to stimulus	3
	Extensor response to stimulus	2
	No response to any stimulus	1
Verbal response	Oriented, conversant	V5
	Conversation confused	4
	Inappropiate speech	3
	Incomprehensible sounds	2
	No response to any stimulus	1

Coma score: E + M + V = possible score of 3–15.
Source: From ref. [16].

represents a severe head injury. Lower scores correlate with worse functional outcome (see Chapter 22).

After passively observing the patient and assessing arousal by stimulation, additional examination should be undertaken. Since brainstem lesions frequently result in impaired consciousness, brainstem function should be carefully assessed by evaluating the cranial nerves. The cranial nerves are first evaluated by noticing the pupillary size and configuration and their response to light stimulation. The fundi should also be observed. Note if the eyes scan spontaneously. The head can next be turned to the left and right to elicit an oculocephalic or "doll's eyes" response. The presence of this sign suggests functional integrity of the brainstem and implies that impaired consciousness is due to abnormalities of the diencephalon or cerebral hemispheres. Reference is made to the excellent text on the comatose patient by Drs. Plum and Posner for a detailed description of this maneuver, as well as the comprehensive examination of the patient in coma [18]. If necessary, the caloric or ear ice water test may be utilized to produce an oculovestibular response. It should be remembered that with an intact brainstem, ice water placed into an external ear canal will produce a tonic deviation of the eyes toward the stimulated ear. With a low brainstem lesion, no ocular response will be seen. Warm water stimulation may also be used, but usually does not give as vigorous a response. If a response is seen, the features are the opposite of the ice water caloric test. A summary of the ocular responses and their significance is shown in Figure 2 [18].

If the eyes are open, a threatening movement toward each eye from the lateral field may elicit a blink response in all but the patient in deep coma. A unilateral lack of response may be an indication of an hemianoptic field defect.

The fifth cranial nerve can be passively tested by touching the corneas with a wisp of cotton, taking care to approach the eye from the far lateral field to avoid a defensive blink reaction. A blink or aversive response indicates an intact sensory pathway via the ophthalmic branch of the trigeminal nerve. The absence of a response may be the only indication of a hemisensory loss. Of course a focal lesion of the ophthalmic branch of the trigeminal nerve must be ruled out, as must paralysis of the facial muscles, which also could lead to no noticeable blink response. If the eyes cannot be accurately tested due to forced eye closure or instilled ophthalmic ointment, the next most sensitive way to determine intact trigeminal sensory function is to test the nasociliary response. This is performed by tickling the nares or nasal hairs with a fine wisp of cotton and observing if there is an aversive head movement or a "wiggling" movement of the nose and upper lip. A more dramatic response would include the elevation of a hand to rub the nose and, in a more

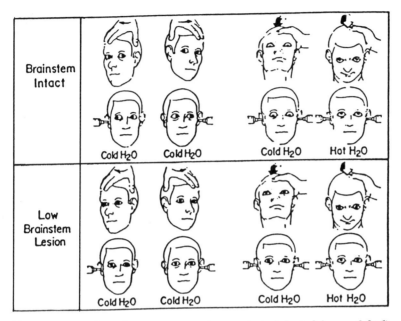

Figure 2 Ocular reflexes in unconscious patients (adapted from ref. [17]).

widespread response, the patient may sneeze. For these responses to occur, coma cannot be too deep.

Facial strength can be assessed by observing for facial symmetry and for a flattened nasolabial fold, drooping of one corner of the mouth, or an asymmetry in the palpebral fissures. Tearing from one eye may indicate a laxness of that orbicularis oculi muscle. Pressure (with the examiner's thumb) over a supraorbital nerve as it exits the supraorbital foramina will produce a grimace in all but patients in the deepest of coma. Both sides should be tested; any asymmetry of facial movement may indicate unilateral facial muscle weakness.

A gross test of hearing in the nonresponsive patient is to clap the hands or click the fingers beside one ear, then the other. Care should be taken that the hands are out of the patient's sight to avoid a visual stimulus that can confuse the test interpretation. A positive response would be a blink or startle reaction to the noise at each ear.

Stimulating the pharynx with a tongue depressor to elicit a gag reflex may demonstrate a loss of sensation (if there is no response at all) or unilateral pharyngeal paralysis, if the gag response pulls the uvula to one side because of unilateral weakness. Movement of the uvula is toward the intact side. In a patient with suspected persistent vegetative state, the presence of "reflexive" chewing and swallowing should be sought.

The motor examination consists of observation, followed by passive movement of the extremities to determine if they are flail or exhibit increased tone. Look for spontaneous movement or posturing such as decorticate (arms flexed, legs extended) or decerebrate (arms extended, legs extended) posturing. Stimulation may provoke or cause such posturing. Painful stimulation that elicits withdrawal indicates a grossly intact sensory system in the area stimulated in addition to the ability to move.

At the end of the examination of the patient with impaired consciousness, the rehabilitation clinician should be able to identify which portions of the central nervous system are impaired. It is more important that residual functional abilities be identified to determine the intensity of further rehabilitation efforts and to assist in planning rehabilitation strategy.

Mental Status Examination

A description of the mental status examination has already been presented. A full mental status examination need not be performed on every patient; however, many patients with neurological illness or injury have impaired cognition, which may be the most important factor in successful rehabilitation. Therefore, certain aspects of the mental status evaluation may deserve special emphasis. If the mental condition of the patient assumes great importance, a more detailed examination, including formal neuropsychological testing, should be done. An excellent reference for the mental status examination is the text by Strub and Black [18]. A cognitive assessment can be invaluable, not only for the education of family and staff but also for planning a rehabilitation program that can fully utilize the patient's remaining cognitive abilities. The frequency of behavioral aberrations following such conditions as stroke, traumatic brain injury, encephalitis, and brain surgery makes it mandatory that the rehabilitation physician develop considerable skill in this area of evaluation. Behavioral observations are crucial in the proper diagnosis of acute confusional states, frontal lobe syndromes, and denial/neglect syndromes [20].

Because of the propensity for frontal contusions following head trauma, frontal lobe syndromes are ubiquitous among patients with traumatic brain injury. There are basically two such syndromes: the inferior orbitofrontal and dorsolateral frontal syndromes. The first is manifested by disinhibition, impulsiveness, and childlike behavior; and the second by a flattened affect and lack of initiation. In addition, the patient may have impairment of frontal executive function as manifested by poor judgment, lack of insight, and denial of illness. Patients with frontal lobe syndromes may show psychomotor slowing, little or no initiation, and an apathetic appearance. This may be easily confused with depression, and the term pseudodepression has frequently been applied. Some tests for frontal lobe impairment rely on the perseveration seen in these patients. Evaluation, therefore, should utilize rapidly alternating physical moves or changes in mind set. Examples would include the "slap-fist-cut" test (wherein the patient is asked to strike repetitively a knee or a desk top with his or her hand in this sequence) [21] or the Trails A and B tests in formal neuropsychological evaluation [22].

With nondominant parietal lobe lesions, contralateral neglect and denial syndromes are common. Simple tests to assess neglect include asking the patient to bisect a line, asking the patient to mark each of many lines drawn on a sheet of paper, or asking the patient to draw a clock or other design. Many more complex neuropsychological tests are also available. However, the behavioral manifestations of neglect or denial may be immediately evident by observing the patient during functional activities. A person with severe neglect may fail to read words on the left side of a page, or even the letters on the left side of individual words. The food on the neglected side may remain uneaten. The patient may consistently bump into objects on one side when propelling a wheelchair. Based on such observations, strategies to encourage attention toward the side of neglect can be implemented. Anosognosia of Babinski, or the inability to recognize a paretic arm or hemiparesis, may be seen. In extreme form there may be a useless hand or alien hand syndrome.

Another common behavioral manifestation of cerebral injury is impaired attention. While often a feature of frontal lobe impairment, it is nonspecific and frequently seen with diffuse or multifocal lesions as well. Patients are often noted to be highly distractable and unable to attend to a task when other environmental stimuli are present. Even in a quiet environment, a patient may be unable to concentrate on an activity for more than brief periods of time. Since learning, memory, and other cognitive activities are dependent on attention, identification of this problem is crucial. If attention is impaired, the patient's rehabilitation program should then be designed to minimize distracting stimuli and to limit the time of individual training sessions.

Characteristic patterns of cognitive dysfunction often accompany lesions in specific brain regions. Easy distractibility, impulsivity, impaired insight, poor judgment, impaired abstraction ability, impaired planning and problem solving, and regressive behavior often signify frontal lobe injury. Signs of temporal lobe dysfunction include receptive aphasia, amnestic syndromes, focal seizures, upper quadrantopsia, and auditory hallucinations. Parietal lobe dysfunction includes impaired cortical sensory and perceptual discrimination as measured by such perceptual tests as tactile localization, two-point discrimination, stereognosis (tactile agnosia), and graphesthesia. Unilateral neglect and disorders of body schema are also seen in parietal lobe lesions, especially of the nondominant hemisphere. Dominant hemisphere parietal lesions result in language disturbances, including receptive aphasia and alexia. Finger agnosia may be identified, which can be seen in association with dyscalculia, dysgraphia, and left–right disorientation, as in the Gerstmann syndrome. Occipital lobe dysfunction would include field defects, cortical blindness, visual agnosia, and the interesting syndrome of prosopagnosia, or an inability to recognize faces. Occasionally, pure word blindness may also occur.

Recognition of these various cortical dysfunctions is not merely an exercise in behavioral neuropsychology. These syndromes are frequently not recognized and are a cause of consternation to the family and therapists when the patient's expected level of function is not realized. For example, neglect syndromes can dramatically impede such activities as dressing when the patient seems alert and strong enough to perform such tasks.

SUMMARY

The rehabilitation physician has an important and difficult task in performing this evaluation. He or she must first delineate the nature, location, and extent of the neurological lesion(s) producing clinical impairment and disability. While this is often the result of motor deficits, the physician must also recognize the extent of sensory impairment and identify and understand the patient's cognitive and higher cortical functional losses in order to guide the rehabilitation process appropriately and to explain to the family the full scope of the patient's injuries. To the extent that he or she can understand, the patient should also be apprised of his or her condition, the rehabilitation plan, and the goals of therapy. All of this information, including the cognitive and behavioral changes that are identified, must also be explained to the staff so that proper therapeutic steps are taken and unreasonable expectations are minimized. To gain this information the physician must rely primarily on the physical examination. Ancillary studies such as magnetic resonance imaging, computed tomographic scans, electroencephalography, electromyography, and evoked potentials are certainly of value, but the physical examination and its assessment of function are critical to understanding the patient and setting the rehabilitation program.

From a neurological perspective, the rehabilitation physician must have a good working knowledge of neuroanatomy and functional clinical neurology. He or she must have a full understanding of the changes brought about by the underlying neurological lesions(s) and the potential for recovery. Furthermore, he or she must have a good sense of the sequence and rate at which neurological recovery can be anticipated. Such knowledge, much of which is gained from the clinical examination, is mandatory to manage the patient's care effectively and communicate with staff, patient, and family. For example, anticipating the agitation phase of brain injury recovery (Rancho level IV) can help allay a great deal of anxiety, not only in the patient but also the staff and family. It can only be hoped that this brief chapter, within its limited scope, will assist the reader in the development of these essential neurorehabilitation examination skills.

The complete neurorehabilitation evaluation, of necessity, must go beyond the neurological examination. It must include a musculoskeletal assessment as well as a general medical examination. This latter aspect of the evaluation has assumed even greater importance with the recent trend toward earlier referral to rehabilitation of patients who are sicker and with an increased incidence of comorbidity. Factors of comorbidity and potential higher complication rates can only make the task of the rehabilitation specialist more difficult. Critical in the management of these patients will be the ability to make accurate and meaningful clinical observations. This means that the rehabilitation physician must possess good medical examination skills. This chapter primarily focused on the neurological aspect of the evaluation. However, this should not be construed to mean that other aspects are irrelevant. The physician who plans to practice neurorehabilitation, therefore, must also develop and maintain expertise in performing a comprehensive medical history and examination.

REFERENCES

1. R.N. De Jong, *The Neurological Examination*, Harper & Row, New York (1967).
2. W. Haymaker, *Bing's Local Diagnosis in Neurological Diseases*. C.V. Mosby, St. Louis (1969).
3. W. Pryse-Phillips and T.J. Murray, *Essential Neurology*, 2nd edition, Medical Examination Publishing Co., Garden City, NY (1982).
4. J.C. Chusid, *Correlative Neuroanatomy and Functional Neurology*. Lange Medical Publications, Los Altos, CA (1973).
5. A.B. Baker and R.J. Joynt, *Clinical Neurology*. Harper and Row, Philadelphia (1987).
6. World Health Organization, *International Classification of Impairments, Disabilities and Handicaps: A Manual of Classification Relating to the Consequences of Disease*. World Health Organization, Geneva, Switzerland (1980).
7. M.F. Folstein, S.E. Folstein, and P.R. McHugh, *J. Psychiatr. Res.*, 12:189–198 (1975).

8. Medical Research Council, *Aids to the Investigation of Peripheral Nerve Injuries. War Memorandum No. 7.* (revised second edition, 1943). Her Majesty's Stationery Office (1970).

9. H.L. Frankel, et al. *Paraplegia,* 7:179 (1969).

10. B. Ashworth, *Practitioner,* 162:540 (1964).

11. R.K. Daniel, E.J. Hall, and M. McCleod, *Ann. Plast. Surg.,* 1:53–63 (1979).

12. C.V. Granger, G.L. Albrecht, and B.B. Hamilton, *Arch. Phys. Med. Rehabil.,* 60:145 (1979).

13. F.I. Mahoney and D.W. Barthel, *MD State Med. J.,* 14:61 (1965).

14. C.V. Granger and B.B. Hamilton, *Am. J. Phys. Med. Rehabil.,* 71:108 (1992).

15. Professional Staff Association, Rancho Los Amigos Hospital, *Rehabilitation of the Head Injured Adult: Comprehensive Management.* Downey, CA (1976).

16. ANA Committee on Ethical Affairs, *Ann. Neurol.,* 33:388–390 (1993).

17. B. Jennett and G. Teasdale, *Management of Head Injuries.* F.A. Davis, Philadelphia (1981).

18. F. Plum and J.B. Posner, *The Diagnosis of Stupor and Coma.* F.A. Davis, Philadelphia (1980).

19. R.L. Strub and F.W. Black, *The Mental Status Examination in Neurology.* F.A. Davis, Philadelphia (1985).

20. R.L. Strub and F.W. Black, *Neurobehavioral Disorders.* F.A. Davis, Philadelphia (1988).

21. D.F. Benson and D.T. Stuss, *Neurology,* 32(12):135 1353–1357 (1982).

22. D.T. Stuss and D.F. Benson, *The Frontal Lobes.* Raven Press, New York (1986).

2

Gait Disturbances and Analysis

Rodger J. Elble

Center for Alzheimer Disease and Related Disorders and
Southern Illinois University School of Medicine
Springfield, Illinois

PHYSIOLOGY OF WALKING

The locomotor capacity of spinalized mammalian quadrupeds has been known since the experiments of T. Graham Brown [1]. Normal locomotion emerges from spinal pattern generators that are under the control of supraspinal motor centers. The neuronal networks that make up these spinal pattern generators are poorly defined [2]. Gordon Holmes [3] observed that the lower extremities of a few soldiers with spinal cord injuries occasionally exhibited involuntary rhythmic movements that resembled the locomotor movements of spinal cats. Postmortem studies revealed that the ventral columns of the spinal cord in these soldiers were spared. Sparing the ventral columns is also sufficient and necessary for spontaneous or treadmill-induced locomotion in laboratory primates [4] and for spontaneous locomotion in cats [5]. These observations suggest that reticulospinal and possibly vestibulospinal pathways are crucially important in the activation of spinal locomotor networks.

Studies of locomotion in decerebrate and intact cats and rats have revealed that the spinal pattern generators are controlled by two parallel motor pathways, one involving the cerebellum and the other involving mesencephalic and diencephalic nuclei (Fig. 1). This organization of the motor system emphasizes an important principle of locomotor control: Normal locomotion requires the proper control and integration of limb movement,

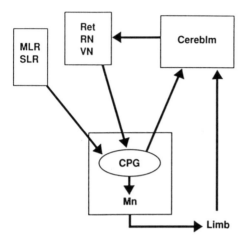

Figure 1   The spinal central pattern generator (CPG) is under the influence of two parallel control systems, one involving the cerebellum (Cereblm) and the other involving the mesencephalic and subthalamic locomotor regions (MLR, SLR) of the midbrain and diencephalon. Ret, lateral pontomedullary reticular nuclei; RN, red nucleus; VN, lateral vestibular nucleus; Mn, spinal motoneurons.

posture and balance. The experimental basis for this fundamental principle will be reviewed here and emphasized repeatedly in subsequent discussions of clinical gait assessment.

Under the influence of the cerebellum, the rubrospinal, lateral ponto-medullary reticulospinal, and vestibulospinal (Dieter's nucleus) pathways are believed to control the rhythmicity of locomotion and phasic coordination of bodily segments. Neurons in these brainstem nuclei fire phasically with the locomotor rhythm, and this phasic firing requires an intact cerebellum [6–8]. The ventral spinocerebellar pathway carries output from the spinal pattern generators to the cerebellum. This efference copy of the spinal pattern generator is compared with peripheral sensory feedback carried by the dorsal spinocerebellar pathway. The cerebellum may thereby participate in the adjustment of motor outflow to suit environmental and musculoskeletal constraints.

Studies of locomotion in decerebrate and intact cats and rats have revealed four anatomical loci in the brainstem and diencephalon that appear to underlie the initiation of gait and the control of postural tonus (Fig. 2) [8, 9]. The subthalamic locomotor region (SLR) is the most poorly defined and is located in the lateral hypothalamic area [10]. Stimulation of this site in intact cats produces stooped, stealthy locomotion, as though the animals were

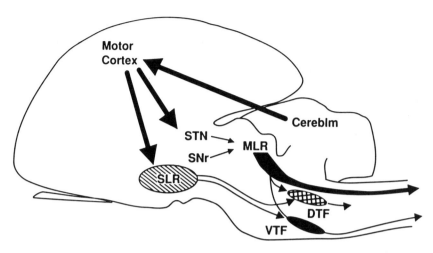

Figure 2   The locations and interconnections of the mesencephalic locomotor region (MLR), subthalamic locomotor region (SLR), ventral tegmental field (VTF), dorsal tegmental field (DTF), subthalamic nucleus (STN), substantia nigra pars reticulata (SNr), motor cortex, and cerebellum (Cereblm) are shown in this sagittal view of the brain.

pursuing prey. The mesencephalic locomotor region (MLR) corresponds to the nucleus cuneiformis and the cholinergic pedunculopontine nucleus of the dorsolateral midbrain. Brief stimulation of the MLR induces rapid walking, followed by running. The ventral tegmental field (VTF) corresponds to the rostral nucleus raphe magnus of the caudal midline pons. Stimulation of the VTF increases antigravity muscle tone. The dorsal tegmental field (DTF) corresponds to the caudal nucleus raphe centralis superior of the caudal midline pons. Stimulation of the VTF suppresses antigravity muscle tone and prevents walking when the SLR or MLR is stimulated.

The MLR is integrated with ipsilateral basal ganglia function [11]. The pedunculopontine nucleus has ipsilateral reciprocal connections with the substantia nigra pars reticulata (SNr; GABAergic) and the globus pallidus interna (GPi; GABAergic). These GABAergic inputs to the MLR are believed to have an inhibitory influence on locomotion [12]. It is therefore noteworthy that destruction of the nigrostriatal dopaminergic pathway with 1-methyl-4-phenyl-1,2,5,6-tetrahydropyridine (MPTP) produces increased neuronal activity in both SNr and GPi [13]. The MLR (pedunculopontine nucleus) receives excitatory glutaminergic inputs from the subthalamus and the motor cortex. The MLR has N-methyl-D-aspartate (NMDA) and substance-P receptors, the stimulation of which promotes locomotion [12]. The MLR also receives cholinergic input from the adjacent laterodorsal tegmental nucleus and the contralateral pedunculopontine nucleus [12]. This cholinergic input (probably muscarinic) has an inhibitory effect on locomotion. Cholinergic cells in the pedunculopontine nucleus and adjacent laterodorsal tegmental nucleus also project to the cerebral cortex, thalamus, cerebellar nuclei, locus ceruleus, pontine nuclei, vestibular nuclei, and throughout the descending reticular nuclei of the caudal pons and medulla [11, 14–17].

The MLR and SLR project to both the VTF and DTF [8]. Cholinergic agonists, excitatory amino acid agonists, GABAergic antagonists, and substance P facilitate locomotion when injected into the VTF [18] and inhibit locomotion when injected into the DTF. Neurons in the DTF fire tonically during locomotion, and the DTF and VTF are probably involved in control of postural tonus [7]. The motor cortex is involved in the initiation of gait and in the modification of gait to suit environmental and psychological needs [6, 19]. This influence of motor cortex is accomplished, at least in part, through its projections to the MLR and SLR. The motor cortex can also participate with the cerebellum in the control of locomotor rhythmicity since the deep cerebellar nuclei project to the contralateral motor cortex via the ventrolateral thalamus, and the motor cortex projects to the contralateral cerebellum via the pontine and olivary nuclei. Hence, the cerebellum is ideally suited for the feedforward control of movement.

PHYSIOLOGY OF POSTURAL CONTROL

Postural Reflexes

The control of posture and balance is part and parcel of walking. The line of gravity for normal erect posture is normally 3–8 cm anterior to the ankles and fluctuates within narrow limits [20] (Fig. 3). These fluctuations, called postural sway, are reflected in the center of pressure of the feet, as measured with floor-mounted force plates. Postural sway is measured more directly with accelerometers, potentiometers, and photogrammetric techniques. Comparison of force-plate data with motion analysis data is difficult because motion of the center of pressure deviates significantly from motion of the center of mass at frequencies greater than 0.5 Hz [21]. Studies using both methods have shown that postural sway is increased in people over age 65, but this increase is largely, if not entirely, due to a variety of pathological conditions, not to age per se [22–24].

The somatosensory (muscle, joint, and cutaneous receptors), vestibular, and visual systems provide the nervous system with sensory inputs that are utilized in the control of posture and locomotion. Studies of postural sway have provided only limited insight into the manner in which these sensory

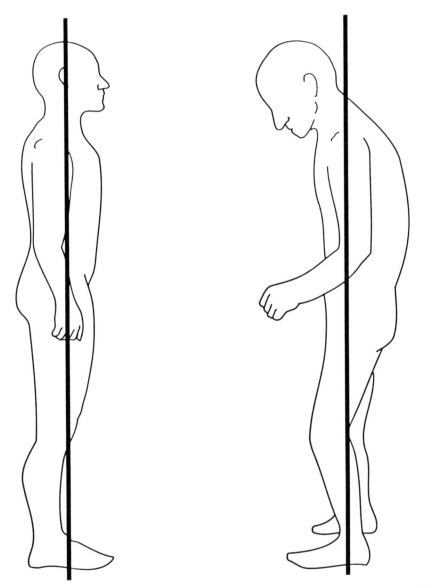

Figure 3   The line of gravity for a normal young adult (left) is 3–8 cm anterior to the ankles. The line of gravity may shift posteriorly (right) with the development of abnormal spinal curvature and pelvic rotation, resulting in a tendency to fall backward.

modalities are used. Normal individuals exhibit little or no increase in postural sway when their eyes are closed (Romberg test) [25]. However, a rotating visual image increases postural sway in the frequency range of 0–1 Hz [26, 27]. Absent or distorted vision does not increase postural sway in people with loss of somatosensory input from the feet and ankles [25], but postural sway increases greatly when there is additional loss of somatosensory input from the leg muscles [28]. Patients with bilateral vestibular loss exhibit little or no increase in postural sway with eyes open or closed, but their postural sway increases profoundly when both visual and somatosensory inputs are lost or distorted [25]. Clinical measures of visual, vestibular, and pedal somatosensory function correlate poorly with the magnitude of postural sway, even in older people [22].

Nashner [29, 30] and co-workers [31] have extensively examined the strategies used by normal people in maintaining erect stance. They found surprising stereotypy in the kinematic and electromyographic reactions to specific postural perturbations delivered by a mobile platform upon which the people were standing. Muscles in the legs respond through monosynaptic reflexes to such perturbations within 45–50 msec, but these short-latency reflexes contribute little to postural control [29]. More important is that muscles in the lower extremities and trunk respond with long-latency somatosensory reflexes, called functional stretch reflexes, at approximately 100 msec and with visual and vestibular reflexes at 180 msec or greater [29, 32]. The coordination of the 100 msec responses among proximal and distal limb muscles and truncal muscles occurs so quickly (within 10–12 msec) and stereotypically that their synergistic activation must be preprogrammed by the nervous system and triggered by the initial perturbation of the ankle. If triggered inappropriately, functional stretch reflexes can impair balance rather than restore it [29]. These triggered responses are modulated by supraspinal locomotor centers and are accompanied by cerebral evoked potentials [33].

The functional stretch reflexes combine to produce rather stereotypical patterns of movement in response to postural perturbation [34]. Small or slow postural perturbations are usually counteracted by motion of the body about the ankles, resembling an inverted pendulum. For example, a small force to the sternum elicits the so-called ankle strategy in which a distal-to-proximal activation of the ventral musculature of the lower extremities and torso creates a forward movement about the ankles (Fig. 4). A force to the back is likewise counteracted by a distal-to-proximal activation of the dorsal musculature, which produces a backward movement about the ankles. The hip strategy occurs when the support surface is shorter than the feet, when large postural perturbations are encountered, or when there is somatosensory loss from the feet and ankles. Under these circumstances, a person bends forward

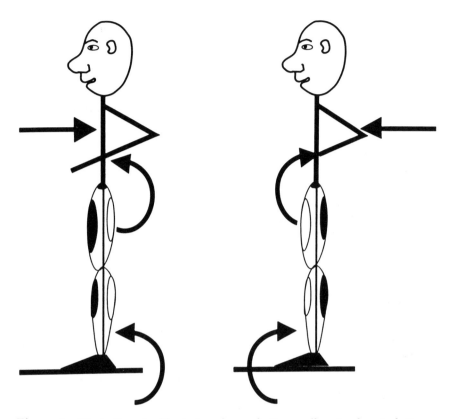

Figure 4   Illustration of ankle strategy for combating small postural perturbations. Synergistic activation of the ventral musculature (shaded muscles of the left figure) produces a forward movement (torque) about the ankles, in response to a sternal push. Synergistic activation of the dorsal muscles produces a backward movement about the ankles, counteracting a push from the rear.

at the waist and hips to counteract the postural disturbance. Finally, a person may squat to lower the center of mass in response to postural perturbations in the vertical direction. In general, various combinations of these three strategies are used to combat the variety of perturbations encountered by most people.

Vision and vestibular information subserve complex mechanisms of postural control. Nashner and co-workers [25, 35] examined postural stability in patients with vestibular lesions who received distorted visual and somatosensory inputs through a mobile balance platform and visual surround. These patients exhibited postural responses that were sufficiently normal to maintain balance unless they were exposed to conflicting visual and somatosensory inputs. Normal people were able to resolve such conflicting sensory inputs and maintain their balance, although older people had more difficulty than young adults [36]. These observations led Nashner and co-workers to hypothesize that vestibular inputs are used to modulate postural reflexes and to serve as an orientational reference against which visual and somatosensory inputs are compared and interpreted. Patients with vestibular loss exhibit a 70% reduction in the electromyographic (EMG) and ankle torque responses of the ankle strategy [37] and cannot deploy the hip strategy when it is required to maintain equilibrium [25]. Nashner and Berthoz [38] found that visual inputs can attenuate involuntary postural adjustments by 100 msec. This modulation of functional stretch reflexes probably occurs through central mechanisms, because direct recordings from muscle spindle afferents revealed no change in discharge rates with eye closure or head tilting [39]. The contribution of vision to postural reflexes is particularly important when there is impaired vestibular and somatosensory function.

Preparatory Postural Adjustments

Perturbation of posture occurs during most volitional movements such as suddenly raising the upper extremities overhead. Numerous studies have shown that the normal nervous system anticipates, through prior experience, the postural perturbation that results from volitional movement and initiates a coordinated neuromuscular response before the postural perturbation occurs. Thus, postural control and movement are integrated into a coordinated motor act. For example, Belen'kii and co-workers [40] found that muscles of the lower extremities and trunk were activated or inactivated 40–50 msec *before* activation of the deltoid when normal subjects raised an upper extremity during quiet stance (Fig. 5). Bouisset and Zattara [41, 42] showed that this preparatory muscle activity produced anticipatory accelerations of the body that counteracted the opposing accelerations caused by raising the upper extremities [43, 44]. In these preparatory postural adjustments, the distal muscles closest to the base of support are activated first, followed in rapid sequential succession by more proximal muscles. These adjustments are a preprogrammed component of the volitional movement, not a reflex response to postural perturbation [45]. Without these preparatory postural adjustments, reliance upon an excessively slow stretch-reflex response to the postural disturbance produced by arm movement could result in loss of balance. Preprogrammed preparatory postural activity is also an integral part of forward and backward bending of the human torso, and the muscular synergies involved in these maneuvers are so effective that they limit sagittal displacement of the center of gravity to approximately 1 cm [46].

Pal'tsev and El'ner [47] found that when patients with frontal lobe or

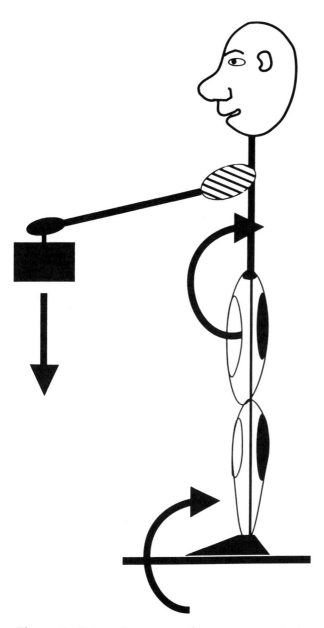

Figure 5 Volitional movement of an upper extremity is preceded by anticipatory postural adjustments. In this example, the deltoid is activated to lift a weight that will perturb the body forward. The dorsal muscles of the lower extremities and torso are activated before the deltoid to produce an anticipatory postural adjustment.

cerebellar lesions raised their upper extremities, the preparatory postural activation of muscles in the lower extremities was abolished or delayed by more than 50 msec. By contrast, Traub and co-workers [48] found that patients with cerebellar ataxia exhibited reduced preparatory postural activities with normal latencies. Based upon studies of 225 patients with frontal lobe lesions, Gurfinkel' and El'ner [49] determined that the supplementary motor cortex was the critical site of frontal lobe pathological involvement in patients with suppressed or delayed preparatory postural activity. The supplementary motor cortex is a major site of projection from the basal ganglia through the ventrolateral thalamus. One might predict, therefore, that the effect of basal ganglia pathology on preparatory postural activity would resemble the effect of supplementary motor cortex lesions. In this regard, Dick and co-workers [50] found that preparatory postural activity in patients with Parkinson's disease was reduced in amplitude but not delayed.

In summary, normal balance and posture are not maintained by simple reflex responses to somatosensory, visual, and vestibular inputs to the nervous system. Normal balance requires anticipatory postural adjustments (i.e., feedforward motor control) that are an integral part of the motor strategy for a particular voluntary movement. Similar integration of postural control and movement occurs in all aspects of locomotion.

Effects of Aging

Older people frequently have impaired vision, vestibular function, and somatic sensation in the legs and feet. Such impairments reduce postural stability, particularly when there is concomitant disease-related impairment of central sensory processing. Woollacott and co-workers [32] found that older people, but not young adults, lost their balance when visual feedback was eliminated or distorted concomitantly with a reduction in somatosensory feedback. Tobis et al. [51] found that visuospatial perception is impaired in many older people who fall. Visuospatial perception may be particularly important in the anticipatory formulation of postural adjustments for a specific environmental hazard.

The functional stretch-reflex response to postural perturbation is delayed and reduced in many older people, and the responses of individual muscles are not as tightly coupled as in younger controls [52, 53]. Hence, many older people exhibit greater variability in their postural responses to perturbations. Furthermore, preparatory postural control and movement are loosely integrated in many older people [54]. These changes in functional somatosensory reflex latencies and preparatory postural latencies are most evident when a perturbation or volitional movement produces backward postural sway [36, 53, 55]. Finally, the prolongation of choice reaction times in older people [56] indicate a slowing of central motor programming that may impede anticipatory locomotor adjustments to environmental hazards.

The extent to which these changes in postural control are attributable to normal aging is unclear. Many studies of elderly control subjects probably contained significant numbers of older people with unrecognized illness. For example, Inglin and Woollacott [55] examined the preparatory postural activity in older (mean age, 71 years) adults during voluntary push and pull maneuvers with the dominant upper extremity and found delayed onset of preparatory postural activity in the lower extremities and delayed voluntary muscle activity in the upper extremity. However, these changes were largely attributable to 2 of the 15 older people who were found by a neurologist to have abnormal neurological signs [57]. Many older people have compared favorably with young adults in studies of postural control [58].

KINEMATICS OF NORMAL WALKING

Normal Adults

Human locomotion has been studied for 100 years with high-frequency photogrammetric techniques [59, 60]. The accuracy and efficiency of photogrammetric methods have increased considerably during the past 30 years [61]. Consequently, a large volume of data has accrued that describes the kinematics, kinetics, and electromyographic characteristics of human gait. These data are reviewed in many fine books [62, 63] and in an excellent set of videocassettes by Koerner [64].

Walking is a cyclical movement with two dimensions: the time and length of stride [62, 63]. The gait cycle is defined arbitrarily as the time between successive heel–floor contacts with the same foot (Fig. 6). Consequently, one gait cycle consists of two steps. From right heel–floor contact to left toe-off is a period of double-limb support (stance) that lasts approximately 10% of the total gait cycle. This phase of the cycle is followed by the left swing phase, which is simultaneous with and equal to the right single-limb support phase. The time from left heel–floor contact to right toe-off comprises the second of two double-limb support phases in a gait cycle and is followed by the right swing phase and left single-limb support phase. Stride length and cadence (2 ÷ time of stride) are generally regarded as the independent variables of walking, which determine the velocity of walking (stride length × cadence ÷ 2) and the magnitudes of other kinematic characteristics of gait such as arm swing, toe–floor clearance, hip and knee rotations, and time in double-limb stance [65–67]. Detailed pictorial reviews of the patterns of muscle activation during the gait cycle are provided elsewhere [62, 68].

During normal walking, the center of mass oscillates vertically at a fre-

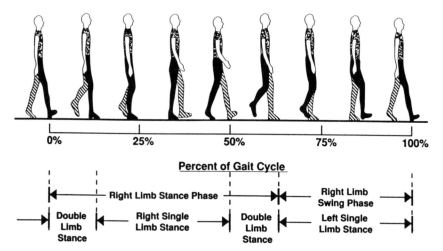

Figure 6   The phases of a normal adult gait cycle are expressed as percentages of stride. The percentage of total time spent in double-limb stance is inversely proportional to the speed of walking.

quency equal to the cadence and horizontally at a frequency of one-half the cadence [62]. During a gait cycle, the two maxima in vertical oscillation occur in the middle of right and left single-limb stance, and the two minima of vertical oscillation occur in the middle of the two phases of double-limb stance. The left- and rightmost horizontal excursions of the center of mass occur at the times of midleft and right single-limb stance. These vertical and horizontal excursions of the center of mass are optimized in such a way that the center of mass moves forward with the least amount of expended energy [62, 69].

Saunders and co-workers [70] defined the six major determinants of human gait efficiency.

1. Pelvic rotation of approximately 8 degrees about the vertical axis elevates and smoothes the minima of vertical oscillation of the center of mass and reduces the need for hip rotation at a given length of stride.
2. Pelvic tilt of approximately 5 degrees in the coronal plane reduces the maxima of vertical oscillation.
3. Knee flexion during the stance phase reduces the maxima of vertical oscillation. This and the two determinants above all serve to increase the effective length of the lower limb by 220%.
4. Rotation of the foot from the time of initial heel contact to ultimate toe-off

smoothes the minima of vertical oscillation of the center of mass, thus reducing energy expenditure.

5. Coordination of knee flexion with foot rotation during stance phase also serves to smooth the minima of vertical oscillation of the center of mass.

6. Lateral displacement of the pelvis is needed to position the center of mass over the stance limb. This displacement is minimized by the tibio-femoral angle.

When a neurological or musculoskeletal disease affects one or more of these determinants, the remaining normal determinants will be modified in such a way that balance and conservation of energy are maximized [60, 70]. Many characteristics of abnormal gaits are dictated by this principle of energy conservation and by the biomechanical constraints of the body [71]. Reduced stride and gait velocity are seen in most patients, regardless of cause, and many abnormalities of gait are attributable to these nonspecific kinematic changes.

Effects of Aging

Many studies have examined quantitatively the kinematics of walking in elderly people with the principal goal of defining the changes in walking that can be attributed to normal aging [62, 72–78]. Most quantitative studies have found that healthy elderly people walk more slowly than young adults. In addition, elderly people exhibit a shorter stride, which necessitates a faster cadence for a given speed of walking [72–79].

When assessing an elderly person's pattern of walking, the effects of reduced stride and velocity on the other characteristics of gait must be considered. Increased time spent in double-limb stance and reduced arm swing, toe–floor clearance, and rotation of the hip and knee are expected to occur when the velocity of walking is reduced [65, 67, 80–83]. Elble and co-workers [84] used computerized infrared stroboscopic photometry to quantify the kinematic profiles of fast and natural walking in 20 young adults (10 men and 10 women; mean age, 30.0 ± 6.1 years) and 20 elderly people (9 men and 11 women; mean age, 74.7 ± 6.6 years) who had no history of falling, fear of falling, or abnormal neurological signs other than reduced vibratory sensation in the feet and absent ankle reflexes. The average natural and fast velocities of walking in the elderly were, respectively, 20% and 17% less than in the young. These differences in gait velocity were produced by comparable differences in stride length. Cadence did not differ between the young and old for fast or natural walking.

Kinematic data from the studies of Elble and co-workers [84] are summarized in Table 1. Velocity (m/sec), cadence (steps/min.) percentage of stride in double-limb stance, stride length (m), maximum vertical toe–floor

Table 1 Kinematics of Natural Walking in Young and Older Adults

Variable	Young Adults (N = 20)	Older Adults (N = 19)	Patients (N = 0)
Age (years)	30.0 (6.1)[a]	76 (6)[b]	79 (4)
Velocity (m/sec)	1.18 (0.15)	0.96 (0.15)[b]	0.338 (0.16)[c]
Stride length (m)	1.32 (0.12)	1.08 (0.11)[b]	0.49 (0.17)[c]
Cadence (steps/min)	107 (7.3)	106 (10)	80 (18)[c]
Step width (m)	0.109 (0.041)	0.11 (0.03)	0.14 (0.04)[c]
Double-limb stance (%)	23.8 (4.09)	26.0 (3.9)	47.0 (7.5)[c]
Minimum toe displacement (m)	0.014 (0.004)	0.015 (0.006)	0.013 (0.01)
Maximum toe displacement (m)	0.069 (0.009)	0.055 (0.008)[b]	0.025 (0.01)[c]
Wrist displacement (m)	0.081 (0.018)	0.068 (0.03)[b]	0.036 (0.01)[c]
Minimum hip flexion (degrees)	−4.21 (7.79)	−2.9 (6.5)	7.7 (12.0)[c]
Maximum hip flexion (degrees)	31.2 (6.28)	30.0 (6.4)	27.7 (7.6)
Hip Rotation (degrees)	35.4 (4.88)	32.9 (4.3)	20.8 (7.7)[c]
Minimum knee flexion (degrees)	−0.50 (2.93)	2.2 (5.3)[b]	8.7 (9.3)[c]
Maximum knee flexion (degrees)	61.2 (4.38)	56.3 (5.0)[b]	43.9 (10.5)[c]
Knee rotation (degrees)	61.7 (4.19)	54.1 (4.5)[b]	30.8 (17.0)[c]

All kinematic measures except step width were taken in the sagittal plane.
[a]Values given as mean (SD).
[b]Different from young adults at $p < 0.05$ (two-tailed Student's t test).
[c]Different from normal older adults at $p < 0.05$.
Source: From ref. 142.

displacement (m; occurs at initial heel contact), minimum vertical toe–floor displacement (m; occurs in midswing phase), maximum vertical wrist displacement (a measure of arm swing in meters), maximum and minimum hip and knee flexions (degrees; rotation = maximum − minimum flexions) were measured in the sagittal plane, and step width (i.e., base; distance in meters between the heel markers at successive heel–floor contacts) were measured in the coronal plane. Although the healthy young and older people differed in several aspects of gait, analysis of covariance revealed that these differences were statistically attributable to the reduced stride of the elderly. Cadence, height, and age did not contribute. This dependence of kinematic variables on stride was similar to that reported by Kirtley and co-workers [67] and explains why stride and gait velocity are useful, albeit nonspecific, measures of disability [85–87].

The nonspecific influence of stride on the other kinematic characteristics of gait must be considered in the clinical evaluation of gait disturbances in elderly patients. Clinicians must remain mindful of the role of the musculoskeletal, circulatory, and respiratory systems in determining stride length and gait velocity. The need to minimize energy expenditure largely dictates the cadence–stride relationship exhibited at a particular velocity of walking [62, 88–94]. In addition, reduced stride and velocity could result from nonneurological causes such as increased stiffness or reduced muscular power at the hips and knees. Just as patients with stiff lungs or weak muscles breathe most efficiently by taking frequent breaths at a reduced volume, people with stiff joints or weak muscles, by analogy, are likely to minimize energy expenditure by taking shorter, more frequent steps to accomplish a particular velocity and distance of walking. In addition, elderly people with reduced cardiopulmonary reserve [95] will be forced to adopt a reduced natural velocity of walking, with an associated reduction in stride and cadence. Critchley [96] warned that "an abnormal gait in the aged is frequently the result of disease outside the nervous system." Schenkman and co-workers [97, 98] stressed the importance of biomechanical constraints in the impairment of ambulation. Musculoskeletal stiffness of the limbs, spine, and pelvis can make sitting, standing, turning and rolling over very difficult. Maintenance of joint flexibility and range of motion are therefore critical to normal balance and mobility. To illustrate the importance of lumbopelvic mobility to balance and ambulation, Schenkman and Butler [97] challenged their readers to assume a stooped posture (i.e., lumbothoracic kyphosis with the pelvis rotated posteriorly, as illustrated in Fig. 3) and attempt to walk, sit, stand, turn, and adjust to a postural disturbance such as a nudge to the chest.

Age-related degeneration in monoaminergic pathways is frequently proposed as a mechanism of gait senescence. Age-related loss of nigrostriatal dopaminergic input occurs at an estimated rate of 8% per decade of life. This loss would not be clinically significant in most people before the tenth decade of life [99–101]. There is an average 20% reduction in cells of the locus ceruleus by age 85 [102], but this degree of cell loss is not likely to have an appreciable effect on locomotor behavior [103]. Age-related cholinergic cell loss in the pedunculopontine and dorsolateral tegmental nuclei has not been demonstrated, although loss of these cholinergic cells may play a role in the gait disturbances of Parkinson's disease and progressive supranuclear palsy [104–106]. Cell loss in the neocortex and cerebellum occurs with aging [107, 108] and could contribute to locomotor impairment in the elderly [109, 110].

Ventricular size in healthy controls increases significantly after age 60 [111]. The mechanism(s) and clinical significance of this ventriculomegaly is unclear. Fisher [112] suggested that hydrocephalus may play a role in many older people with symmetrical impairment of gait. Fisher [112] and Sudarsky and Ronthal [113] found that the distance across the frontal horns of the lateral ventricles frequently exceeded 38 mm in patients with impaired walking but not in the normal elderly. Koller and co-workers [114] also found that enlargement of the ventricular system correlated with the presence of gait impairment, but this ventriculomegaly was not sufficient in most cases to warrant the diagnosis of hydrocephalus. In many elderly people the causes and clinical significance of ventriculomegaly are never determined.

Type II (fast twitch) muscle fiber atrophy is a well-documented accompaniment of aging [115, 116]. This is a nonspecific phenomenon caused by reduced activity, toxins, systemic metabolic disturbances, and endocrine disorders. This form of muscle atrophy is seen more frequently in elderly patients who fall [115, 117] and is reversed by exercise, which results in improved ambulation [118].

A loss of vibratory sensation is common in the elderly, particularly in their toes and fingers [119, 120]. Delwaide and Delmotte [121] found that 15% of older people with disturbed ambulation exhibited greatly reduced vibratory sensation in the feet and ankles. Loss of vibratory sensation is attributable in many older people to a loss of cutaneous sensory receptors and to arthritic joint disease [122, 123]. Proprioception, by contrast, is well preserved in healthy older people [124], and vibratory sensation may be absent in the feet of healthy older people who have no abnormality of walking [84]. Therefore, the clinical significance of vibratory loss per se is questionable in many older people, and clinicians should carefully consider all possible diagnoses before dismissing locomotor impairment as due to a senile neuropathy that is seemingly manifested by poor vibratory sensation in the feet.

This discussion of putative age-related neurological and musculoskeletal changes must be concluded with the important caveat that there is no generally accepted definition of normal aging. Until the unavoidable consequences of aging are rigorously defined, no abnormality of posture or locomotion should be attributed to aging per se. While there may be an age beyond which abnormalities of posture and locomotion are inevitable, this age is not defined.

NONSPECIFIC NEUROLOGICAL SYNDROMES OF IMPAIRED WALKING

Senile Gait (Cautious Gait)

Newman and co-workers [119] examined 260 elderly residents of Durham, North Carolina, aged 60–93 (mean, 70). Fifteen percent had some abnormality of gait, which most commonly consisted of a shortened stride and shuffling. Prakash and Stern [120] examined 100 medical inpatients, average age 81.8 (range, 69–94), with no history of neurological disease and found evidence of impaired ambulation in 22. Most of these patients exhibited a nonspecifically slow, wide-based, cautious gait.

Older patients who complain of impaired ambulation exhibit a pattern of gait that deviates significantly from their neurologically healthy peers [75,

125]. These patients exhibit a guarded or restrained pattern of walking that resembles someone walking on a slippery surface [78]. Stooped posture, reduced arm swing, increased time with both feet on the floor (double-limb stance), loss of the normal heel–toe sequence of foot–floor contact, disturbed coordination of cyclical limb movements, decreased toe–floor clearance, and reduced hip and knee rotations are observed in most elderly people with locomotor impairment [126–128]. This kinematic profile of walking in an older person is referred to as senile gait [129].

Many clinicians reserve the term senile gait for those elderly patients with a symmetrical gait disturbance of unknown cause [129]. However, these patients exhibit a pattern of walking indistinguishable from that of many patients with a variety of neurological, musculoskeletal, and systemic diseases. Patients with bilateral subdural hematomas [130], Binswanger's disease [131], normal pressure hydrocephalus [112, 132–138], Parkinson's disease [139, 140], and high cervical myelopathy [141] exhibit gait disturbances that are heavily veiled by the characteristics of senile gait.

Elble and co-workers [142] reasoned that senile gait is a nonspecific syndrome of abnormal walking in older people, not a specific disease, and warned that the characteristics of senile gait may be largely compensatory effects of reduced stride and velocity. Support for this notion came from a comparison of the gait characteristics in 19 healthy older people with those of 10 elderly patients with a mixture of neurological conditions, including vascular dementia, shunt-responsive normal pressure hydrocephalus (NPH), dementia of Alzheimer's type (DAT), levodopa-resistant parkinsonism, and sensorimotor polyneuropathy. All patients walked with the characteristics of senile gait. Quantitatively, their kinematic characteristics of gait differed greatly from those of elderly controls, far more than the differences between young and elderly controls (Table 1). Nevertheless, an analysis of covariance revealed that these differences were statistically attributable to reduced stride.

In sum, senile gait is a syndrome characterized largely by nonspecific, stride-dependent characteristics of gait. This profile of walking is not a specific entity and is not peculiar to older people. Cautious gait is a more general term, and its characteristics heavily veil the patterns of walking produced by a wide variety of neurological illnesses. Consequently, symmetrical gait disturbances due to many causes have a similar appearance.

Paraplegia in Flexion and Senile Paraplegia

Paraplegia in flexion occurs in patients with advanced chronic myelopathies and bilateral cerebral disease. Pathologically enhanced flexor reflexes and hypertonia in the lower extremities are associated with extreme flexion and adduction of the hips, flexion of the knees, and extension of the ankles, which ultimately lead to musculoskeletal contractures [143, 144]. Patients with paraplegia in flexion due to bilateral cerebral disease usually have severe damage to both frontal lobes. The original descriptions of this syndrome were mainly in patients with advanced vascular degeneration of the centrum semiovale and basal ganglia. However, this syndrome also occurs in patients with advanced primary degenerative dementias (e.g., Alzheimer's disease and Pick's disease), general paresis, multiple sclerosis, posttraumatic encephalopathy, and other acquired encephalopathies not limited to the elderly [145]. This syndrome in an elderly patient has been called senile paraplegia [146].

Yakovlev [145] noted that paraplegia in flexion begins with the development of paratonic rigidity (gegenhalten), followed by flexion attitude. Paratonia is a form of hypertonia that occurs when the patient attempts to relax during passive range of motion of a limb by an examiner. Despite the patient's sincere effort to relax, the limb seems to resist passive movement actively. Paratonia increases when the patient becomes frustrated or excited. Paratonia is frequently associated with hyperactive tendon reflexes, Babinski signs, emotional apathy, perseveration, poor attention span, and reduced avoidance reaction to pain despite normal sensation. Flexion attitude consists of a flexion of the torso, neck, hips, knees; adduction of the shoulders and thighs; cupping of the hands with thumbs in apposition to the forefingers; and postural instability. Facial masking, drooling, bradykinesia, lethargy, reduced spontaneous movement, and tremor of the lips, tongue, and fingers are common. The gait of these patients is hesitant and unstable and characterized by short shuffling steps. The repertoire of movement becomes limited. Interaction with the environment becomes less purposeful, and negotiation with obstacles is less effective. Pseudobulbar palsy and affect may be present. The similarities between this nonspecific syndrome and advanced Parkinson's disease are obvious and were emphasized by Yakovlev [145]. Based upon postmortem studies of six patients, Yakovlev concluded that the critical lesion in this syndrome was damage to the frontal lobes and basal ganglia, but Yakovlev also noted that his patients exhibited degeneration in fiber tracts that originated from brainstem nuclei. The role of brainstem pathological damage, therefore, could not be excluded.

The characteristics of senile gait are contained in the earliest stage of paraplegia in flexion (i.e., paratonic rigidity). The syndrome of paraplegia in flexion illustrates the important fact that stooped unstable posture, paratonic rigidity, and hesitancy depend as much on the stage of an illness as on the type of pathology.

Apraxia of Gait and Frontal Ataxia

Many neurologists of the 19th and early 20th centuries recognized that lesions of the frontal lobe were capable of producing contralateral clumsiness (ataxia) of the limbs similar to that produced by lesions of the ipsilateral cerebellum [147, 148]. This phenomenon is referred to as frontal ataxia. Gerstmann and Schilder [149] were the first authors to suggest that the gait disturbance of bilateral frontal lobe disease also could be due to apraxia of the lower limbs. Van Bogaert and Martin [150] concurred with this notion. However, patients with bilateral frontal lobe disease rarely, if ever, fulfill Wilson's strict definition of apraxia as an "inability to perform certain subjectively purposive movements or movement-complexes, with conservation of motility, of sensation, and of coordination" [151]. Denny-Brown [152] observed that patients with lesions of the mesial frontal lobes exhibited impaired performance of purposive motor acts with the affected extremities, an instinctive grasp with the fingers and toes, instinctive suck, and paratonia. He attributed all of these phenomena to perseveration of abnormal postures that resulted from bodily contact. When his patients attempted to walk, he noted that the toes flexed onto the floor and the lower extremities stiffened. He reasoned that perseveration of abnormal posture of stance caused his patients to walk with short, hesitant, halting steps, as though their feet were "glued" to the floor. Denny-Brown acknowledged S. A. K. Wilson's strict definition of apraxia, but he believed that his patients had sufficient preservation of motility, sensation, and coordination to justify the term magnetic apraxia in describing the gait disturbance of his patients.

In their frequently quoted 1960 paper in *Brain*, Meyer and Barron [147] differentiated frontal ataxia from gait apraxia. They defined apraxia of gait as "the loss of ability to properly use the lower limbs in the act of walking which cannot be accounted for by demonstrable sensory impairment or motor weakness." They characterized gait apraxia as a hesitant, slow, short-stepped, shuffling gait in which the feet seemed to stick to the ground. Postural instability, including retropulsion, was common. They emphasized that this type of gait disturbance could readily be differentiated from frontal ataxia and cerebellar ataxia. Meyer and Barron's description of gait apraxia was based upon clinical data from seven patients, none of whom was autopsied. Their patients had cerebral vascular disease (3), general paresis (1), parasagittal meningioma (1), metastatic squamous cell carcinoma of the cervix (1), and cerebral vascular disease with pickwickian syndrome (1). These patients exhibited various combinations of postural instability, hypertonia, perseveration of posture, bradykinesia, reduced spontaneous movement, hyperreflexia, and Babinski signs. Volitional movements of the lower extremities were executed hesitantly, slowly, and inaccurately, in contrast to the cases reported by Denny-Brown [152].

The principal problem with the term "gait apraxia" is that most patients do not have sufficient preservation of motor and sensory function to justify use of this terminology. Therefore, gait apraxia is a misnomer in most instances and does not differ significantly from the advanced stages of paraplegia in flexion, described by Yakovlev.

SPECIFIC NEUROLOGICAL CONDITIONS THAT CAUSE GAIT ABNORMALITIES

Arteriosclerotic Parkinsonism

Patients with multiple vascular lesions of the frontal lobes and basal ganglia frequently exhibit a pattern of walking that resembles the gait disturbance of Parkinson's disease. Macdonald Critchley [154] defined arteriosclerotic parkinsonism as a generalized weakness, slowness of movement, and rigidity of a nonpyramidal type. Patients with this condition exhibit a gait disturbance characterized by shortened stride and slow uncertain steps. As the disease progresses, foot–floor clearance is reduced, and posture becomes stooped. There is a tendency to fall backwards, and the toes may flex excessively as though they were gripping the floor. The gait also becomes hesitant and halting. Turns are made stiffly and with multiple steps. Dejerine and Marie referred to this gait as *marche á petits pas*. Patients with this syndrome are diffusely hypertonic, but the hypertonia is often distinct from typical spasticity and parkisonian rigidity. The variable hypertonus in these patients frequently has the characteristics of paratonia (gegenhalten). Perseveration of posture is sometimes seen, particularly in advanced cases. There is little or no loss of muscle strength, and the lower extremities are usually affected more than the upper extremities, hence the term lower-half parkinsonism. Muscle stretch reflexes are usually brisk, and Babinski signs are frequently present. During walking, the upper extremities are frequently abducted, in contrast to the adducted, flexed posture in patients with Parkinson's disease.

Thompson and Marsden [131] described the patterns of gait in 12 patients with the clinical diagnosis of Binswanger's disease. In those patients who were able to stand and walk without assistance, the pattern of gait was characterized by a wide base, "parkinsonian" steps, and mild axial instability. By contrast, the more advanced patients exhibited, in addition, loss of truncal mobility, marked axial instability, stooped posture, inability to initiate steps (feet sticking to the floor), hesitation when turning, and freezing. Festination was conspicuously absent, and facial expression and arm swing were relatively preserved in comparison to patients with Parkinson's disease. These observations suggest that the degree to which the feet stick to the floor (the so-called magnetic foot response) is a function of the extent of gait impairment and not a specific indication of apraxia. The degree to which the gaits of these patients resemble frontal ataxia versus apraxia may depend upon the relative proportions of axial instability versus stiff, shuffling immobility.

Thompson and Marsden [131] noted that the characteristics of gait in Binswanger disease were similar to those in many patients with normal pressure hydrocephalus, bilateral frontal lobe disease, Parkinson's disease, multiple system atrophy, progressive supranuclear palsy, and cryptogenic senile gait. They proposed that dysfunction of pathways to and from the supplementary motor cortex and mesial motor cortex (leg area) may be the critical pathological changes. The symptoms and signs of arteriosclerotic parkinsonism are largely contained within the syndrome of paraplegia in flexion and are not peculiar to patients with multiple vascular lesions of the frontal lobes and basal ganglia.

Normal Pressure Hydrocephalus

McHugh [135] described seven patients in whom symptomatic hydrocephalus occurred in adulthood. McHugh's description of the gait disturbance in his patients could not be differentiated from the gait disturbance of paraplegia in flexion. Adams and co-workers [132] reported their three "most striking examples" of patients with normal pressure hydrocephalus who responded dramatically to cerebrospinal fluid shunting. These three cases and subsequent reports by other authors [112, 133, 134, 136–138] document the variability and nonspecificity of the associated gait disturbance. Mildly affected patients typically exhibit a nonspecific unsteadiness, shortened stride, normal or mildly widened base, and reduced velocity. As the gait disturbance progresses, these characteristics become increasingly severe, postural instability increases, and the gait becomes more hesitant and halting, creating the impression of motor apraxia.

The characteristic gait disturbance of normal pressure hydrocephalus is frequently referred to as gait apraxia [155], despite the admittedly nonspecific abnormalities of gait in this syndrome and the nearly invariable presence of generalized motor dysfunction. Estanol argued that the gait disturbance of communicating hydrocephalus is due to a release of proprioceptive supporting reactions. This notion is congruent with the observation that voluntary motion in the lower limbs of mildly impaired patients is relatively normal except when the patients stand up. This characteristic of lower limb function suggests that a postural disturbance, not apraxia, underlies this and similar disturbances of gait.

The nonspecificity of the gait disturbance in normal pressure hydrocephalus (NPH) has been lamented by many other authors. Sudarsky and Simon [138] measured the kinematics of gait in six patients with NPH and in eight elderly patients with a mixture of gait disorders. The characteristics of gait did not differ between the two groups except that a greater reduction in foot–floor clearance and pelvic rotation was observed in the patients with

NPH. Goto and co-workers [130] found that the kinematic characteristics of gait did not differ among 10 patients with chronic bilateral subdural hematoma and 10 patients with normal pressure hydrocephalus. The similarities in gait between patients with NPH and vascular dementia are probably not fortuitous because both illnesses impair frontal lobe function [156], vascular disease may cause NPH [157–160], and many characteristics of gait in both conditions are probably compensatory [142].

Knutsson and Lying-Tunell [161] and Sudarsky and Simon [138] found the EMG activity in the lower extremities of patients with NPH was less phasic, and there was increased coactivation of antagonistic muscles. However, similar patterns of EMG are seen in patients with Parkinson's disease and vascular dementia (personal observations), and this abnormality of EMG is probably a nonspecific manifestation of the associated hypertonia and postural instability. Conrad and co-workers [162] demonstrated that similar abnormalities in EMG occur in normal people who are attempting to walk while blindfolded. Therefore, steady coactivation of EMG in antagonistic muscle groups of the lower extremities can be a normal sign of physiological adaptation to environmental uncertainties.

Many authors emphasized that the upper extremities were not affected in NPH or were affected less than the lower extremities [132, 135, 163]. The greater impairment of the lower extremities was attributed to greater stretching of fibers from the paracentral cerebral cortex [163]. This region of the motor-sensory cortex contains neurons that control the lower extremities, and this region also contains the supplementary motor cortex, which is involved in basal ganglia function. Similar differential involvement of the upper and lower extremities was described, but not emphasized, by Yakovlev in his essay on paraplegia in flexion [145]. NPH causes mild weakness, clumsiness, postural tremor, paratonia, increased tendon reflexes, and bradykinesia in the upper extremities [137], similar to that described by Yakovlev [145], and impairment of oculomotor control may also occur [164]. Therefore, NPH, like paraplegia in flexion, is a generalized disturbance of motor control. The characteristics of paraplegia in flexion, as described by Yakovlev, are sufficiently broad to describe many patients with the syndrome of NPH. Keep in mind that many patients with NPH exhibit a nonspecific unsteadiness, shortened stride, normal or mildly widened base, and reduced velocity of gait, which provide no clue to the underlying pathology.

Parkinson's Disease

Sudarsky and Ronthal [113] found that hesitation, festination, en bloc turning, flexed posture, and reduced accessory movements were more common in 5 patients with Parkinson's disease than in 45 elderly patients with other disturbances of gait. With the possible exception of festination, these charac-teristics of gait are seen in advanced gait disturbances of many causes. Knutsson [139] performed a quantitative kinematic analysis of gait in 2 patients with postencephalitic parkinsonism and 19 patients with Parkinson's disease and found increased time in double-limb stance, increased minimum knee flexion, and reduced gait velocity, cadence, stride length, sagittal rotation of the hips and knees, toe–floor clearance, and arm swing. None of these abnormalities is specific for Parkinson's disease. Murray and co-workers [140] quantitatively examined the kinematics of gait in 44 patients with Parkinson's disease and obtained results similar to those of Knutsson. Murray and co-workers found that the reduced gait velocities of their patients were entirely attributable to reductions in stride length. Neither Knutsson nor Murray and co-workers examined the extent to which the parkinsonian profile of walking was attributable to reduced stride. Nevertheless, the characteristics of senile gait and paraplegia in flexion are prominent features in patients with Parkinson's disease, and additional, more specific signs (e.g., rest tremor and festination) are necessary to allow one to make this diagnosis with certainty.

Hemiparesis, Spastic Diplegia, and Myelopathy

Patients with pyramidal tract lesions usually exhibit various combinations of paralysis, hypertonia, and segmental reflex enhancement. The effect of a hemiparesis on locomotion will depend upon the relative magnitudes of these three characteristics. Coexistent sensory deficits may also contribute. There-fore, the gait abnormalities caused by unilateral and bilateral pyramidal tract lesions vary considerably among adults, and the effects of such lesions in adults may differ from those in children.

In general, patients with hemiplegia exhibit reduced gait velocity, stride and cycle duration [165]. Reduced balance and impaired ability to shift weight between limbs may contribute as much to locomotor impairment as weakness and spasticity. Abnormal hip flexion, knee extension, and ankle plantar flexion occur in conjunction with circumduction of the lower extrem-ity during the swing phase of gait. Abnormal hip flexion and hyperextension of the knee occur in the stance phase [165, 166]. Knutsson [167] found that one-third of patients with a hemiparesis exhibited premature activation of the triceps surae during the single-limb stance phase of the gait cycle. Spasticity seemed to be the critical source of locomotor impairment in these patients. This impeded rotation of the leg over the supporting foot and caused hyperextension of the knee. Enhanced activation of the hip adductors oc-curred in some patients during the transition from stance to swing phase. Abnormally enhanced and poorly modulated stretch-reflex responses in these muscles were believed to underlie, at least in part, these abnormal muscle patterns. The stretch reflex is normally carefully modulated during the gait cycle [168, 169]. In another third of hemiparetic patients, Knutsson found low or complete absence of activity in two or more muscle groups. Paresis was the principal problem in these patients, with spasticity playing little or no role in locomotor impairment. Approximately 15% of patients exhibited abnormal coactivation of antagonistic muscle groups and loss of normal phasic activity in individual muscles. The remaining patients exhibited combinations of paresis, spasticity, and abnormal coactivation. In contrast to these abnormalities in adult patients, pathologically sustained coactivation of antagonistic muscles was the predominant feature in children with cerebral palsy [167].

Combinations of abnormalities, similar to those of hemiparesis, are seen in patients with myelopathy. Although the abnormalities are bilateral, asymmetries are common. Patients with cervical myelopathies may exhibit restricted movement and posturing of the upper extremities, which are often poorly coordinated with the lower extremities. Stiff, scissoring, mechanical movements of the lower extremities are usually associated with equinovarus posturing of the foot, causing abnormal foot–floor contact during the stance phases of gait. However, some patients with cervical myelopathy are predominantly affected by posterior column dysfunction, such that their gait is characterized more by nonspecific clumsiness. As discussed previously, a nonspecific pattern of walking is frequently observed in older people with cervical spondylosis.

The characteristics of gait in spastic diplegia also vary significantly. Asymmetries are common. In addition to the usual reductions in stride and gait velocity, patients typically exhibit variable combinations of increased flexion of the hips, flexion of the knees, abnormal ankle plantar flexion during the stance and swing phases of gait, malrotation of the feet, abnormal tilt and limited rotation of the pelvis, and excessive adduction and internal rotation of the hips. Mechanical limitation of joint rotation due to muscle spasticity and contracture is common. Misguided surgical lengthening of the Achilles tendon without prior attention to hip and knee contractures will exacerbate this pattern of walking [170]. Quantitative motion analysis with electromyography is particularly useful in planning and evaluating the surgical treatment of gait abnormalities due to cerebral palsy [170, 171].

Myopathic, Neuropathic, and Biomechanical Disturbances of Gait

The effect of a myopathic disease on gait depends upon the distribution of weakness, making it impossible to generalize among patients with different

illnesses [170]. Hip-girdle weakness, which is characteristic of many myopathies, impairs rotation and lateral displacement of the pelvis. The consequences of this weakness are illustrated classically in Duchenne type muscular dystrophy [170]. As hip girdle weakness increases, the gait becomes
increasingly wide-based. The stride shortens, and the hips begin to rotate
internally during the stance phases of the gait cycle. Lumbar lordosis is
exaggerated as the pelvis develops an anterior tilt. Lateral shoulder sway and
arm abduction occur in response to weakness of the gluteus medius. Pelvic
obliquity increases, and the foot–floor strike becomes flat-footed. These
changes produce an awkward, waddling gait. Loss of ankle dorsiflexion and
knee stability occur in the final stages.

The consequences of peripheral polyneuropathy also vary among diseases
and depend upon the magnitude and distribution of sensory loss and weakness
[170]. The steppage gait of hereditary polyneuropathies, such as Charcot-
Marie-Tooth disease, is the prototypic example of neuropathic gait. The early
development of weakness in the anterolateral leg muscles produces a foot
drop and ankle inversion, which is particularly noticeable during the mid to
late stages of the swing phases of the gait cycle. Foot–floor strike is slapping
and flat–footed. The foot becomes externally rotated during the stance phase,
as weakness develops in the posteromedial muscles of the leg. Push-off into
swing phase with the triceps surae becomes progressively limited, as does flexion of the knee during stance phase. Sensory impairment disturbs limb coordination and balance, producing an increased base during gait and stance.

The importance of Saunder's six determinants of efficient walking (see
above) is illustrated nicely by mechanical impairments of the hip, knee, or
ankle, as discussed by Inman and co-workers [62]. Physicians and rehabilitation therapists must remain mindful of the biomechanical complications of
myopathic and neuropathic diseases. Muscle contractures and arthropathies
may contribute greatly to the impairment of balance and locomotion. Spinal
and pelvic deformities restrict the ability to position the torso and center of
mass purposefully, impairing balance and the ability to sit, stand, turn, and
roll over. Finally, musculoskeletal and neuropathic illnesses generally produce both direct and compensatory changes in gait. The resulting pattern of
gait may deviate considerably from normal but usually serves to minimize
energy expenditure and tissue strain. As a consequence, misguided attempts
to correct a patient's gait with orthotics or surgery can lead to inefficient
walking and musculoskeletal trauma. The planning of a successful rehabilitative program must be guided by a careful evaluation of the patient's gait
mechanics. Quantitative motion analysis with photogrammetric techniques,
floor-mounted force transducers, and electromyography is being used with
increasing frequency [170, 171].

Cerebellar Ataxia

Patients with cerebellar damage exhibit impaired balance, limb coordination, and rhythmicity of gait. The timing and magnitude of limb movement are incorrect, resulting in considerable cycle-to-cycle variability in the kinematic features of gait. Hence, the gait disturbance of cerebellar ataxia is frequently described as wide-based, reeling, and lunging. Start hesitation is not a characteristic, even though locomotion may be initiated incorrectly. Damage to the vermis, flocculonodular lobe, and fastigial nuclei are particularly deleterious to locomotion and postural control, but damage to the cerebellar hemispheres may also produce ataxia [172].

FALLS

Lipsitz and co-workers [173] found that recurrent falling was attributable to a primary cause in 73% of elderly patients. Stroke, parkinsonism, visual impairment, drug-induced hypotension, and severe arthritis were the most common causes. However, the majority of these patients had multiple contributing medical conditions, and the remainder of Lipsitz's patients had multiple pathological factors that could not be differentiated in explaining the falls. Impaired vision [53, 163], orthopedic problems including foot impairment [79, 174, 175], cognitive and emotional disorders [176–180], systemic disorders, and medication effects [181, 182] must be considered in all patients, including those with an obvious neurological diagnosis. Treatment of these coexisting conditions may improve ambulation, even when the principal neurological condition is not treatable.

Environmental hazards and errors in judgment were responsible for 35–50% of falls in some studies [181] and for very few falls in other studies [173]. Nevertheless, a safety evaluation of the home by an experienced occupational therapist is important. The bedroom and bathroom are particularly common sites for hazards such as loose rugs and clothing, slippery floors and bathtubs, and poor lighting. Installation of handrails, raised toilet seats, adequate lighting, and rubber floormats; elimination of electrical cords, clutter, and throw rugs; and repair of uneven floors and cracked sidewalks are important considerations. Shoes with slippery soles or high heels should be avoided.

Increased immobility may occur for no apparent reason following a serious fall [178]. This postfall syndrome should be treated early and aggressively. Reduced mobility may also occur as a result of prolonged bedrest. Unnecessary restriction of activities (e.g., bedrest) should be avoided in all hospitalized and home-bound patients. Nurses provide a great service by regularly walking elderly inpatients in hallways.

GENERAL APPROACH TO EVALUATING PATIENTS WITH IMPAIRED MOBILITY

Accurate diagnosis and treatment of disturbed locomotion require careful attention to details of the patient's history, a diligent search for localizing neurological signs, and a comprehensive, performance-oriented evaluation of functional deficits (Table 2). The presence of multiple contributing illnesses of systemic, neurological, or psychiatric origin is often emphasized in the evaluation of older people [174, 183–186], but this clinical guideline is worth remembering in the evaluation of all patients, young and old.

The profile of walking in older patients is often heavily veiled by nonspecific stride-dependent characteristics of gait, which comprise the syndrome of senile gait. Patients with senile gait may not exhibit glaringly diagnostic signs such as parkinsonian rest tremor and hemiparesis, and an exhaustive evaluation of these patients commonly leaves the clinician with multiple abnormalities of uncertain significance. As in the treatment of dementia, a compulsive correction of all treatable conditions is necessary.

Table 2   Performance-Oriented Measures of Gait
and Posture

Posture and balance during quiet stance
   Curvature of spine
   Head position
   Pelvic tilt
   Flexion of knees and hips
   Romberg test
Sitting and arising from a chair
Initiation of gait
Turning 360 degrees
Step length, width, rhythmicity, and symmetry
Coordination of upper and lower limbs
Foot–floor clearance
Walking path
Nature of foot–floor contact
Spontaneity of gait (freezing and hesitancy)
Bending over and reaching up while standing
Leaning back while standing
Gait velocity
Walking on heels and toes
Tandem walking
Response to active and passive neck motion while standing
Response to a nudge on chest or back

Until normal aging is rigorously defined, no abnormality of gait should be dismissed as due to old age.

Smidt [86] and others have lamented that gait analysis per se is rarely if ever sufficient to diagnose a disease entity. This is true, regardless of the methodology used. Quantitative gait analysis in a modern motion analysis laboratory is neither practical nor necessary in most patients. However, there is an increasing consensus of opinion regarding the usefulness of quantitative gait analysis with EMG before and following the surgical treatment of biomechanical abnormalities [170, 171]. Measures of stride length, cadence, and gait velocity are useful and sufficient quantitative adjuncts to a purely observational assessment of gait in most patients. Measures of preferred and maximal gait velocity are particularly useful indicators of walking ability [86].

SUMMARY

Successful locomotion requires the normal control and integration of posture and movement. Abnormalities of both are encountered in most patients with neurological impairment of gait. The characteristics of a patient's gait typically reflect the direct effects of neurological damage and the indirect effects of compensatory changes that occur within the biomechanical and energy constraints of the body. These constraints must be considered in the diagnosis and treatment of every patient. Saunders' [70] six biomechanical determinants of gait are particularly applicable to patients with musculoskeletal and peripheral neuropathic diseases, but are also relevant to patients with lesions of the central nervous system. Biomechanical considerations are especially important when one is considering the use of orthotic and surgical interventions. Most patients, young and old, have multifactorial impairment of locomotion, which includes the musculoskeletal changes that result from primary neurological disease. A comprehensive, performance-oriented assessment of each patient is crucial to the formulation of a successful rehabilitative program.

ACKNOWLEDGMENTS

Supported by a grant from the Whitaker Foundation and by grant P30 AG08014 from the National Institute on Aging.

REFERENCES

1. T.G. Brown, *J. Physiol.* (*London*), 48:18–46 (1914).
2. S. Grillner, *Handbook of Physiology: The Nervous System, Motor Control* (V.B. Brooks, ed.), Williams & Wilkins, Baltimore, pp. 1179–1236 (1981).

3. G. Holmes *Br. Med. J.*, 2:815–821 (1915).

4. E. Eidelberg, J.G. Waldin, and L.H. Nguyen, *Brain*, 104:647–663 (1981).

5. E. Eidelberg, J.L. Story, J.G. Walden, and B.L. Meyer, *Exp. Brain Res.*, 42:81–88 (1981).

6. D.M. Armstrong, *J. Physiol. (London)*, 405:1–37 (1988).

7. K. Kawahara, S. Mori, T. Tomiyama, and T. Kanaya, *Brain Res.*, 341:377–380 (1985).

8. S. Mori, *Prog. Neurobiol.*, 28:161–195 (1987).

9. S. Mori, T. Sakamoto, Y. Ohta, K. Takakusaki, and K. Matsuyama, *Brain Res.*, 505:66–74 (1989).

10. M. Marciello and H.M. Sinnamon, *Behav. Neurosci.*, 104:980–990 (1990).

11. E. Garcia-Rill, *Brain Res. Rev.* 11:47–63 (1986).

12. E. Garcia-Rill, N. Kinjo, Y. Atsuta, Y. Ishikawa, M. Webber, and R.D. Skinner, *Brain Res. Bull.*, 24:499–508 (1990).

13. M.R. DeLong, *Trends Neurosci*, 13:281–285 (1990).

14. N.S. Canteras, S.J. Shammah-Lagnado, B.A. Silva, and J.A. Ricardo, *Brain Res.*, 513:43–59 (1990).

15. A. Jourdain, K. Semba, and H.C. Fibiger, *Brain Res.*, 505:55–65 (1989).

16. D. Paré, M. Steriade, M. Deschênes, and D. Bouhassira, *J. Neurosci.*, 10:20–33 (1990).

17. J.D. Steeves and L.M. Jordan, *Brain Res.*, 307:263–276 (1984).

18. N. Kinjo, Y. Atsuta, M. Webber, R. Kyle, R.D. Skinner, and E. Garcia-Rill, *Brain Res. Bull.*, 24:509–516 (1990).

19. T. Drew, *Brain Res.*, 457:181–187 (1988).

20. Y. Brenière, and M.C. Do, and J. Sanchez, *J. Biophys. Méd. Nucl.*, 5:197–205 (1981).

21. E.V. Gurfinkel, *Agressologie*, 14:9–14 (1973).

22. J.C. Brocklehurst, D. Robertson, and P. James-Groom, *Age Ageing*, 11:1–10 (1982).

23. A.J. Sinclair and U.S.L. Nayak, *Compr. Ther.*, 16:44–48 (1990).

24. H.H. Thyssen, J. Brynskov, E.C. Jansen, and J. Münster-Swendsen, *Acta Neurol. Scand.*, 66:100–104 (1982).

25. F.B. Horak, L.M. Nashner, and N.C. Diener, *Exp. Brain Res.*, 82:167–177 (1990).

26. J. Dichgans, K.H. Mauritz, J.H.J. Allum, and T. Brandt, *Agressologie*, 17:15–24 (1976).

27. F. Lestienne, J. Soechting, and A. Berthoz, *Exp. Brain Res.*, 28:363–384 (1977).

28. H.C. Diener, J. Dichgans, B. Guschlbauer, and H. Mau, *Brain Res.*, 296:103–109 (1984).

29. L.M. Nashner, *Exp. Brain Res.*, 26:59–72 (1976).

30. L.M. Nashner, *Exp. Brain Res.*, 30:13–24 (1977).

31. L.M. Nashner, M. Woollacott, and G. Tuma, *Exp. Brain Res.*, 36:463–476 (1979).

32. M.H. Woollacott, A. Shumway-Cook, and L. Nashner, *The Aging Motor System*, (J.A. Mortimer, F.J. Pirozzolo, and G.J. Maletta, ed.), Praeger, New York, pp. 98–119 (1982).

33. V. Dietz, J. Quintern, W. Berger, and E. Schenck, *Exp. Brain Res.*, 57:348–354 (1985).
34. L.M. Nashner and G. McCollum, *Behav. Brain Sci.*, 8:135–172 (1985).
35. L.M. Nashner, F.O. Black, and C. Wall, *J. Neurosci.*, 2:536–544 (1982).
36. M.H. Woollacott, A. Shumway-Cook, and L.M. Nashner, *Int. J. Aging Hum. Dev.*, 23:97–114 (1986).
37. E.A. Keshner, J.H.J. Allum, and C.R. Pfaltz, *Exp. Brain Res.*, 69:77–92 (1987).
38. L. Nashner and A. Berthoz, *Brain Res.*, 150:403–407 (1978).
39. A.M. Aniss, H-C Diener, J. Hore, S.C. Gandevia, and D. Burke, *J. Neurophysiol.*, 64:661–670 (1990).
40. V.Y. Belen'kii, V.S. Gurfinkel', and Y.I. Pal'tsev, *Biofizika*, 12:135–141 (1967).
41. S. Bouisset and M. Zattara, *Neurosci. Lett.*, 22:263–270 (1981).
42. S. Bouisset and M. Zattara, *J. Biomech.*, 20:735–742 (1987).
43. M. Zattara and S. Bouisset, *J. Neurol. Neurosurg. Psychiatry*, 51:956–965 (1988).
44. P.J. Cordo and L.M. Nashner, *J. Neurophysiol.*, 47:287–302 (1982).
45. R. Forget and Y. Lamarre, *Brain Res.*, 508:176–179 (1990).
46. P. Crenna, C. Frigo, J. Massion, and A. Pedotti, *Exp. Brain Res.*, 65:538–548 (1987).
47. Y.I. Pal'tsev and A.M. El'ner, *Biofizika*, 12:142–147 (1967).
48. M.M. Traub, J.C. Rothwell, and C.D. Marsden, *Brain*, 103:393–412 (1980).
49. V.S. Gurfinkel and A.M. El'ner, *Neirofiziologiya*, 20:7–15 (1988).
50. J.P.R. Dick, J.C. Rothwell, A. Berardelli, P.D. Thompson, M. Gioux, R. Benecke, B.L. Day, C.D. Marsden, *J. Neurol. Neurosurg. Psychiatry*, 49:1378–1385 (1986).
51. J.S. Tobis, S. Reinsch, J.M. Swanson, M. Byrd, and T. Scharf, *J. Am. Geriatr. Soc.*, 33:330–333 (1985).
52. J.D. Brooke, R. Singh, M.K. Wilson, P. Yoon, and W.E. McIlroy, *Neurobiol. Aging*, 10:721–725 (1989).
53. G.E. Stelmach, J. Phillips, R.P. DiFabio, and N. Teasdale, *J. Gerontol.*, 44:B100–106 (1989).
54. G.E. Stelmach, L. Populin, and F. Müller, *Neurosci. Lett.*, 117:188–193 (1990).
55. B. Inglin and M. Woollacott, *J. Gerontol.*, 43:M105–M113 (1988).
56. A.T. Welford, *Ann. N.Y. Acad. Sci.*, 515:1–17 (1988).
57. M.H. Woollacott, B. Inglin, and D. Manchester, *Ann. N.Y. Acad. Sci.*, 515:42–55 (1988).
58. F.B. Horak, C.L. Shupert, and A. Mirka, *Neurobiol. Aging*, 10:727–738 (1989).
59. J.V. Basmajian and C.J. De Luca, *Muscles Alive. Their Functions Revealed by Electromyography*. Williams & Wilkins, Baltimore (1985).
60. R. Ducroquet, J. Ducroquet, and P. Ducroquet, *Walking and Limping. A Study of Normal and Pathological Walking*. J.B. Lippincott, Philadelphia (1968).
61. R.W. Man and E.K. Antonsson, *Bull. Hosp. Joint Dis. Orthop. Inst.*, 43:137–146 (1983).
62. V.T. Inman, H.J. Ralston, and F. Todd, *Human Walking*. Williams & Wilkins, Baltimore (1981).

63. D.A. Winter, *The Biomechanics and Motor Control of Human Gait.* University of Waterloo Press, Waterloo, Ontario (1987).

64. I. Koerner, *Observation of Human Gait.* Health Sciences Consortium, Chapel Hill, North Carolina (1986).

65. M.P. Murray, B.H. Kory, R.C. Clarkson, and S.B. Sepic, *Am. J. Phys. Med.*, 45: 8–24 (1966).

66. S. Grillner, J. Halbertsma, J. Nilsson, and A. Thorstensson, *Brain Res.*, 165: 177–182 (1979).

67. C. Kirtley, M.W. Whittle, and R.J. Jefferson, *J. Biomed. Eng.*, 7:282–288 (1985).

68. R. Shiavi, In *Gait in Rehabilitation* (G.L. Smidt, ed.), Churchill Livingstone, New York, pp. 97–119 (1990).

69. T.A. McMahon, *Muscles, Reflexes, and Locomotion.* Princeton University Press, Princeton, New Jersey (1984).

70. J.B.deCM. Saunders, V.T. Inman, and H.D. Eberhart, *J. Bone Joint Surg.*, 35: 543–558 (1953).

71. R. Waters, and J. Yakura, In *Gait in Rehabilitation* (G.L. Smidt, ed.), Churchill Livingstone, New York, pp. 65–96 (1990).

72. D.J. Blanke and P.A. Hageman, *Phys. Ther.*, 69:144–148 (1989).

73. F.R. Finley, K.A. Cody, and R.V. Finizie, *Phys. Med. Rehab.*, 50:140–146 (1969).

74. P.A. Hageman and D.J. Blanke, *Phys. Ther.*, 66:1382–1387 (1986).

75. F.J. Imms and O.G. Edholm, *Age Ageing*, 10:147–156 (1981).

76. E.C. Jansen, D. Vittas, S. Hellberg, and J. Hansen, *Acta. Orthop. Scand.*, 53: 193–196 (1982).

77. D.D. Larish, P.E. Martin, and M. Mungiole, *Ann. N.Y. Acad. Sci.*, 515:18–31 (1988).

78. M.P. Murray, R.C. Kory, and B.H. Clarkson, *J. Gerontol.*, 24:169–178 (1969).

79. B. Lundgren-Lindquist, A. Aniansson, and A. Rundgren, *Scand. J. Rehab. Med.*, 15:125–131 (1983).

80. S. Hirokawa, *J. Biomed. Eng.*, 11:449–456 (1989).

81. L-E. Larrson, P. Odenrick, B. Sandlund, P. Weitz, and P.A. Oberg, *Scand. J. Rehab. Med.*, 12:107–112 (1980).

82. M.P. Murray and B.H. Clarkson, *J. Am. Phys. Ther. Assoc.*, 46:585–589 (1966).

83. M.P. Murray, S.B. Sepic, and E.J. Barnard, *J. Am. Phys. Ther. Assoc.*, 47:272–284 (1967).

84. R.J. Elble, S.S. Thomas, C. Higgins, and J. Colliver, *J. Neurol.*, 238:1–5 (1991).

85. R. Nakamura, T. Handa, S. Watanabe, and I. Morohashi, *Tohoku J. Exp. Med.*, 154: 241–244 (1988).

86. G.L. Smidt, In *Gait in Rehabilitation* (G.L. Smidt, ed.), Churchill Livingstone, New York, pp. 301–315 (1990).

87. D.T. Wade, V.A. Wood, A. Heller, J. Maggs, and R.L. Hewer, *Scand. J. Rehab. Med.*, 19:25–30 (1987).

88. R.McN. Alexander, *Physiol. Rev.*, 69:1199–1227 (1989).

89. G.A. Cavagna and P. Franzetti, *J. Physiol. (London)*, 373:235–242 (1986).

90. G.A. Cavagna, H. Thys, and A. Zamboni, *J. Physiol. (London)*, 262:639–657 (1976).

91. N.C. Heglund and C.R. Taylor, *J. Exp. Biol.*, 138:301–318 (1988).

92. J. Nilsson and A. Thorstensson, *Acta Physiol. Scand.*, 129:107–114 (1987).

93. H.J. Ralston, *Int. Z. Angew. Physiol.*, 17:277–283 (1958).

94. M.Y. Zarrugh, F.N. Todd, and H.J. Ralston, *Eur. J. Appl. Physiol.*, 33:293–306 (1974).

95. E.R. Buskirk and J.L. Hodgson, *FASEB J.*, 46:1824–1829 (1987).

96. M. Critchley, *Lancet*, 1:1221–1230 (1931).

97. M. Schenkman and R.B. Butler, *Phys. Ther.*, 69:932–943 (1989).

98. M. Schenkman, J. Donovan, J. Tsubota, M. Kluss, P. Stebbins, and R.B. Butler, *Phys. Ther.*, 69:944–955 (1989).

99. J. De Keyser, G. Ebinger, and G. Vauquelin, *Ann. Neurol.*, 27:157–161 (1990).

100. P.L. McGeer, S. Itagaki, H. Akiyama, and E.G. McGeer, In *Parkinsonism and Aging* (D.B. Calne, D. Crippa, G. Comi, R. Horowski, and M. Trabucchi, eds.), Raven Press, New York, pp. 25–34 (1989).

101. D. Scherman, C. Desnos, F. Darchen, P. Pollak, F. Javoy-Agid, and Y. Agid, *Ann. Neurol.*, 26:551–557 (1989).

102. B. Marcyniuk, D.M.A. Mann, and P.O. Yates, *Neurobiol. Aging*, 10:5–9 (1989).

103. R.H.B. Fishman, J.J. Feigenbaum, J. Yanai, and H.L. Klawans, *Prog. Neurobiol.*, 20:55–88 (1983).

104. E.C. Hirsch, A.M. Graybiel, C. Duyckaerts, and F. Javoy-Agid, *Proc. Natl. Acad. Sci.*, 84:5976–5980 (1987).

105. K. Jellinger, *J. Neural Transm.*, 24:109–129 (1987).

106. K. Jellinger, *J. Neurol Neurosurg. Psychiatry*, 51:540–543 (1988).

107. P.D. Coleman and D.G. Flood, *Neurobiol. Aging*, 8:521–545 (1987).

108. D.G. Flood and P.D. Coleman, *Neurobiol. Aging*, 9:453–463 (1988).

109. M.E. Scheibel, U. Tomiyasu, and A.B. Scheibel, *Exp. Neurol.*, 56:598–609 (1977).

110. A.B. Scheibel, *Clin. Geriatr. Med.*, 1:671–676 (1985).

111. J.L. Stafford, M.S. Albert, M.A. Naeser, T. Sandor, and A.J. Garvey, *Arch. Neurol.*, 45:409–415 (1988).

112. C.M. Fisher, *Neurology*, 32:1358–1363 (1982).

113. L. Sudarsky and M. Ronthal, *Arch. Neurol.*, 40:740–743 (1983).

114. W.C. Koller, R.S. Wilson, S.L. Glatt, M.S. Huckman, and J.H. Fox, *Ann. Neurol.*, 13:343–344 (1983).

115. A. Aniansson, C. Zetterberg, M. Hedberg, and K.G. Henriksson, *Clin. Orthop.*, 191:193–201 (1984).

116. E.J. Bassey, M.J. Bendall, and M. Pearson, *Clin. Sci.*, 74:85–89 (1988).

117. R.H. Whipple, L.I. Wolfson, and P.M. Amerman, *J. Am. Geriatr. Soc.*, 35:13–20 (1987).

118. M.A. Fiatarone, E.C. Marks, N.D. Ryan, C.N. Meredith, L.A. Lipsitz, and W.J. Evans, *JAMA*, 263:3029–3034 (1990).

119. G. Newman, R.H. Dovenmuehle, and E.W. Busse, *J. Am. Geriatr. Soc.*, 8:915–917 (1960).

120. C. Prakash and G. Stern, *Age Ageing*, 2:24–27 (1973).
121. P.J. Delwaide and P. Delmotte, In *Parkinsonism and Aging* (D.B. Calne, D. Crippa, G. Comi, R. Horowski, and M. Trabucchi, eds.), Raven Press, New York, pp. 229–237 (1989).
122. H.W. Newman and K.B. Corbin, *Proc. Soc. Exp. Biol.*, 35:273–276 (1936).
123. C.F. Bolton, R.K. Winkelmann, and P.J. Dyck, *Neurology*, 16:1–9 (1966).
124. E. Kokmen, R.W. Bossemeyer, and W.J. Williams, *J. Gerontol.*, 33:62–67 (1978).
125. F.J. Imms and O.G. Edholm, *Age Ageing*, 8(suppl):261–267 (1979).
126. P.I. Spielberg, In *Investigations on the Biodynamics of Walking, Running, and Jumping.* (N. A. Bernstein, ed.), Moscow, pp. 72–76 (1940).
127. M. Tinetti, *J. Am. Geriatr. Soc.*, 34:119–126 (1986).
128. L. Wolfson, R. Whipple, P. Amerman, and J.N. Tobin, *J. Gerontol. [Med. Sci.]*, 45:M12–M19 (1990).
129. W.C. Koller, S.L. Glatt, and J.H. Fox, *Clin. Geriatr. Med.*, 1:661–668 (1985).
130. I. Goto, Y. Kuroiwa, and K. Kitamura, *J. Neurosurg. Sci.*, 30:123–128 (1986).
131. P.D. Thompson and C.D. Marsden, *Mov. Disord.*, 2:1–8 (1987).
132. R.D. Adams, C.M. Fisher, S. Hakim, R.G. Ojemann, and W.H. Sweet, *N. Engl. J. Med.*, 273:117–126 (1965).
133. P.McL. Black, *J. Neurosurg.*, 52:371–377 (1980).
134. C.M. Fisher, *Clin. Neurosurg.*, 24:270–284 (1977).
135. P.R. McHugh, *Q. J. Med.*, 33:297–308 (1964).
136. B. Messert and B.B. Wannamaker, *Neurology*, 24:224–231 (1974).
137. P.S. Sorensen, E.C. Jansen, and F. Gjerris, *Arch. Neurol.*, 43:34–38 (1986).
138. L. Sudarsky and S. Simon, *Arch. Neurol.*, 44:263–267 (1987).
139. E. Knutsson, *Brain*, 95:475–486 (1972).
140. M.P. Murray, S.B. Sepic, G.M. Gardner, and W.J. Downs, *Am. J. Phys. Med.*, 57: 278–294 (1978).
141. P.K. Murray, *J. Am. Geriatr. Soc.*, 32:324–330 (1984).
142. R.J. Elble, C. Higgins, and L. Hughes, *J. Neurol.*, 239: 71–75 (1991).
143. L.E. Daniels, *Arch. Neurol. Psychiatry*, 43:736–764 (1940).
144. P. Stewart, *Senile paraplegia.* In *A System of Medicine* (T.C. Allbutt, ed.), Macmillan, New York, pp. 805–809 (1910).
145. P.I. Yakovlev, *J. Neuropathol. Exp. Neurol.*, 13:267–296 (1954).
146. M. Critchley, *Geriatrics*, 3:364–370 (1948).
147. J.S. Meyer and D.W. Barron, *Brain*, 83:261–284 (1960).
148. E.B. Montgomery, *Arch. Neurol.*, 40:422–423 (1983).
149. J. Gerstmann and P. Schilder, Wien Med. *Wochenschr.*, 76:97–102 (1926).
150. M.M.L. Van Bogaert and P. Martin, *Encephale*, 24:11–18 (1929).
151. S.A.K. Wilson, *Brain*, 31:164–216 (1908).
152. D. Denny-Brown, *J. Nerv. Ment. Dis.*, 216:9–32 (1958).
153. I. Petrovici, *J. Neurol. Sci.*, 7:229–243 (1968).
154. M. Critchley, *Brain*, 52:23–83 (1929).
155. B. Messert, T.K. Henke, and W. Langheim, *Neurology*, 16:635–649 (1966).
156. N. Ishii, Y. Nishihara, and T. Imamura, *Neurology*, 36:340–345 (1986).

157. M. Casmiro, R. D'Alessandro, F.M. Cacciatore, R. Daidone, F. Calbucci, and E. Lugaresi, *J. Neurol. Neurosurg. Psychiatry*, 52:847–852 (1989).
158. M.P. Earnest, S. Fahn, J.H. Karp, and L.P. Rowland, *Arch. Neurol.*, 31:262–266 (1974).
159. N.R. Graff-Radford and J.C. Godersky, *Neurology*, 37:868–871 (1987).
160. A. Koto, G. Rosenberg, L.H. Zingesser, D. Horoupian, and R. Katzman, *J. Neurol. Neurosurg. Psychiatry*, 40:73–79 (1977).
161. E. Knutsson and U. Lying-Tunell, *Neurology*, 35:155–160 (1985).
162. B. Conrad, R. Benecke, J. Carnehl, J. Höhne, and H.M. Meinck, In *Motor Control Mechanisms in Health and Disease* (J.E. Desmedt, ed.), Raven Press, New York, pp. 717–726 (1983).
163. P.I. Yakovlev, *Am. J. Ment. Defic.*, 51:561–576 (1947).
164. V. Estanol, *J. Neurol. Neurosurg. Psychiatry*, 44:305–308 (1981).
165. C.A. Giuliani, In *Gait in Rehabilitation* (G.L. Smidt, ed.), Churchill Livingstone, New York, pp. 253–266 (1990).
166. E. Knutsson and C. Richards, *Brain*, 102:405–430 (1979).
167. E. Knutsson, *Scand. J. Rehab. Med.*, 12:47– 52 (1980).
168. M. Edamura, J.F. Yang, and R.B. Stein, *J. Neurosci.*, 11:420–427 (1991).
169. J.F. Yang and R.B. Stein, *J. Neurophysiol.*, 63:1109–1117 (1990).
170. D.H. Sutherland, *Gait Disorders in Childhood and Adolescence*. Williams & Wilkins, Baltimore (1984).
171. J.R. Gage and S. Ounpuu, In *Adaptability of Human Gait*. (A.E. Patla, ed.), Elsevier, North-Holland, pp. 359–385 (1991).
172. S. Gilman, J.R. Bloedel, and R. Lechtenberg, *Disorders of the Cerebellum*. F.A. Davis, Philadelphia, pp. 197–198 (1981).
173. L.A. Lipsitz, P.V. Jonsson, M.M. Kelley, and J.S. Koestner, *J. Gerontol.*, 46: M114–122 (1991).
174. M.I. Collyer, *Geriatr. Med.*, 11:27–30 (1981).
175. B. Wyke, *Age Ageing*, 8:251–258 (1979).
176. B.E. Maki, P.J. Holliday, and A.K. Topper, *J. Gerontol.*, 46:M123–131 (1991).
177. J.M. Mossey, *Clin. Geriatr. Med.*, 1:541–552 (1985).
178. J. Murphy and B. Isaacs, *Gerontology*, 28:265–270 (1982).
179. L. Sloman, M. Berridge, S. Homatidis, D. Hunter, and T. Duck, *Am. J. Psychiatry*, 139:94–97 (1982).
180. H. Visser, *Age Ageing*, 12:296–301 (1983).
181. L.Z. Rubenstein, A.S. Robbins, B.L. Schulman, J. Rosado, D. Osterweil, and K.R. Josephson, *J. Am. Geriatr. Soc.*, 36:266–278 (1988).
182. L. Sudarsky, *N. Engl. J. Med.*, 322:1441–1446 (1990).
183. J.W. Davie, M.D. Blumental, and S. Robinson-Hawkins, *Arch. Gen. Psychiatry*, 38:463–467 (1981).
184. B.C. Perry, *J. Am. Geriatr. Soc.*, 30:367–371 (1982).
185. D. Prudham and J.G. Evans, *Age Ageing*, 10:141–146 (1981).
186. M.E. Tinetti, T.F. Williams, and R. Mayewski, *Am J. Med.*, 80:429–434 (1986).

3

Physical Conditioning in the Elderly

James R. Couch, Jr.

The University of Oklahoma Health Sciences Center
Oklahoma City, Oklahoma

ACTIVITY IN THE ELDERLY

It is well known that elderly people, as a group, are not as active as young people. Nevertheless, we all have recollections of individual elderly subjects who remain very active and productive despite advanced age. It is for this reason that a firm definition of the term "elderly" is difficult to state. From the standpoint of neurorehabilitation, it is more practical to attempt to understand the factors that relate to the level of general physical conditioning and activity and how they change with age. Following the format proposed by Shepard [1], this will consider elderly patients as "young" elderly, age 65–74; "middle" elderly, age 75–84; and "old" old, age 85+.

On examining the reasons for diminished activity in the elderly, it is immediately apparent that this is a multifactorial problem. A review of these problems is presented in Table 1. Medical problems, psychiatric problems, or even cultural dictums that are perceived by the patient to require limiting certain types of activity, may lead to inactivity. Additionally, inactivity tends to breed further inactivity. The deconditioning of inactivity rapidly reduces physical stamina and reserve, as will be discussed, and can result in complications on this basis alone.

Bone and joint problems are major contributors to diminished activity. In general, the joints lose some of their range of motion and flexibility with aging [2,3]. Similar loss of flexibility occurs in muscle. These two problems by

Table 1 Causes of Inactivity in Elderly People

Bone and joint problems	Medication side effects
Osteoarthritis	Neurological problems
Rheumatoid arthritis	Central nervous system focal lesions
Osteoporosis	Dementia
Fracture	Peripheral neuropathy
Medical problems	Focal radiculopathy or mononeuritis multiplex
Pulmonary	Myopathy
Cardiac	Neuromuscular junction problems
Anemia	Psychiatric conditions
Endocrine	Cultural dictums
Metabolic	
Hepatic failure	
Renal failure	

themselves will slow movement in the elderly and require an increase in time and energy output to perform a task over that required by a younger subject. The problems of osteoarthritis and rheumatoid arthritis are common in the elderly patient [2,3]. These further compromise joint function and may require further increase in energy output to compensate for abnormal joint function. Finally, the component of pain on movement is added in these patients with arthritis, which, in turn, can lead to further decreased mobility.

A number of general medical problems may contribute to diminished activity in the aging. These problems would result in diminished activity in the patient at any age but are more common in the aging individual. These include pulmonary disease, cardiac disease, anemia, renal failure, hepatic failure, and endocrinopathy. This area is reviewed in greater detail in Chapter 18.

Anemia will limit activity by diminishing capability for oxygen transport to tissue and muscle. At hematocrit levels below 20%, young and otherwise healthy patients may have enough energy only for minimal activities of daily living due to compromised oxygen transport and diminished aerobic power. Elderly subjects would have significantly less reserve and could become symptomatic at hematocrits higher than 20.

Endocrine problems including hypothyroidism or Addison's disease will produce diminished overall energy and activity. Hyperthyroidism and Cushing's disease can be associated with myopathic processes and exhaustion that may eventually led to diminished activity. Hypoparathyroidism leads to diminished psychic energy and relative weakness. Hyperparathyroidism leads to sedation and eventually coma from the hypercalcemia.

Renal and hepatic failure produce obvious multisystem problems that lead to diminished activity. Hypertension and diabetes can result in decreased activity from their secondary complications.

The problem of therapy for medical diseases must be considered in this context. Many classes of drugs lead to sedation, diminished energy, and overall diminished activity [4]. The antihypertensive medications, histamine H-2 receptor blockers, and drugs that affect gastrointestinal motility such as metaclopramide and urinary tract motility such as oxybutanone or imipramine all may produce varying degrees of sedation, loss of energy, loss of drive, and subsequently, inactivity.

Neurological problems will have a very significant effect upon patients' activity. A common neurological problem is the distal symmetrical neuropathy which may be associated with many metabolic or vascular diseases. In its very mild form, this may only produce minimal difficulty with balance. Nevertheless, such difficulty may result in modest decrease of activity. In its more severe form, neuropathy produces greater interference with the patient's balance resulting in significant increase in the difficulty of getting in and out of a chair or bed and in ambulating. The neuropathy may also be painful and further diminish the desire to carry out activity. Weakness may also be due to motor neuron disease such as amyotrophic lateral sclerosis that will limit activity and produce muscle atrophy in conjunction with the progress of the disease. Diseases of the neuromuscular junction, myasthenia gravis and myasthenic syndrome, will lead to increasing impairment of mobility as disease severity increases. Myopathic processes with a definable pathological basis can result in primary loss of muscle strength such as polymyositis, late onset dystrophy, or type II fiber atrophy with metabolic myopathies. In more severe forms, these diseases all lead to rapid exhaustion with exercise and marked decrease in mobility.

A problem of grave import in the elderly is that muscle weakness may lead to falling. Falling was studied by Whipple et al. [5] by evaluating muscle power and frequency of falling. In this study, they compared 17 patients, averaging age 84, with a history of falling to 17 age-matched patients without a history of falling. They measured the peak power for knee extensors, knee flexors, ankle plantar flexors, and ankle dorsiflexors in nursing home patients. Patients with a history of falling were found on the average to have approximately 50% of the strength of those without a history of falling. The authors concluded that leg muscle weakness, especially if it involves ankle dorsiflexors, is a very important factor in poor balance and falling.

Central nervous system lesions produce diminished activity in many ways. Parenchymal disease may give rise to focal paralysis or ataxia. Patients may also develop lesions that produce an organic mental syndrome or dementia with loss of drive and energy or with neglect.

Body weight, itself, may become a major problem in mobility. Mobility depends on the strength of the muscles to carry out activity. Obese individuals may lose mobility due to inadequate strength relative to body mass. Even when the so-called ideal body weight is maintained, there may still be a problem if the lean body mass is replaced by fat [6]. In this situation, the loss of muscle contributes significantly to the loss of lean body mass. Decrease in lean body mass is usually associated with decrease in overall muscle strength [6].

Psychiatric problems, may occur in the elderly. Of these, depression is the most common. These problems may lead to diminished interest in surroundings and diminished activity. Finally, there is a cultural imperative that older individuals should be more sedate and not attempt activities carried out by younger people. This is a much less prevalent idea now than it was previously. Nevertheless, these cultural factors may interfere with development of exercise programs for elderly patients.

ENERGY PRODUCTION AND CONSUMPTION

The concepts of oxygen consumption (VO_2) and exhaustion are very useful in understanding the contribution of disease processes to diminished exercise tolerance. The maximum oxygen intake per minute (VO_2 max.) has also been termed by exercise physiologists as aerobic power [1,7,8]. VO_2 max. varies with age, weight, and muscle mass, however, it is mainly dependent on muscle mass. In young, healthy males VO_2 max. may equal or exceed 50 ml/kg/min [8,9]. In women VO_2 max. is usually 77% of that of men with this difference due to greater relative body fat in women [8,9].

Exhaustion occurs when requirements for energy from muscle exceed aerobic and anaerobic metabolic capacity for a prolonged period [1,8]. Exhaustion intervenes if an individual works at a level exceeding 40% of aerobic power (VO_2 max.) for an extended time [1]. The minimal activities of daily living such as standing or slow walking require an oxygen consumption (VO_2) of 5.7 ml/kg/min. (or 0.4 L/min. for a 70 kg. subject) [1,8,9]. In the healthy individual, there is a large reserve of aerobic power. However, in an elderly subject with VO_2 max. of 14.3 ml/kg/min. (or 1 L/min.) then carrying out minimal ADL with a VO_2 demand of 5.62 ml/kg/min. (40% of 14.3 ml/kg/min) will lead to exhaustion. Greater activity such as that associated with a rehabilitation program will rapidly produce to exhaustion in the patient with a VO_2 max. of 15 ml/kg/min.

Aerobic power decreases by approximately 5% per decade from age 25–65 leading to a loss of 20% by age 65 [1]. After age 65, the process may accelerate. The effect of disease and deconditioning can be to accelerate the normal decline in aerobic power. Conditioning, however, can increase muscle mass and can enhance the aerobic power by 15–20% [8]. If, in an individual, patient exercise and conditioning could add an additional 4–7 ml/kg/min of aerobic power, this would shift the decline of the strength curve and aerobic power curve to the right and could add another 8–15 years before institutionalization related to loss of strength and aerobic power based on the aging process by itself would be necessary.

The comments above bear heavily on the situation for rehabilitation subjects. These patients usually are on the acute neurology service for 1–3 weeks before being transferred to the rehabilitation service. During their time on the acute neurology service, patients very likely have markedly diminished activity from their normal pattern. This can produce a significant deconditioning of the neurologically intact side and loss of muscle mass before the patient reaches the rehabilitation ward. Part of the rehabilitation program must be directed at reconditioning muscles of the intact side, even to the extent of increasing their level of conditioning beyond that prior to the stroke. This extra conditioning and strengthening will likely be needed to help the patient compensate for deficit on the involved side as well as adding to aerobic power.

Other factors that influence the patients' status when they reach the rehabilitation ward (a) extent of physical activity prior to the stroke, (b) patients' premorbid habits including the use of alcohol, cigarettes, or exposure to other toxins that could be deleterious to cardiovascular or neuromuscular function, (c) drugs or medication that could interfere with cardiovascular function, muscle function, neuromuscular transmission, or produce sedation thus interfering with mental function. The problem of excess body weight requires attention and possibly treatment with a weight-reduction program. In the case of the wasted patient, a high protein diet may be necessary to help in increasing muscle mass. It is also necessary to recognize the patient with stable weight, but with relative decrease in lean body mass (muscle), who has replaced lost lean mass with fat.

MUSCLE CONDITIONING IN THE ELDERLY

As indicated, the rehabilitation potential of a patient is dependent on many factors. An important factor is the status of the musculoskeletal system and potential for muscles and limbs to perform maximally for the degree of control available to the damaged nervous system. The potential for aged muscle to increase function in terms of power and VO_2 becomes a critical issue in whether there is potential benefit in rehabilitation therapy for a patient.

There have been a number of studies on changes in muscle with aging and activity which have led to conflicting results [7,10–15]. Early studies concluded aging was associated with loss of Type II muscle fiber [11]. In general, the clinical maxim was "type II muscles: use them or lose them." In Larsson et al.'s study, 55 untrained but healthy men were subjected to muscle biopsy and evaluation of percentage of type I and type II fibers as well as the average of type I and II fiber area in the muscle [11]. These data are summarized in Table 2. In this sample, the percentage of type I fibers in vastus lateralis was 41% in patients under age 40, rising to 55% in those above

Table 2 Muscle Fiber Parameters in 55 Untrained
Healthy Men

Age (yrs)	N	Percentage Type I	Area Type I (μm)	Area Type II (μm)
20–29	7	41	5666	6953
30–39	11	37	6344	6975
40–49	7	48	6754	6627
50–59	9	52	5941	5954
60–65	7	55	5591	5243

Ref. 11

age 60. The amount of cross-sectional area for a type II fibers was greatest in the third and fourth decade but declined after the fifth decade.

Grimby and colleagues restudied this in 1982 and found relatively little change in the ratio of type I of II fibers with age [13]. There was a relative increase in type IA fibers compared with type IIB fibers. Also considering blood supply, Grimby found no change in capillary density with age. He did, however, find that the cross-sectional area of both fiber types decreased with age and was more prominent in type II than type I fibers. The most marked changes were noted in the vastus lateralis. Less intense changes were noted in the biceps.

Another study evaluating muscle fiber type in vastus lateralis muscle of hip fracture patients also concluded there were no differences in muscle fiber type distribution from age 66–100 years [14]. In this and other studies, the author did find smaller fiber area and increasing neuropathic changes in these older subjects, however, myopathic change did not increase with age [15,16].

Frontara et al. looked at muscle biopsies in elderly patients and again found no change in the type II/type I fiber ratio but a decrease in mean cross-sectional area of muscle fiber appeared to be the most important change relating to loss of muscle function with aging [17].

A number of studies have looked at the results of training programs for older and chronic institutionalized patients. Stamford looked at the chronic institutionalized patient and recently institutionalized patient with mean ages of 68 and 67 years respectively and subjected these to a modest training program that produced a stimulus resulting in increase in heart rate to 50% of maximum [18]. He found strength gains in the chronically institutionalized but not in the recently institutionalization group. He postulated that the program was not strenuous enough to allow one to see an effect. In another study, Stamford used a walking paradigm with 70% maximal heart rate as criterion for exercise, and showed significant gains in strength that continued over 12 weeks [19].

Frontara et al. worked with a group of sedentary men between the ages of 60–72 to test the effects of exercise [17,18]. The strength of one repetition maximum (1 RM) for extensors and flexors of the knee joints was used as an outcome measure. These individuals then went through a 12 week training program with retesting at 6 and 12 weeks. Progressive increase in muscle strength was found over the 12 week period during which the training load was reset weekly at 80% of 1 RM. An increase in the muscle cross-sectional area was also found as measured by a computed tomographic scan (CT) of the leg. Urinary excretion of 3-methyl-1-histidine in the urine increased by 40.8% with training. This enzyme reflects the breakdown rate of contractile proteins and increased excretion suggests increase of turnover of muscle protein. VO_2 increased by six percent. In the muscle biopsy specimens, there was an increase in capillary density and oxidative enzymes. Overall, muscle strength increased by 10–20% and this correlated with increase in area of type I and II fibers as well as increase in muscle mass measured by the CT scan. The authors concluded that in the elderly, the response to exercise was multifactorial with increase in muscle mass, oxidative capacity, and capillary density. This latter factor reflects increased blood supply to muscle.

In 1990, Fiatarone et al. looked at high-intensity strength training and nonagenarians [10]. They evaluated 10 subjects with a mean age of 90.2 years who undertook a program of 8 weeks of high-intensity resistance training. The training paradigm was similar to that used by Frontara et al. [17]. With the load set to 80% of 1 RM, patients performed 3 sets of 8 repetitions of lifting and lowering the leg against the load with 1–2 minute rest periods between. Before the program, 4 subjects required minimum assistance activities of daily living for ADL and 6 needed moderate assistance. Eight of the subjects had a history of falls and seven used an ambulatory assistive device consistently. Nine subjects completed the protocol. One was unable to complete it because of problems with an inguinal hernia. After 8 weeks, strength increased by 174 ± 31% for the entire group. Subjects were tested on their ability to rise from a chair and time needed to walk 50 feet. This time diminished significantly and 2 subjects were able to walk without using canes showing improvement in strength and balance. Muscle mass in the leg as measured by the CT scan showed a 9.0 ± 4.7% increase which was significant (P = 0.05). Following the experimental protocol, the patients returned to their sedentary lifestyle. After 4 weeks of detraining, there was an average 32% loss in muscle strength from peak performance noted above.

In another study, Fischer et al. [21] evaluated a group of 18 impaired elderly subjects who were nursing home residents. Study selection criteria were (1) ability to walk at least 5 steps, (2) transfer to the exercise bench, and (3) flex knees to at least 45 degrees. Subjects were put through a program in which they exercised 3 times per week for 6 weeks with emphasis on leg muscles. The program started with a resistance of 10% and increased to a maximum of 50% of the subject's strength. The authors found an improvement in strength and endurance, and seventy-five percent of the patients indicated that they enjoyed the program and it benefited them. Two-thirds of the patients felt better and could walk, stand and rise out of a chair more easily. The patients in the study maintained a higher level of activity following the study. This was reflected in relative maintenance of the improved muscle strength for up to 4 months after the study.

Studies by these and other authors [22,23] have shown that diminished activity and immobility can be improved in elderly subjects with a strength-training program. Programs of this type have shown clear increase in patients' strength, which, in turn, is reflected by an increase in mobility, improved balance, and improvement in activities of daily living. In addition, the patients have a better psychological "mind set" as result of the exercise program. There is some disagreement in the literature as to the extent of gains that may be achieved with lower intensity training. There is agreement that higher intensity training produced better results. Concern was expressed in all of these studies as to whether musculoskeletal system might be injured by the training program. This, in fact, did not occur in these patients who completed the program. There were drop-outs in all of the studies, but none related to injuries.

From a practical standpoint, it is necessary to look at the intact as well as the impaired side following stroke. Conditioning programs will have a beneficial effect on both sides and need to be stressed for both. Strong benefits to the patient may result in terms of increased mobility, better balance, and improved activities of daily living. On the other hand, the patient must maintain a program of increased activity in order to maintain the gains. If the activity returns to its former levels, the gains are apparently quickly lost.

Shepard [1] reviewed the problem in detail and made the following recommendations regarding an exercise program.

1. Outdoor exercise should be avoided in extremes of heat and cold and in the driest conditions.
2. Exercise prescriptions should be advanced gently.
3. Activity should never make the patient more than pleasantly tired the next day.
4. Activity should be halted for angina, arrhythmia, or excessive breathlessness.
5. Warm-up and cool-down periods should be instituted and be of adequate duration.
6. Sudden twisting movements should be avoided.
7. Vigorous activity should not be carried out if a patient has an acute viral infection.

8. Older individuals should always exercise in pairs so that one may assist the other.

The exercise program will often need to individualized for each patient to some extent. Nevertheless, the factors of the program remain relatively constant and patients will usually show definite gains from a program of encouraged and enforced training including increased mobility, better balance, improved mood, and fewer medical complications.

REFERENCES

1. R.J. Shepard, Physical training for the elderly. *Clin. Sports. Med.*, 5:515–532 (1986).
2. G.V. Ball, and W.J. Koopman, Rheumatoid arthritis. In *Textbook of Internal Medicine*, vol. 2 (W.N. Kelley, ed.), J. B. Lippincott, Philadelphia, pp. 974–981 (1989).
3. G.G. Bole, Osteoarthritis. In *Textbook of Internal Medicine*. vol. 2 (W.N. Kelley, ed.), J. B. Lippincott, Philadelphia, pp. 981–986 (1989).
4. J.W. Rowe, Aging in the major organ systems. In *Textbook of Internal Medicine*. vol. 2. (W.N. Kelley, ed.), J. B. Lippincott, Philadelphia, pp. 2584–2590 (1989).
5. R.H. Whipple, L.L. Wolfson, and P.M. Amerman, The relationship of knee and ankle weakness to falls in nursing home residents: an isokinetic study. *J. Am. Geriatr. Soc.*, 35:13–20 (1987).
6. G.A. Borkan, D.E. Hults, S.G. Gerzof, A.H. Robbins, and C.K. Silbert, Age changes in body composition revealed by computed tomography. *J. Gerontol.*, 38:673–677 (1983).
7. C.N. Meredith, W.R. Frontera, E.C. Fisher, V.A. Hughes, J.C. Herland, J. Edwards, and W.J. Evans, Peripheral effects of endurance training in young and old subjects. *J. Appl. Physiol.*, 66:2844–2849 (1989).
8. K. Wasserman, J.E. Hansen, D.Y. Sue, B.J. Whipp, In *Principles of Exercise Testing and Interpretation*. Lea & Febiger, Philadelphia, pp. 72–86 (1986).
9. D.Y. Sue and J.E. Hansen, Normal values in adults during exercise testing. *Clin. Chest. Med.*, 5:89–98 (1984).
10. M.A. Fiatarone, E.C. Marks, N.D. Ryan, C.N. Meredith, L.A. Lipsitz, W.J. Evans, High-intensity strength training in nonagenarians. *JAMA*, 263:3029–3034 (1990).
11. L. Larsson, B. Sjodin, and J. Karlsson, Histochemical and biochemical changes in human skeletal muscle with age in sedentary males, age 22–65 years. *Acta Physiol. Scand.*, 103:31–39 (1978).
12. L. Larsson, Histochemical characteristics of human skeletal muscle during aging. *Acta Physiol. Scand.*, 117:469–471 (1983).
13. G. Grimby, B. Danneskiold-Samoe, K.H., and B. Saltin, Morphology and enzymatic capacity in arm and leg muscles in 78–81 year old men and women. *Acta Physiol. Scand.*, 115:125–134 (1982).
14. A. Aniansson, C. Zetterberg, M. Hedberg, and K.G. Henriksson, Impaired

muscle function with aging: a background factor in the incidence of fractures of the proximal end of the femur. *Clin. Orthop.*, *191*:193–201 (1984).

15. A. Aniansson and E. Gustafsson, Physical training in elderly men with special reference to quadriceps muscle strength and morphology. *Clin. Phys.*, *1*:87–98 (1981).

16. A. Aniannson, P. Ljungberg, A. Rundgren, and H. Wetterqvist, Effect of a training programme for pensioners on condition and muscular strength. *Arch. Gerontol. Geriatr.*, *3*:229–241 (1984).

17. W.R. Frontera, C.N. Meredith, K.P. O'Reilly, H.G. Knuttgen, and W.J. Evans, Strength conditioning in older men: skeletal muscle hypertrophy and improved function. *J. Appl. Physiol.*, *64*:1038–1044 (1988).

18. W.R. Frontera, C.N. Meredith, K.P. O'Reilly, and W.J. Evans, Strength training and determinants of VO_2 max in older men. *J. Appl. Physiol.*, *68*:329–333 (1990).

19. B.A. Stamford, Physiological effects of training upon institutionalized geriatric men. *J. Gerontol.*, *27*:451–455 (1972).

20. B.A. Stamford, Effects of chronic institutionalization on the physical working capacity and trainability of geriatric men. *J. Gerontol.*, *28*:441–446 (1973).

21. N.M. Fisher, D.R. Pendergast, and E.C. Calkins, Maximal isometric torque of knee extension as a function of muscle length in subjects of advancing age. *Arch. Phys. Med. Rehabil.*, *71*:729–734 (1990).

22. T.L. Kauffman, Strength training effect in young and aged women. *Arch. Phys. Med. Rehabil.*, *66*:223–226 (1985).

23. D.R. Pendergast, E.E. Calkins, N.M. Fisher, and R. Vickers, Muscle rehabilitation in nursing home residents with cognitive impairment: a pilot study. *Am. J. Alzheimer Care Rel. Disorders Res.*, *July-August*:pp. 20–25 (1987).

SELECTED READINGS

B. Benson and M. Hogstel, *J. Gerontol. Nursing*, *12*(12):8–16 (1986).

Council on Scientific Affairs: Exercise programs for the elderly. *JAMA*, *252*(4):544–546 (1984).

L. Larsson, G. Grimby, J. Karlsson, Muscle strength and speed of movement in relation to age and muscle morphology. The American Physiological Society *46*(3):451–456 (1979).

L. Larsson L, *Acta Physiol. Scand.*, *117*:469–471 (1983).

R.F. Thompson, D.M. Crist, M. March, M. Rosenthal, Effects of physical exercise for elderly patients with physical impairments. The American Geriatrics Society *36*(2):130–135 (1988).

J.A. Work, *Physician Sportsmed.*, (1989).

4

Recovery of Locomotion Following Spinal Cord Injury: New Concepts and Approaches in Rehabilitation

Hugues Barbeau

McGill University
Montreal, Quebec, Canada

Joyce Fung

R.S. Dow Neurological Sciences Institute
Portland, Oregon

INTRODUCTION

One of the major motor functions that is lost or compromised following spinal cord injury (SCI) is walking. The degree of disability varies with the level and the extent of the lesion, as well as with the magnitude of residual motor and sensory deficits. In a large-scale national study, Young et al. [1] reported that 20.3% of 2769 paraplegic and 16.4% quadriplegic patients regained the ability to walk. In a regional study, Burke et al. [2] reported that 63% of 262 discharged patients who had sustained SCI could walk, but only 39% were functional walkers while the remaining 24% resorted to the wheelchair for daily locomotion.

It has long been known from animal studies that the spinal cord, severed from supraspinal structures, can generate alternating motor activity useful for locomotion [3,4]. Even after deafferentation or paralysis by curarization, efferent nerve activity from the "fictive" locomotor state can still be monitored and largely retains the same characteristics as in the intact animal [5,6]. Thus it is now accepted that the basic act of locomotion is generated centrally within the spinal cord circuitry, generally termed central pattern generator [7]. This is the same circuitry of interneurons upon which inputs from supraspinal centers and peripheral afferents converge and interact to refine the output, thus giving rise to a final expression of the locomotor pattern that is goal-oriented, functional, and adaptive.

The serious consequence of a spinal cord transection, in most adult mammals, is that the spinal network of pattern generation can no longer be activated at will. Previous studies have nonetheless shown that this can be activated in the spinal cat by some pharmacological means, such as intravenous injection of L-dopa, a noradrenergic (NA) precursor, or clonidine, an NA agonist, depending on the time after spinal injury [8–13]. Moreover, cats with complete spinal cord transection can be trained to bear weight and to walk on the treadmill, and, to a certain extent, to adapt to the changes in speed [11,14]. These animal studies have paved the way for some exciting work in the development of novel rehabilitation strategies to improve locomotion in humans with SCI, the preliminary findings of which will be presented and discussed in this chapter.

NORMAL GAIT

Since the gait pattern of each individual is uniquely adapted through the processing and interaction of internal and external constraints, it can be debated whether a norm really exists. However, certain quantitative characteristics are consistent within a normal range. The commonly used gait descriptors include temporal distance measurements such as speed, cadence, or step length; kinematic measurements such as joint angular displacements or point trajectories; and electromyographic (EMG) profiles. These descriptors will be briefly reviewed, to provide a template against which spastic paretic gait can be compared.

The normal angular displacements of the hip, knee and ankle joints, together with the EMG patterns of the medial hamstrings, vastus lateralis, tibialis anterior, and medial gastrocnemius are shown in Figure 1. The gait cycle is typically normalized to 100% from one foot–floor contact to the next. There are several critical gait events: heel strike (foot–floor contact), occurring at 0% and 100% of the gait cycle; midstance, period of single limb support with the other limb in midswing, occurring at around 20%; period of push-off to toe-off, occurring from 50 to 60%; and midswing, with the knee reaching maximal flexion. The stance to swing ratio at comfortable speed is approximately 60:40%.

While locomotion involves complex limb and trunk displacements in a three-dimensional manner, kinematic description is generally comprised of two-dimensional joint angular displacement in the sagittal plane of motion [15–19]. As shown in Figure 1A, the hip undergoes one phase of extension and flexion in a stride. Maximum flexion occurs just prior to heel strike, after which there is extension until push-off, as the leg rotates about the pivot of the foot and the trunk passes over the foot. This is followed by flexion as the limb swings forward for the next heel strike. The knee undergoes two phases of

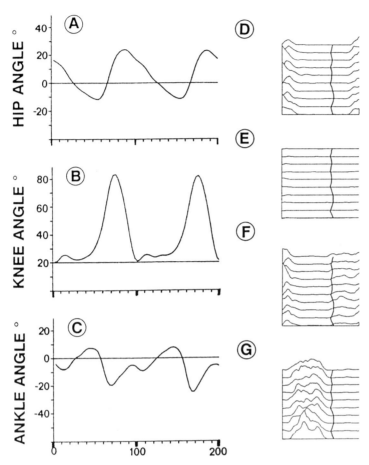

Figure 1   The kinematic (A–C) and EMG (D–G) profiles of a normal subject walking on the treadmill at a comfortable speed of 0.90 m/sec. Illustrated are two consecutive cycles of hip (A), knee (B), an ankle (C) angular displacements, normalized to the gait cycle from one foot–floor contact (0%) to the next (100%). All angles were calculated with respect to the neutral standing position (0%), with flexion or dorsiflexion taken as upward displacements, and extension or plantarflexion taken as downward displacements. Also shown are 10 consecutive cycles of EMG activity in the MH (D), VL (E), TA (F), and GA (G) normalized to 100% of the gait cycle. Solid line across the cycles depicts stance–swing transition.

flexion–extension in one stride. The knee flexes slightly after heel strike to prepare the limb for weight acceptance, then extends during single limb support while the contralateral limb is swinging forward. Flexion occurs again prior to toe-off, reaching a maximum at midswing, after which extension occurs again to prepare for heel strike. The ankle joint also has two phases of extension–flexion in one stride. From the neutral position in heel strike, the ankle plantarflexes slightly until the foot becomes flat on the ground, after which dorsiflexion occurs as the limb rotates over the foot. A greater and more rapid excursion of plantarflexion occurs from push-off to toe-off, followed by dorsiflexion to enable foot-floor clearance in swing.

The EMG activity from the lower limb muscles, averaged across 10 consecutive cycles in the same normal subject, is also shown in Figure 1 (D–G). The medial hamstrings (Figure 1D) are active in late swing to decelerate the swinging leg, and remain active through early and midstance to provide knee stability and hip extension, respectively. A second, inconsistent burst is sometimes seen at stance–swing transition (not seen in this particular subject). The vastus lateralis is normally activated in late swing, with a peak in early stance, and remains active in midstance to provide knee stability during weight acceptance. However, its activity can also be minimally detectable in some normal subjects, as shown in the figure (Figure 1E). The tibialis anterior and the triceps surae (soleus and gastrocnemius) exhibit a reciprocally active pattern. A lengthening contraction of the tibialis anterior occurs immediately after heel strike, after which the muscle is relatively silent until toe-off, at which instance a shortening contraction occurs as the foot clears the ground in swing. The medial gastrocnemius (Figure 1G) is active in stance, initially being stretched due to the forward rotation of the leg over the ankle, followed by a shortening contraction to generate momentum at push off.

SPASTIC GAIT DYSFUNCTION

One of the major sequelae of spinal cord injury that leads to locomotor impairment is spasticity in different manifestations: hyperreflexia (augmented tendon reflexes); hypertonia (increase in muscular resistance to passive stretch); clonus (variable frequencies of rhythmic, repeated muscle contractions elicited by a rapid but maintained stretch); and impaired control of voluntary movement associated with various degrees of paresis [20,21]. It has been reported by Hussey and Stauffer [22] that, among ambulatory patients who have sustained SCI, the presence of spasticity can confine the boundary of ambulation from community to household. However, no satisfactory functional scale of spasticity exists. If spasticity is to be assessed in a dynamic motor task such as locomotion, a more functionally relevant measurement is necessary.

The definition and underlying mechanisms of spasticity are still the topic of much debate. Lance [23] defined spasticity as "a motor disorder characterized by a velocity dependent increase in tonic stretch reflexes with exaggerated tendon jerks, resulting from hyperexcitability of the stretch reflex, as one component of the upper motoneuron syndrome." This definition, though not without its limitations, reflects the state of the art in neurophysiology for the past decades. Objective quantification relied mainly on electrophysiological testing of the H-reflex, tonic vibration, and stretch reflexes as well as the tendon jerk [24]. It is not an uncommon finding that these reflexes can become depressed by various kinds of therapeutic intervention without any corresponding improvement in motor function [25]. Since reflex testing is subjected to the limitation of testing in a resting position, the findings may not necessarily reflect the dynamic muscle tone during voluntary movement or the extent of functional impairment caused by spasticity. This is substantiated by results showing that the tendon jerk and H-reflex could actually be modified by voluntary movement [26]. In a previous study by Capaday and Stein [27], the human soleus H-reflex amplitude was found to be strongly task-dependent, being greater during standing than during walking at the same effective stimulus intensities. Moreover, Neilson and Andrews [28] have shown in spastic athetotic subjects that the tonic stretch reflex measured during a resting position and during sustained voluntary contraction differed in sensitivity, pattern, duration, and timing. Perry [29] has also shown that the ankle frequency of oscillation could be enhanced markedly by a change in body posture from supine to sitting to standing. Therefore it is essential to evaluate spasticity as a motor disorder in a dynamic and voluntary task such as walking, in order to relate to functional outcomes.

Spasticity could be considered not as a single pathophysiological entity but as a release phenomenon reflecting motor program disorders [30]. To quantify the spastic muscle activation disorder during locomotion, we have previously contrasted the EMG patterns of normal subjects with those of spastic patients who have sustained SCI and proposed an EMG profile index [31]. The index can indicate the degree of abnormal activation of locomotor muscles from their normally relaxed state, as compared to the total recruitment in the active phase. Figure 2 contrasts the locomotor EMG patterns of five normal subjects and four severely spastic patients with SCI, with the range of index values displayed on top of each plot. The relatively silent phase, or "off" bin (demarcated in vertical lines), where the muscle was minimally active in normal subjects, was determined to be 35–85% of the gait cycle for both the medial hamstrings and the vastus lateralis; 20–70% for the tibialis anterior; and 70–20% for the medial gastrocnemius. The index, defined as the ratio of the integrated EMG in the "off" bin(s) of the gait cycle to that in the "on" bin(s), was found to be low in normal muscles and high in

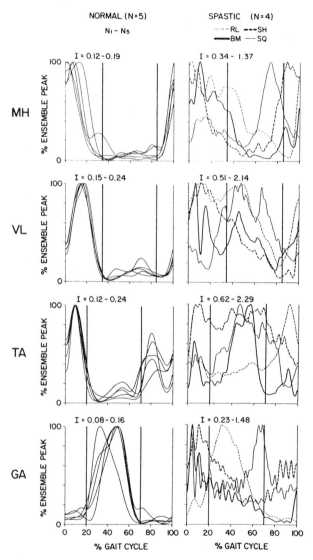

Figure 2 Superimposed EMG ensemble averages of MH, VL, TA, and GA for the two groups of subjects: normal and spastic. The range of index values in the group are displayed on top of each plot (see text) (modified from [31]).

spastic muscles [31]. The index can be highly elevated due to the loss of normal activation in the "on" bins and the presence of abnormal activity in the "off" bins. As shown in Figure 2, in the spastic patients there is a marked increase in EMG activity in the "off" bin(s), such as early stretch activation and clonus in medial gastrocnemius and elevated tonic activity in tibialis anterior.

The angular displacement of lower limb joints characteristic of spastic paretic gait have been briefly described by Conrad et al. [32,33]. These include an overall decrease in the amplitude of knee excursion in conjunction with an increase in knee flexion at foot–floor contact, and an absence of the normal full extension in midstance. The ankle joint was reported to be held in excessive dorsiflexion throughout stance. However, knee hyperextension during stance was reported by Knutsson and Richards [34], which can result from premature activation of triceps surae, and/or as a compensatory mechanism to reduce limb instability due to paresis.

Considerable between-subject variations in the muscle activation patterns of spastic paretic patients during overground walking were reported by Knutsson [35]. In the group of 17 spastic paretic patients studied, a wide range of abnormal coactivation in agonist and antagonist muscle groups was seen, together with mixed signs of stretch-related activation of spastic reflexes and paresis. This renders it difficult to classify the disturbance into any specific types, as done in spastic hemiparetic gait [34]. Knutsson [25] also identified prolonged activation of weight-supporting muscles, quadriceps and abductors, during the stance phase, which could be due to loading and stretch activation. The phenomenon was described as "crutch spasticity," a mechanism to compensate for limb instability during the loading phase. A series of studies by Dietz and colleagues [36,37] demonstrated that the high tension developed at the Achilles tendon correlated poorly with the gastrocnemius EMG activation, which was markedly reduced in the spastic leg. They hypothesized that muscular hypertonia was mainly caused by changes in the mechanical properties of the muscles rather than neuronal mechanisms. However, as these authors also discussed, the natural constraints of the ankle joint and physiological length–tension characteristics of the triceps surae muscle must also be considered as contributing factors. The gait pattern of patients after SCI is further complicated by the presence of both positive symptoms (spasticity) and negative signs (paresis), which may be a result of exaggerated spinal reflex activities and insufficient action of preprogrammed central locomotor activities, rendering dissociation of spasticity from paresis almost impossible. The disturbance can further be confounded by the presence of nonspecific elements such as "protective gait mechanisms" that depended largely on psychological elements, perceived efforts, and consciousness of gait impairment [32,33].

The most common approach in gait analysis involves descriptive–comparative study or visual inspection of EMG and kinematic data. The muscle activation disorder in spastic paretic gait is far from being elucidated. The underlying neurophysiological mechanism is even more obscure. There is much need for quantitative study of spastic gait disorders and a clarification of the underlying mechanisms.

DEFECTIVE MECHANISMS

The presence of abnormal muscle activity in the normally silent phase of the gait cycle, such as triceps surae stretch activation in early stance and clonus in swing, suggests that defective Ia afferent gating mechanisms may be implicated in spastic gait dysfunctions. Injury to the central nervous system (CNS) that interrupts descending input to the spinal cord often results in altered excitability of segmental reflexes (reviewed by Ashby and McCrea [38]). After the initial period of shock due to trauma to the spinal cord, segmental reflexes associated with the muscle spindle (i.e., the tendon jerk and H-reflex) slowly become hyperactive [21,39,40]. The H-reflex, elicited most commonly in the soleus muscle, has been used as a means of indirectly assessing the synaptic efficacy of the monosynaptic stretch reflex. In the normal subject it appears that modulation of the H-reflex during different tasks may be under the control of different mechanisms [27,41]; thus after injury to the spinal cord, the modulation may be controlled differently. It is known that the H-reflex in the normal individual is modulated to a great extent during the gait cycle [27,42]. This modulation appears to be functionally important for achieving smooth locomotion [27,41]. However, it was not known how this reflex activation is affected in patients after SCI during walking and standing. To explore further the defective gating mechanisms of spinal reflexes underlying spastic paretic gait, we examined and contrasted the soleus H-reflex modulation pattern, during standing and walking, in 10 normal subjects and 10 spastic patients [43].

The normal phase-dependent modulation of the soleus H-reflex during walking from one representative subject is shown in Figure 3A. The mean peak-to-peak amplitude together with the standard deviation of the M and H responses across different phases of the gait cycle are shown on the left. The mean trace (averaged across at least 10 responses) in each phase from foot–floor contact to end of swing is displayed from top to bottom on the right side of the plot. It can be seen that with a relatively constant M-response, the soleus H-reflex amplitude was reduced in early stance, progressively increased from midstance to push off, and remained inhibited in swing. Such changes in the soleus motoneuronal excitability were generally related to the soleus muscle activity profile in gait. As compared to the mean control

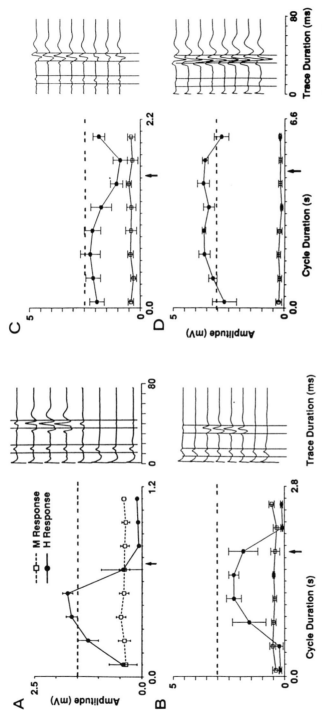

Figure 3 Soleus H-reflex modulation pattern during locomotion in a normal subject and in three spastic paretic subjects: A and B, moderately spastic; C, severely spastic. Note the marked increase in stance and cycle duration in the three patients compared to that in the normal subject. Note also the absence of H-reflex modulation throughout the entire gait cycle in D and the increase in amplitude beyond that observed during quiet standing (indicated by the dotted horizontal line).

81

amplitude in quiet standing (shown as dotted horizontal line across the plot), the H-reflex amplitude was generally reduced in walking, except for the push-off phases when the soleus activity peaked. It should be noted that during quiet standing the soleus activity was kept in a range of 0–10% maximal isometric contraction, which was even lower than the minimal level of EMG activity obtained during walking.

The patterns of soleus H-reflex modulation in spastic paretic patients could be classified into three types (Figure 3B–D), which did not seem to parallel the soleus muscle activity as closely as normal subjects. Figure 3 shows the examples from two moderately impaired patients (Figure 3B–C) who could walk at a comfortable treadmill speed of 0.3 m/sec, and a severely impaired patient (Figure 3D) who could only walk at 0.15 m/sec, with marked clonus elicited. The patient in Figure 3B showed a pattern similar to that of a normal subject (Figure 3A), except for the prolonged stance duration, and an increased response before swing phase. The patient in Figure 3C showed a generally elevated reflex response throughout stance, with a slight degree of inhibition present in swing. The severely spastic patient in Figure 3D showed a consistently elevated and similar H-reflex amplitude through the gait cycle, indicating an entire absence of phasic modulation. The H-reflex amplitude in this patient was elevated even beyond that obtained during standing (see horizontal dotted line).

In a recent study [44], we pooled the data from 21 spastic paretic subjects who had sustained spinal cord and/or head injury and reported that the most common pattern of responses observed (10 of 21) was a lack of H-reflex modulation throughout the stance phase and slight depression of the reflex in the swing phase. In three patients who were able to walk for extended periods, the effect of stimulus intensity was examined. Two of these patients showed a greater degree of reflex modulation at lower stimulus intensities, which suggested that the lack of modulation observed at higher stimulus intensities could be due in part to saturation of the reflex loop. Since phasic modulation of the reflex remained in most patients, this suggests either that the descending fibers that remained were able to generate the reflex modulation or that the modulation was generated by processes within the spinal cord, as in cats. Six patients, however, failed to exhibit any modulation through the step cycle, even at low stimulus intensities. It is unclear whether the mechanisms for rhythmic modulation of reflexes remained intact but were obscured because the reflex loop was saturated by the stimulus input or whether the mechanisms for generating the modulation were indeed impaired.

The plausible mechanisms underlying hyperactive reflexes, which are associated with movement disorders, include a reduction in presynaptic inhibition of primary afferent fibers [21,45], denervation supersensitivity

[46], and altered reciprocal inhibition [47]. The possibility that presynaptic inhibition is reduced is particularly interesting here because the task-specific amplitude of the H-reflex appears to be controlled by presynaptic inhibition [48]. In normal subjects the large reflex amplitude of standing is rapidly switched to a lower amplitude at the initiation phase of walking [49]. These patients appear to retain a higher reflex gain during walking, as would be expected if presynaptic inhibition is impaired or reduced. However, the phasic modulation associated with walking could be observed in many patients by lowering the stimulus intensity. Hence, the mechanisms responsible for generating phasic modulation remain at least partially intact in most of these patients. It is likely that both central and peripheral mechanisms contribute to the cylical modulation of the soleus H-reflex.

ADAPTATION OF THE GAIT PATTERN

Recent studies in normal rats and cats have shown the effects of speed and incline upon the motor output [50,51]. Pierotti and collaborators [51] reported that as speed or incline is increased, the ouput of selective extensor muscles is augmented. They concluded that since the additional power required must be obtained by increasing the number and/or the frequency of firing motor units, speed of locomotion or adaptation to inclines must be accomplished by varying the level of excitation in the relevant extensor motor unit pools.

It has been reported that after recovery cats spinalized at the thoracic level can adapt to the increase in walking speed [14,52,53], but this adaptation is limited to a maximal speed of 0.8–1.0 m/sec; beyond that, the walking pattern becomes disorganized [14,53].

Thus, the spinal cat has a limited capacity to adapt to increases in speed, presumably achieved solely by peripheral influence since all descending tracts have been severed. In spastic paretic humans with incomplete spinal cord injury, the adaptability of the gait to changes in mechanical demands could be greater than in the spinal animal since some descending tracts are preserved. What are the adaptation mechanisms in spastic subjects and how comparable are these mechanisms to those in normal subjects?

Spastic patients walk at speeds considerably lower than the comfortable walking speed of healthy subjects [33,54]. The contributory factors may be a decrease in supraspinal drive due to disruption of the descending tracts; presence of muscle hypertonia [55]; speed-dependent increase in hyperactive stretch reflexes [56]; and an inability to generate force at higher speeds of limb movements [57]. Shiavi et al. [54] reported that the speed and single-limb support duration of hemiplegic subjects were less than normal, while stance and cycle duration were greater than those of normal subjects walking at very low speeds. Asymmetrical involvement of the lower extremities is

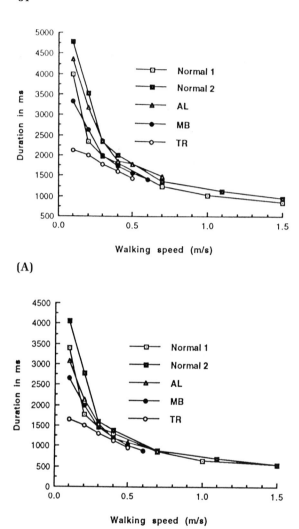

Figure 4   Cycle (A) and stance (B) duration as a function of treadmill speed. These data were recorded in two normal subjects and three spinal cord injured subjects. Each point represents an average of 10–15 measurements.

very often seen in spastic paretic subjects, in which case the less involved limb may play a compensatory role, as observed in hemiplegic patients. A prolonged swing and decreased stance duration is compatible with patients' difficulty in bearing weight on the more affected extremity [34,58]. This is more due to the problem of weakness than spasticity. Thus, it is important to specify when possible whether the more spastic limb or the weaker limb is being evaluated.

The cycle time (Figure 4A) and stance duration (Figure 4B) or two normal subjects and three patients with SCI walking at various treadmill speeds are shown in Figure 4. The prolonged cycle and stance duration observed in the patients' comfortable speed range (0.2–0.3 m/sec) are also present in normal subjects for matched speeds. In the normal subjects, knee flexion during early stance and ankle plantarflexion at push-off were also greatly reduced at low speeds, as observed in the patients. These results suggest that some characteristics of the gait pattern of spastic patients with SCI are associated in part with their limitation in walking speed and cannot be attributed solely to their deficits [59].

Figure 5 compares the EMG activity of a normal subject with that of a spastic subject at three different speeds. As the speed increased from 0.1 to 0.6 m/sec, the EMG activity in the normal subject increased in amplitude with the phasing generally preserved. In the spastic patient (Figure 5B), the increase in EMG amplitude with increased speed was limited, but phasing of activation was changed, with longer burst duration and increased early activation in triceps surae. This stretch-induced bursting pattern is enhanced by increasing the walking speed, but the underlying mechanism needs to be investigated further.

NEW EXPERIMENTAL APPROACHES TO RESTORE LOCOMOTOR FUNCTION

As reviewed above, the recovery of locomotion following spinal cord injury depends on a multitude of factors. Spastic paretic gait is characterized by a spectrum of problems including hyperactive spinal reflexes, altered muscle activation patterns, and the inability to cope with external demands. Conventional treatment efforts have focused on normalizing muscle tone by the use of antispastic medication [60], corrective surgery [61], or physical means such as passive stretching [62] and orthotic devices [63]. While abnormal muscle tone may be corrected in the static or resting position, the response very often cannot be carried over to a dynamic situation such as locomotion. Even in gait rehabilitation, the traditional approach is to progress from standing to walking while individual problems are corrected, rather than retraining all the dynamic components simultaneously in a task-specific manner. Thus, despite

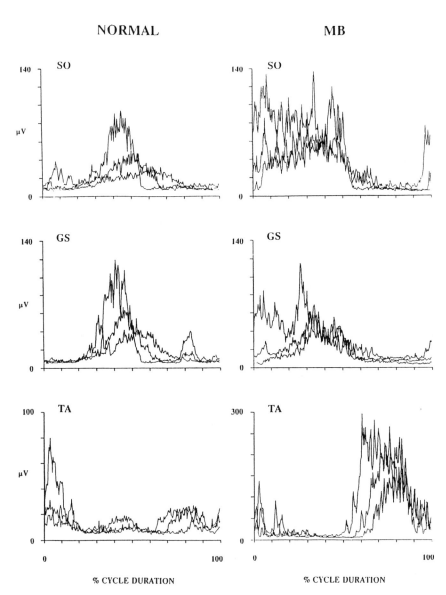

Figure 5   Examples of the effect of increasing speed (0.1, 0.3, and 0.6 m/sec) on EMG activity of soleus (SO), gastrocnemius (GS), and tibialis anterior (TA) in a normal and spinal cord injured subject.

a labor-intensive rehabilitation regimen, many individuals with a central nervous system lesion have persistent gait deviations. Animal research has provided some interesting insights and alternative treatment approaches that are reviewed in the following sections.

Interactive Locomotor Training with Weight Support

Recovery of locomotor function following a spinal cord transection was considered to be largely dependent on the age of the animal at the time of the injury [7,52,64]. Until recently, cats spinalized at maturity were described as poor functional walkers with major deficits in their gait pattern. Although they were capable of producing stepping movements with their hindlimbs, they were unable to support their body weight on their hindquarters up to 8 weeks after transection [65]. However, this concept has recently been re-examined and the importance of training in accelerating the recovery and maximizing the quality of the locomotor pattern in the adult spinal cat has been recognized. Rossignol et al. [11] as well as Barbeau and Rossignol [14] have shown that cats spinalized (T13) as adults could recover a near-normal locomotor pattern following an "interactive locomotor training" program. During interactive locomotor training, the animal was supported by the tail and allowed to bear only a proportion of its weight so that it could walk with proper foot placement (with sole of the foot) on the treadmill. The proportion was increased, as appropriate to the animal's abilities. Following a period of 1–3 months of this training regimen, the animal was capable of walking at different treadmill speeds while completely supporting the weight of its hind-quarters with proper foot placement. Moreover, the gait pattern was comparable in many aspects to that of the intact adult cat [66]. Thus, it was concluded that interactive locomotor training is an important factor in the recovery of locomotion in the adult spinal cat.

Based on the above animal findings, and clinical observations of inadequate weight bearing among neurologically impaired patients, it has been proposed that supporting a percentage of body weight and progressively decreasing the support while retraining gait may be an effective approach. To validate this training strategy, it is important to study the effects of body weight support (BWS) on neurologically impaired gait.

In a preliminary study of seven spinal cord injured subjects, it has been shown that providing body weight support (BWS) during treadmill walking can facilitate the expression of a more normal gait pattern [67]. As the demand of loading and balance decreased, there was also an increase in speed and step length. The advantage of such an intensive locomotor training approach is that all the different dynamic components of gait, as well as external influences such as loading, speed, support, and balance can be addressed simultaneously during gait. When BWS is provided, even severely impaired patients can be assisted to walk on the treadmill at a minimal speed. These patients normally have difficulty just standing between parallel bars and conventional gait training cannot be instituted until a much later stage. This proposed interactive locomotor training program can be initiated almost immediately after injury, provided that the condition is stable and there are no other medical contraindications. However, only patients with chronic disability who had reached a plateau in their rehabilitation were included in the present studies to avoid the confounding influence of natural recovery.

Figure 6 shows an example of the effects of 6 weeks of interactive locomotor training using body weight support on the kinematic pattern in a chronic spastic paretic subject (26 years old) who had sustained a traumatic (C_{7-8}) spinal cord injury. The interactive locomotor training was performed on a treadmill, with the subject mechanically supported in a comfortable overhead harness at different percentages of BWS using a strain gauge transducer [68]. As the subject walks on the treadmill with reduced load on the lower extremities, gait deviations can instantly be corrected and proper muscle activation can be facilitated during both the stance and swing phases [69]. Optimal BWS is initially provided and progressively reduced until the subject can walk at full weight bearing (0% BWS) with minimal gait deviation, coping comfortably with the adjustable treadmill speed. In the present example, the subject was trained for six consecutive weeks, 4–5 times/week for 1 hr per session with intermittent rest periods.

During the pretraining evaluation, the subject presented with severe spasticity in extension and had great difficulty coping with the weight and treadmill speed. Being a nonfunctional walker over ground, he could barely be evaluated at full weight bearing on the treadmill only when the walking speed was as low as 0.13 m/sec. The kinematic pattern showed mainly a knee hyperextension during the loading phase (from 10 to 60% of the gait cycle) with a lack of flexion during the swing period (peaking at 30 and 40 degrees: Figure 6B, dotted line). Hip hiking (an upward displacement of the hip and pelvis to assist swinging the limb through; see arrows in Figure 6A) was also present at the stance–swing transition. Foot–floor contact was made with the plantarflexed forefoot (12 degrees; Figure 6C). A marked plantarflexion up to 50 degrees during the beginning of swing was the result of foot drag on the surface of the treadmill belt. Following 6 weeks of locomotor training, marked changes could be observed in the kinematic profiles (Figure 6A–C, thin line). At the same treadmill speed of 0.13 m/sec, a symmetrical and smooth kinematic pattern with increased hip and knee flexion could be observed. A marked decrease of hip hiking at the stance–swing transition was also noticeable. Heel contact was now clearly present, and a marked decrease of the toe drag during the swing phase could be observed. It was interesting that this spastic paretic subject could now walk at a much faster speed of 0.42

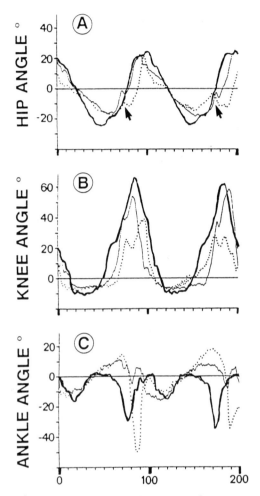

Figure 6   The effects of interactive locomotor training on the kinematic pattern of a spastic paretic subject during treadmill walking. Illustrated are angular displacements of the hip (A), knee (B), and ankle (C) normalized across consecutive gait cycles in pretraining evaluation at minimal speed of 0.13 m/sec (dotted line), posttraining evaluation at 0.13 m/sec (fine solid line), and posttraining evaluation at 0.42 m/sec (bold solid line) Arrows indicate "hiking" response at the hip and knee.

m/sec, with a smoother gait pattern and a near-normal amplitude of excursion at the three joints (compare the bold line in Figure 6A–C with the normal pattern illustrated in Figure 1). The main defect that remained was the knee flexion at foot–floor contact and the absence of yield during the loading phase of stance. The lack of ankle dorsiflexion could also be observed. The appearance of clonus in the gastrocnemius (GA) became evident at that treadmill speed, but did not impede locomotion. An inconsistent burst of activity in the tibialis anterior (TA) at foot–floor contact could also be observed (not illustrated). The temporal pattern was characterized by a more regular pattern with low variability of the stance–swing transition, which is similar in many aspects to the normal gait pattern.

This initially wheelchair-bound spastic paretic patient could now walk over ground at 0.23 m/sec with two Canadian crutches for a distance up to 50 m. Moreover, a marked improvement in his endurance could be noted, as indicated by the walking tolerance on the treadmill, which was more than 10 min after training.

New Experimental Medications

The use of experimental medications such as cyproheptadine (5-HT antagonist) and clonidine (NA agonist) was also based on animal studies [11,13,70]. Following chronic, complete spinal cord transection in the adult cat, in which all the descending systems have degenerated, monoaminergic (5-HT and NA) agents that act on the receptors below the transection site were shown to modify spinal reflex activity and modulate the locomotor pattern. Based on these findings as well as recent clinical trials [71–73], separate clinical trials utilizing a randomized, double-blind, placebo-medication crossover design, have established the effectiveness of each of these medications in reducing clinical signs of spasticity and improving the locomotor function of spastic paretic patients [46,74,75].

The effects of cyproheptadine were first reported in chronic spinal rats [76,77] and chronic spinal cats [11,70]. These effects included a decrease in spastic features such as spasms and clonic activity. Its action was proposed to be mediated through blockage of 5-HT receptors below the transection site, leading to a decrease in neuronal hyperexcitability. Hence the use of cyproheptadine was extended to humans as an antispastic medication [78]. Figure 7 illustrates the effects of pharmacological intervention using cyproheptadine on the recovery of locomotion in a patient with incomplete SCI. The subject, SQ (T_{4-7} traumatic SCI), was initially functionally nonambulatory and wheelchair-bound due to severe spasms and clonus. He had reached a plateau in his rehabilitation 1 year after his spinal cord injury and was stabilized on other antispastic medication before participating in this study. In the premedication trial, he could only manage to step on the treadmill at a minimal speed when 40% BWS was provided by the weight-supporting harness. The

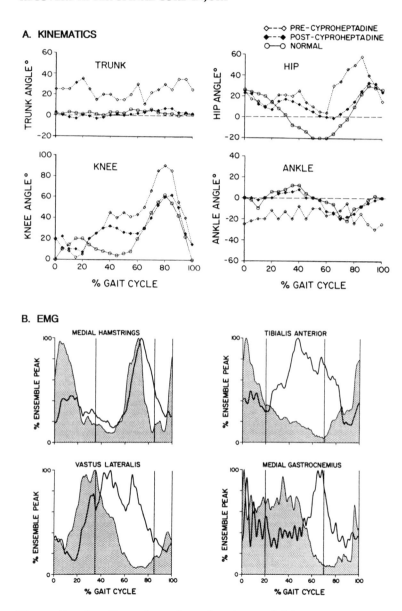

Figure 7 The effects of cyproheptadine (24 mg daily) on spastic paraparetic gait. (A) Kinematics pattern on one representative gait cycle of subject walking on the treadmill before and after cyproheptadine administration compared to a normal subject. (B) Change of EMG profiles in the MH, VL, TA, and GA muscles. The bold curves represent EMG ensemble averages in the precyproheptadine walking and hatched profiles represent those in the postcyproheptadine evaluation (Modified from [31]).

kinematic profiles in Figure 7A reveal a gait pattern characterized by a flexed posture, with marked flexion in the hip and knee during stance, indicating the inability to bear weight efficiently on the lower extremity and to maintain an upright posture while advancing on the treadmill. Furthermore, flexor spasms were encountered frequently as soon as the foot was lifted off the treadmill, giving rise to an excessive flexion in the hip and knee during swing. The initial foot–floor contact was made with the toe, as indicated by the flexed hip and knee, as well as the plantarflexed ankle joint. There was a tendency to hip and knee extension in early stance, but this yielded to flexion immediately on weight acceptance.

Following administration of cyproheptadine, there was, objectively, an improvement in functional outcome and, subjectively, a reduction in spasticity. The patient became functionally ambulatory with crutches and a Klenzac brace for the left lower limb. He was able to walk with full weight bearing on the treadmill with mild assitance for the left lower limb and no assistance on the right, with a marked decrease in flexor spasms and clonus. With cyproheptadine treatment, heelstrike appeared at initial contact with proper ankle dorsiflexion ocurring after midstance. The foot drag disappeared with decreased plantarflexion, resulting in proper foot clearance during swing. The corresponding hip, knee, and ankle angular displacement profiles (Figure 7A) approximated those of a normal subject. Moreover, these findings were related to a better phasing pattern in all four lower limb muscles studied, as shown in the pre- and postmedication EMG ensemble averages in Figure 7B. Before medication, the abnormal burst of activity in the "off" bin of the flexor muscles, medial hamstrings (MH) and TA, that predominated due to flexor spasms, was markedly reduced after medication and replaced by a functional burst in the "on" bin. This change corresponded with the marked decrease in the maximum hip and knee swing angle (Figure 7A, hip: 58–33 degrees, knee: 90–62 degrees). There was also a marked coactivation in the extensor muscles, vastus lateralis (VL) and GA, due to frequent flexor spasms in early swing (at approximately 70% of the gait cycle) before medication, causing a shift of activity into the predetermined "off" bin. The prolonged activation profile of the VL muscle from midstance to midswing before medication, was reduced after medication with an earlier recruitment in stance, and much less activity was present in late stance to midswing (the predetermined "off" bin of 35% to 85% of the cycle). Although early stretch activation of the GA was still evident after medication, the predominantly clonic discharge pattern, leading to a diminished push-off, was substituted by a more functional profile, with decreased clonus and increased activity for push-off in the "on" bin. This was also reflected by the ankle kinematic changes as shown in Figure 7A. These observed changes were depicted by the locomotor spasticity index showing a marked reduction after medication (MH: 1.37–0.82; VL: 2.14–0.66; TA: 1.71–0.41; GA: 0.90–0.71) [31].

A marked modification in locomotor function was also noted with clonidine, a noradrenergic agonist (Figure 8): this patient with SCI no longer utilized a trunk flexion strategy, demonstrating instead a more erect trunk posture while walking. In kinematic terms, the hip, knee, and ankle angular displacements (Figure 8) were characterized by a gradual increase in flexion across the gait cycle while on placebo. During clonidine therapy, both the hip and knee joints moved into progressive extension during stance, followed by a reversal into flexion during the swing phase. The total angular excursion of the hip increased (placebo: 10–30 degrees, clonidine −4 to 30 degrees), due to an increase in extension range during stance. However, the total angular excursion of the knee did not change, and excessive knee flexion at foot–floor contact (FFC) persisted. Ankle plantarflexion at FFC also remained; however, this was followed by a more normal profile, with more dorsiflexion through early/mid stance, and plantarflexion following toe-off (TO). The marked coactivation between antagonistic muscles during the placebo period was replaced by a better phasic activation during the clonidine treatment period (not illustrated).

While receiving placebo, none of the patients with complete SCI were able to initiate independent stepping. Instead, each patient was assisted in stepping passively on the treadmill while completely supported by the harness. The presence of regular flexor bursts is evident in Figure 9A, during assisted locomotion in the placebo session of a patient with complete SCI. Right and left MH showed a consistent alternating pattern (Figure 9A). The timing of this burst was coincident with the stretch applied to the hamstrings in mid and late swing, when the knee was passively extended as the leg was drawn forward by the research assistants in preparation for foot–floor contact. Passive flexion and extension of the knee, with the same patient seated, likewise consistently evoked an MH burst following administration of the placebo. However, during the clonidine session, both stretch reactions were abolished (Figure 9B). Furthermore, during assisted locomotion while the patient was taking clonidine, the research assistants reported a reduction in the resistance previously felt when pulling the leg forward. This reduction in stretch reactions in MH during locomotion was demonstrated in four of six subjects with complete SCI while taking clonidine [75].

The absence of the locomotor pattern in patients with complete SCI could possibly be explained by the chronic state, since they had not experienced locomotion for many years. It is possible that the spinal central pattern generator for locomotion depends more heavily on the presence of supraspinal influences in primates [79,80]. It is also possible that some forms of flexor reflex afferent stimuli are required to trigger spinal locomotion, as demonstrated in spinal cats [81,82]. It can be argued that a higher dosage of clonidine may be necessary to facilitate the expression of the locomotor pattern; however, the presence of adverse side effects is an important limiting

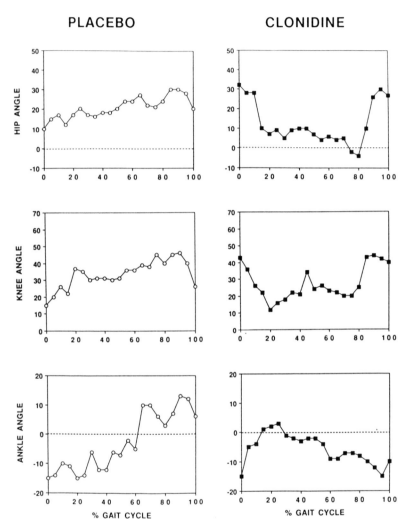

Figure 8   The hip, knee, and ankle joint excursions for an incomplete subject with SCI during placebo period as well as a representative gait cycle during clonidine treatment period are presented. Points represent every 5% of the step cycle. Arrows indicate TO for each gait cycle. Stance–swing transition occurred at 70% ± 22% (placebo) and 84% ± 7% (clonidine) of the gait cycle (modified from [75]).

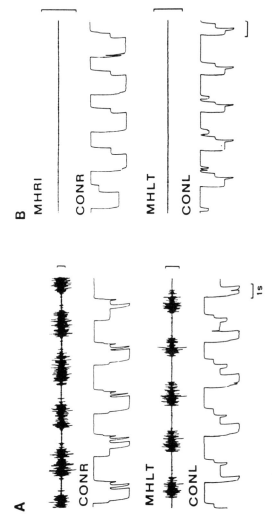

Figure 9 Bilateral MH EMG activity and footswitch traces of a subject with complete SCI during assisted treadmill locomotion recorded during placebo (A) and clonidine (B) sessions (modified from [75]).

factor. An alternative method of drug administration, such as intrathecal injection, which would help to minimize side effects, should also be investigated. Another limiting factor was that three patients were taking other drugs, such as baclofen, at the time of this study. This could possibly interfere with the effect of clonidine.

Functional Electrical Stimulation

Many of the patients seen in our laboratory are already taking medications such as baclofen to reduce spasticity, yet their reflexes remained abnormally high and exaggerated stretch responses could not be eliminated during walking. Additional methods may be necessary to lower the reflex at appropriate phases in the step cycle. Methods that could control the reflex amplitude within 100–200 msec would be particularly desirable. This would allow more flexibility, not only to tailor the reflex excitability for the particular task at hand but also to modify the reflexes at different times in a movement, in such a way that mimics the normal control of the central nervous system. Preliminary results have shown that in the moderately and severely impaired spastic paretic subjects, conditioning cutaneous stimulation delivered to the medial plantar region can selectively inhibit the soleus H-reflex in both the early stance and swing phases during walking [83]. This approach has potential to be incorporated as a regimen of functional electrical stimulation for gait retraining.

Electrical stimulation applied to the sole of the foot may enhance certain reflex pathways such as the flexor reflex afferents (FRA) and inhibit the hyperactive extensor stretch reflex during walking. It may prove beneficial to the proper restoration of locomotion, if the soleus H-reflex can be inhibited in a phase- and task-dependent manner by conditioning cutaneomuscular stimulation of the sole during walking.

Figure 10 shows two examples of severely injured subjects who showed little or no phasic modulation of the soleus H-reflex during walking. These subjects generally had severe clinical signs of spasticity and marked gait deficits. Overground walking was laborious or unstable, hence limited to 5–10 steps per trial, when the subject was provided with a safety body harness and handrails for support. As can be seen from Figure 10, there was no phasic modulation of the H-reflex throughout the entire gait cycle, with little or no inhibition present in early stance or swing. With conditioning cutaneomuscular stimulation, the H-reflex was significantly reduced in the early stance and swing phases, thereby producing a pattern of H-reflex that seemed to be modulated phasically through the step cycle.

All patients reported ease for the limb to swing through and a decreased effort to walk secondary to the reduction in limb stiffness, when the condi-

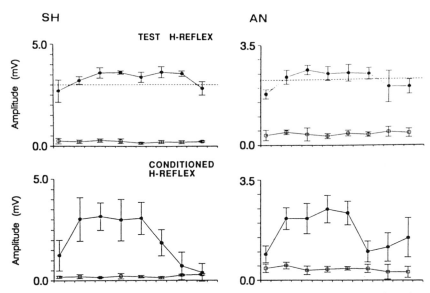

Figure 10 Modulation of the test and conditioned soleus H-reflex (filled circles, mean ± SD) in two severely impaired spastic paretic subjects (SH, AN) during treadmill walking. Note the absence of H-reflex modulation throughout the entire gait cycle and the increase in amplitude beyond that observed during quiet standing (indicated by the dotted line). With cutaneomuscular stimulation, the H-reflex became partially and selectively inhibited in early stance and swing, thereby revealing a more normal modulation pattern. The M-wave (open squares, mean ± SD) remained relatively low and constant.

tioning stimulation is appropriately timed to occur just before or during swing. This was especially true for moderately or severely impaired subjects who had difficulty dorsiflexing the foot, often resulting in toe drag during swing.

Figure 11 shows the effect of FES on the angular excursion of one subject with incomplete SCI on the treadmill. The walking speed for all the graphs is 0.18 m/sec, which represented the comfortable speed at the beginning of the training. The stimulation was triggered by a hand switch. The major difference with FES is the absence of excessive plantarflexion, which could possibly be induced by dragging the toes on the moving treadmill belt. Other differences include increased dorsiflexion and hip flexion. These results are comparable to those described by Kralj and Badj [84], who reported increased knee flexion, increased hip flexion at the stance to swing transition, and a small decrease in plantarflexion during the swing phase due to FES. The present results show only the immediate effect of

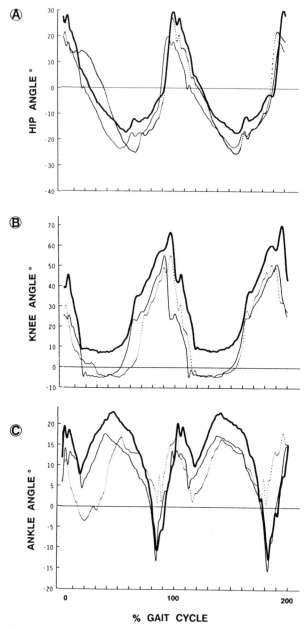

Figure 11   The effects of FES-assisted walking on the kinematic pattern of a subject with incomplete SCI during treadmill walking at 0.18 m/sec. Illustrated are angular displacements of the hip (A), knee (B), and ankle (C) across consecutive cycles in pre-FES evaluation (dotted line), post-FES evaluation (fine solid line), and 6 weeks posttraining evaluation without FES (bold solid line).

FES-assisted walking. As reported for hemiplegics by Liberson [85] and for patients with SCI by Kralj and Badj [84] FES-assisted walking can have a long-term training effect and improve gait to such an extent that FES is no longer necessary. The characterization of those adaptation is a major focus of the studies underway in our laboratory. The maximal speed attained on the treadmill by the SCI subject using FES during a 6 month period increased from 0.25 m/sec at the control stage to 0.6 m/sec during the FES-assisted stage. The speed could be maintained at 0.50 m/sec even without the use of FES at the end of the 6 month period. Figure 11 shows an example of the adaptation observed following 6 weeks of FES-assisted walking. The bold solid line represents a trial without the use of FES after 6 weeks of FES-assisted walking. The major changes apparent when one compares the pretraining trial without FES to the posttraining trial without FES are increased hip flexion, decreased knee hyperextension during stance, increased knee flexion during swing, and increased dorsiflexion at foot contact. However, the passive plantarflexion occurring at the end of the stance period is not suppressed. Meanwhile a multicenter clinical trial has been undertaken to investigate the potential of this approach to improve locomotion in a significant number of patients with SCI across Canada.

CONCLUSIONS AND FUTURE DIRECTIONS

Research is underway to validate these individual and combined approaches, and to identify the optimal period following lesion to initiate each intervention. At present, a clinical trial utilizing a single-subject, randomized, block design has been undertaken to compare and contrast the effects of each of the new medications to the conventional antispastic medication, baclofen, and the results are promising [86]. Eventually, investigations will be undertaken to see if any combination of medications will be superior and offer optimal results. A recent preliminary study [87] has shown that the combination of cyproheptadine and clonidine could restore locomotor function in two chronic spinal cord injured subjects who were previously wheelchair bound. Their locomotor patterns and endurance were further improved after a period of interactive locomotor training. Research studies have been undertaken to identify the patient population who would benefit from such a combined approach. The long-term goal of the proposed experimental approaches is to provide a dynamic, comprehensive, and integrated alternative for the treatment of gait disorders.

Although the new experimental approaches presented in this chapter have only been investigated in subjects with SCI, it is envisaged that the concepts in neuroplasticity can be generalized to the gait rehabilitation of patients with other neurological disorders such as cerebrovascular lesions or cerebral palsy. Treatment strategies have to be adopted and considered in the context of internal constraints such as muscle and joint biomechanics and

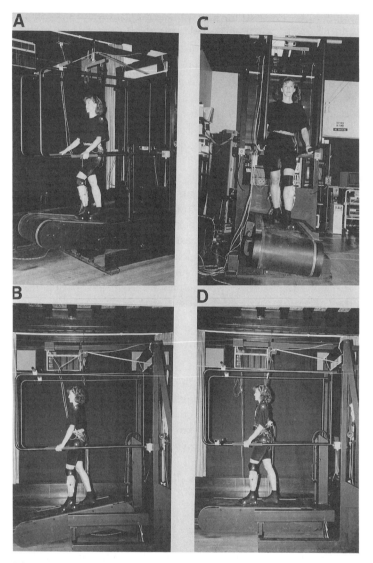

Figure 12 A treadmill that can incline at different degrees in both anteroposterior (0 to 20 degrees; A,B) and the lateral directions (0–10 degrees; C) has been built to allow study of gait adaptation for both normal and neurologically impaired patients.

Also shown is a body weight support system consisting of two padded thigh rings attached in three places to a waist belt supported by shoulder straps. The shoulder straps are in turn connected to a motor-driven pulley system that provides the lift. Transducers are used to quantify BWS provided (D). In these four pictures, some of the EMG recording electrodes and the reflective joint markers are also clearly visible.

external constraints such as adaptation to the environment. A new treadmill that can incline at different degrees in both the anteroposterior (0–20 degrees) and the lateral directions (0–10 degrees) has recently been built to study gait adaptation in both normal and spinal cord injured subjects (Figure 12). Together with the different speed controls and the body weight support system, the various external variables such as speed, inclination, and loading can be manipulated and examined in an integrated manner [59].

ACKNOWLEDGMENTS

This work was supported by grants from the Medical Research Council and the Network of Centres of Excellence for Neural Regeneration and Functional Recovery. H.B. is a Chercheur-Boursier of the Fonds de la Recherche en Santé du Québec and J.F. received a postdoctoral fellowship from the Rick Hansen Man in Motion World Tour Society. The authors wish to thank M. Wainberg, J. Stewart, M. Visintin, R. Blunt, K. Norman, M. Danakas, A. Pepin, M. Ladouceur, and K. Chitre for their original contribution to the different studies quoted in the chapter. Special thanks are due to K. Norman for reviewing earlier versions of the manuscript.

REFERENCES

1. J.S. Young, B.E. Burns, A.M. Bowen, and R. McCutchen, Spinal cord injury statistics. Experience of the regional spinal cord injury system. Good Samaritan Medical Center, Phoenix, Arizona.
2. D.C. Burke, H.T. Burley, and G.H. Ungar, *Aust. N.Z. J. Surg.*, 55:377–382 (1985).
3. C.S. Sherrington, *J. Physiol.*, *40*:28–121 (1910).
4. T.G. Brown, *J. Physiol Lond.*, *44*:4818–4846 (1914).
5. S. Grillner, *Handbook of Physiology. The Nervous System*, vol II (V.E. Brooks, ed.), American Physiological Society, Bethesda, pp. 1179–1236 (1981).
6. S. Grillner and P. Wallén, *Annu. Rev. Neurosci.*, 8:233–261 (1985).
7. S. Grillner, *Control of Posture and Locomotion* (R.B. Stein, K.G. Pearson, R.S. Smith, and J.B. Redford, eds.), Plenum Press, New York, pp. 515–535 (1973).
8. E. Jankowska, M.G.M. Jukes, S. Lund, and A. Lundberg, *Acta Physiol. Scand.*, 70:389–402 (1967).
9. H. Forssberg and S. Grillner, *Brain Res.*, 50:184–186 (1973).
10. A. Lundberg, *The Nervous System, The Basic Neurosciences* (D.B. Tower, ed.), Raven Press, New York, pp. 253–265 (1975).
11. S. Rossignol, H. Barbeau, and C. Julien, *Development and Plasticity of the Mammalian Spinal Cord*, (M.E. Goldberger, A. Gorio, and M. Murray, eds.), Springer Verlag, Spoleto, Italy, pp. 323–346 (1986).
12. H. Barbeau, C. Julien, and S. Rossignol, *Brain Res.*, 437:83–96 (1987).
13. H. Barbeau and S. Rossignol, *Brain Res.*, 546:250–260 (1991).
14. H. Barbeau and S. Rossignol, *Brain Res.*, 412:84–95 (1987).

15. M.P. Murray, A.B. Drought, and R.C. Kory, *J. Bone Joint Surg.*, 46:334–360 (1964).

16. D.H. Sutherland, L. Cooper, and D. Daniel, *J. Bone Joint Surg.*, 62A(3):354–363 (1980).

17. V.T. Inman, H.J. Ralston, and F. Todd, *Human Walking*. Williams & Wilkins, Baltimore (1981).

18. D.A. Winter, *J. Motor Behav.*, 15:302–330 (1983).

19. D.A. Winter, *The Biomechanics and Motor Control of Human Gait*. University of Waterloo Press, Waterloo, Ontario, Canada (1987).

20. C.E. Chapman and M. Weisendanger, *Physiother. Can.*, 34(3):125–135 (1982).

21. P. Ashby, E. Stalberg, T. Winkler, and J.P. Hunter, *Exp. Brain Res.*, 69:1–6 (1987).

22. R.W. Hussey and E.S. Stauffer, *Arch. Phys. Med. Rehab.*, 54:544–547 (1973).

23. J.W. Lance, *Spasticity: Disordered Motor Control* (R.G. Feldman, R.R. Young, W.P. Koella, eds.), Year Book, Chicago, pp. 485–494 (1980).

24. P.J. Delwaide, *Clinical Neurophysiology in Spasticity* (P.J. Delwaide and R.R. Young, eds.), Elsevier, Amsterdam, pp. 185–203 (1985).

25. E. Knutsson, *Motor Control Mechanisms in Health and Disease* (J.E. Desmedt, ed.), Raven Press, New York, pp. 1013–1034 (1983).

26. G.L. Gottlieb and G.C. Agarwal, *J. Neurol. Neurosurg. Psychiatry*, 36:529–546 (1973).

27. C. Capaday and R.B. Stein, *J. Neurosci.*, 6(5):1308–1313 (1986).

28. P.D. Neilson and C.J. Andrews, *J. Neurol. Neurosurg. Psychiatry*, 36:547–554 (1973).

29. J. Perry, *Spasticity: Disordered Motor Control* (R.G. Feldman, R.R. Young, and W.P. Koella, eds.), Year Book, Chicago, pp. 87–100 (1980).

30. R.J. Grimm, *Adv. Neurol.*, 39:1–11 (1983).

31. J. Fung and H. Barbeau, *EEG Clin. Neurophysiol.*, 73:233–244 (1989).

32. B. Conrad, R. Benecke, J. Carnehl, J. Hohne, and H.M. Meinck, *Motor Control Mechanisms in Health and Disease* (J.E. Desmedt, ed.), Raven Press, New York, pp. 717–726 (1983).

33. B. Conrad, R. Benecke, and H.M. Meinck, *Clinical Neurophysiology in Spasticity* (P.J. Delwaide and R.R. Young, eds.), Elsevier, Amsterdam, pp. 155–174 (1985).

34. E. Knutsson and C. Richards, *Brain*, 102:405–439 (1979).

35. E. Knutsson, *Scand. J. Rehab. Med.*, 12(Suppl. 7):47–52 (1980).

36. V. Dietz and W. Berger, *Exp. Neurol.*, 79:680–687 (1983).

37. V. Dietz, J. Quintern, and W. Berger, *Brain*, 104:431–449 (1981).

38. P. Ashby and D. McCrea, *Handbook of the Spinal Cord* (R.A. Davidoff, ed.), Marcel Dekker, New York, pp. 119–143 (1987).

39. S. Taylor, P. Ashby, and M. Verrier, *J. Neurol. Neurosurg. Psychiatry*, 47:1102–1108 (1980).

40. J.W. Little and E.M. Halar, *Arch. Phys. Med. Rehab.*, 66:19–22 (1985).

41. C. Capaday and R.B. Stein, *J. Physiol. Lond.*, 392:513–522 (1987).

42. P. Crenna and C. Frigo, *Exp. Brain. Res.*, 66:49–60 (1987).

43. J. Fung, R. Blunt, and H. Barbeau, *Disorders of Posture and Gait*, (T. Brandt, W. Paulus, W. Bles, M. Dieterich, S. Krafczyk, A. Straube, eds.), Thieme, New York, pp. 398–401 (1990).
44. J.F. Yang, J. Fung, M. Edamura, R. Blunt, R.B. Stein, and H. Barbeau, *Can. J. Neurol. Sci.*, *18*:443–452 (1991).
45. D. Burke and P. Ashby, *J. Neurol. Sci.*, *15*:321–326 (1972).
46. M. Wainberg, H. Barbeau, and S. Gauthier, *J. Neurol.*, *233*:311–314 (1986).
47. P. Ashby and M. Wiens, *J. Physiol (Lond.)*, *414*:145–157 (1989).
48. C. Capaday and R.B. Stein, *J. Neurosci. Methods*, *21*:91–104 (1987).
49. E. Edamura, J.F. Yang, and R.B. Stein, *J. Neurosci.*, *11*:420–427 (1991).
50. D.L. Hutchinson, R.R. Roy, J.A. Hodgson, and V.R. Edgerton, *Brain Res.*, *502*: 233–244 (1989).
51. D.J. Pierotti, R.R. Roy, R.J. Gregor, and V.R. Edgerton, *Brain Res.*, *481*:57–66 (1989).
52. H. Forssberg, S. Grillner, and J. Hallbertsma, *Acta. Physiol. Scand.*, *108*:269–281 (1980).
53. M. Bélanger, Ph.D. thesis (nonpublished), Département de Physiologie, Faculté de Médecine, Université de Montréal (1990).
54. R. Shiavi, H.J. Bulge, and T. Limbird, *J. Rehab. Res. Dev.*, *24*:24–30 (1987).
55. V. Dietz, *Disorders of Posture and Gait*, (W. Bles, T.H. Brandt, eds.), Elsevier Science Publishers, Amsterdam, pp. 243–252 (1986).
56. D.C. Burke and J.W. Lance, *New Developments in Electromyography and Clinical Neurophysiology*, vol. 3 (J.E. Desmedt, ed.), Karger, Basel, pp. 475–495 (1973).
57. E. Knutsson and A. Mariensson, *Scand. J. Rehab. Med.*, *12*:93–106 (1980).
58. M.E. Brandstater, H. de Bruin, C. Gowland, and B.M. Clark, *Arch. Phys. Med. Rehab.*, *64*:583–587 (1983).
59. A. Pepin and H. Barbeau, *Soc. Neurosci. Abstr.*, *18*:860 (1992).
60. R.R. Young and P.J. Delwaide, *N. Engl. J. Med.*, *304*:28 (1981).
61. J.R.E. Close, *Motor Function In The Lower Extremity*. C.C. Thomas, Springfield IL (1964).
62. I. Odeen and E. Knutsson, *Scand. J. Rehab. Med.*, *13*:117–121 (1981).
63. F. Tremblay, F. Malouin, C.L. Richards, and F. Dumas, *Scand. J. Rehab. Med.*, *22*:171–180 (1990).
64. J.L. Smith, L.A. Smith, R.F. Zernicke, and M. Hoy, *Exp. Neurol.*, *16*:393–413 (1982).
65. E. Eidelberg, J.L. Story, B.L. Meyer, and J. Mystel, *Exp. Brain Res.*, *40*:241–246 (1980).
66. I. Engberg and A. Lundberg, *Acta Physiol. Scand.*, *75*:614–630 (1969).
67. M. Visintin and H. Barbeau, *Can. J. Neurol. Sci.*, *16*:315–325 (1989).
68. H. Barbeau, W. Wainberg, and L. Finch, *Med. Biol. Eng. Comput.*, *25*:341–344 (1987).
69. L. Finch and H. Barbeau, *Physiother. Can.*, *38*:36–41 (1985).
70. H. Barbeau and S. Rossignol, *Brain Res.*, *514*:55–67 (1990).
71. J. Tuckman, D.S. Chu, C.R. Petrillo, and N.E. Naftchi, *Spinal Cord Injuries* (N.Z.E. Naftchi, ed.), Spectrum Publications, New York, pp. 133–136 (1983).

72. F.M. Maynard, *Paraplegia*, *24*:175–192 (1986).
73. P.W. Nance, A.H. Shears, and D.M. Nance, *Can. Med. Assoc. J.*, *133*:41–42 (1985).
74. M. Wainberg, H. Barbeau, and S. Gauthier, *J. Neurol, Neurosurg. Psychiatry*, *53*:754–763 (1990).
75. J.E. Stewart, H. Barbeau, and S. Gauthier, *Can. J. Neurol. Sci.*, *18*:321–331 (1991).
76. P. Bédard, H. Barbeau, G. Barbeau, and M. Filion, *Brain Res.*, *169*:393–397 (1979).
77. H. Barbeau and P. Bédard, *Neuropharmacology*, *20*:611–616 (1981).
78. H. Barbeau, C. Richards, and P. Bedard, *J. Neurol. Neurosurg. Psychiatry*, *45*: 923–926 (1982).
79. E. Eidelberg, J.G. Walsen, and L.H. Nguyen, *Brain*, *104*:647–663 (1981).
80. A.J. Vilensky, *Neurosci. Biobehav. Rev.*, *11*:263–274 (1987).
81. H. Forssberg, *J. Neurophysiol.*, *42*:936–953 (1979).
82. H. Forssberg, *Muscle Receptors and Movement* (A. Taylor and A. Prochazka, eds.), Macmillan, London, pp. 403–412 (1981).
83. J. Fung and H. Barbeau, *Soc. Neurosci. Abstr.*, *16*:1262 (1990).
84. A. Kralj and T. Badj, Functional Electrical Stimulation Standing and Walking after a Spinal Cord Injury. CRC Press, Boca Raton, FL (1989).
85. W.T. Liberson, H.J. Holmquest, D. Scott, and M. Dow, *Arch. Phys. Med. Rehab.*, *42*:101–105 (1961).
86. K.E. Norman and H. Barbeau, *Soc. Neurosci. Abstr.*, *18*:860 (1992).
87. J. Fung, J.E. Stewart, and H. Barbeau, *J. Neurol. Sci.*, *100*:85–93 (1990).

II
OUTCOME MEASURES AND THE REHABILITATION PROCESS

5

Outcome Assessment in Chronic Neurological Disease

David C. Good

Bowman Gray School of Medicine
Wake Forest University
Winston-Salem, North Carolina

IMPORTANCE OF OUTCOME ASSESSMENT AND MEASUREMENT

Predicting and measuring outcome has always been important in the delivery of health care. However, perhaps never in the history of medicine have these areas been studied as intensively as they are today.

Outcome assessment has many applications. Third party payers, both public and private, desire the best return for their health care dollars. Accrediting agencies are increasingly interested in outcome measures as markers of quality for an institution. Individual health care providers are evaluated by hospitals and clinics on the basis of outcome. Society in general has shown increased awareness and interest in measurement of outcome.

However, the need for outcome prediction and assessment goes much deeper than the desire to contain health care costs or societal concerns about quality. Clinical researchers must have reliable measures of outcome in order to evaluate the effectiveness of therapies. The choice of an appropriate outcome measure is critical for the design of any research study. Clinicians want the best possible outcomes for their patients and clients. Clinicians also want to direct their interventions where the most good can be accomplished, and want to avoid painful or costly interventions where the outlook is hopeless. In fact, it is virtually impossible to consider medical treatment without also considering outcome. Practioners therefore must know the "natural" range of outcomes for a given medical condition, commonly referred to as "prognosis." With this information, interventions can be designed to alter outcome, and a "treatment plan" proposed.

Finally, patients and families must understand potential clinical outcomes, so that realistic expectations can be established and plans made for the future.

DIFFERENCES BETWEEN ACUTE AND CHRONIC MEDICAL CONDITIONS

What is the role of outcome assessment and measurement in chronic neurological disease? First of all, "outcome" in this context must be defined, since there are obvious differences compared to other medical settings. In acute conditions, favorable outcomes are usually easy to define and measure. Survival, the medical cure of an illness, a successful surgical result, and the proper healing of a fracture are all examples of desirable outcomes that are evident to both physicians and patients. Implicit in most outcome measures for acute medical conditions is the assumption that the condition is self-limited and that the patient will return to his or her previous level of health.

In chronic conditions, full recovery is unlikely, and long-term impairment is expected. Outcomes such as return home, independence in basic activities of daily living, independence in ambulation or mobility, and, most importantly, a satisfying lifestyle, become more important. Other appropriate outcomes for persons with chronic conditions might include ability to function in the community, ability to drive, or satisfactory family adjustment. It is evident that these outcomes are very different from those of patients with acute medical conditions. In chronic illness, outcomes are much less "medically" oriented and more "patient" oriented. Outcomes are also more subject to differences of opinion and therefore more difficult to measure. The definition of an important outcome may vary from person to person. Clinician and patient may even disagree on the importance of various outcomes, resulting in misunderstandings or noncompliance. At times the collective beliefs of the health care system may come into conflict with those of the individual.

Outcomes in chronic illness are often interdependent, or at least interrelated. For example, independence in activities of daily living may be one (but not the only) prerequisite for returning home. Finally, a positive outcome in one area does not guarantee positive outcomes in other important areas. For example, a person may return home, be independent in all activities of daily living, but still have an unsatisfactory lifestyle.

OUTCOME MEASURES FOR CHRONIC NEUROLOGICAL CONDITIONS

General Overview

As implied above, there is no single "right" or "correct" measurement of outcome for chronic neurological conditions. All the outcome measures discussed in this chapter have an appropriate role in the assessment of persons with chronic neurological disease. The intent of this chapter is not to discuss in detail each specific outcome measure, but to provide a framework to assist the reader in using them. The use of a particular measurement depends on the type of underlying condition and the specific motive for obtaining the measure. In addition, different outcome measures may be appropriate for a patient or group of patients at different stages of their illness. For an excellent comprehensive discussion of outcome assessment in chronic neurological disease, the reader is referred to work by Wade [1].

This chapter will not discuss simple measures, such as returning home or returning to work after a neurological illness or injury. The validity and importance of these outcomes are self-evident, and they are easily measured. Instead, outcome measures that provide special insight into adaptation to chronic neurological disorders will be discussed. Many of these are "intermediate" to the "final outcomes" of return home or return to work. Examples include measures of motor function or activities of daily living, and are very applicable to the rehabilitation process. Outcome measures may assess impairment, disability, or handicap, as defined by the World Health Organization (WHO) in 1980 [2] (Table 1). Table 2 includes the general categories of outcome measures appropriate for chronic neurological disease that will be discussed in this chapter.

Assessment Scales

Many outcome measures require an instrument or "tool." In chronic neurological conditions, the tool is often a scale. Scales are not unique to the evaluation of neurological disorders, and their usefulness is appreciated by practitioners in many medical disciplines. For example, all physicians are familiar with Apgar scores in newborn infants [3] and tumor grading scales [4]. Assessment scales can provide structure to diverse, but related, data and allow an overall summary "at a glance." Clinical impressions of clinicians may be false or misleading [5,6]. By focusing attention on key parameters, assessment scales highlight information that might otherwise be overlooked. Scales are ideal for following change in groups of patients over time, and provide standardization among different examiners and institutions.

Table 1 Impairments, Disabilities, and Handicaps: WHO Definitions

	Definition	Characteristics	Examples
Impairment	Loss or abnormality of structure or function	Reflects disturbances at the level of the organ	Aphasia, paraplegia, incontinence
Disability	Restriction or lack of ability to perform an activity in the manner considered normal	Reflects disturbances at the level of the person	Inability to ambulate, bathe, or communicate
Handicap	Inability to fulfill a role normal for a specific individual	Represents the socialization of an impairment or disability	Inability regarding occupation, social integration, economic self-sufficiency

Most scales used in medicine are ordinal scales [1,7,8], with categories of dysfunction, as opposed to interval scales, which are linear. This is an important concept, because change in one portion of an ordinal scale may not be equivalent to change in another portion [8]. Powerful parametric statistical tests (Student's t or analysis of variance) should not be applied to ordinal scales [1,9]. The potential pitfalls and misapplications of ordinal scales have been emphasized by Merbitz [8].

A bewildering number of scales have been designed to assess outcome in chronic neurological conditions [1,7]. Two caveats are important when choosing a scale to measure outcome. First, the scale must be applied appropriately [5,7,10,11]. In other words, the criteria used in the development of the scale must match the user's purpose [7,12]. The choice of the wrong scale can lead to misleading, or even erroneous, information. Second,

Table 2 Categories of Outcome Measures

Isolated parameters
Functional systems
Overall neurological function
Activities of daily living
Instrumental living skills
Global outcome measures
Quality of Life

care must be chosen to use a scale that is reliable, valid, and appropriately responsive [1,5,7,10,11]. This is especially important, because many scales were not designed according to strict psychometric standards, and have not been critically evaluated. Excellent reviews of scale design are available elsewhere [1,12,13].

Any useful scale must be reliable. All measurement involves some degree of error, which must be minimized if the score is to be stable and reproducible. Three types of reliability are measurable for assessment scales [7,12]. Test–retest reliability requires stability of scores on serial administration by the same rater. Interrater reliability is calculated from correlations between scores obtained by different raters. Statistical formulas, (for example, the kappa statistic) are available to assess each type of reliability [9,12]. Internal consistency is a third measure of reliability, which describes the degree to which different scale items are measuring the same content.

Although reliability is required for validity, additional evidence is needed that a scale measures what it is designed to measure [7,9]. Criterion validity can be assessed when a "gold standard" exists with which to compare a new measure. This is difficult when assessing outcome in chronic neurological conditions, since the nature of the parameters being measured results in differences in viewpoint and philosophy. Validity is always a difficult concept when applied to variables such as behavior or performance on a test maneuver. Content validity is more applicable for scales that assess this type of information, and refers to how adequately sampling questions reflect the aims of the index. However, there is no statistical test for content validity, which must be assessed by systematic use of expert opinion [9]. Scales often "weight" some parameters more than others. Weighting can profoundly affect scale validity and must be carefully considered.

Any scale must be responsive to clinical change. This can be a problem, since many scales used in rehabilitation miss subtle but important changes. Many scales are significantly responsive to change only in the midportion of the scale. Such scales should not be applied to patients or populations who are at one extreme of the scale (either the "best" or "worst" end), where change is more difficult to detect [14]. In addition, some scales may be appropriate for assessing change in some illnesses but not others.

Many other practical considerations are critical in scale design and utilization [7]. The number and type of parameters chosen are obviously important. A small number of variables contributes to simplicity of measurement, but may result in loss of completeness. On the other hand, an excessive number of variables may lead to reduncency of measurement and inefficiency. There are advantages and disadvantages to different modes of administration, including direct observation, interview, or self-administered questionnaire [5,7]. The degree of imposition or burden on study participants, the time of administration, and the degree of staff training required are all important features that will have an impact on the usefulness of any assessment instrument.

Another decision that must be made when choosing an assessment scale is whether a disease-specific or a more general scale best meets the purpose of the user. Disease-specific scales are widely used in neurological disease. Examples include the Kurtzke Expanded Disability Status Scale (EDSS) for multiple sclerosis [15]; the Unified Parkinson's Disease Rating Scale [16] and the Hoehn and Yahr Scale [17] for Parkinson's disease; and the Mathew Scale [18], the NIH Stroke Scale [19], and the Toronto Stroke Scale [20] for stroke. Other scales have been developed to have wide applicability regardless of medical diagnosis. This is especially characteristic of scales that assess functional status, such as the Barthel Index [21], or quality of life, for example, the Sickness Impact Profile [22]. Disease-specific scales often have a predominantly medical focus on impairment. This is often inadequate to meet the broader goals of rehabilitation, where the focus is on function and quality of life irrespective of diagnosis. Disease-specific scales have found their widest use in disease treatment studies, whereas more general scales have found favor as outcome measures in rehabilitation.

As previously noted, many scales have been designed for the assessment of chronic neurologic disease [1,7]. However, not all have undergone thorough validity and reliability studies. In addition to the need to choose a scale that is psychometrically sound, it should be stressed again that any scale should be used only in the context for which it was designed. Although no scale is perfect, it is generally better to use a well-established scale rather than to attempt to design a new scale [1,23,24].

Specific Outcome Measures

Isolated Parameters

The simplest outcome measures are isolated parameters. Examples applicable to chronic neurological illness include isolated muscle strength, position sense testing, or performance on a specific task. Using motor function as an example, physicians often grade individual muscle strength on a scale of 0–5, using the Medical Research Council Scale [25]. Several scales have been developed to assess spasticity. The best known is the Ashworth Scale [26], which is also easy to score clinically.

Specific parameters are often easily measured, and improvement readily followed over time. However, performance on a highly circumscribed parameter is often totally unrelated to other important outcome variables. For example, motor strength in the biceps muscle may have only the remotest correlation with return home. Thus, while isolated parameters have a place in outcome assessment, the parameter must be carefully chosen with a specific goal in mind.

Functional Systems

A functional system can be defined as a group of related individual parameters that are closely integrated and important in the performance of a set of activities. An obvious example is the motor system, which includes the complex integrated activity of multiple muscles mediated by central mechanisms. The ability of this system to accomplish tasks important for an independent lifestyle can be measured by a variety of measurement tools, including the timed nine-hole peg test (for assessing upper extremity function), the Fugl-Meyer Scale (for assessing motor function in hemiparesis) [27], or the Motor Assessment Scale [28].

The Fugl-Meyer Scale has been widely used as a clincial research assessment tool following stroke. It is a comprehensive evaluation of motor function in hemiparesis, and includes sections to evaluate upper extremity function, lower extremity function, balance, sensation, and range of motion. The maximum score for the sum of the sections is 226. However, upper extremity and lower extremity may be assessed using subscales. The validity and reliability for the entire scale and subscales have been demonstrated [29,30]. The disadvantages of the Fugl-Meyer Scale are that it must be administered by a skilled therapist, and takes 20–30 min to perform accurately [29]. It has also been criticized for containing a high degree of redundancy and oversampling [9].

A more abstract example of a functional system is the whole repertoire of feelings, attitudes, and vegetative functions that are components of mood or affect. Again, a large number of measurement tools are available to assess affect, including the commonly used Beck Depression Inventory [31], Hamilton Scale [32], and Zung Self-Rating Scale [33]. Other examples of tools to measure other functional systems include multiple scales to measure aspects of neurophyschological function (global scales of dementia, memory scales, aphasia batteries, etc.), or aspects of behavior (many pain scales).

The advantage of tools that assess functional systems is their ability to target quickly a specific group of activities of great importance to a patient, caregiver, or clinician. Many of these activities are amenable to specific strategies of intervention, and the efficacy of the intervention may be monitored by the assessment tool. For example, the efficacy of a program to improve motor function might be monitored by the Fugl-Meyer Scale or the treatment of depression monitored by the Beck Depression Inventory.

Most measurements of functional systems assess impairments. Some measures correlate with other important outcomes. For example, following stroke, higher scores of motor function are associated with independence in self-care [30,34–38], whereas depression [6,7,39] and dementia [36] both correlate with dependence in self-care and lower probability of returning home. At times, an intensive therapeutic effort directed toward one functional system can substantially improve a patient's quality of life.

However, functional systems do not *always* correlate with other important outcomes, especially those related to disability. For example, simple motor assessment does not always correlate with ability to perform more complex activities. All clinicians have seen patients who are very functional in daily life despite severe motor deficits. Another example is the use of intelligence tests to assess the cognitive abilities of individuals who have sustained head injuries. Although these tests are widely performed in this setting, the results relate only broadly to an individual's ultimate ability to function in society, or even the ability to return to work (see Chapter 22).

Use of assessment tools related to a single functional system carries the risk of focusing on a small component of a complex picture, to the detriment of other issues that may be equally important.

Overall Neurological Function

Many outcome measures have been developed that assess overall neurological function. Most of these are aggregate scales that attempt to quantify physical deficit by allocating points for various components of the traditional neurological examination [9]. Most such scales are "weighted," with items thought to be important by the scale designers given a higher relative score. The subscores are then added to give a single number to represent global neurological function.

Most scales of this type are disease-specific, and the weighting of various components of the scale is heavily influenced by the clinical features of the specific neurological condition. Most of these scales measure impairment, or combinations of impairment and disability. These include the Mathew Scale [18] and NIH Scale [19] used for stroke, and the Kurtzke EDSS [15] for multiple sclerosis.

Scales that measure overall neurological function have been widely used in evaluating the effects of therapeutic interventions on the course of specific illnesses. While these scales are intuitively attractive, the assumptions made in the design of these instruments limit their usefulness. Critics have maintained that the neurological examination cannot logically be adapted for use as a global instrument of neurological function. The major strength of the neurological examination is the diagnosis and localization of abnormalities of the nervous system. Although it is an accurate description of a single patient at a given time, it is ill-suited for describing groups of patients over an extended period of time. The "weighting" of individual scale components has been criticized as arbitrary, even when the scale designers are experts in the evaluation of the condition for which the scale was designed. Furthermore, most scales of this type are aggregate in nature, with a sum presented as the "degree of impairment." An aggregate score may conceal as much information as it reveals. As a specific example, the same score could be obtained by persons with very different combinations of neurological deficits. While there clearly is an association between some features of the neurological examination and other measures of outcome, this relationship is not always strong. For example, the Hoehn and Yahr Scale for Parkinson's disease does not correlate well with scales based on activities of daily living, especially for grades I–III [40].

Activities of Daily Living

Most clinicians and patients would agree that the ability to perform everyday activities such as bathing, dressing, eating, and moving from one place to another are important outcomes in chronic neurological disease. Such activities require the integration of a number of functional systems, as well as interaction between the individual and the surrounding environment. On an everyday basis, considerable time and effort are spent in rehabilitation programs teaching patients to perform individual functional activities.

At times, the ability to accomplish a specific functional task important to the patient is a very appropriate outcome measure. Performance on a specific task may be improved by a highly directed intervention such as intensive training. An example might include learning to push a specific button to call for help. While ability to perform individual tasks can be very important, it is often more relevant to use a global measure of functional abilities.

The most widely used scales to assess persons with chronic neurological disease are those based on activities of daily living (ADLs) and functional abilities. These are designed to measure disability, rather than impairment, and are therefore less medically oriented than most scales previously discussed [11]. Since disabilities are not unidimensional, and cannot be defined in terms of a single variable, outcome measures of this type are usually multifaceted and cover a wide range of abilities [41]. Although many different abilities could be measured, almost all scales include measures of proficiency in ADLs and mobility. Because there is a widespread consensus that these abilities are central to the rehabilitation of chronic neurological disease, these scales have been very popular in assessing outcome [24]. Because ADL-based scales originate from the perspective of the individual as the unit of analysis, and emphasize function, they are useful for assessing outcome in many different conditions.

Functionally based scales are also attractive because of their strong correlation with other outcome measures, especially the ability to live independently [42–44] and to experience a satisfactory "quality" of life [43–45].

Many ADL scales have been designed [41], including the well-known Kenny Self-Care Evaluation [46] and Katz Activities of Daily Living Scale [47]. The score on each ADL scale correlates highly with scores on the others, and all classify the overall degree of independence in ADLs in a very similar manner [48]. Undoubtedly, the best known and most extensively studied ADL scale is the Barthel Index (BI) (Table 3), initially introduced in 1965 [21]. The BI is an aggregate scale with a total score of 100. It consists of 15 items, 9 of

Table 3 Barthel Index

Category	Evaluation	Score
Feeding	Totally dependent	0
	Needs help (i.e., for cutting)	5
	Independent	10
Bathing	Cannot perform without assistance	0
	Performs without assistance	5
Grooming	Needs assistance	0
	Washes face, combs hair, brushes teeth	5
Dressing	Totally dependent	0
	Needs help but does at least half of task within reasonable period of time	5
	Independent: ties shoes, fastens fasteners, applies braces	10
Bowel control	Frequent accidents	0
	Occasional accidents or needs help with enema or suppository	5
	No accidents: able to use enema or suppository if needed	10
Bladder control	Incontinent or needs indwelling catheter	0
	Occasional accidents or needs help with device	5
	No accidents, able to care for collecting device, if used	10
Toilet transfers	No use of toilet, bedridden	0
	Needs help for balance, handling clothes or toilet paper	5
	Independent with toilet or bedpan	10
Chair/bed transfers	Completely bedridden, use of chair not possible	0
	Able to sit, but needs maximum assistance to transfer	5
	Minimum assistance or supervision	10
	Independent, including locks of wheelchair and lifting footrests	15
Ambulation/ mobility	Sits on wheelchair, but cannot wheel self	0
	Independent with wheelchair 50 yards, only if unable to walk	5
	Ambulates with help for 50 yards	10
	Independent for 50 yards, may use assistive devices, except for rolling walker	15
Stair-climbing	Cannot climb stairs	0
	Needs help or supervision	5
	Independent: may use assistive devices	10
Total score = (100 maximum)		

which relate to self-care and 6 to mobility. Virtually all basic variables of ADL are included. The BI is especially important in predicting other important outcomes, especially the need for personal assistance in daily living. Granger and his associates have shown that following stroke, a BI score of over 60 generally correlates with ambulation and care with assistance [44,49]. This is the point at which a spouse or caregiver can reasonably manage a patient at home. A BI score of over 95 correlates well with independence in ambulation and self-care activities [42]. The BI and other scales mentioned above have repeatedly been shown to be psychometrically valid and reliable [23,50], and are widely used outcome measures for rehabilitation. However, they have been criticized as being insensitive to small changes in function [41], and therefore inadequate for tracking the clinical course of an individual patient.

Recently, more comprehensive scales have been developed that are more directly applicable to traditional multidisciplinary rehabilitation. Examples include the Functional Independence Measure (FIM) [51], the Level of Rehabilitation Scale [LORS] [52], and the Patient Evaluation and Conference System (PECS) [53,54]. These more comprehensive scales have expanded the number of subcategories found in earlier ADL scales, and have increased the number of scoring possibilities for each individual subcategory. For example, the FIM scale is basically an expanded Barthel Index, incorporating additional measures of cognitive and communication skills and social integration. In addition to additional measurement parameters, the number of scoring possibilities increases from two to four per category for the BI, to seven per category for FIM. The net effect is to increase the sensitivity of the scale to small changes in function, but also to decrease the reliability, or confidence, in any given value. Because of the additional categories and increased sensitivity, expanded ADL scales have been used to follow the clinical progress of individual patients undergoing rehabilitation.

The FIM scale has been incorporated into a national data base, and is used to compare outcomes between institutions with similar patient mix. This information can provide valuable feedback to clinicians and institutions. For example, subcategory scores are sometimes used within institutions to provide feedback to practitioners of individual rehabilitation disciplines. Physical therapy can follow long-range institutional trends for patient abilities in ambulation and mobility skills, and occupational therapy can track trends in ADLs for a given set of patients. Although caution must be exercised in overinterpreting information of this sort [8], many institutions use functional scales to assist in internal program evaluation and quality assessment [5,52,55]. On a much larger scale, it has been proposed that patients be selected for intensive rehabilitation on the basis of functional abilities, and that reimbursement for services be based on documentation of improvement in function [56]. Therefore, it is likely that the already intense interest in functional assessment scales will escalate in the future.

Despite the widespread acceptance of functionally based scales as assessment measures for neurological conditions, they have limitations. Most are aggregate scales (a notable exception is the Katz Activities of Daily Living Scale), with a total score reached by summing subscores. Therefore, they possess the drawbacks of other scales of this type, as discussed previously. These disadvantages are partially counterbalanced by a tendency for functional scales to be hierarchical [41]. In other words, for many diseases individual abilities are lost or recovered in a fairly predictable sequence. For example for persons with stroke, ability to bathe and dress are lost first and recovered last. On the other extreme, ability to feed oneself is usually regained early. Thus, a single aggregate score is usually a fair representation of a set of abilities. Nonetheless, functional scales are not interval (linear) scales, and changes in function in one part of the scale are not equivalent to changes in another [8].

Another potential problem with this group of assessment instruments stems from the fact that they are primarily designed for persons who have an "intermediate" level of disability: the type of person participating in a comprehensive rehabilitation program. The BI has shown greater sensitivity in the midportion of the scale, and is not as useful at the "high end." In addition, a "perfect score" of 100 on the BI does not mean the individual has normal neurological function, but only that the person is independent in the self-care tasks included in the scale. This leads to another limitation: that a high score on a functional scale does not ensure a satisfying lifestyle. Although independence in these activities correlates well with return to independent living and other important outcomes, the association with satisfaction with life is not complete. In fact, occasionally a person's life is more satisfying with a degree of assistance with functional tasks, rather than to struggle to be totally independent.

Instrumental Living Skills

Functioning in the community represents a far greater degree of independence than providing for one's basic self-care. Skills important for community living include shopping, meal preparation, use of private or public transportation, basic laundry and housekeeping skills, ability to use the telephone, and ability to handle finances. This set of activities is collectively termed instrumental living skills. A number of assessment scales have been designed to measure the degree of disability and handicap in a community living setting, including the Instrumental Activities of Daily Living Scale (Lawton) [57] and Pfeffer Functional Activities Questionnaire [58]. Some scales, including the Pfeffer Scale, include measures heavily dependent on cognition, including tracking current events, remembering appointments, and participating in skilled games or hobbies. Scoring for subcategories of instrumental scales is usually ordinal. For example, each item in the Pfeffer Scale is scored according to whether someone else has taken over an activity, whether advice or assistance is required, whether the activity can be performed but with more difficulty than previously, or whether the activity is performed without difficulty. Although many instrumental living skills are aggregate, a great deal of information about ability for community living can be obtained by looking at subcategory scores. Strengths and weaknesses are quickly identified, and some deficits identified may not be obvious to the clinician. The primary purpose of instrumental living scales is to highlight areas of disability or handicap in which a person may need assistance, and to assist in identifying the optimum living situation [23]. While having the widest application to an elderly population, instrumental living measurement tools are also appropriate for assessing younger persons with a variety of chronic neurological conditions. Scales combining ADLs and instrumental living skills have also been described [23].

An advantage of instrumental living scales is that they may be scored by either telephone or personal interview. The disadvantages of this type of scale are similar to those that assess basic ADLs. The specific parameters included in instrumental living scales are perhaps more controversial and arbitrary than those chosen for ADL scales. For example, there may not be uniform agreement that ability to use the telephone is equivalent to the ability to do the laundry. Any weighting of parameters is also controversial for the same reason, and the validity of an aggregate score may be seriously questioned.

Global Outcome Measures

Global outcome scales are simple ordinal scales that assign patient function to one of a small number of broad classifications [9].

One of the earliest to be developed was the Rankin Scale (Table 4), which was the first used for stroke in 1957 [59]. This five-point global scale categorizes a patient from no significant disability to severe disability requiring constant attention. Another commonly used global scale is the Glasgow

Table 4 Rankin Scale

Score	Evaluation
0	No symptoms at all
1	Symptoms only, no significant disability; can perform all usual activities
2	Slight disability; cannot carry out all previous activities, but able to provide all basic self-care
3	Moderate disability; able to ambulate independently, but requires assistance with some other activities
4	Moderately severe disability; cannot ambulate independently and requires assistance for basic activities of daily living
5	Severe disability; requires constant care with all activities, bedridden, incontinent

Outcome Scale [60], which was designed for use with head injury. This also utilizes five outcomes ranging from death to good recovery.

The advantages of global scales are that they are simple to use, reliable, and allow patients to be compared in a "worse than/better than" fashion [9]. Because the categories are few and easy to score, retrospective scoring is readily performed. The major disadvantage is that global scales paint disability only in broad brush strokes. Thus, they lack the sensitivity to detect small but very important changes in function.

Quality of Life

The ultimate outcome for all patients with chronic neurological disease is a good quality of life. Quality of life can be broadly defined as an individual's overall satisfaction with life, and one's general sense of well-being. A more precise definition of quality of life is difficult because of the highly personal judgments inherent in the term. Thus, although it is probably the most important outcome measure from the perspective of the patient, it is certainly the most difficult to measure. It is also furthest conceptually from traditional medicine, since physical status and functional abilities, although important, are only two contributors to overall quality of life.

Scales attempting to measure quality of life generally assess each of the following categories (domains) of quality of life: physical status and functional abilities, psychological well-being, economic status, and social integration [61]. Since these categories are interdependent, this makes measurement difficult. Despite methodological problems in scale design, and no uniform consensus on what quality of life is, a number of scales have been devised. Some apply to specific illnesses [10], but others have been used for diverse conditions, including total hip arthroplasty, low back pain, and cardiac rehabilitation. An example of a scale that has found applicability to a variety of conditions is the Sickness Impact Profile [22]. This is a psychometrically sound, comprehensive, 130 item questionnaire that contains 12 subscales. Quality of life scales are usually cumbersome and time-consuming to administer, but may show important changes in psychological function and social integration that are missed by medically or functionally oriented outcome measures. Some quality of life scales are more limited in scope. For example, the Rand Social Health Battery [62] primarily assesses social interaction. The general trend to include measures of quality of life in clinical research trials indicates the growing awareness of the importance of this type of outcome measure.

APPLICATION TO SPECIFIC NEUROLOGICAL CONDITIONS

Although a comprehensive discussion of all measures of outcome assessment that may be applicable for all chronic neurological conditions is beyond the scope of this chapter, some concrete examples of outcome measures used in common conditions are instructive. The reader is also referred to other chapters in this book, which discuss specific neurological illnesses, and to the text by Wade [1].

For each of the conditions discussed below, one may choose from a "menu" of assessment tools to measure outcome. The tool chosen depends on the specific purpose of the clinician or investigator.

Stroke

Stroke is certainly the most common neurological condition requiring rehabilitation. Many types of outcomes are of clinical and research interest, and a large repertoire of assessment tools is available. Simple outcomes such as return home or return to work are easy to measure and important. Other outcomes of great importance to the patient and society include independence in activities of daily living, and instrumental living skills. The patient with stroke is ultimately interested in maintaining a satisfactory quality of life.

Regardless of which outcome measure is of interest, much has been written about the prediction of outcome. For any outcome measure chosen, many independent variables may interact to influence the final outcome. The most important of these is the severity of the neurological deficit [38,42]. However, this is insufficient, since many other variables have been correlated with outcome, including age, history of prior stroke, concurrent medical illness, and social support systems [36,63–66]. Dementia and poststroke depression also correlate with the degree of independence and social integration attained [36,39,67]. Although these variables correlate individually with stroke outcome, none has shown a correlation strong enough to predict outcome precisely for an individual patient. Attempts to identify a group of variables that could collectively predict outcome using multivariate analysis have had only limited success [63,66,68–72]. Variables identified differ from study to study. The problems in predicting stroke outcome have been summarized elsewhere [72,73]. Simple clinical variables such as level of consciousness early after stroke and state of urinary continence have been shown to have as much predictive value for outcome as complex models based on a discriminant function of multiple regression formula [74].

The heavy emphasis on independence in ADLs as a major goal of rehabilitation has resulted the widespread use of ADL scales. The Barthel Index has certainly been the most intensively studied. The BI score at discharge from the hospital correlates strongly with ability to function independently and return home [75]. A score over 90 generally ensures that a person with stroke can function at home independently without major assistance [42]. A score over 60 correlates with ambulation and care with assistance, and is generally the cut off point at which a person with stroke can function at home with the reasonable assistance of a spouse or caregiver

[42,49]. A BI score of less than 20 correlates with total dependence. In addition, low BI hospital admission scores following stroke correlate with low BI discharge scores [49], and patients with low BI scores recover more slowly than those with higher scores [42,76]. Low BI discharge scores are correlated with lower satisfaction with life on long-term follow up [77]. Despite the value of functional assessment scales in the rehabilitation of stroke, it is important to remember that ability to perform ADLs is not the only measure of outcome. A high BI score is not specific enough to be the sole selection criterion to identify which patients will benefit from rehabilitation services, return home, or experience a satisfactory lifestyle [77].

In addition to their value for outcome prediction, functional scales have found widespread acceptance in stroke rehabilitation settings to track patient progress, and to assist therapists in setting goals. Scales with more scoring possibilities for each scale subcategory are generally used, especially the FIM.

Scales based on overall neurological function have not found widespread clinical use in stroke rehabilitation, but have been used in clinical research trials. On the other hand, measures of specific functional systems have been widely used for stroke rehabilitation, both to track clinical progress and for research purposes [30]. The applicability of depression rating scales to the geriatric stroke patient has been recently reviewed [78]. Other examples of functional systems measures include the many available aphasia batteries, neuropsychological scales, and the Fugl-Meyer and Motor Assessment Scales for motor function.

Relatively few studies have evaluated quality of life following stroke [79]. Those that have suggested a high degree of dissatisfaction and sense of deterioration in quality of life domains [43,45,80,81]. High scores on neurological scales and functional scales are correlated with greater satisfaction with life. However, even those who regain independence frequently do not return to their previous level of well-being and social integration [80,81]. The implication for those involved in the rehabilitation of stroke patients is that improvement in neurological status and functional abilities is not enough. Emphasis must also be placed on the postdischarge environment, community reintegration, and psychological support.

Traumatic Brain Injury

Outcome assessment in traumatic brain injury (TBI) may use any of a wide variety of assessment tools, depending on the purpose of the user. Acute assessment traditionally has used the Glasgow Coma Scale (GCS) [82], a multifaceted scale based on several key features of the neurological examination including level of consciousness, best motor response, and eye signs. The GCS is often used to assess acute intervention soon after head injury. The initial score on the GCS correlates with survival, but not with outcome in survivors [83]. However, the GCS becomes a predictor of permanent disability with time [83–85]. Another commonly used scale is the Glasgow Outcome Scale [60], a simple global outcome measure similar to the Rankin Scale.

Many studies of head-injured patients have focused on their special chronic problems, especially disorders of cognition, memory, and behavior. Multiple scales related to these functional systems are available, and are largely used to document patients' progress or to assist in directing interventions for specific deficits. Changes in personality and behavior are frequently seen in persons with head injury, and a variety of global rating scales have been developed. Examples include the commonly used Rancho Los Amigos Scale [86,87] and the Neurobehavioral Rating Scale [88]. More comprehensive scales, comprised of multiple behavorial indicators, are also available, an example being the Coma Recovery Scale [83].

Measures of activity of daily living and instrumental living skills discussed earlier are certainly applicable to persons with TBI. Quality of life indicators and other measures of handicap including social integration and family functioning have been extensively used in studies of TBI. For example, the Katz Adjustment Scale is a 127 item scale for relatives that assesses behavior and life situation adjustments [89]. For additional information regarding outcome assessment and measurement in persons with head injury, refer to Chapter 22.

Multiple Sclerosis

Compared to stroke and head injury, in which there is an acute onset followed by a slow, gradual recovery, multiple sclerosis (MS) has a highly variable clinical course. Outcome prediction is therefore difficult, although predictive models of outcome have been proposed [90]. The major use for clinical outcome measures has been to assess the efficacy of treatment trials. The most commonly used tool is a disease-specific scale, the Kurtzke Expanded Disability Status Score (EDSS) [15]. Possible scores range from 0 to 10, with higher scores reflecting more severe disease. The score for each individual is obtained by considering scores derived from "functional systems" subscales, which are based on areas of neurological function commonly affected by MS (pyramidal functions, cerebellar functions, brainstem functions, etc.). As with all assessment instruments, it has advantages and disadvantages. It tends to measure impairment, and is based primarily on the neurological exam, but heavily emphasizes ambulation at the upper level of the scale. However, ambulation is often considered a disability rather than an impairment, so the scale tends to assess disability in persons with more advanced disease [91].

Theoretical design problems of the EDSS have been outlined by Willoughby and Paty [91]. These include difficulty with interobserver reliability [92,93], especially for lower scores, and a bimodal frequency distribution in unselected patients with MS, with a relative lack of patients at intermediate scale levels, especially at grade 5 [91].

Many non-disease-specific scales are also applicable for use in multiple sclerosis, including those already discussed that assess ADLs, community living skills, functional systems (e.g., depression), and quality of life.

Other Neurologic Conditions

Although these diseases will not be discussed in detail here, the assessment and outcome tools discussed earlier can be applied to many other neurological diseases. For some conditions, for example, Parkinson's disease [94], disease-specific scales are widely used, but more general scales have also been used successfully [40]. The frequent variations in symptoms make quantification of Parkinson's disease difficult [95]. Applicability of scales to conditions such as spinal cord injury are discussed elsewhere [1,96]. Finally, most of the functionally based or quality of life measures previously mentioned are also applicable.

SUMMARY

A wide variety of outcome measures are applicable for the rehabilitation of neurological conditions. The most important caveat in choosing a specific measure is to be sure that the instrument is valid and reliable for the purpose for which it is chosen.

Although simple outcomes such as survival and return home are important, multifaceted assessment scales are available for measuring a wide variety of outcomes, and are useful for synthesizing diverse information into a meaningful overview. These scales have found wide acceptance as outcome measures in neurological rehabilitation.

The importance of using appropriate assessment instruments in clinical research, patient care, and clinical program evaluation has been stressed. In the future, it is likely that assessment instruments will also be used to guide reimbursement. For the physician interested in the rehabilitation of neurological diseases, a basic understanding of outcome assessment and its measurement is crucial.

REFERENCES

1. D.T. Wade, *Measurement in Neurological Rehabilitation*. Oxford University Press, Oxford (1992).

2. World Heath Organization, *The International Classification of Impairments, Disabilities, and Handicaps*. World Health Organization, Geneva (1980).

3. V. Apgar, *Anesth. Analg.*, 32:260–267 (1953).

4. M. H. Harmer (ed.), *Classification of Malignant Tumours*, 3rd ed. International Union Against Cancer, Geneva (1978).

5. W. B. Applegate, J. P. Blass, and J. F. Williams, *N. Engl. J. Med.*, 322:1207–1214 (1990).

6. E. M. Pinholt, K. Kroenke, J. F. Hanley, M. J. Kussman, P. L. Twyman, and J. L. Carpenter, *Arch. Intern. Med*, 147:484–488 (1987).

7. R. R. Turner, *Quality of Life Assessments in Clinical Trials* (B. Spilker, ed.), Raven Press, New York, pp. 247–267 (1990).

8. C. Merbitz, J. Morris, and J. C. Grip, *Arch. Phys. Med. Rehab.*, 70:308–312 (1989).

9. P. D. Lyden and G. T. Lau, *Stroke*, 22:1345–1352 (1991).

10. G. H. Guyatt and R. Jaeschke, *Quality of Life Assessments in Clinical Trials* (B. Spilker, ed.), Raven Press, New York, pp. 37–46 (1990).

11. K. M. Jette, *Functional Assessment in Rehabilitation Medicine* (C. V. Granger and G. E. Gresham, eds.), Williams & Wilkins, Baltimore, pp. 46–64 (1984).

12. M. V. Johnston, R. A. Keith, and S. R. Hinderer, *Arch. Phys. Med. Rehab.*, 73: S-3–S-12 (1992).

13. B. Kirshner and G. Guyatt, *J. Chron. Dis.*, 38:27–36 (1985).

14. C. R. MacKenzie and M. E. Charlson, *Br. Med. J.*, 292:40–43 (1986).

15. J. F. Kurtzke, *Neurology*, 33:1444–1452 (1983).

16. A. E. T. Lang and S. Fahn, *Quantification of Neurologic Deficit* (T. L. Munsat, ed.), Butterworth, Stoneham, MA, pp. 285–309 (1989).

17. M. M. Hoehn and M. D. Yahr, *Neurology*, 17:427–42 (1967).

18. N. T. Mathew, V. M. Rivera, J. S. Meyer, J. Z. Charney, and A. Hartmann, *Lancet*, 2:1327–1329 (1972).

19. T. Brott, H. P. Adams, C. P. Olinger, et al., *Stroke*, 20:864–870 (1989).

20. J. S. Norris, *Arch. Neurol.*, 33:69–71 (1976).

21. F. I. Mahoney and D. W. Barthel, *MD Med. J.*, 14:61–65 (1965).

22. M. Bergner, R. A. Bobbitt, W. B. Carter, and B. S. Gilson, *Med. Care*, 19:787–805 (1981).

23. W. D. Spector, *Quality of Life Assessments in Clinical Trials* (B. Spilker, ed.), Raven Press, New York, pp. 115–129 (1990).

24. R. A. Keith, *Arch. Phys. Med. Rehab.*, 65:74–78 (1984).

25. Medical Research Council, *Aids to the Examination of the Peripheral Nervous System*. Her Majesty's Stationery Office, London (1976).

26. B. Ashworth, *Practitioner*, 192:540–542 (1964).

27. A. R. Fugl-Meyer, L. Jaasko, L. Leyman, S. Olsson, and S. Steglind, *Scand. J. Rehab. Med.*, 7:13 (1975).

28. J. H. Carr, R. B. Shepherd, L. Nordholm, and D. Lynne, *Phys. Ther.*, 65:175–180 (1985).

29. P. W. Duncan, M. Propst, and S. G. Nelson, *Phys. Ther.*, 63:1606–1610 (1983).

30. S. L. Wood-Dauphinee, J. I. Williams, and S. H. Shapiro, *Stroke*, 21:731–739 (1990).

31. A.T. Beck, C.H. Ward, M. Mendelson, J.E. Mock, and J.K. Erbaugh, *Arch. Gen. Psychiatry*, 4:561–571 (1961).

32. M. Hamilton, *Br. J. Soc. Psychol.*, 6:278–296 (1967).

33. W.W.K. Zung, *Arch. Gen. Psychiatry*, 12:63–70 (1965).

34. P.W. Duncan, L.B. Goldstein, D. Matchar, G.W. Divine, and J. Feussner, *Stroke*, 23:1084–1089 (1992).

35. M. Newman, *Stroke*, 3:702–710 (1972).

36. M. Kotila, O. Waltimo, M. Niemi, M.A. Laaksonen, and M. Lempinen, *Stroke*, 15:1039–1044 (1984).

37. T.S. Olsen, *Stroke*, 21:247–251 (1990).

38. B. Bernspang, K. Asplund, S. Eriksson, and A.R. Fugl-Meyer, *Stroke*, 18:1081–1086 (1987).

39. Y. Bacher, N. Korner-Bitensky, M. Mayo, R. Becker, and H. Coopersmith, *Can. J. Rehab.*, 4:27–37 (1990).

40. L. Henderson, C. Kennard, T.J. Crawford, S. Day, B.S. Everitt, S. Goodrich, F. Jones, and D.M. Park, *J. Neurol. Neurosurg. Psychiatry*, 54:18–24 (1991).

41. A.R. Feinstein, B.R. Josephy, and C.K. Wells, *Ann. Intern. Med.*, 105:413–420 (1986).

42. M.J. Reding and E. Potes, *Stroke*, 19:1354–1358 (1988).

43. M. Viitanen, K.S. Fugl-Meyer, B. Bernspang, and A.R. Fugl-Meyer, *Scand. J. Rehab. Med.*, 20:17–24 (1988).

44. C.V. Granger, B.B. Hamilton, and G.E. Gresham, *Arch. Phys. Med. Rehab.*, 69:506–509 (1988).

45. M. Astrom, K. Asplund, and T. Astrom, *Stroke*, 23:527–531 (1992).

46. H.A. Schoening, L. Anderegg, D. Bergstrom, M. Fonda, N. Steinke, and P. Ulrich, *Arch. Phys. Med. Rehab.*, 46:689–697 (1965).

47. S. Katz, A.B. Ford, R.W. Moskowitz, B.A. Jackson, and M.W. Jaffe, *JAMA*, 185:914–919 (1963).

48. G.E. Gresham, T.F. Phillips, and M.L.C. Labi, *Arch. Phys. Med. Rehab.*, 61:355–358 (1980).

49. C.V. Granger, L.S. Dewis, N.C. Peters, C.C. Sherwood, and B.A. Barrett, *Arch. Phys. Med. Rehab.*, 60:14–17 (1979).

50. G.E. Gresham, T.E. Phillips, and M.L.C. Labi, *Arch. Phys. Med. Rehab.*, 61:355–358 (1980).

51. C.V. Granger, B.B. Hamilton, and F.S. Sherwin, *Guide for the Use of the Uniform Data Set for Medical Rehabilitation.* Uniform Data System for Medical Rehabilitation Project Office, Buffalo General Hospital, Buffalo, New York (1986).

52. R.G. Carey and E.J. Posevac, *Arch. Phys. Med. Rehab.*, 59:330–337 (1978).

53. R.F. Harvey and H.M. Jellinek, *Arch. Phys. Med. Rehab.*, 62:456–461 (1981).

54. N. Silverstein, K.M. Kilgore, W.P. Fischer, J.P. Harley, and R.F. Harvey, *Arch. Phys. Med. Rehab.*, 72:631–637 (1991).

55. M.V. Johnston, R.A. Keith, and S.R. Hinderer, *Arch. Phys. Med. Rehab.*, 73:S-12–S-23 (1992).

56. D.L. Wilkerson, A.I. Batavia, and G. DeJong, *Arch. Phys. Med. Rehab.*, 73:111–120 (1992).

57. M.P. Lawton and E.M. Brody, *Gerontologist*, 9:179–186 (1969).
58. R.I. Pfeffer, M.S. Kurosaki, C.H. Harrah, J.M. Chance, and S. Filos, *J. Gerontol.*, 37:323–329 (1982).
59. J. Rankin, *Scott. Med. J.*, 2:200–215 (1957).
60. B. Jennett and M. Bond, *Lancet*, 1:480–484 (1975).
61. H. Schipper, J. Clinch, and V. Powell, *Quality of Life Assessments in Clinical Trials* (B. Spilker, ed.), Raven Press, New York, pp. 11–24 (1990).
62. C.A. Donald, J.E. Ware, R.H. Brook, and A. Davies-Avery, *Conceptualization and Measurement of Health for Adults in the Health Insurance Study: Vol. IV. Social Health*. Rand Pub No. R-1987/4-HEW, Santa Monica, CA (1978).
63. S. Shah, F. Vanclay, and B. Cooper, *Stroke*, 20:766–769 (1989).
64. M. Kelly-Hayes, P.A. Wolf, W.B. Kannel, P. Sytkowski, R.B. D'Agostino, and G.E. Gresham, *Arch. Phys. Med. Rehab.*, 69:415–418 (1988).
65. N.B. Lincoln, M. Blackburn, S. Ellis, J. Jackson, J.A. Edmans, E.M. Nouri, M.F. Walrer, and H. Haworth, *J. Neurol. Neurosurg. Psychiatry*, 52:493–496 (1989).
66. C.M.C. Allen, *J. Neurol. Neurosurg. Psychiatry*, 47:475–480 (1984).
67. R.M. Parikh, R.G. Robinson, J.R. Lipsey, S.E. Starkstein, J.P. Fedoroff, and T.R. Price, *Arch. Neurol.*, 47:785–789 (1990).
68. G. Howard, J.S. Till, J.F. Toole, C. Matthews, and B.L. Truscott, *JAMA*, 253:226–232 (1985).
69. S. Shah, F. Vanclay, and B. Cooper, *Stroke*, 21:241–246 (1990).
70. D.H. Barer and J.R.H. Mitchell, *Q. J. Med.*, 261:27–39 (1989).
71. M. Kelly-Hayes, P.A. Wolf, C.S. Kase, G.E. Gresham, W.B. Kannel, and R.B. D'Agostino, *J. Neuro. Rehab.*, 3:65–70 (1989).
72. D.B. Hier and G. Edelstein, *Stroke*, 22:1431–1436 (1991).
73. L. Jongbloed and W. Jones, *Can. J. Rehab.*, 2:87–92 (1988).
74. J.R.F. Gladman, D.M.J. Harwood, and D.H. Barer, *J. Neurol. Neurosurg. Psychiatry*, 55:347–351 (1992).
75. C.V. Granger, C.C. Sherwood, and D.S. Greer, *Arch. Phys. Med. Rehab.*, 58:555–561 (1977).
76. C.E. Skillbeck, D.T. Wade, R. Langton Hewer, and V.A. Wood, *J. Neurol. Neurosurg. Psychiatry*, 46:5–8 (1983).
77. C.V. Granger, B.B. Hamilton, G.E. Gresham, and A.A. Kramer, *Arch. Phys. Med. Rehab.*, 70:100–103 (1989).
78. B. Agrell and O. Dehlin, *Stroke*, 20:1190–1194 (1989).
79. R. de Haan, N. Aaronson, M. Limburg, R. Langton Hewer, and H. van Cregvel, *Stroke*, 24:320–327 (1993).
80. G. Santus, A. Razenigo, R. Caregnato, and M.R. Inzoli, *Stroke*, 21:1019–1022 (1990).
81. M. Niemi, M.A. Laaksonen, M. Kotila, and O. Waltimo, *Stroke*, 19:1101–1107 (1988).
82. G. Teasdale and B. Jennett, *Lancet*, 2:81–84 (1974).
83. J.T. Giacino, M.A. Kezmarsky, J. DeLuca, and K.D. Cicerone, *Arch. Phys. Med. Rehab.*, 72:897–901 (1991).

84. H.S. Levin, A.L. Benton, and R.G. Grossman, *Neurobehavioral Consequences of Closed Head Injury*. Oxford University Press, New York (1982).

85. S. Dikmen, J. Machamer, N. Temkin, and A. McLean, *J. Clin. Exp. Neuropsychol.*, *12*:507–517 (1990).

86. Professional Staff Association, Rancho Los Amigos Cognitive Scale, Rancho Los Amigos Hospital, Downey, CA.

87. P.W. Duncan, *Rehabilitation of the Adult and Child with Traumatic Brain Injury*, 2nd ed (M. Rosenthal, E.R. Griffith, M.R. Bond, and J.D. Miller, eds.), F.A. Davis, Philadelphia, pp. 264–283 (1990).

88. H.S. Levin, W.M. High, K.E. Goethe, R.A. Sisson, J.E. Overall, H.M. Rhoades, H.M. Eisenberg, Z. Kalisky, and H.E. Gary, *J. Neurol. Neurosurg. Psychiatry*, *50*:183–193 (1987).

89. M.M. Katz and S.B. Lyerly, *Psychol. Rep.*, *13*:503–535 (1963).

90. B.G. Weinshenker, G.P.A. Rice, J.H. Noseworthy, W. Carriere, J. Baskerville, and G.C. Ebers, *Brain*, *114*:1045–1056 (1991).

91. E.W. Willoughby and D.W. Paty, *Neurology*, *38*:1793–1798 (1988).

92. D.A. Francis, P. Bain, A.V. Swan, and R.A.C. Hughes, *Arch. Neurol.*, *48*:299–301 (1991).

93. M.P. Amato, L. Fratiglioni, C. Groppi, G. Siracusa, and L. Amaducci, *Arch. Neurol.*, *45*:746–748 (1988).

94. R.S. Wilson and C.G. Goetz, *Quality of Life Assessments in Clinical Trials* (B. Spilker, ed.), Raven Press, New York, pp. 347–356 (1990).

95. A.E.T. Lang and S. Fahn, *Quantification of Neurologic Deficit* (T.L. Munsat, ed.), Butterworths, Boston, pp. 285–309 (1989).

96. M. Stambrook, C. Psych, S. MacBeath, A.D. Moore, L.C. Peters, E. Zubek, and I.C. Friesen, *Paraplegia*, *29*:318–323 (1991).

6

Depression and Cognition as Factors in Recovery

David N. Alexander

Daniel Freeman Hospital
Inglewood, and
UCLA School of Medicine
Los Angeles, California

INTRODUCTION

Depression and disorders of higher cortical function are frequent accompaniments of stroke, traumatic brain injury, and other chronic neurological illness. They achieve particular importance during the rehabilitation phase because of the limitations they create in a patient's functional abilities. This chapter will explore the frequency, assessment, prognosis, and treatment of patients with depression and cognitive disorders. It is not a primer on neurobehavior, but explores the impact of depression and disorders of cognition on rehabilitation. Because of the frequent occurrence of depression and disorders of cognition in patients who have sustained stroke and traumatic brain injury, the chapter will focus on these conditions.

DEPRESSION

Reactive depression is frequent in all patients undergoing rehabilitation, and was the most common diagnosis in a review of psychiatric consultations in a rehabilitation hospital [1]. Patients with spinal cord injury (SCI) are frequently depressed [2], primarily because of the loss of function, with its far-reaching implications of chronic disability in multiple spheres. Poststroke depression (PSD) has been studied extensively in the past 10 years and is the subject of numerous reviews [3–10]. PSD is common, has a deleterious effect on recovery, and effective treatment is available. It can cause cognitive impairment ("pseudodementia"), and is a major factor in quality of life after stroke [11–13] (see Figure 1). PSD is different from that seen after SCI in that it is more likely to be associated with anxiety, and probably has a significant organic cause [14]. Depression after closed head injury (CHI) may have both an organic and a reactive component, but has been less extensively studied than PSD.

Depression following stroke historically was regarded as a regrettable but understandable grief reaction to the loss of health [15,16]. It was thought to resolve spontaneously as the patient improved and required minimal intervention. Pharmacological medication was not considered useful, and was possibly deleterious [17]. Less than 5% of more than 1800 patients (1983–1986) enrolled in the stroke data bank received antidepressants during their hospitalization or at discharge [18]. Clinical depression was considered by some to be overdiagnosed.

Recognition that PSD may have an organic, neuroanatomical, and neurophysiological basis (a neurobiological depression or organic depression), rather than "simply" being a reactive depression (grief reaction, psychological depression) has led to more study. Depressive symptoms do occur as a grief reaction following stroke and are not unimportant, but minor or major depression (by *Diagnostic and Statistical Manual, 3rd ed.*, [DSM III] criteria) are common and benefit from more aggressive treatment.

Problems in Clinical Assessment

Depression in patients with stroke or head injury is difficult to assess, and is part of the reason for earlier underestimates of its frequency. The most

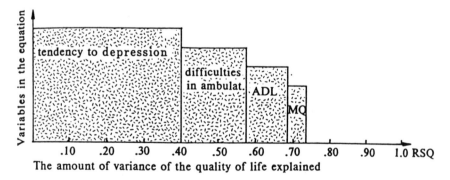

Figure 1   The subjective tendency to depression is the most important variable predicting quality of life after stroke, when compared with difficulties with ambulation, difficulties with ADLs, and memory quotient (MQ) [12].

obvious example is that of aphasia. Patients unable to communicate effectively may not be able to communicate complex internal mood states. As a consequence, patients with right hemispheric lesions have been treated more often for depression than patients with left hemispheric lesions, despite evidence linking the degree and severity of depression to left anterior hemispheric lesions [19]. Patients with right hemispheric lesions can complain verbally about depression whereas aphasic patients may not be able to.

Assessment of a patient's mood (internal subjective feeling state) is partly accomplished by an examination of affect. Yet a depressed affect may not necessarily reflect a depressed mood. Pseudobulbar palsy is associated with emotional incontinence. Poorly controlled crying or laughing induced by minor stimuli occurs but is not necessarily associated with a corresponding emotional feeling of sadness or happiness. "Pathologic emotionalism" occurs in 21% of patients in some reports, but there is only a slight association with depression [20]. Antidepressants are frequently used to treat emotional lability [21]. Amitriptyline and fluoexitine may be effective, but other medications are also available, such as the dopamine agonists [22,23].

Changes in the affective component of behavior and verbal communication can be seen with structural central nervous system (CNS) damage, particularly to the right parietal region. Patients with aprosodia may have such modulation in their voice that their reports of dysphoria are not convincing. Careful attention to the presence of vegetative signs of depression such as anorexia and insomnia is important in diagnosing depression in such patients. Conversely, an aprosodic voice pattern may mimic a flattened affect of depression when, in fact, the patient is not depressed [24].

Depression is difficult to diagnose in patients who are hospitalized, ill, or elderly [25,26]. Patients with CHI or stroke may have deficits in attention, arousal, or concentration, and are difficult to test for depression. Many somatic symptoms of depression such as weight loss, change in appetite, constipation, difficulty sleeping, and fatigue can be seen in patients due to physical and environmental reasons and may complicate an analysis of somatic signs of depression. Most depression scales cannot differentiate depression from the effects of physical illness [27]. Because noisy, unfamiliar rooms make sleeping difficult in the hospital, it may be difficult to determine if complaints of insomnia are truly due to depression. Motor impairments impose restriction of activities that automatically narrow the scope of a patient's interests. Patients may be psychologically inhibited in complaining about depression. Even healthy elderly patients in primary care settings tend not to report emotional distress to their physicians, and physicians may unconsciously collude with this by being unwilling to face the issue [28].

Assessment of depression in patients with neurological injury must also take into account the patient's premorbid personality, tendency to depression, coping styles, history of psychiatric illness, and history of alcohol or drug abuse (both of which are more frequent in head and spinal cord injured patients). In summary, assessment of depression in patients with stroke and head injury is complicated by multiple neurological, medical, and environmental factors.

Incidence

Despite these difficulties with the assessment of depression, a number of studies have indicated a substantial frequency of depression in patients who have had a stroke, generally 30–50%, using a variety of clinical methods of diagnosis (see Table 1). In an assessment of mood and vegetative disturbance in 25 randomly selected patients who sustained stroke, using a modification of the Hamilton depression rating scale, Finklestein et al. found moderate to severe depression in 48% [29]. When comparison was made to a similar group with physical impairment but without stroke, the prevalence of depression was far greater in the stroke patients. In addition, patients with depressed mood tended to be those with involvement of the left (69%) rather than the right (25%) hemisphere. Reding found a 49% incidence of depression using a combination of the Zung self-rated depression score, a modified Hamilton Depression Scale, and the dexamethasone suppression test [30]. Robinson found a 50% incidence of PSD, with 25% having a major depression by the DSM III criteria and 25% having a minor depression [31]. Retrospective studies report a lower incidence, closer to 30% [21].

Table 1 Incidence of Poststroke Depression

Author and Reference	Assessment Tool	Severity	Incidence (%)
Finklestein [29]	Hamilton, modified	Moderate to severe	48
Reding [82]	DSM III, DST, Zung, Ham-D modified	Major	39
Malec [32]	RDC	Major depression	30
Robinson [46]	DSM III, PSE, Hamilton, Zung	Moderate to severe	47
Lim [21]	Required treatment with antidepressants (retrospective)	Not assessed	30
Robinson [19]	Visual analog mood scale, Hamilton, Zung, nurses' rating scale	Moderate to severe	60
Feibel [119]	Nurses' observation	Not assessed	26

Because of the heterogeneous nature of some initial reports on the frequency of PSD, a prospective study of patients admitted to a stroke rehabilitation unit at the Mayo Clinic was undertaken. The study included patients over 55 years who had sustained unilateral stroke within 6 weeks of inclusion in the study, and excluded patients with any history of brain injury, substance abuse, prior stroke, or major affective or thought disorder. Despite these strict criteria and a patient population from a different socioeconomic stratum than Robinson's, the study demonstrated a 30% incidence of major depression by research diagnostic criteria (RDC) [32].

Major depression after stroke tends to last 6–12 months (see Figure 2) [33,34], with minor depressions lasting longer [35]. Suicide is rare [36]. To appreciate fully these high rates of depression in patients with stroke, a comparison with the rate of depression in medically ill geriatric patients is

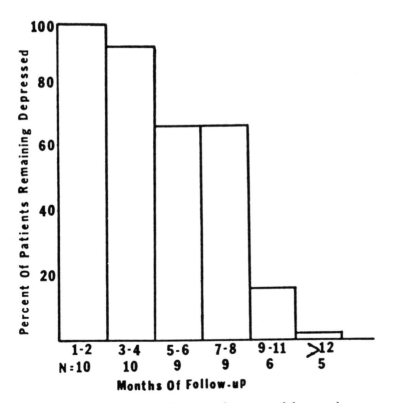

Figure 2 The percentage of patients who remained depressed at various intervals following the initial interview: poststroke depression tends to last less than a year [45].

necessary. Koening found an incidence of major depression in medically ill geriatric patients over the age of 70 of 11.5% [4]. The incidence of major depression in the community of elderly patients is 1–2%, with an additional 2% experiencing a dysthymic disorder or minor depression [37].

Major depression, as measured by the Hamilton Rating Scale for depression, was found in one-quarter of patients with CHI [38]. Those with major depression had a higher frequency of premorbid psychiatric illness and poorer social functioning. Depression is one of constellation of neuropsychiatric changes seen after CHI. Patients with CHI tend to be depressed, angry, and confused [39,40]. A prospective study of 71 patients with SCI found an incidence of major depression (DSM III) of 20%, although the majority of patients with SCI had no clear evidence of depression [41].

Biological Role

Depression, in the absence of CNS injury, is related to altered catecholamine or serotonergic function. This is supported by the pharmacological effects of drugs that cause or alleviate depression. Reserpine depletes presynaptic terminals of serotonin and norepinephrine by inhibiting storage, resulting in depression. Many tricyclic antidepressants (TCAs) block amine reuptake (particularly serotonin) from the synaptic cleft, which may relieve a relative serotonin deficiency causing depression [42]. In addition, TCAs work by downregulating central beta-adrenoreceptors.

Initial evidence for a biological role in the production of PSD came from a study of hospitalized patients with stroke. It demonstrated that 45% of patients with stroke were depressed compared with only 10% of hospitalized orthopedic patients with comparable disability [43]. Later work consistently failed to show any direct relationship between the degree of impairment and frequency or severity of depression (a "dose–response curve"), which would be expected if depression was directly related to impairment [34]. Depression did not correlate with motor strength, aphasia, or disability as measured by the Barthel index [6,31,34,44]. This implies the existence of an organic or biological cause of depression, related to direct injury to the brain.

A relationship between lesion location and the severity of depression has been identified by Robinson et al. [19]. In right-handed patients with no previous psychiatric history, they found that the severity of depression was related to the proximity of lesions to the left frontal pole. First reported in 1981, this has been confirmed by subsequent work [31,35,45–49] but disputed by others [6,21,32,50]. Some have hypothesized that patients with right hemispheric lesions plus anosognosia and neglect would not become depressed, but this finding has been reported [51,52].

Biological Tests

No satisfactory biological tests exist for the diagnosis of depression in neurologically injured patients. The desirability of a biochemical marker or biological test for depression is clear; depression is difficult to diagnose in the rehabilitation population and hard to quantitate. Until recently the most frequently used test has been the dexamethasone suppression test (DST). This is performed by giving an oral dose of 1 mg dexamethasone at 11:00 p.m. and then measuring serum cortisol levels at 8:00 a.m. and 4:00 p.m. on the following day. Levels greater than 5 μg/dl are considered to be nonsuppressed or positive, indicative of depression. Interference with the results can occur due to concurrent use of sedative medications, steroids, anticonvulsant drugs, as well as acute intercurrent medical illnesses. These factors alone limit the use of the test. Early reports indicated that the DST was an adjunct to the diagnosis of depression in patients who had sustained stroke [29]. It was found to be a marker for depression although it did not predict rehabilitation outcome [30]. The limitations of this test restrict its use in making clinical decisions regarding treatment of depression [53]. It has also been reported to lack specificity [32]. For example, in one study a positive DST was associated with disorientation and lesion proximity to the frontal pole, but not to depression [54].

Other biological tests for depression have included the thyrotropin-releasing hormone (TRH) stimulation test, measurement of plasma and urinary MHPG, cerebrospinal fluid (CSF) 5-HIAA, and other measurements of amine degradation products. These have not been found to be useful in depression in general and have not been studied in the rehabilitation setting [55]. Accurate prediction of a positive therapeutic response to tricyclic antidepressants would be particularly useful, because it takes several weeks to ascertain the response to TCAs. A trial of methylphenidate has been used to predict response to imipramine or desipramine [56], and was found to be safe and effective in the treatment of poststroke depression in one small uncontrolled trial [57].

Assessment Scales

Given the lack of a specific and reliable biochemical marker of depression, clinical evaluation is essential. A number of screening devices and rating scales used for endogenous depression have been employed in the evaluation of depression in the rehabilitation setting. These provide quantitative data for use in research and are used as assistive devices in clinical decision-making regarding depression.

The Zung Self-Rating Depression Scale (SDS) is a short, simple, quantitative test for the symptoms of depression [58]. It requires a response to 20 statements, such as "I feel downhearted and blue" (see Table 2). The patient must state whether he or she feels this a little of the time, some of the time, a good part of the time, or most of the time. The Beck Depression Inventory (BDI) assesses the behavioral manifestations of depression [59]. It has a 63 point scoring system for 21 questions, and a score of 21 or more is considered a sensitive screen for moderately severe depression in hospitalized patients [60]. Limitations of the BDI are that it emphasizes the somatic and vegetative signs of depression. Both the Zung and Beck scales are self-administered, which is a limitation for patients who are aphasic or compromised in their writing abilities. The Hamilton Depression Scale (Ham-D) was developed for patients already diagnosed with depression and is the most commonly used research-oriented tool for quantifying depression in psychiatric studies. It is particularly useful for assessing treatment [61]. It consists of 21 questions that require a skilled psychiatric examiner and is partially dependent on the skill of the examiner.

The DSM III-R lists nine symptoms associated with major depression [62] (see Figure 3). These include depressed mood most of nearly every day, a loss of interest or pleasure in all activities (also characterized as apathy or lack of joy); a significant appetite or weight change (weight change of 5% in 1 month); sleep disturbance: hypersomnia, insomnia, or early morning awakening; psychomotor slowing often associated with a poverty of speech or a soft monotone voice; fatigue; feelings of guilt or worthlessness; inability to concentrate or think, feeling of being indecisive or distractible; suicidal thoughts or recurrent thoughts of death. For the diagnosis of a major depression by DSM III-R criteria, a patient must have 5 of these 9 criteria for a period of 2 weeks. At least one of the symptoms must be depressed mood or loss of

Table 2 Zung Self-Rating Depression Scale

1. I feel downhearted and blue.	12. I find it easy to do the things I used to.
2. Morning is when I feel the best.	
3. I have crying spells or feel like it.	13. I am restless and can't keep still.
4. I have trouble sleeping at night.	14. I feel hopeful about the future.
5. I eat as much as I used to.	15. I am more irritable than usual.
6. I still enjoy sex.	16. I find it easy to make decisions.
7. I notice that I am losing weight.	17. I feel that I am useful and needed.
8. I have trouble with constipation.	18. My life is pretty full.
9. My heart beats faster than usual.	19. I feel that others would be better off if I were dead.
10. I get tired for no reason.	
11. My mind is as clear as it used to be.	20. I still enjoy the things I used to do.

Note: A "Major Depressive Syndrome" is defined as criterion A below.

A. At least five of the following symptoms have been present during the same two-week period and represent a change from previous functioning; at least one of the symptoms is either (1) depressed mood, or (2) loss of interest or pleasure. (Do not include symptoms that are clearly due to a physical condition, mood-incongruent delusions or hallucinations, incoherence, or marked loosening of associations.)

(1) depressed mood (or can be irritable mood in children and adolescents) most of the day, nearly every day, as indicated either by subjective account or observation by others

(2) markedly diminished interest or pleasure in all, or almost all, activities most of the day, nearly every day (as indicated either by subjective account or observation by others of apathy most of the time)

(3) significant weight loss or weight gain when not dieting (e.g., more than 5% of body weight in a month), or decrease or increase in appetite nearly every day (in children, consider failure to make expected weight gains)

(4) insomnia or hypersomnia nearly every day

(5) psychomotor agitation or retardation nearly every day (observable by others, not merely subjective feelings of restlessness or being slowed down)

(6) fatigue or loss of energy nearly every day

(7) feelings of worthlessness or excessive or inappropriate guilt (which may be delusional) nearly every day (not merely self-reproach or guilt about being sick)

(8) diminished ability to think or concentrate, or indecisiveness, nearly every day (either by subjective account or as observed by others)

(9) recurrent thoughts of death (not just fear of dying), recurrent suicidal ideation without a specific plan, or a suicide attempt or a specific plan for committing suicide

Figure 3 DSM III-R diagnostic criteria for a major depressive episode [62].

interest and pleasure. A minor depression or dysthymic disorder is a slightly less severe form of depression. By DSM III-R requirements, it requires depressed mood for at least 2 years, making it problematic to apply this to patients in the acute phase of their illness. By DSM III-R criteria, all depression associated with stroke or brain injury is included under the heading "organic affective disorder," however, major or minor depression is frequently used to describe this condition if all the other criteria are fulfilled [35].

Treatment

Depression clearly interferes with the patient's functional progress in rehabilitation. It has been associated with longer hospital stays [32], slower recovery of walking [63], impaired cognition [64], and slower gains in performing activities of daily living (ADLs) [65]. An inhospital diagnosis of depression (either major or minor) in a patient with stroke correlates significantly with both impaired physical abilities and language functioning compared with nondepressed patients with stroke [66]. More important is that this disparity between depressed and nondepressed patients persists for 2 years following stroke (see Figure 4). These findings suggest that maximum recovery may not be achievable if depression remains untreated.

Treatment consists of interpersonal psychotherapy in its various forms and pharmacological treatment. Problem-centered psychotherapy has been shown to be effective in alleviating depression [67]. On inpatient rehabilitation services the supportive, therapeutic environment should always be emphasized. It is provided by all who come into contact with the patient including nurses, doctors, and therapists. More direct and specific treatment is provided by the social worker, psychologist, or psychiatrist on a continuing basis.

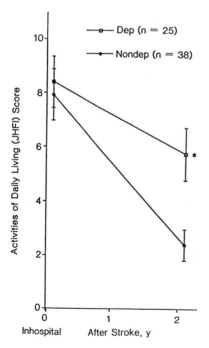

Figure 4   Depressed patients (Dep) had greater impairment in ADLs (measured as a higher score on the Johns Hopkins Functioning Index [JHFI]) than nondepressed patients (Nondep), and this persisted at the 2 year follow-up evaluation [66].

The rehabilitation physician often plays a role in the medical management of depression. This includes a careful analysis of the patient's medical history to ascertain possible pre-existing medical causes of depression, such as hypothyroidism, and a careful review of the patient's medications [68]. Propranolol, methyldopa, clonidine, benzodiazepines, and sedatives have all been identified as potential causes of depression.

Medications for Depression

When antidepressants are prescribed, the patient's general medical condition, cognitive functioning, level of arousal, bladder, bowel, and cardiac function all relate to the specific choice of antidepressants used. The most frequently used and extensively studied medications are the tricyclic antidepressants (TCAs). The TCAs are classified into the tertiary amines, which have three substituents on the terminal nitrogen of the aminopropyl side chain; and the secondary amines, which are derivatives of the parent tertiary amines through demethylation (see Figure 5). The tertiary amines are amitriptyline, imipramine, and doxepin. They have prominent serotonergic and anticholinergic properties. The secondary amines are nortriptyline, desipramine, and protriptyline, and they share primarily noradrenergic properties.

Tertiary and secondary amines have different side effects. The tertiary amines (imipramine, amitriptyline, and doxepin) can cause a sense of tiredness and sleepiness. They often calm the patient, decrease nighttime awakenings, decrease the amount of rapid eye movement (REM) sleep, and increase the amount of stage IV sleep. Sedation is caused by receptor blockade of H1 receptors [69]. Postural hypotension is caused by blockade of alpha-1 adrenergic receptors. Blurred vision, exacerbation of narrow-angle glaucoma,

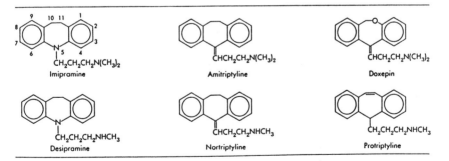

Figure 5 The tricyclic antidepressants are classified into the tertiary amines (imipramine, amitriptyline, and doxepin) and the secondary amines (desipramine, nortriptyline, and protriptyline) [69].

dry mouth, constipation, and urinary retention are attributed to the anti-muscarinic effects [60]. Amitriptyline is most likely to cause tachycardia and is best avoided in the elderly. The secondary amines (nortriptyline, desipramine, and protriptyline) are more activating than the tertiary amines and can be effectively used in patients who show psychomotor slowing.

The therapeutic effectiveness of all antidepressants is relatively similar. Therefore, a frequent strategy is to choose a medication based on its side effect profile. For agitated patients, a more sedating tertiary amine is indicated. For patients who need more activation, typically a secondary amine or other heterocyclic compound (such as trazodone, amoxapine, or buproprion) can be used [70].

Fluoxetine and sertraline are new selective inhibitors of neuronal serotonin (5-hydroxytryptamine [5-HT]) uptake, and are structurally unrelated to the TCAs or other antidepressants. Fluoxetine has minimal affinity for dopaminergic, histaminic, noradrenergic, and muscarinic receptors, giving it a highly specific action, and therefore, fewer side effects [71–73]. Occasional side effects include insomnia, nausea, headache, anxiety, rash (with desquamation), seizures (0.2%), hyponatremia, and syndrome of inappropriate antidiuretic hormone release (SIADH) [71]. Fluoxetine may be useful in patients who want to avoid the weight gain that can be seen with tricyclic antidepressants.

Sertraline, like fluoxetine, tends to have a stimulant effect on the CNS and is not sedating. The most frequent adverse side effects include agitation, nervousness, insomnia, headache, tremor, nausea, and diarrhea. Sertraline may be particularly useful in patients taking medications requiring hepatic metabolism (e.g., warfarin) because it does not significantly inhibit the cytochrome P-450 enzyme system [74]. Both selective serotonin reuptake inhibitors (SSRIs) can be given once a day (20 mg/day for fluoxetine and 50 mg/day for sertraline) which makes it easier to achieve compliance upon discharge. Neither of the SSRIs cause electrocardiographic (ECG) changes, which are sometimes associated with the TCAs.

In addition to the TCAs and the SSRIs, several other medications or treatments may be considered. Trazodone is an effective antidepressant that is moderately sedating and can be used in patients who are anxious or need some sedation. It has little anticholinergic effect or cardiac toxicity. On rare occasions in men, it can cause priapism, which limits its use. Amoxapine may have extrapyramidal side effects. Buproprion has been associated with seizures, and it is best avoided in patients already at risk for seizures. Occasionally other medications, such as the monoamine oxidase (MAO) inhibitors can be used, particularly if the patient has a previous history of a positive response to such medications. Use of MAO inhibitors such as phenelzine should be undertaken with care because of the multiple dietary restrictions required.

Nonpharmacological treatment of depression (electroconvulsive therapy [ECT]) has been used and may be beneficial in selected patients [75,76].

Effectiveness of Treatment

Depression associated with chronic neurological illness can be effectively treated pharmacologically. The first double-blind randomized controlled trial of antidepressant treatment of stroke was reported by Lipsey in 1984 [77]. Patients treated with nortriptyline improved compared to patients receiving placebo (see Figure 6). Depression was assessed with an overall depression score using a combination of the Hamilton Depression Score, the Zung Depression Score, and the Present State examination score. Therapeutic serum levels of nortriptyline were achieved (serum concentration of 50–100 ng/ml) but delirium, confusion, drowsiness, or agitation occurred in 3 of 17 patients. The high dosages used in this study and vigorous initiation of TCA treatment have been criticized. Others have suggested that improvement in outcome with nortriptyline can be achieved by starting at a low dosage and increasing it more slowly [78,79]. A daily dose of 30 mg of nortriptyline may be optimal [70,80].

The measurement of plasma levels of TCAs is problematic. There is a 10–30-fold variation in individual metabolism, which, combined with the

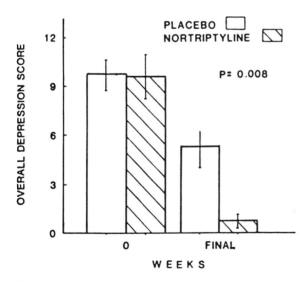

Figure 6 Nortriptyline was compared to placebo in this randomized double-blind trial of the treatment of poststroke depression in 32 patients. Treatment was significantly more effective than placebo in alleviating the symptoms of depression [77].

high lipid solubility and tight protein binding of the TCAs, makes interpretation of levels difficult [42]. The concept of a therapeutic window has been established for nortriptyline [60]. Some relationship exists between blood level and clinical response for imipramine and amitriptyline [81], but no studies relating clinical effect to levels are available in neurologically compromised patients.

Another randomized trial examined the treatment of 27 patients with PSD using trazodone, with a target dosage of 200 mg/day [82]. Treatment with trazodone showed greater improvement in ADLs, as measured by the Barthel Index, in the treated group compared with those given placebo.

Retrospective studies on select stroke populations seen by psychiatrists in a rehabilitation setting have shown that tricyclic antidepressants can be useful in certain subpopulations at relatively low dosages (70 mg/day of imipramine) [44]. Amitriptyline has been shown to be useful in the treatment of pathological laughing and crying (pseudobulbar affect) [23]. Doxepin was shown in a double-blind study to be useful in depressed geriatric rehabilitation patients. These patients had a variety of diagnoses beside stroke, but responded to a low dosage of doxepin (10–20 mg daily) in a double-blind study of 24 patients on an inpatient geriatric rehabilitation unit [83]. Although depression after CHI is common, few studies specifically address the medication choices and outcome of treatment of depression in patients with CHI. The choice of antidepressants should pay close attention to the side effect profile, particularly as it relates to the common occurrence of confusion, agitation, and restlessness [84].

COGNITION

Cognition is defined as "the mental process or faculty by which knowledge is acquired, or that which comes to be known through perception, reasoning, or intuition" [85]. Alterations in cognition involve the basic processes of language, attention, and memory, and may profoundly affect the rehabilitation course. An extraordinary number and variety of subtle and gross cognitive changes can occur in patients with stroke, TBI, multiple sclerosis, or other neurological illnesses seen on the rehabilitation service.

Cognitive changes are often more important to the patient and subsequent functioning in the community than are physical impairments, such as hemiparesis. Cognitive and behavioral changes are generally the primary limitation in patients with TBI [86,87]. Cognitive impairments affect the patient's safety, mobility, communication, and self-care, as well as vocational and avocational pursuits.

Recognition and identification of cognitive changes are important for the rehabilitation process, since this knowledge directs treatment and helps

Table 3 Cognitive and Perceptual Deficits
Frequently Encountered in Patients with Stroke and
Head Injury Undergoing Rehabilitation

Stroke	Head injury
Aphasia	Attention disturbance
Apraxia	Confusion
Anosognosia	Memory loss
Dementia	Changes in
Memory loss	Judgment
Neglect	Problem solving
Visuoperceptual deficits	Reasoning
	Insight
	Perseveration
	Concentration
	Personality and behavior
	Apathy
	Irritability
	Impulsivity
	Decreased motivation

to explain the totality of a patient's disability. The patient and the family will be easily frustrated and confused if the behavioral and cognitive effects of stroke and head injury are not clearly identified. Just as education about the nature of motor deficits promotes understanding by the patient and family, identification of cognitive deficits may make these deficits easier to deal with.

Cognitive impairments are of the utmost significance for stroke and head injury rehabilitation. The pattern of impairments and range of deficits for stroke and head injury are different, although overlapping (see Table 3). In general, the cognitive deficits in head injury tend to be more "global" in nature, whereas those in stroke are more "focal." Cognitive changes have been described after SCI [88,89] but are likely the result of concomitant CHI.

Head Injury

A more detailed discussion of the cognitive deficits associated with head injury is included in Chapter 22. Head injuries frequently impair frontal lobe functions such as judgment, motivation, problem solving, reasoning, impulsivity, and insight. Memory, particularly short-term and verbal memory, are impaired, as well as attention span. The cognitive disturbances found after head injury depend on the timing of the evaluation, the severity of the injury, premorbid traits, premorbid intellectual abilities, and the age of the patient.

Initially, coma or poor arousal may be the dominant neurobehavioral consequence of TBI. This usually resolves, followed by a phase of posttraumatic amnesia (PTA). Resolution of PTA occurs when day-to-day memory is restored. As the patient becomes more aroused, there is a stage of confusion, agitation, and possible aggression. Subsequent to that there are a variety of cognitive problems including difficulty with planning, reasoning, problem-solving, and initiation. Integral to cognitive functioning are a host of noncognitive behavioral disturbances that include socially inappropriate behavior, disinhibition, apathy, aggression, depression, and irritability. The patient may show little initiation, drive, or motivation [86]. Families complain that they are caring for a "different" person.

The severity of the initial injury, as measured by the Glasgow Coma Scale (GCS), correlates with the rate of improvement as well as the degree of residual cognitive impairment 2 years after CHI. Rapid improvement occurs between the 6th and 12th months following moderate to severe CHI, as measured by the WAIS [90]. Unlike stroke, specific or focal dysfunction such as aphasia and constructional apraxia is less common or less dominant. Such dysfunctions may occur, particularly with focal contusions, but generally are not the major or dominant cognitive dysfunction.

Stroke

The focal deficits following stroke are more familiar to most physicians and include disturbances of language in its various forms. The reader is referred to Chapter 13 and a recent review of aphasia by Damasio [91]. Visual–spatial dysfunction, apraxis, agnosias, and neglect are seen commonly. Neglect occurs in 20–31% of patients with stroke, and cognitive disturbance in 35–48%, based on an analysis of more than 1800 patients in the stroke data bank (personal communication, R. Sacco, M.D.). Gradual spontaneous resolution is the rule, with most recovery seen in the first 6 months [92]. The effectiveness of treatment, (i.e., cognitive remediation) must be measured against this background of spontaneous recovery.

Specific cognitive deficits, such as apraxia and neglect, have been found to influence a patient's functional outcome. Apraxia is a disorder of learned movement that cannot be explained by deficits in the patient's strength, coordination, sensation, or lack of comprehension [93]. Apraxia can impair a patient's abilities to produce or copy designs (constructional apraxia), dress him- or herself (dressing apraxia), or perform complex automatic learned acts (e.g., light a match). These deficits found on neuropsychological examination have real functional implications for patients with stroke. Constructional apraxia, as tested by having the patient reproduce a drawing or a model, correlates with dressing impairment [94]. Perceptual performance, particularly constructional praxis, as tested by a large battery of perceptual tasks, correlates with activities of daily living [95]. Others have found that apraxia and perceptual abnormalities predict dependency in self-care skills [96,97].

The rehabilitation of a patient with a moderately severe pure motor left hemiparesis caused by a lacunar infarct in the internal capsule is a reasonably straightforward task. Add hemispatial neglect, however, and the rehabilitation task becomes quite challenging. For example, safety in ambulation is now a more complex issue. Independent ambulation may not be possible because of the need for assistance with environmental hazards on the left side. The difficulties encountered during dressing and self-care because of hemiparesis are likewise now compounded by inattention to the paretic side. Unlike a patient with pure motor hemiparesis, the patient with neglect may be unaware of or unconcerned about his or her deficit, and the motivation to learn, improve, and cooperate will be diminished. Neglect has been associated with poor functional recovery as well as higher mortality in patients with stroke [98].

Higher cortical functioning is assessed by testing a patient's fund of knowledge, ability to do calculations, interpret proverbs, assess similarities, and complete conceptual series. Deficits in these areas are related to eventual functional outcome. Mysiw found that the patient's attention, calculation abilities, and judgment were the best predictors of improvement in the Barthel Index in patients with stroke [99]. Early cognitive scores correlated with later ability to perform ADLs, indicating that cognitive skills are important for functional outcome in stroke [100]. Poor ADL scores also correlate with poor visual recall [101].

A variety of screening devices have been used to test for cognitive impairment in patients with stroke, including the Neurobehavioral Cognitive Status Examination (NBCSE) [99], Cognitive Capacity Screening Examination (CCSE) [102], Mini-Mental Status Examination (MMSE), and the Stroke Unit Mental Status Examination (SUMSE) [103].

Treatment of Visual–Perceptual Deficits After Stroke

Visual–perceptual deficits are very common in the rehabilitation setting, and there is evidence that treatment (cognitive retraining) is effective in alleviating the deficits following a stroke. Weinberg showed improvement in visual scanning in a randomly controlled trial [104]. Carter performed a randomized control trial using stroke patients in a community hospital [105]. Patients were randomly assigned to specific treatment (3 hr/week) in three areas of cognitive skill. These included visual scanning (tested by a letter cancellation test), visuospatial orientation (tested by matching pictures), and a time judgment skill (tested by having the patient estimate a 1 min epoch of time). Patients in the treatment group improved their scores on these pen and paper tests when compared with a control group who received only standard rehabilitation. In a posthoc analysis of their earlier data, Carter attempted to show that cognitive skill remediation was generalizable to ADL function and was not simply task-specific [100]. The analysis showed significant improvement in ADL function in certain specific areas (personal hygiene, bathing, and toilet activities), but training did not generalize to all aspects of self-care.

Gordon showed improvement in perceptual functioning in patients with right brain damage treated with a comprehensive program to improve visual–perceptual deficits [106]. Patients were studied in a "quasirandom design" to receive remediation involving visual scanning, somatosensory awareness, size estimation training, and complex visual–perceptual organization. The experimental group improved relative to the control group. However, after discharge the experimental group plateaued in response and the control group continued to improve. This suggests that the process of cognitive remediation may speed up or activate the process of rehabilitation. A randomized trial showed that "intellectual training" improved function in some areas compared with a control rehabilitation program [107]. However, maintenance of the training effect was not seen in the long term. Taylor found no improvement in self-care with perceptual and cognitive treatment compared with controls [108].

The treatment of neglect has received considerable attention. Cueing has been reported by some [109,110] to help unilateral neglect, but not by others. A single subject design study with alternating treatment found no support for the hypothesis that stimulation of the right hemisphere would decrease neglect [111]. Computerized scanning and attention training did not improve left visual neglect [112]. An interesting pharmacological study reported that dopamine agonist therapy with bromocriptine is useful in treating neglect [113].

Memory and Dementia

Decreased memory and inability to learn new material are common following stroke. Physicians working in a rehabilitation unit frequently underestimate the frequency of cognitive impairment [102]. In England, a community-based epidemiological study on memory disturbance after stroke found an inability to learn new material in 14% of patients [101]. The Framingham study showed a decline in the MMSE when done before and after stroke in 39 patients evaluated over 4 years, but there was no change among controls [114]. A greater incidence of depression also followed stroke, suggesting that post-stroke depression may have accounted for some of the change in mental status.

The prevalence of dementia in a large cohort study of patients with stroke shows a prevalence ranging from 10% at age 60 to 25% at age 80 [115] (see Figure 7). This is important in rehabilitation because dementia is associated with lower ability to return home and a worse functional outcome. In a review of patients in the stroke data bank, dementia correlated with age as well as atrophy and hydrocephalus on computed tomographic (CT) scans. The relationship between ischemic cerebral vascular disease and dementia is, however, complex. Evidence of dementia should be sought in the history and physical examination. No direct correlation with size or number of infarcts has been possible, and no specific CT or magnetic resonance imaging (MRI) profile will predict dementia. Subcortical ischemic disease (Binswanger's) may produce dementia. Single infarctions in certain critical areas of the brain such as the anterior thalamus, midbrain, or hippocampus can also be associated with dementia. In the age group of patients with stroke, Alzheimer's disease can coexist. The diagnosis of dementia soon after a stroke is difficult because arousal and attentional deficits may interfere. Later, focal lesions can reduce the MMSE score to less than 24 without a true global cognitive decline [116].

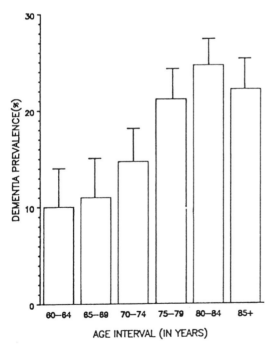

Figure 7   The rising incidence of dementia with increasing age seen in 726 patients 60 years of age or older with ischemic stroke, in the Stroke Data Bank [115].

Complex learning has been achieved in single case studies in patients with organic amnesia. A patient with amnesia following encephalitis was trained, using vanishing cues, to perform complex computer tasks that eventually allowed the patient to return to the workplace [117]. Techniques to increase memory by visual associations can improve performance in formal learning tasks, but have not been shown to be generalizable to practical situations [118].

SUMMARY

Depression and cognitive changes are frequently seen in patients undergoing neurorehabilitation. They are common, disabling, and influence functional gains. They require recognition, identification, and treatment. Treatment, both pharmacological and based on cognitive training, has been found to be effective and should be used.

REFERENCES

1. J. Gans, *Arch. Phys. Med. Rehab.*, 62:386–389 (1981).
2. F.K. Judd, D.J. Brown, G.D. Burrows, *Paraplegia*, 29:91–96 (1991).
3. J. Clothier and J. Grotta, *Clin. Geriatr. Med.*, 7:493–406 (1991).
4. H.G. Koenig and S. Studenski, *Gen. Intern. Med.*, 3:509–517 (1988).
5. A. House, *Br. Med. J.*, 294:76–78 (1987).
6. R.A. Stern and D.L. Bachman, *Am. J. Psychiatry*, 148:351–356 (1991).
7. R.M. Dupont, C.M. Cullum, and D.V. Jeste, *Psychiatr. Clin. North Am.*, 11: 133–149 (1988).
8. P.P. Coll, *J. Fam. Pract.*, 28:153–155 (1989).
9. F. Catapano and S. Galderisi, *J. Clin. Psychiatry*, 51:9 (suppl):9–12 (1990).
10. T.R. Price, *Stroke*, 9:3 (1990).
11. B. Ahlsio, M. Britton, V. Murray, and T. Theorell, *Stroke*, 15:886–890 (1984).
12. M.L. Niemi, R. Laaksonen, M. Kotila, and O. Waltimo, *Stroke*, 19:1101–1107 (1988).
13. J.H. Feibel, S. Berk, and R.J. Joynt, *Neurology*, 29:592 (1979).
14. J.P. Fedoroff, J.R. Lipsey, S.E. Starkstein, A. Forrester, T.R. Price, and R.G. Robinson, *J. Affect. Disord.*, 22:83–88 (1991).
15. J. Sharpless, *Problem-Oriented Approach to Stroke Rehabilitation*. Charles C. Thomas, Springfield, IL (1982).
16. L. Holland and M. Whalley, *Br. J. Psychiatry*, 138:222–229 (1981).
17. S. Horenstein, *Behavior Changes in Cerebrovascular Disease* (L. Benton, ed.), Harper & Row, New York (1970).
18. M. Foulkes, P. Wolf, T. Price, J. Mohr, and D. Hier, *Stroke*, 19:547–554 (1988).
19. R.G. Robinson and B. Szetela, *Ann. Neurol.*, 9:447–453 (1981).
20. A. House, M. Dennis, A. Molyneux, C. Warlow, and K. Hawton, *Br. Med. J.*, 298:991–994 (1989).

21. M.L. Lim and S.B.J. Ebrahim, *Postgrad. Med. J.*, 59:489–491 (1983).
22. G.M. Seliger and A. Horstein, *Neurology*, 39:1400 (1989).
23. R.B. Schiffer, R.M. Herndon, and R.A. Rudick, *N. Engl. J. Med.*, 312:1480–1482 (1985).
24. E.D. Ross and A.J. Rush, *Arch. Gen. Psychiatry*, 38:1344–1354 (1981).
25. J.F. McGreevey, Jr. and K. Franco, *J. Gen. Intern. Med.*, 3:498–507 (1988).
26. A.F. Schatzberg, B. Liptzin, A. Satlin, and J.O. Cole, *Psychosomatics*, 25:126–131 (1984).
27. W. Applegate, J. Blass, and T. Williams, *N. Engl. J. Med.*, 322:1207–1214 (1990).
28. L. Eisenberg, *N. Engl. J. Med.*, 326:1080–1084 (1992).
29. S. Finklestein, L.I. Benowitz, R.J. Baldessarini, G.W. Arana, D. Levine, E. Woo, D. Bear, K. Moya, and A.L. Stoll, *Ann. Neurol.*, 12:463–468 (1982).
30. M. Reding, L. Orto, P. Willensky, I. Fortuna, N. Day, S.F. Steiner, L. Gehr, and F. McDowell, *Arch. Neurol.*, 42:209–212 (1985).
31. R.G. Robinson, K.L. Kubos, L.B. Starr, K. Rao, and T.R. Price, *Brain*, 107:81–93 (1984).
32. J.F. Malec, J.W. Richardson, M. Sinaki, and M.W. O'Brien, *Arch. Phys. Med. Rehab.*, 71:279–284 (1990).
33. S.E. Starkstein, R.G. Robinson, and T.R. Price, *Stroke*, 19:1491–1496 (1988).
34. H. Dam, H.E. Pedersen, and P. Ahlgren, *Acta Psychiatr. Scand.*, 80:118–124 (1989).
35. R.G. Robinson, P.L. Bolduc, and T.R. Price, *Stroke*, 18:837–843 (1987).
36. F.H. Garden, S.J. Garrison, and A. Jain, *Arch. Phys. Med. Rehab.*, 71:1003–1005 (1990).
37. D. Blazer, *N. Engl. J. Med.*, 320:164–166 (1989).
38. J.P. Fedoroff, S.E. Starkstein, A W. Forrester, F.H. Geisler, R.E. Jorge, S.V. Arndt, and R.G. Robinson, *Am. J. Psychiatry*, 149:918–923 (1992).
39. T.W. McAllister, *Psychiatr. Clin. North Am.*, 15:395–413 (1992).
40. M. Stambrook, A.D. Moore, L.C. Peters, E. Zubek, S. McBeath, and I.C. Friesen, *J. Clin. Exp. Neuropsychol.*, 13:521–530 (1991).
41. F.K. Judd, J. Stone, J.E. Webber, D.J. Brown, and G.D. Burrows, *Br. J. Psychiatry*, 154:668–671 (1989).
42. L.E. Hollister, *N. Engl. J. Med.*, 299:1106 (1978).
43. M. Folstein, R. Maiberger, and P. McHugh, *J. Neurol. Neurosurg. Psychiatry*, 40:1018–1020 (1977).
44. S.P. Finklestein, R.J. Weintraub, N. Karmouz, C. Askinazi, G. Davar, and R.J. Baldessarini, *Arch. Phys. Med. Rehab.*, 68:772–776 (1987).
45. R.G. Robinson and T.R. Price, *Stroke*, 13:635–641 (1982).
46. R.G. Robinson, L. Starr, K.L. Kubos, and T.R. Price, *Stroke*, 14:736–741 (1983).
47. R. Robinson, L. Starr, and T. Price, *Br. J. Psychiatry*, 144:256–262 (1984).
48. R.G. Robinson, J.R. Lipsey, K. Rao, and T.R. Price, *Am. J. Psychiatry*, 143(10):1238–1244 (1986).
49. S. Yamaguchi, S. Kobayashi, A. Murata, K. Yamashita, J. Koide, J. Fukuda, and T. Tsunematsu, *J. Cereb. Blood Flow Metab.*, 7:S218 (1987).

50. D. Sinyor, P. Jacques, D.G. Kaloupek, R. Becker, M. Goldenberg, and H. Coopersmith, *Brain*, 109:537–546 (1986).

51. T. Danel, D. Leys, A. Destee, M. Goudemand, and J. Parquet, *Neurology*, 41: 951 (1991).

52. S.E. Starkstein, M.L. Berthier, P. Fedoroff, T.R. Price, and R.G. Robinson, *Neurology*, 40:1380–1382 (1990).

53. B.J. Carroll, *J. Clin. Psychiatry*, 43:11 (section 2): 44–48 (1982).

54. T. Olsson, M. Astrom, S. Eriksson, and A. Forssell, *Stroke*, 20:1685–1690 (1989).

55. A. Roy, D. Pickar, and S. Paul, *Psychosomatics*, 25:443–451 (1984).

56. H.C. Sabelli, J. Fawcett, J.I. Javaid, and S. Bagri, *Am. J. Psychiatry*, 140:212–214 (1983).

57. L.W. Lazarus, D.R. Winemiller, V.R. Lingam, I. Neyman, C. Hartman, M. Abassian, U. Kartan, L. Groves, and J. Fawcett, *J. Clin. Psychiatry*, 53:447–449 (1992).

58. W.W.K. Zung, *Arch. Gen. Psychiatry*, 12:63–66 (1965).

59. A.T. Beck, C.H. Ward, M. Mendeson, J. Moch, and J. Erbaugh, *Arch. Gen. Psychiatry*, 4:561–571 (1961).

60. J.W. Richardson, III and E. Richelson, *Mayo Clin. Proc.*, 59:330–337 (1984).

61. M. Hamilton, *J. Neurol. Neurosurg. Psychiatry*, 23:56–62 (1960).

62. *Diagnostic and Statistical Manual of Mental Disorders: (DSM-III-R)*. American Psychiatric Association, Washington D.C. (1987).

63. N.E. Mayo, B.N. Korner, and R. Becker, *Am. J. Phys. Med. Rehab.*, 70:5–12 (1991).

64. K. Bolla-Wilson, R.G. Robinson, S.E. Startstein, J. Boston, and T.R. Price, *Am. J. Psychiatry*, 146(5):627–634 (1989).

65. D. Schubert, C. Taylor, L. Suk, A. Mentari, and W. Tamaklo, *Gen. Hosp. Psychiatry*, 14:69–76 (1992).

66. R.M. Parikh, R.G. Robinson, J.R. Lipsey, S.E. Starkstein, J.P. Fedoroff, and T.R. Price, *Arch. Neurol.*, 47:785–789 (1990).

67. W. Potter, M. Rudorfer, and H. Manji, *N. Engl. J. Med.*, 325:633–642 (1991).

68. D. Bishop, *Stroke Rehabilitation* (M. Brandstater and J. Basmajian, eds.), Williams & Wilkins, Baltimore, pp. 369–392 (1987).

69. L. Goodman and A. Gilman, *The Pharmacologic Basis of Therapeutics*. Macmillan, New York (1971).

70. G.W. Small, *J. Clin. Psychiatry*, 50:27–33 (1989).

71. G.L. Cooper, *Psychiatry*, 153:77–86 (1988).

72. M. Lader, *Br. J. Psychiatry*, 153:51–58 (1988).

73. R.F. Bergstrom, L. Lemberger, N.A. Farid, and R.L. Wolen, *Br. J. Psychiatry*, 153:47–50 (1988).

74. *Med. Lett.*, 34:47–48 (1992).

75. W. Karliner, *Psychomatics*, 19:781–783 (1978).

76. G.B. Murray, V. Shea, and D.K. Conn, *J. Clin. Psychiatry*, 47:258–260 (1986).

77. J.R. Lipsey, R.G. Robinson, G.D. Pearlson, K. Rao, and T.R. Price, *Lancet*, i: 297–300 (1984).

78. A. G. Fullerton, *Lancet*, *i*:519 (1984).
79. M. Agerholm, *Lancet*, *i*:519–520 (1984).
80. G.W. Small, *J. Clin. Psychiatry*, 52:11–22 (1991).
81. C. Salzman, *N. Engl. J. Med.*, 512 (1985).
82. M. Reding, L. Orto, S. Winter, I. Fortuna, P. DiPonte, and F. McDowell, *Arch. Neurol.*, 43:763–765 (1986).
83. M. Lakshmanan, L.C. Mion, and J.D. Frengley, *J. Am. Geriatr. Soc.*, 34:421–425 (1986).
84. M.M. Brooke, K.A. Questad, D.R. Patterson, and K.J. Bashak, *Arch. Phys. Med. Rehab.*, 73:320–323 (1992).
85. *The American Heritage Dictionary of the English Language*. The American Heritage Publishing Co., New York (1971).
86. M.P. Alexander, *Neurobehavioral Recovery from Head Injury*. (H.S. Levin, J. Grafman, and H.W. Eisenberg, eds.), Oxford University Press, New York, pp. 191–205 (1987).
87. N. Namerow, *Neurol. Clin.*, 5:569–583 (1987).
88. G.N. Davidoff, E.J. Roth, J.S. Haughton, and M.S. Ardner, *Arch. Phys. Med. Rehab.*, 71:326–329 (1990).
89. G.N. Davidoff, E.J. Roth, and J.S. Richards, *Arch. Phys. Med. Rehab.*, 73:275–284 (1992).
90. H. Levin, and F. Goldstein, *Traumatic Brain Injury* (P. Bach-y-Rita, ed.), Demos, New York, pp. 53–72 (1989).
91. A. Damasio, Review Articles 326:531–540 (1992).
92. D. Hier, J. Mondlock, and L. Caplan, *Neurology*, 33:345–350 (1983).
93. R. Strub and F. Black, *The Mental Status Examination in Neurology*. F.A. Davis, Philadelphia (1985).
94. M. Warren, *Am. J. Occup. Ther.*, 35:431–437 (1981).
95. M. Titus, N. Gall, E. Yerxa, T. Roberson, and W. Mack, *Am. J. Occup. Ther.*, 45:410–418 (1991).
96. E. Bjorneby and I. Reinvang, *Scand. J. Rehab. Med.*, 17:75–80 (1985).
97. B. Bernspang, K. Asplund, S. Eriksson, and M.A. Fugl, *Stroke*, 18:1081–1086 (1987).
98. D. Smith, A. Akhtar, and W. Garraway, *Age Ageing*, 12:63–69 (1983).
99. W.J. Mysiw, J.G. Beegan, and P.F. Gatens, *Am. J. Phys. Med. Rehab.*, 68:168–171 (1989).
100. L. Carter, D. Oliveria, J. Duponte, and S. Lynch, *Am. J. Occup. Ther.*, 42:449–455 (1988).
101. D. Wade, V. Parker, and R. Hewer, *Int. Rehab. Med.*, 8:60–64 (1986).
102. J. Luxenberg and F. LZ, *Arch. Phys. Med. Rehab.*, 67:796–798 (1986).
103. V.E. Hajek, D.L. Rutman, and H. Scher, *Arch. Phys. Med. Rehab.*, 70:114–117 (1989).
104. J. Weinberg, L. Diller, W. Gordon, L. Gerstman, A. Lieberman, P. Lakin, G. Hodges, and O. Ezrachi, *Arch. Phys. Med. Rehab.*, 58:479–486 (1977).
105. L. Carter, B. Howard, and W. O'Neil, *Am. J. Occup. Ther.*, 37:320–326 (1983).

106. W. Gordon, M. Hibbard, S. Egelko, L. Diller, M. Shaver, A. Lieberman, and K. Ragnarsson, *Arch. Phys. Med. Rehab.*, 66:353–359 (1985).
107. I. Soderback, *Scand. J. Rehab. Med.*, 20:47–56 (1988).
108. O. Taylor, J. Schaeffer, F. Blumenthal, and J. Grisell, *Arch. Phys. Med. Rehab.*, 52(4):163–169 (1971).
109. M. Riddoch and G. Humphreys, *Neuropsychologia*, 21:589–599 (1983).
110. S. Ishiai, M. Sugishita, N. Odamima, M. Yaginuma, S. Gono, and T. Kamaya, *Neurology*, 40:1395–1398 (1990).
111. S. Cermak, C. Trombly, J. Hausser, and A. Tiernan, *Occup. Ther. J. Res.*, 11 (1991).
112. I. Robertson, J. Gray, B. Pentland, and L. Waite, *Arch. Phys. Med. Rehab.*, 71: 663–668 (1990).
113. W. Fleet, E. Valenstein, R. Watson, and K. Heilman, *Neurology*, 37 (1987).
114. C. Kase, P. Wolf, M. Kelly-Hayes, W. Kannel, D. Bachman, R. Linn, and R. D'Agostino, *Neurology*, 37:119 (1987).
115. T. Tatemichi, M. Foulkes, J. Mohr, J. Hewitt, D. Hier, T. Price, and P. Wolf, *Stroke*, 21:858–866 (1990).
116. A. Hijdra, M.M. Derix, S. Teunisse, G.W. van, and I. H. Kwa, *Stroke*, 22:416 (1991).
117. E. Glisky and D. Schacter, *Neuropsychologia*, 27:107–120 (1989).
118. J.T. Richardson, *Neurology*, 42:283–286 (1992).
119. J. Feibel and C. Springer, *Arch. Phys. Med. Rehab.*, 63:276–278 (1982).

7

Interdisciplinary Team Approach to Rehabilitation

Patricia B. Jozefczyk

University of Pittsburgh School of Medicine
Pittsburgh, Pennsylvania

Medical rehabilitation is defined as the restoration of a patient to a prior state of health through treatment and retraining. In some illnesses and injuries, restoration may be complete. However, in many neurological diseases, complete recovery is not possible. The aim of neurological rehabilitation is to achieve optimal physical, psychological, cognitive, and social functioning consistent with the residual physiological or anatomical impairment.

Patients with neurological illnesses such as stroke, spinal cord injuries, traumatic brain injuries, multiple sclerosis, parkinsonism, and muscular disorders have long-term care problems and benefit from comprehensive care [1]. In rehabilitation, this care is traditionally delivered by a team of professionals. Although the efficacy of the team approach to health care is not proven, a number of studies suggest that patients with chronic diseases receiving coordinated team care show improved outcome [2]. Research in the area of rehabilitation is difficult because of the number of variables that affect patient selection, differences in rehabilitation practices, and nonuniform outcome measures. For example, much has been written specifically about stroke rehabilitation in an attempt to determine its benefits, but results of these studies vary [3]. It does appear however, that selected patients can make functional improvements in the rehabilitation setting that may make the difference between institutionalization and return to home [4].

THE TEAM CONCEPT

Focused patient care is a concept that should not be limited to medical specialties, individual diseases, or specific facilities. The goal of the entire health care system should be the best possible outcome for every patient. Historically, medical care had been provided primarily by a physician and nurse. However, as technology developed and medical science grew, specialization in patient care emerged, with the development of new disciplines like physical therapy and social work. In addition, physicians became more specialized and focused on a smaller portion of the patient's overall problems. The development of the team approach arose in an attempt to bridge specialization and the need for comprehensiveness and continuity of care [5].

A team is an organized group of professionals who share common values and work toward common objectives. In health care, the team goal is comprehensive patient care. In rehabilitation medicine, it should be obtaining optimum function for each patient despite persistent pathological conditions or disease.

The structure, organization, and approaches of a given team may vary depending on the purpose. Medical teams can be organized by specialty (trauma), body system (cardiovascular), or health care delivery system (outpatient therapy). One feature common to all teams is that each member has a special area of expertise that contributes to the overall success of the team in accomplishing the predetermined goal. A team structure may be multidisciplinary or interdisciplinary. A multidisciplinary team is defined as one in which each professional specialty provides its own unique contribution, and the output of the group is the sum of the efforts of each discipline. An interdisciplinary team is one in which there is a common defined goal. In addition to providing the skills of their own discipline, each team member contributes to the common goal through a group effort. Thus, the total group output is greater than the sum of the individual parts [6].

Classic organizational structure involves the principle of vertical integration. The organization is a pyramid with the base formed by those who perform specialized tasks. These individuals are organized by department, and a hierarchy of command develops with fewer numbers of personnel as one rises up the pyramid. No communication is necessary within a level, since each person performs his or her assigned job. Specialists at one level concentrate on their own goals and may lose sight of the fact that their goals are not ends in themselves, but a means of reaching the broader goals of the organization.

Newer theories of organizational structure propose a more integrated system in which all parts are interrelated and departmentalization occurs along functional lines. This type of "project" structure can be superimposed on a more traditional structure to create a matrix design, resulting in an organization with both horizontal and vertical dimensions. This format allows goals to be reached across specialty lines [7].

In medical rehabilitation, a vertical organization framework does not achieve the goal of comprehensive patient care. The matrix approach adds a "project" orientation and meshes with the problem-oriented approach to patient care. Each team member has the opportunity to determine how a problem may affect the outcome within his or her own discipline. For example, the spinal cord injured patient may develop a urinary tract infection that will require care from a physician and nurse. However, the physical therapist needs to be aware of the problem also, since it may be reflected by increased leg spasticity during therapy sessions. In the matrix system of team care, each person representing a specific discipline is responsible for making decisions to achieve his or her own specialized goals, but also contributes to the total team goal. This requires planning and communication.

TEAM DEVELOPMENT

The interdisciplinary model of health care delivery is not unique to medical rehabilitation. Although the disciplines involved and the goals of specialized teams may vary, all share a similar organizational structure and the problems inherent in this approach. A working, responsible, and productive team requires time and effort to develop and manage.

In discussing the development of an outpatient health care team in Harlem, Wise [8] identified problems focusing on the individuality of each professional, conflicts in "turf," and poor communication. He noted: "It is naive to bring together a highly diverse group of people and expect that, by calling them a team, they will in fact behave as a team."

A team must define their goal. In the case of medical rehabilitation the goal is to achieve the best overall functioning of the patient at multiple levels (physical, emotional, social, vocational). In simplest terms, once the objectives are understood, everyone on the team must participate. A team leader is needed to guide the group forward, without domination, toward the goal.

A new team begins slowly by establishing a working relationship between members. The development of a facilitative emotional climate is imperative. The team must be adaptable and able to change structure as necessary. It must continually reassess itself by establishing feedback mechanisms between team members, and also by seeking the observations of those outside the team. Disagreements are to be expected at times and each member must feel free to express critical opinions and conflicts. In addition to identifying conflicts or problems, each member should actively contribute in working toward a solution. Decisions must be made by the group as a whole, not by a dominant personality or the team leader [9]. The group process is a dynamic one and communication in a "round table" type of setting is psychosocially most productive. Some professionals may not be team players and they need to be identified and re-educated in team organization.

Success of a team depends primarily on communication but also on encouraging new ideas. Team members should avoid complaisance and keep abreast of new developments in their disciplines. Professional and educational contacts outside the group should be encouraged. Each member must contribute within his or her own discipline and between disciplines.

Several general reviews of team development are available [5,10]. By its very nature, any organization has an inherent structural hierarchy influenced by profession, age, power, status, and gender. In the ideal team, everyone is an equal, but this psychosocial hierarchy often persists on an unconscious level and may result in failure or inefficiency of the team approach. Osborne [11] reviewed the structure of the mental health care system in which professionals from different disciplines are involved. He noted that even in an apparent interdisciplinary team, team dynamics may be influenced by the traditional medical hierarchy model involving the interrelationship of physician, psychology nurse, and paraprofessionals. Persons at the highest levels of an organization often develop and maintain programs that reflect the tradition of their own profession rather than the inclusion of the varied skills of other disciplines. He recommended a social-action model in which there was no interpersonal hierarchial structure, and proposed that the change be made by educating physicians in organizational structure and by encouraging and rewarding achievements of the other professionals.

Gaston [12] reported attempts to convert a "back ward" of a psychiatric hospital to an active rehabilitation unit and stressed the importance of an organizational climate in which staff motivation is improved by promoting personal esteem and self-development. This was accomplished by developing and improving competence in the staff and by recognizing their achievements.

Despite the best efforts, it may be difficult to develop a truly functional interdisciplinary team. Rothberg [5] describes interpersonal and interprofessional barriers to team participation. At the interpersonal level, frustration may develop when members are asked to be independent in their own discipline yet interdependent in the team. Ego satisfaction may suffer and some personalities may never be able to accept this dichotomy of responsibility. This apparent role ambiguity may appear to cause incongruous expectations. Personal qualities necessary for team membership include the ability to function interdependently and form new attitudes and perspectives toward other team members. One must accept personal differences and differences of opinion, be able to tolerate review, and be challenged by new ideas. A team member must maintain personal identity yet be able to negotiate role boundaries with the other team members. If a member does not or cannot accept the team philosophy of care, the entire approach will fail.

On an interprofessional level, problems arise when one team member demonstrates a lack of trust in the professional judgment of other members. This usually results from a lack of knowledge of the responsibilities and scope of the other disciplines. By definition, educational preparation for each discipline is undisciplinary, and implicit in this training is the concept that one's own discipline may be the most important one. This leads to disputes of a territorial nature and may lead to inappropriate expectations of other team members.

Team leadership may be another area of conflict [7]. Leadership is the ability to inspire and influence others to contribute to the attainment of objectives [13]. Successful leadership does not depend necessarily on the personal traits of the leader, but develops as a result of the interaction of the leader and team members. An autocratic leadership style is not conducive to a successful rehabilitation team. A leader who makes all the decisions defeats the team concept. A more democratic type of leadership, by which the team is guided without being dominated, allows for maximal individual team member expression and support.

In most cases, a physician assumes the leadership role and coordinates strategy, but should be aware that authority is a position and not a person, and that power is bestowed by the group. To avoid domination, leadership often needs to be "passed around" during team meetings and the physician must see him or herself as an equal member of the professional team.

In summary, an effective rehabilitation team must give its members time to work on developing the team, not simply to work on their own individual discipline. Patterns of professional interaction need to be established and there must be mutual respect toward team members' skills and knowledge. Individual team member roles should be defined and utilized to their fullest potential. A mechanism for accountability of each member needs to be developed and members must recognize that leadership and authority may shift as the team matures. Maintaining communication and working on developing and assessing the team's function are imperative for success. In realizing that conflict is inevitable in any group, efforts must be made to recognize problems early and develop a mechanism to deal with them promptly.

NEUROLOGICAL REHABILITATION TEAM MEMBERS

As is now obvious, various professionals need to be involved in the neurological rehabilitation team to help return an ill or injured patient to the most independent and productive lifestyle possible.

Physician

The physician plays a dual role in managing the medical issues and supervising the rehabilitation program of the patient. The physician evaluates the patient's present problem in the context of the overall medical condition. The experienced physician will recognize if the patient's neurological condition is reversible or not, and help guide rehabilitation along either restorative or adaptive lines. It is the responsibility of the physician to recognize potential medical complications associated with specific neurological conditions, and to prescribe prompt and appropriate treatment.

Psychologist

The psychologist assists in determining the patient's personality, problem solving abilities, and tolerance for stress, and works with the team in preparing the patient for full participation in rehabilitation. In selected cases it is necessary to determine intellectual functioning, memory, cognitive, and perceptual functioning using a series of neuropsychological tests. Neuropsychological testing helps to identify the nature and extent of emotional and cognitive deficits, and can guide in the development of an individualized behavioral and cognitive program to aid in rehabilitation and social reintegration after the patient is discharged from the hospital. Psychologists provide counseling in the emotional aspects of the patient's new limitations, including acceptance of disability and altered body image, and concerns about death and dying. They also interact with family members in coping with their own responses to the patient's physical and emotional changes. Psychologists are also invaluable in helping to identify conflicts and their solutions within the interdisciplinary team.

Physical Therapist

Physical therapy improves function using an individually tailored exercise program to improve range of motion, muscle strength, balance, and endurance. Specific activities addressed include bed mobility, transfers, wheelchair training, and ambulation, if possible. Equipment needs are addressed including wheelchair specifications, seat cushion design, and assistive devices including ankle-foot orthoses (AFOs), canes, and walkers.

Occupational Therapist

Occupational therapy focuses on range of motion, strength, and functional use of the upper extremities for activities of daily living (ADLs) including feeding, bathing, grooming, dressing, toileting, and home management skills. Adaptive equipment may be recommended to help with arm positioning and improved function in ADLs. The occupational therapist may assist with development of new skills to help compensate for motor, sensory, or perceptual loss and development of vocational and avocational interests. If dysphagia is identified, the occupational therapist may assist the speech therapist in training the patient to use compensatory techniques for feeding. Home or workplace visits are sometimes done to adapt these environments for the patient, and to ensure maximum safety and independence.

Rehabilitation Nurse

The nursing staff provides physical care and helps the patient achieve short- and long-term goals. Responsibilities include monitoring patients for medical complications including bowel and bladder dysfunction, skin problems, and venous thrombosis. The rehabilitation nurse must be attentive to small changes in the patient's skills and relay these to other team members to help adjust rehabilitation goals as necessary. The nurse teaches the patient and family about the care they are receiving while hospitalized, and helps prepare them for discharge by teaching any special care techniques that must be continued at home.

Speech–Language Pathologist

The speech–language pathologist deals with problems in communication by evaluating and retraining patients with speaking, listening, writing, or reading problems. If the patient cannot speak, alternative means of communication are explored. In addition, speech–language pathologists evaluate patients for swallowing and cognitive problems and assist with retraining in these areas. Family counseling is provided to help instruct caregivers and family in the best ways of communication.

Recreational Therapist

This specialist assesses the patient's resources and interests in order to use recreation to promote growth and development along physical, emotional, and social lines. The recreational therapist assesses the patient's social capabilities, designs adaptive equipment if necessary, and helps the patient explore alternatives to his or her previous lifestyle. Activities are used to increase independence, help with family adjustment, and improve the patient's attention span. Community reintegration and the identification of community resources are also pursued.

Prosthetist and Orthotist

Certified prosthetists and orthotists, along with the therapists and physician, identify the need for assistive devices. They fabricate these devices according to the patient's deficits, with the goals of improving function and independence.

Social Worker

The social worker acts as an advocate for patients and their families in financial matters, questions about insurance, and by helping other team members communicate with the family. The social worker arranges for family training and identifies community resources for continued care after hospital discharge. Personal and family concerns are also addressed in general counseling sessions and alternative living arrangements are made, if necessary.

Vocational Counselor

Vocational counselors help plan for return to work or school after discharge by identifying the patient's skills, aptitude, and interests. They organize job interviews, conduct group support sessions, and counsel the patient if a change in vocation is necessary. They serve as a liaison between the patient and employer to help adjust the work environment and help to educate potential employers.

Nutritionist

The nutritionist evaluates the patient's nutritional requirements and develops a balanced dietary intake to meet them. The nutritionist helps to determine if the patient's caloric and protein intake is sufficient and works with the speech therapist if a modified-consistency diet is necessary. Parenteral nutritional needs are assessed if indicated. Educating the patient and family about healthy eating patterns and specific dietary restrictions at home is essential.

Patient and Family

The patient and the family are important team members and need to be encouraged to participate and take an active role in the recovery and rehabilitation process. Family members are encouraged to participate in "hands-on" training with team members in order for them to feel comfortable and competent in continuing these activities at home. If possible, the patient must also assist in these activities, including learning home exercise programs and following dietary, medical, and medication guidelines as instructed by various team members. The traditional passive role of the patient needs to be discouraged, and patients undergoing rehabilitation should be trained to be active and responsible for their rehabilitation [14]. Techniques learned in the therapy gym should be practiced in the patient's hospital room. As they become more adept in ambulation or wheelchair propulsion, patients should be given the responsibility of following their daily schedules and getting themselves to the appropriate therapy session on time.

TEAM MEETINGS

Since communication is the key to effective teamwork, a format to enhance and promote communication needs to be developed. The team meeting is a necessary activity of the rehabilitation team. Once all of the team members have had the opportunity to evaluate the patient, they should meet as a group to discuss their individual impressions and set team rehabilitation goals. This is usually done within the first week of the patient's admission, and repeated every 1–2 weeks during hospitalization to report progress, update goals, and work toward discharge planning. All team members need to attend and contribute to the meeting. Meetings should be goal-oriented and productive. Various approaches can be used. Team members may give progress reports according to their discipline and organize their own set of problems and goals. Another approach is problem-oriented: an issue is identified and all team members contribute to its resolution according to their individual expertise. Often these two approaches are combined by beginning the session with discipline reports, but encouraging other members to contribute their own observations. For example, the physical therapist's report on poor progress in wheelchair propulsion in a patient with stroke can be expanded by the occupational therapist's observation of neglect or a field cut on the affected side, and the speech therapist's observation of a receptive aphasia leading to poor understanding of new tasks. Thus, the multifactorial basis of a single issue is identified and appropriate team goals are set to help resolve the problem.

The report of the team meetings should include recognition and explanation of specific issues, identification of team member's contribution to resolution of the issues, goals set, and anticipated time frame to reach those goals. Each subsequent team meeting reanalyzes the issue, notes progress if any, and redefines goals and discharge planning if necessary.

TEAM TREATMENT GOALS

Approach to the treatment of the neurologically impaired patient includes a number of strategies. These include preventing complications, promoting recovery from the neurological deficit, or teaching adaptation to the deficit [9]. The physician must be certain that the primary disability is not compounded by additional medical problems. Observation for potential complications helps to prevent additional disability and improves rehabilitation outcome. Control of hypertension, diabetes, or other pre-existing medical conditions is obviously important. Maintenance of nutrition and prevention of aspiration is required in patients who are dysphagic. Bowel and bladder care should be meticulous to prevent complications such as urinary tract infections and fecal impaction. Observation of skin for pressure points and breakdown is important. Some neurological deficits, such as significant plegia or decreased level of consciousness, increase the risk of deep venous thrombosis, pulmonary embolism, urinary tract infections, and aspiration pneumonia. Patients with spinal cord injury are at risk for autonomic dysreflexia, urinary tract infections, decubiti, venous thrombosis, and heterotopic ossification. Any disease resulting in increased muscle tone and spasticity can result in contractures or painful spasms. Preventive stretching and range-of-motion exercise are important in the care of these patients.

Improving the deficit to the extent possible by progressive exercises to strengthen weakened muscles will aid in the recovery. Visual feedback may be used to compensate for sensory deficits. Rehabilitation strategy should also address parts not affected by the pathological condition. These include exercise and strengthening of the uninvolved extremities. When complete recovery from a deficit is not possible, functional improvement is an important goal. Depending on individual needs, functional recovery may require adaptive equipment or assistive devices such as wheelchairs, AFOs, prostheses, shoe modifications, ADL equipment, or hand controls for wheelchair or automobile adaptation. The home and work environment may require adaptations. Family and social education may be necessary for the patient's successful reintegration into society.

SUMMARY

Recovery from a neurological disability requires the expertise of many professionals. However, beyond achieving as much as possible within a specific discipline, the patient as a whole must be considered. The care from each discipline must be integrated into an interdisciplinary team in which the efforts of one team member enhance those of the others. When all professionals involved work together as a team, maximum goals can be achieved.

In many cases, neurological diseases cause long-term deficits and the fragmented care from multiple specialists and professionals fails to serve the patient's overall needs. The coordinated interdisciplinary team approach is more effective in caring for patients with these types of disabilities, and ensures the best possible functional status when recovery from a pathological condition is incomplete.

The team care approach has been criticized by some because of the increased utilization of health care services and subsequently increased health care costs it involves. However, one may argue that maximizing functional abilities and independence is less costly, in the long run, than lifelong custodial or maintenance care.

REFERENCES

1. N. Namerow and L. Scheinberg, *J. Neuro. Rehab.*, 2:91–94 (1987).
2. L. Halstead, *Arch. Phys. Med. Rehab.*, 57:507–511 (1976).
3. M. Dombovy, B. Sandok, and J. Basford, *Stroke*, 17:363–369 (1986).
4. K. Lind, *J. Chron. Dis.*, 35:133–149 (1982).
5. J.S. Rothberg, *Arch. Phys. Med. Rehab.*, 62:407–410 (1981).
6. J.L. Melvin, *Arch. Phys. Med. Rehab.*, 61:379–380 (1980).
7. B.B. Longest, Jr., *Management Practices for the Health Professional* (3rd ed), Reston Publishing Co., Reston, VA (1984).
8. H. Wise, *Arch. Intern. Med.*, 130:438–444 (1972).
9. J.A. DeLisa, G.M. Martin, and D.M. Currie, *Rehabilitation Medicine Principles and Practice* (J.A. De Lisa, ed.), J.B. Lippincott, Philadelphia, pp. 3–24 (1988).
10. B. Given and S. Simmons, *Nursing Form*, 16:165–184 (1977).
11. O.H. Osborne, *Hosp. Commun. Psychiatry*, 26:207–213 (1975).
12. E. Gaston, *Hosp. Commun. Psychiatry*, 31:407–412 (1980).
13. L. Lundborg, *J. Nursing Admin.*, 12:32–33 (1982).
14. T.P. Anderson, *Medical Rehabilitation* (J.V. Basmajian and R.L. Kirby, eds.), Williams & Wilkins, Baltimore, pp. 144–151 (1984).

8

Social Concerns and Discharge Planning

Laura Lennihan

College of Physicians and Surgeons of Columbia University
New York, and
Helen Hayes Hospital
West Haverstraw, New York

Planning the discharge of a neurologically disabled patient from a rehabilitation service is an interdisciplinary collaboration to make a plan that provides for appropriate independence, assistance and safety, and continuing care. The development of the discharge plan begins before the patient's admission to the rehabilitation service and continues throughout the rehabilitation stay. The patient's neurological impairments, functional capacities, social and financial circumstances, and home and community environments are the elements considered in making the discharge plans. The process of discharge planning involves the collaboration of the rehabilitation treatment team, social worker, patient, and family.

Discharge planning is a formal responsibility of hospitals mandated by government regulations. This chapter does not focus on the regulatory and fiscal aspects of discharge planning, which are constantly changing, nor does it attempt to outline the hospital administrative perspective on discharge planning, which is well described in texts on the subject [1]. This chapter introduces physicians new to neurorehabilitation to the thinking behind discharge planning and illustrates how discharge planning reflects the goals of rehabilitation.

THE ELEMENTS

Neurological Impairments and Functional Status

A major purpose of rehabilitation is to maximize independence through improvements in functional capacity. Neurological impairments due to a nervous system disorder interfere with a patient living independently and being an active member of a community. The rehabilitation team aims to reduce the neurological impairments and teach adaptive techniques to compensate for persistent impairments, in order to increase an individual's capacity for independent living. In discharge planning, the team observes the response to therapy and predicts what level of functional independence will be achieved by the time of discharge.

Cognition

Cognitive impairment may interfere considerably with independent living. The individual with reduced memory may, for example, be unsafe if left alone for even a short period of time or be unable to take medication as directed. Reduced retention of new information and difficulty with problem solving may impede management of financial and legal matters and restrict the patient's community activities and employment.

During the course of neurorehabilitation, the treatment team observes the individual's need for supervision and capacity to make decisions and manage personal affairs. The occupational therapist tests the patient's ability to do tasks such as paying bills, preparing a meal, or shopping at a grocery store. The physical therapist notes whether the patient can learn safe techniques or needs step-by-step reminders during every maneuver. The rehabilitation nurse determines if the patient can remember the medication schedule and dosages. If, despite cognitive therapy, intellectual impairments persist, the team must make a realistic recommendation about how much and what type of supervision and assistance the individual needs.

Communication

Aphasic disorders may affect the individual's safety, learning capacity, and ability to manage personal affairs. Global or severe mixed aphasias lead to dependence in many spheres and prevent the patient from living alone.

Impaired comprehension can have an impact similar to memory impairment by interfering with learning new information, following directions, and participating in decision making. However, the individual who understands one-step commands and simple, self-related, yes–no questions, but whose comprehension fails on multistep directions, may need less supervision than the individual who does not understand even simple questions and instructions.

The individual with good comprehension but impaired verbalization may be capable of functioning quite independently, needing only a nonverbal system for calling for help and assistance with matters requiring verbal or written communication. Speech therapists assess the capacity of the aphasic individual to communicate about basic needs and to call for help in an emergency. They may also evaluate language function necessary for employment or community activities. The discharge plan will reflect impairments of communication, particularly with regard to the patient's safety when alone.

Psychology and Behavior

Disturbances of mood and behavior contribute to functional incapacity and loss of independence, in part by interfering with full participation in the rehabilitation process. These disturbances may be biological effects of the neurological disorder or be psychological reactions to the disabilities caused by the neurological disorder. In planning discharge, a particular concern is the individual's ability to understand or accept physical and cognitive impairments. The inability to understand impairments may lead to unsafe behavior due to overestimation of physical and cognitive capacity. For example, the individual with hemineglect after nondominant hemisphere injury may dismiss advice not to drive. For patients with unsafe behavior, the discharge plan includes supervision by a caregiver and education of the caregiver about the unsafe behavior.

Difficulty in accepting impairments, which, for some, creates a tremendous drive to improve through hard work in therapy, for others contributes to depression, anger, poor cooperation, and lack of motivation. When this bleak mood prevails during the course of rehabilitation, achievable goals are not met and functional capacity stagnates. When depression and denial continue after discharge, the patient and caregivers suffer as functional capacity declines and caregivers are burdened physically and psychologically. If, despite psychiatric treatment during rehabilitation, depression persists until discharge, the caregiver is educated about how to deal with the denial and the discharge plan may include continued psychological counseling for the patient and caregiver and referral to a respite program [2,3].

Mobility

Maximizing mobility is an important goal of rehabilitation. Impairment of any type of mobility, including repositioning in bed, transferring, propelling a wheelchair, walking, and climbing stairs, may reduce independence and increase the amount of help needed from others. Home and community barriers may add to the restriction of mobility caused by neurological impairment. For example, an individual who cannot walk unassisted but operates a wheelchair and transfers independently may live alone in a one-level, wheelchair-accessible residence, while an individual who walks unassisted but needs help with stairs may need help available all day while living in a home with interior and exterior stairs.

The rehabilitation team tailors the mobility program to the individual's physical impairments, while taking into account barriers in the home and community. Discharge planning incorporates the individual's projected mobility at the time of discharge, equipment needs, modification of residence, and training of caregivers to maximize functional mobility.

Self-Care

Achievement of the greatest possible capacity for self-care is another of the important goals of rehabilitation. The neurologically disabled individual who can accomplish without help the familiar morning routine of toileting, bathing, grooming, dressing, preparing breakfast, and cleaning up afterward is highly independent at home and may be mobile and employable in the community, depending on the community's readiness for the disabled.

When an individual needs assistance with these activities of daily living, the reason that help is needed has implications for the whole discharge plan. If physical disability prevents independence, the individual may need assistance for only brief periods of time intermittently during the day but have the cognitive and social skills for employment and an active social life. For example, the individual with hemiparesis after a stroke might need only a few minutes of help each morning with bathing and putting a brace and shoe on the paretic foot. On the other hand, 24 hr a day supervision for safety may be needed if cognitive impairment interferes with independence in daily tasks. This might be true for the person with memory impairment but normal motor function after head trauma who can bathe and dress independently, but forgets to turn off the stove and gets lost in a familiar neighborhood. The individual with bladder and bowel incontinence needs help available 24 hr a day, while the continent individual may need considerably less attention from a caregiver.

During the course of inpatient rehabilitation, the treatment team observes the progress toward independence in activities of daily living and projects the level of independence and types of assistance needed at the time of discharge.

Community Activities

The kind and extent of assistance needed with activities of daily living in the home are informative about the individual's capacity for independence outside the home. In a community accessible to the disabled, an individual with physical but not cognitive disability may have unlimited participation in the community including employment, social activities, education, shopping, and driving or other types of transportation. Although legislation mandating elimination of barriers to public transportation is gradually improving access by the disabled, the automobile remains the primary mode of transportation in many parts of the country. Driving evaluation and training may be important parts of a rehabilitation program for the disabled individual who will need to drive to work, to shop, or to participate in community activities. If the rehabilitation program does not have driving training, the discharge plan can include referral to an outpatient driving program.

Individuals with cognitive impairment and those living in communities with barriers to access by the disabled will need a discharge plan that provides for assistance with the community activities essential for that individual. For most such individuals, this will include help with shopping and transportation to medical appointments. Others may need transportation to school, job training, job, or religious services.

Social and Financial Status

Social and financial factors contribute substantially to the achievement of maximum independence and community integration. Although the rehabilitation team may not be able to alter these factors significantly, the discharge plan reflects the patient's functional capacity in the context of social and financial circumstances.

Caregivers

Most individuals receiving inpatient neurorehabilitation will need at least some help after discharge. Those who will provide this assistance are identified by the social worker and asked to participate in the discharge planning process early, ideally even before the patient is admitted to the rehabilitation service. Usually these caregivers are family members, especially spouse, children, parents, and siblings, or, occasionally, more distant relatives. Sometimes close friends are prepared to become very involved as caregivers. It may be necessary to plan for assistance from professional caregivers, the need for which will depend on the involvement of family or friends and their capacity to provide the kind of assistance required. The assessment of this need is based on information gained by interviewing patient, family, and friends to learn about their willingness and availability, and on training sessions with potential caregivers and patient. The treatment team advises patient and caregiver whether and how to obtain professional caregiver services.

Although family caregivers may be physically capable of providing assistance, such a responsibility often takes a considerable physical and emotional toll on caregivers, the disabled individual, and other family members, especially if there is only one caregiver and the disabled individual needs help with all activities. Just getting out of the house to the bank or grocery store may be difficult, and visiting with friends impossible. The social worker may anticipate this type of stress and give the caregiver information about community services, such as respite care, to provide some relief [2,3].

Health Insurance

The type of health insurance will determine extent of coverage for inpatient and outpatient rehabilitation, equipment, and home care services. The individual with a policy that restricts the number of days of inpatient rehabilitation may reach that limit when progressing steadily toward independence in mobility and activities of daily living, but still needing considerable help. Although the rehabilitation service may sometimes convince the insurance company to extend the stay, if this petition is unsuccessful, the discharge plan will have to reflect the continuing dependence on others for assistance. The timing of discharge cannot be determined solely by the number of insured days of rehabilitation, however. Since discharge should occur only when a safe plan can be implemented, the period of inpatient rehabilitation may have to be extended beyond the period covered by insurance in order for the patient to reach certain functional levels.

Insurance policies, including Medicare, generally provide little coverage for home care services. Medicaid, in some states, covers up to 24 hr per day of care at home, although, with current fiscal constraints, this coverage is being reduced. Uninsured persons who need inpatient rehabilitation will have to pay the cost themselves, which is impossible for all but wealthy individuals, or those who qualify for Medicaid. The individual with health insurance that limits duration of inpatient rehabilitation or does not cover home care services may also need Medicaid. In discharge planning, this need should be identified early, even before the patient's admission to the rehabilitation service, so that the application can be completed and Medicaid coverage approved in time for discharge. It is financially costly for hospitals and emotionally draining for the patient and family to have the hospitalization prolonged while they wait for Medicaid approval.

Many insurance policies, as well as Medicare and Medicaid, cover the cost of equipment such as wheelchairs, canes, and hospital beds, subject to approval after review of a detailed justification prepared by the rehabilitation therapist and physician. Some equipment is usually not covered by insurance policies, including commodes, tub benches, and ramps. When the rehabilitation team determines what equipment to prescribe for a patient, the social worker can consult with the insurance company to establish what equipment will not be covered by the insurance policy so that the patient and family can plan to meet this expense.

Money

The financial position of the neurologically disabled individual may have a significant impact on the discharge plan. Important components of the financial position include disability insurance, personal savings, and income. The need for rehabilitation and the loss of functional independence and employment make neurologically disabling disorders expensive. Health insurance may soften the financial blow of rehabilitation, but personal financial resources bear the impact of long-term functional disability, sometimes leading to dependence on public assistance.

Most people hospitalized for neurological rehabilitation have their employment interrupted long enough to exhaust medical leave and stop receiving income. With information about short- and long-term disability policies and projections about future employability, the social worker can help the patient and family to estimate their financial reserves and future needs. If permanent disability is expected, the patient and family can be advised to apply for Social Security Disability Insurance or Supplemental Security Income.

Residence

Individual homes and multiunit residences usually have physical barriers to access by the neurologically disabled. The rehabilitation treatment team needs a description and measurements of the patient's residence in order to plan the rehabilitation program, order appropriate equipment, recommend modifications in the home, and train caregivers. The description of the patient's home is usually provided by a family member, but on occasion a therapist visits the home before discharge to make measurements and identify ways to improve home safety, such as installation of grab bars in bathrooms and removal of thick rugs.

Employment

When a neurological disorder interrupts employment, the patient may need advice and training from the rehabilitation team before returning to work. The vocational rehabilitation counselor considers physical and cognitive requirements of the job, physical barriers on the job site, type of transportation available, as well as the type of work the disabled individual can be expected to perform. If the neurological disability prevents return to the original occupation, the discharge plan can include referral to the State Office of Vocational Rehabilitation for enrollment in programs such as job training, driving training, job placement, and sheltered workshops.

Community Services

Community services are different in each town, city, county, and state. State and local health departments, special state agencies such as the Office for the

Aging, and religious organizations will provide information about community services. Examples of services that may benefit the disabled include meals delivered to home, door-to-door transportation, and adult day care centers. The rehabilitation team's social worker helps the patient and family to identify services in their community, based on the treatment team's recommendations of services needed.

THE PROCESS

Discharge planning begins before the patient's admission to the rehabilitation service and continues until the time of discharge. The plan is constantly changed and refined as the treatment team learns about the disabled individual and observes his or her progress. From the time an application for admission to the rehabilitation service is received, goals are projected and then modified. The whole team—therapists, nurses, physicians, social workers, utilization review coordinators, and other health care professionals—in collaboration with patient and caregivers contributes to the development of a detailed, individualized, workable discharge plan.

The ideal discharge plan returns the disabled individual to residence and community with services that maximize his or her functional capacities and meet his or her needs. Ideal arrangements are often not possible because of limitations on services due to personal, societal, or financial constraints. The rehabilitation team endeavors to make the best possible plan within these constraints.

Review of Applications

The fundamental question to be answered at this stage is "Will this rehabilitation program be of benefit to the applicant?" In other words, will participation of the applicant in the rehabilitation program result in changes in mobility, self-care, communication, and other abilities that will have a real impact on the individual's functional status and level of independence? In answering this question, it is recognized that the degree of functional change expected will vary from individual to individual and benefit each individual differently. For example, only modest functional improvement combined with appropriate prescription of equipment and proper training of caregivers may make the difference between discharge to home and discharge to a long-term care facility. This can be an enormous benefit for patient and family, both psychologically and financially.

In answering this question, it is also recognized that unstable medical conditions, cognitive and behavioral problems, or social and financial problems may interfere with full participation and maximum benefit from a rehabilitation program. For this reason, the admission screener will want to know the patient's medical diagnoses and treatment, review documentation by the referring hospital's nursing staff and therapists that the applicant is alert and attentive enough to participate in therapy, and learn about potential caregivers, finances, and long-term residential plans. Although a detailed plan for rehabilitation cannot be made at this stage, it is possible to differentiate between those likely to live independently, those who will need some help at home, and those who will probably need care for most or all of the day. Concerning the latter, it is particularly helpful at this stage to start considering with caregivers and the disabled applicant the social and financial planning necessary to provide continuous or nearly continuous care after rehabilitation. The recognition that neurological disabilities or social circumstances will require care in a skilled nursing facility may result in a recommendation for referral to a skilled nursing facility with rehabilitation services instead of admission to an intensive inpatient rehabilitation program.

Setting Goals

At the first encounter with a new patient, each member of the rehabilitation team begins the process of setting goals for the hospitalization and devising an individualized program to achieve them. Each discipline is responsible for assessing certain aspects of function and, based on a detailed evaluation of the patient during the first few days of hospitalization, makes an initial projection of what will be achieved during the hospital stay. An interdisciplinary conference shortly after admission establishes long-term goals of hospitalization that reflect the team's assessment of the patient including the cause, extent, and severity of neurological impairment and the expected rate and degree of neurological recovery and functional improvement. These goals also incorporate the expectations and plans of the patient and caregivers, and data about health insurance, finances, residence, and other elements described above.

   As rehabilitation proceeds, the team observes the patient's progress and revises goals to reflect more precise estimates of the expected functional levels and the time necessary to reach those levels. When progress is slower than initially predicted, the team institutes strategies to improve progress, discusses whether goals can be achieved with a longer period of treatment, and considers setting lower functional levels as goals of the hospital stay. Reviewing progress and revising goals continue throughout the rehabilitation stay.

   The patient and caregivers are informed about and contribute to the setting of goals. It is often helpful for members of the rehabilitation team to have a conference with patient and caregivers early in the hospitalization to review what goals are likely to be realized during inpatient rehabilitation treatment. This discussion of goals may be very difficult when the team projects long-term functional limitations and the disabled individual and family expect full recovery. Informing the patient and family about the process of setting and then revising goals as treatment proceeds offers important reassurance that snap judgments and rigid opinions are not being formed. Including the patient and family in the process by soliciting their observations about progress and conducting patient–caregiver training sessions may help to dispel some of the mistrust and frustration that often occur when hopes for full recovery are disappointed. Psychological counseling may be essential to help the patient and caregivers cope with these disappointments, so that they can participate in making realistic and timely discharge plans.

In light of the patient's functional goals and social and financial circumstances, the rehabilitation team considers what type of living arrangement will be suitable after discharge. Although most disabled individuals return home, some require more help than is available at home, either because they live alone and lack the financial resources to obtain professional help, or because available caregivers cannot provide the necessary care. On occasion, the home is no longer suitable because of barriers such as stairs or because of insufficient space to accommodate caregivers. Some alternatives to home include skilled nursing facilities, adult homes, and housing for the disabled. When the rehabilitation team makes its housing recommendation to the patient and family, the social worker assists them in obtaining suitable housing.

Role of Caregivers

Most neurologically disabled individuals need some assistance from other people after being discharged from a rehabilitation program. Caregivers, usually family members, help the disabled individual further by participating in the discharge planning process. The caregivers provide information about the residence, such as number of stairs, bathroom location, and doorway widths. Based on these data and the recommendations of the treatment team to improve safety and access in the home, the caregivers can undertake these improvements during the rehabilitation period.

Caregivers review health insurance and financial information with the rehabilitation team social worker. Together with the patient they can decide about applications for Medicaid, disability insurance, and other options. Caregivers then do the footwork and paperwork to complete the applications. The caregivers may help the patient or entirely assume responsibility for budgeting the cost of equipment not covered by insurance, hiring a home health aide, and modifying the home. As soon as the treatment team can make confident recommendations about amount of care needed after discharge, home improvements, and other needs, the patient and caregivers can be informed and encouraged to start their work.

When a patient is ready in physical therapy to do caregiver-assisted transfers to toilet and car, caregivers can be trained in these transfers. It is often psychologically beneficial to the disabled individual to take trips out of the rehabilitation hospital some time before being discharged. A trip home for a few hours also serves to enlighten the patient and caregiver about access and safety problems in the home. For example, it may lead to a decision to remove rugs in the living room or to build a ramp to enter the house.

Training of caregivers to help the disabled individual is an important step in preparation for discharge. The caregivers learn from therapists and nurses how to give assistance correctly and safely to encourage independence while avoiding injury. At the time of discharge, the patient trusts the caregivers and the caregivers have confidence in their capacity to provide safe assistance.

Sometimes caregivers or patients overestimate or underestimate the amount of help that will be needed at home. Caregivers fearful of taking the disabled individual home without other help or who doubt the functional independence reported by the treatment team may be reassured by participating in sessions with therapists and patient. When the need for assistance is underestimated, caregiver–patient training sessions may be convincing about the need for professional help at home or even care in a skilled nursing facility. During training the rehabilitation team evaluates the caregiver's capacity to provide care and advises the patient and caregiver about the emotional and physical exhaustion that may result if there is no outside help.

When a caregiver is to be hired to provide home care services, it is preferable to identify that person before the patient is discharged, so that the therapists can train this person as well. This can be especially helpful when the disabled individual needs considerable assistance or when the hired aide is the only caregiver.

Timing of Discharge

Length of stay may be estimated at the time of admission, but unless the health insurance policy strictly limits the number of days of inpatient rehabilitation, day of discharge is set only 1 or 2 weeks in advance. During interdisciplinary conferences when the rehabilitation team reviews progress and sets new goals, the team also estimates the time needed to reach the long-term goals of the inpatient rehabilitation. The accuracy of the estimate increases as the patient nears the goals. Sometimes, progress may exceed expectations, leading to a delay in discharge to permit achieving even greater functional independence than originally planned. As an alternative, if progress slows and some long-term goals become unrealistic, the stay may be shortened. When little or no progress is made over a 2 week period, or progress is made in only one discipline, such as physical therapy, coverage for inpatient rehabilitation will be terminated by most health insurers, including Medicare and Medicaid. Unless discharge planning occurs promptly at that point, the patient may be financially liable for many days of expensive hospitalization. However, discharge can be delayed until a safe discharge plan can be executed [4].

Some rehabilitation programs have developed intensive outpatient programs that provide all but the hotel services of inpatient programs. A disabled individual who lives within commuting distance of the program, has transportation, and has the assistance of family or other caregivers, may prefer to leave the inpatient program long before achieving maximum functional capacity but as soon as caregivers are trained and the residence is accessible.

Preparing for Discharge

In the last week or so of hospitalization, final preparations are made for discharge. Caregivers continue their training and may participate in many aspects of daily care. The social worker advises the patient and caregiver about how to hire a home attendant or contacts the County Social Services Department to arrange for home health care for Medicaid recipients. Referrals are made to appropriate community services. It is often helpful to have a conference with patient, caregivers, and treatment team members to answer questions and to review the patient's functional gains, need for assistance after discharge, and other aspects of the discharge plan.

Therapists prepare prescriptions and order equipment with features specified to meet the requirements of the disabled individual, such as a wheelchair with special seat and back cushions and lapboard. Other special treatments and devices are ordered now, for example, oxygen and suction equipment. Disabled individuals who will be alone for periods of time at home may rent or purchase an emergency notification device such as Medicalert to use in case of a fall out of reach of the telephone.

If the patient understands and can remember the indications for his medications, the nursing staff teaches medication recognition, side effects, dosage and schedule, and the patient gradually assumes responsibility for administering the medications. Diabetic patients review their insulin dosages, one-handed techniques for administration if necessary, and monitoring of glucose levels with finger-stick blood tests.

Usually the treatment team recommends outpatient rehabilitation therapy after discharge. For patients whose progress has slowed but who are expected to continue to improve gradually in a particular discipline, such as occupational therapy, outpatient treatment a few times a week is prescribed to sustain the improvement. Often the team recommends beginning the outpatient rehabilitation in the home if the health insurance policy permits. The patient and caregiver then practice with the therapists on the terrain and among the obstacles of the home, rather than in the large, well-lighted, barrier-free space of the hospital therapy room, which does not simulate most homes.

Before discharge, it is advisable for the patient and caregiver to make arrangements for subsequent medical care. The rehabilitation physician can then provide important medical information to the outpatient physician at the time of discharge to ensure continuity of medical care.

Although the patient and family eagerly anticipate the return home, the adjustment to home life may be difficult. Professional staff are no longer constantly available to provide assistance, answer questions, or solve problems. The disabled individual and caregiver may find daily activities quite exhausting at first despite having received extensive training before discharge. Therapists and professional caregivers coming to the home may fall short of expectations, especially in comparison to the familiar staff of the rehabilitation unit to whom strong attachments persist. If the disabled individual has significant cognitive or behavioral problems, the caregiver may become socially isolated and emotionally exhausted [5]. The rehabilitation team may diminish these problems somewhat by informing the patient and caregiver about what to expect, by remaining available to answer questions, and by scheduling an outpatient visit a few weeks after discharge. Patient and caregiver can be encouraged to join community groups and clubs for the disabled and to resume favorite activities and avocations appropriate to their functional capacity.

REFERENCES

1. P.A. O'Hare and M.A. Terry, *Discharge Planning. Strategies for Assuring Continuity of Care*, Aspen Publishers, Rockville, MD (1988).
2. E.W. Hamm, *Geriatric Nursing*, July/August:188–190 (1991).
3. M.A. Pearson and S.L. Theis, *J. Commun. Health Nursing*, 8:25–31 (1991).
4. J.D. Levesque, *Social Work Health Care*, 13:49–63 (1988).
5. B. Snyder and K. Keefe, *Social Work Health Care*, 10:1–14 (1985).

III
TREATMENT

9

Physical Therapy Philosophies and Strategies

Steven J. Price

Appleton Medical Center, Novus Health Group
Appleton, Wisconsin

Michael J. Reding

Cornell University Medical College
The Winifred Masterson Burke Rehabilitation Hospital, Inc.
White Plains, New York

Physical therapy, along with occupational and speech therapy, is the major treatment prescribed by clinicians in the field of neurorehabilitation. Its goal is to promote recovery of motor functions, and its use in treating disability of neurological origin is generally well accepted.

There are different schools of thought in physical therapy, and each may lead to a different approach to therapeutic exercise. This inevitably leads to areas of controversy, most notably in the rehabilitation of adult hemiplegia, where there is a lack of consensus as to which approach is most effective. This in turn results from a lack of consensus as to how one measures effectiveness. Should one be concerned with the quality of movement, or with the utility of movement?

Physical therapists have traditionally been more concerned with the quality of movement, that is, how closely it approximates normal. One may argue that more normal movement is inherently more functional. One may also argue that "normal" movement is not a realistic expectation.

In some persons with hemiplegia, there is great potential for recovery. This results in an expectation for return of highly organized, normal control of movement. Contrast this with the example of spinal cord injury, after which permanent impairment is expected, and the emphasis of therapy is on teaching alternative means of accomplishing a functional goal; for example, wheelchair propulsion rather than ambulation. In patients with hemiplegia, such compensatory strategies are encouraged by some therapists, and actively and explicitly discouraged by others.

This chapter will focus on the history and current application of these differing philosophies, particularly as they apply to rehabilitation of the hemiplegic patient.

HISTORICAL DEVELOPMENT

The current practice of physical therapy had its origins in the 1940s, 1950s, and 1960s. From 1946 to 1951, Knott and Voss developed the concepts and techniques of proprioceptive neuromuscular facilitation (PNF) [1]. Beginning about this same time, and continuing through the 1960s, Bobath and Brunnstrom were developing their approaches to the hemiplegic patient, resulting in the publication of their respective books in 1970 [2,3]. In the years that followed, an "integrated" approach that combined PNF with techniques from both Bobath and Brunnstrom was described by Sullivan and colleagues [4].

All of these methods have been classified as neurophysiological treatment approaches. They have been differentiated from "conventional" treatment approaches, which address disability by teaching patients to compensate for their neurological deficits. Neurophysiological approaches claim restoration of neurological control, and thus amelioration of the impairment itself, rather than amelioration of disability through the use of compensatory techniques.

After the methods of Bobath and Brunnstrom were published, still another approach was proposed by Carr and Shepherd and published in 1982 [5]. Their method is "neurophysiological" in the sense that the authors imply recovery of neurological control of movement, yet conventional in the sense that the emphasis is on performance of functional tasks, or motor skills.

To date, none of these methods has been proven more effective than the others. The following sections will describe each in greater detail.

PROPRIOCEPTIVE NEUROMUSCULAR FACILITATION

Knott and Voss [1], physical therapists at the California Rehabilitation Center, defined the techniques of PNF as "methods of promoting or hastening the response of the neuromuscular mechanism through stimulation of the proprioceptors." Their methods, as published in 1956, are still taught in physical therapy programs.

PNF is essentially a technique for strengthening groups of muscles. It does not employ functional activities per se, and some may not regard it as a distinct philosophy or approach to physical therapy. It is, however, a well-defined approach to therapeutic exercise, and may be incorporated into many therapeutic programs.

The techniques described by Knott and Voss use mass movement patterns, which, they determined, are always spiral and diagonal. Physiological groups of muscles are activated, and "overflow" may allow stronger muscles to assist weaker muscles in producing movement. This, in turn, allows strengthening through repetition.

The "spiral and diagonal" pattern is the basis of PNF. This pattern of movement can be applied to the limbs, neck, or trunk.

As an example, consider the technique recommended for the upper extremity. The extremity (shoulder, elbow, and wrist) is placed in extension, abduction, and internal rotation. It is then moved through flexion, adduction, and external rotation, aided as necessary by the therapist (see Figure 1). The starting position, with the arm rotated and diagonally extended from the body, places the flexors at their greatest length, allowing for greatest mechanical advantage. The position at finish can be used as the starting point for strengthening extensors.

Additional key components of PNF include the techniques of "slow reversal" and "rhythmic stabilization." These techniques were developed when Knott and Voss discovered that activation of antagonist muscle groups seemed to augment or facilitate the response of the agonist groups. "Slow reversal" uses sequential iso*tonic* contractions of the agonist and antagonist muscle groups, and "rhythmic stabilization" uses simultaneous iso*metric* contractions.

To illustrate these techniques with the example given above, the therapist would place the patient's arm in internal rotation and extension. She would then help the patient to flex his arm. She may add the technique of slow reversal by asking the patient first to flex his arm, then extend his arm against her resistance, then switch back to flexion. She may also employ rhythmic stabilization by asking the patient to hold his arm still while she applies resistance in either direction. The therapist thus attempts to elicit first alternating activation, and then coactivation, of the agonist group and its antagonists in an effort to stimulate a stronger response in the upper-extremity flexors.

The reader is encouraged to refer to Knott and Voss's text for further discussion. A tabular summary of these PNF techniques and others can be found in their book.

NEURODEVELOPMENTAL TREATMENT (BOBATH)

The neurodevelopmental treatment approach, commonly referred to as NDT or "Bobath," is based entirely on the philosophy of Berta Bobath and her husband, Dr. Karel Bobath. It evolved from her experience as a physical therapist at the Western Cerebral Palsy Center in London beginning in the 1940s. It is perceived as a rigorous method through which the patient is

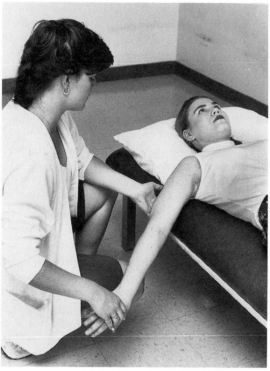

(a)

Figure 1   An example of the spiral and diagonal pattern of PNF applied to the upper extremity. (a) The patient's arm is first placed in extension, abduction, and internal rotation. (b and c) It is then moved through flexion, adduction, and external rotation.

helped to proceed through "normal" developmental motor milestones. NDT is now taught through courses that offer additional certification to physical therapists, and is regarded as the treatment of choice for children with neurological disability.

Mrs. Bobath applied her knowledge and experience to the adult patient with hemiplegia, and her book devoted to this topic was published in 1970 [2], with a second edition in 1978 [6]. In the preface to the second edition, she writes "the treatment process has been enlarged and elaborated, and a more functional application of treatment has been evolved." Nonetheless, the Bobath approach to adult hemiplegia remains the epitome of emphasizing quality over utility.

Bobath based her approach to hemiplegia on the assumption that "spasticity is caused by the release of an abnormal postural reflex mechanism." Bobath put forth this view after considering contemporary physiology,

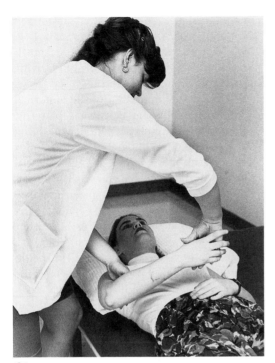

(b)

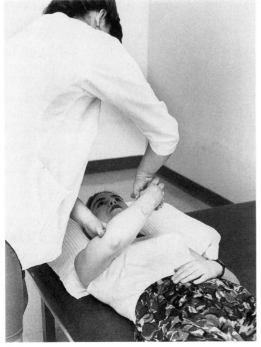

(c)

including the work of Sherrington, Magnus, and Twitchell. She acknowledged that the approach was developed empirically, and the underlying
theory was developed "as a working hypothesis to explain the observed facts."

Based on this theory, Bobath emphasizes inhibition of the abnormal
reflex patterns, and facilitation of normal, volitional movement patterns.
Bobath suggests that proper handling of the hemiplegic patient will direct
such patterns "into the channels of the higher integrated and complex
patterns of more normal coordination." Again, there is a belief in the potential
for *neurological* recovery. Bobath writes "Experience has shown that there is
in every patient some untapped potential for more highly organized activity."

How is this philosophy applied in the clinical setting? Assessment of the
patient with hemiplegia emphasizes analysis of motor patterns and reflex
responses, rather than weakness (weakness or paralysis is considered a
consequence of deficient postural reflex patterns). Proper assessment should
generate a list of missing or inadequate normal motor patterns, and a list of the
interfering, abnormal patterns.

Treatment is then planned to restore (facilitate) the normal patterns, and
to eliminate the *ab*normal patterns. Exercises that take advantage of overflow,
associated reactions, synergy, or any "pathological" reflex or pattern, are
strictly avoided. In NDT, such methods are viewed as a cause of spasticity,
and are believed to interfere with recovery.

The resulting exercises are intended to put the patient through "reflex-
inhibiting movement patterns" with the twofold purpose of suppressing
spasticity and facilitating normal voluntary movement. These exercises are
guided and assisted by the therapist from "key points of control," usually
proximal locations believed to have the most influence on the overall pattern
and spasticity (Figure 2).

Specific therapeutic exercises depend on whether the patient's hemiplegia is flaccid, spastic, or resolving with relative recovery. Treatment in the
flaccid stage consists largely of positioning and activities intended to prepare the patient for sitting, standing, and ambulation. (When NDT was
originally applied to hemiplegic adults, treatment required a progression
through a "developmental" sequence: rolling before sitting before kneeling
before standing before walking. This is still followed by some practitioners.)
As tone returns, treatment begins to incorporate activities carried out while
the patient is sitting or standing. If spasticity interferes, it is viewed as a
consequence of abnormal postural reflexes. The therapist must inhibit these
reflexes, or defer the activity involved until the patient is better prepared.

The goal of treatment is a normal quality of gait and upper extremity
movement. Emphasis is placed on bearing weight and using the extremities
on the affected side to prevent learning to compensate with the intact side.
As gait training begins, walking is accomplished with the aid of the therapist
but *without* devices or bracing, encouraging the patient to bear weight and
walk symmetrically.

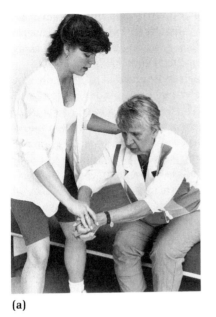 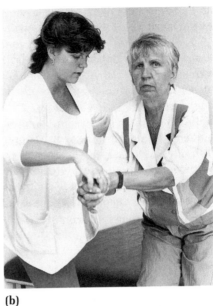

(a)   (b)

Figure 2   The therapist assists this patient with a right hemiparesis in a sit-to-stand transfer, using NDT techniques. Note the hands-on guidance from "key points of control," encouraging the patient to bear weight on the involved side and inhibiting associated reactions (i.e., flexion) of the upper extremity.

The philosophy of NDT is summarized in Berta Bobath's statement that "it must always be remembered that the aim of this type of treatment is to improve the quality of movement on the affected side." The application of this philosophy is summarized by her statement that "In order to prepare for a reasonably normal gait, balance, stance, and weight transfer should be practiced. If all this is first practised while in the standing position, [the patient] will develop a better walking pattern than if he is made to walk immediately without the necessary control of his leg."

BRUNNSTROM'S APPROACH

Signe Brunnstrom's [3] approach to the hemiplegic patient is in many ways the antithesis of Bobath's approach. Brunnstrom recommends and indeed emphasizes the use of mass movement patterns, called synergies, to develop movement, strength, and function. She developed her philosophy during the 1950s and 1960s while an instructor of physical therapy at Columbia University, working specifically with patients who had sustained hemiplegic stroke.

Brunnstrom, like Bobath, proposed a theoretical basis for her approach after reviewing the literature on physiology. She concluded that "the basic limb synergies of hemiplegic patients are primitive spinal cord patterns which have been retained throughout the evolutionary process." She further reasoned that these so-called pathological movement patterns are in fact normal patterns, which are released or exaggerated in the presence of injury to higher neurological centers.

Brunnstrom was also aware of the nascent controversy in her field. She acknowledged the opposing point of view that no pathological movements or patterns should be utilized in therapy, since they will ultimately interfere with recovery of normal movement. She then argued that "Far from preventing further improvement, the synergies appear to constitute a necessary intermediate stage for further recovery," citing Twitchell's work [7] to support her argument. On this basis she developed her rationale for therapeutic exercise in patients with hemiplegia.

In outlining her strategy, Brunnstrom classifies the process of recovery from stroke into six stages. Therapeutic exercises are then recommended for each stage. Stage I, when present, occurs immediately following the stroke and is essentially the period of flaccid paralysis. Stage II begins with the development of movements in a pattern of synergy, usually flexor, and the emergence of spasticity (Figure 3). Stage III indicates voluntary activation of the limb synergies sufficient to produce movement across joints, and spasticity may become more prominent (Figure 4). Stage III may be the point of maximal recovery for patients who are more severely affected. Stage IV begins when the spasticity begins to decrease and the patient is able to initiate movements outside the flexion and extension patterns of synergy. In other words, the patient is now able to activate a single muscle or joint "in isolation" from the physiological group of muscles that produces a mass movement pattern (Figure 5). Stage V indicates developing control of individual or isolated movements, and stage VI suggests a return to near-normal control of the affected limb(s).

Recommended exercises for the leg, hand, and arm are described in detail for each stage of recovery. Brunnstrom's "training procedures" begin with proper positioning in bed, and move quickly to head and trunk control in the sitting position. As the patient progresses to stage II, exercises are intended to aid the patient in voluntary initiation and control of synergistic movement patterns. If the patient continues to improve, exercises shift toward more skilled "isolated" movements (as in Figure 5).

Unlike Bobath, Brunnstrom regards weakness as a problem in and of itself, and encourages exercises for strengthening: activation of the upper extremity flexor synergy pattern to strengthen the biceps, or forcefully activating muscles on the *intact* side to augment muscle activation on the paretic side (as in Figure 4), thus taking advantage of mass movement patterns and associated reactions. Like Bobath, Brunnstrom recommended that walk-

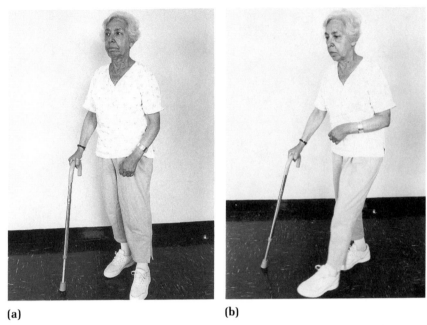

(a)   (b)

Figure 3   Patient with a left hemiparesis demonstrates a component of Brunn-strom's stage II of recovery. The elbow flexion component of the upper extremity flexor synergy pattern appears as an associated reflex or response to the effort of walking.

ing should be delayed and that time be devoted to preparation for walking, so that patients will not learn an unsatisfactory gait pattern before becoming capable of a more normal gait.

THE "MOTOR RELEARNING" APPROACH

The current trend in physical therapy of the adult hemiplegic patient is based on the rationale and techniques advocated by Carr and Shepherd, as a *Motor Relearning Programme for Stroke*, first published in 1982 [5]. Their approach departs from the previous "neurophysiological" techniques, shifting the emphasis from exercise and facilitation to learning and practice of specific functional skills.

Carr and Shepherd have applied contemporary theories of learning and acquiring motor skills to the process of recovery in brain-injured adults [8]. In so doing, they attribute that process to "reorganization and adaptation" within the brain. Whether this is accurate or not (recent evidence supports

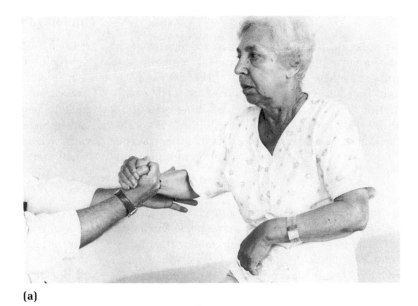

(a)

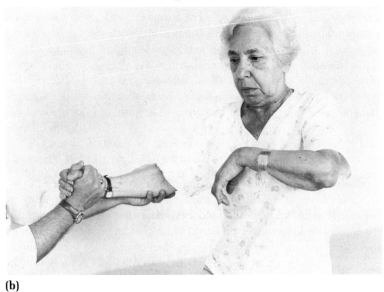

(b)

Figure 4   The same patient as in Figure 3 demonstrates the upper extremity flexor synergy pattern of Brunnstrom's stage III of recovery. (a) She is able to initiate flexion of the left elbow. (b) Then, by pulling forcefully with her intact right arm, she can utilize the associated reaction of the left arm to enhance abduction of the shoulder. Spasticity of the pronators prevents development of the full pattern with supination of the forearm.

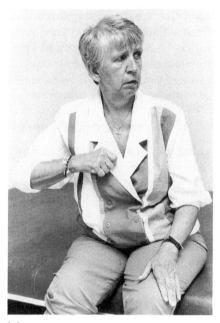

(a)

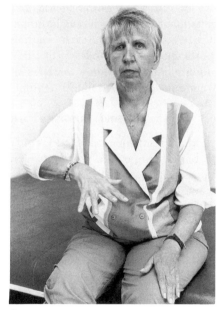

(b)

Figure 5 (a) This patient with right hemiparesis lifts her arm in a pattern of flexor synergy. (b) She then extends her fingers in isolation from the synergy pattern.

this assertion in at least one type of stroke [9]), their application of learning theory is reasonable and deserving of further discussion.

The Motor Relearning Programme (MRP) begins with the concept that the ability to carry out any useful or functional physical task is essentially a motor skill. The MRP then assumes that factors normally useful in learning a motor skill are essential in learning, or relearning, such skills after a stroke. Four such factors are explicitly stated: "elimination of unnecessary muscle activity, feedback, practice, and the interrelationship between postural adjustment and movement."

Unnecessary muscle activity and its elimination assumes particular importance in the philosophy of the MRP, because the authors believe it is a major cause of abnormal muscle tone and spasticity. Thus patients are encouraged to learn to control activation of specific muscles needed for a task, and to avoid activation of muscles not directly involved. This concept directly contradicts the Brunnstrom approach of utilizing mass movement patterns, or synergies. Furthermore, the MRP discourages strengthening per se, since this requires activation of muscles outside the context of a specific task, encourages unnecessary muscle activity, and consequently results in abnormal tone.

The principles of feedback and practice, while straightforward, require an additional comment or two. Feedback should be, in the opinion of Carr and Shepherd, provided primarily through verbal and visual means, not through somatosensory (i.e., proprioceptive and tactile) means as has been historically emphasized. Practice should be "task specific," not simply a movement or exercise that the patient is expected to generalize into a variety of day-to-day activities. Also, practice (and the rehabilitation program in general) should not include compensatory techniques, since the patient may learn "nonuse" of the affected limbs. As an example, Carr and Shepherd suggest that patients should not walk with a quad cane, since they may learn to *not* bear weight on the affected leg, and thus they may never learn to walk without a cane.

The concept of postural adjustments to gravity can be summarized by the statement that "Balance training should . . . not be considered as separate from training of everyday tasks." Under normal circumstances, postural adjustments occur automatically and often in anticipation of movement. As a consequence, postural or balance training cannot be effective if it only entails reacting to perturbations. Again, balance training should be task-specific: balance in sitting does not necessarily improve balance in standing.

In applying these principles, the MRP classifies therapeutic exercise into seven categories: upper limb function; orofacial function; motor tasks performed while sitting, standing up, sitting down; motor tasks performed while standing; and walking. For each activity, a four-step plan is followed: the therapist analyzes the patient's performance of the chosen task, explains or demonstrates the goal to be accomplished and guides the patient in practicing "missing components" of the task, instructs the patient in performing and practicing the task as a whole, and encourages the patient to practice the task throughout the day, and not just in therapy. In steps two and three, practice and verbal and visual feedback are emphasized.

The authors of the MRP recommend no specific order or progression through the seven sections, suggesting instead that activities be chosen from any or all of the sections for each treatment session. They maintain that practice must be task-specific, and that patients do not learn by progressing through a series of steps, because each step requires learning a new skill; for example, walking with a walker is a different skill from walking with a cane. Furthermore, they suggest that each treatment session should include a number of goals that challenge the patient yet can be reached within that session. In contrast to Bobath, and, to some degree Brunnstrom, Carr and Shepherd argue that the primary treatment "technique" employed by the therapist should be a thorough explanation of the task and goal, followed by verbal and visual feedback, rather than hands-on manipulation and facilitation.

BIOFEEDBACK AND FUNCTIONAL ELECTRIC STIMULATION

Unlike the philosophies discussed above, biofeedback is not a complete approach to rehabilitation of the hemiplegic patient. However, it is a technique about which much has been written, and a few words are in order here. The history and application of electromyographic (EMG) biofeedback have been reviewed elsewhere [10].

Biofeedback simply serves as a method of providing feedback in addition to somatosensory, visual, and verbal sources, although it also requires visual and/or auditory processing on the part of the patient. Its theoretical advantage is the potential for greater sensitivity. In the model proposed by Bach-y-Rita, it is intended to improve the signal-to-noise ratio in the information the patient is receiving [11]. It may also provide additional motivation for some patients [12].

Although early reports on biofeedback were encouraging, a later review and a subsequent, well-designed study by Basmajian and colleagues report no statistically significant benefit from the addition of EMG biofeedback to more traditional therapeutic exercise [12,13]. These later studies demonstrate functional gains in patients receiving either type of therapy. Some earlier studies also suggest that patients 1 year or more after stroke may benefit from reinstitution of physical therapy with or without EMG techniques [14,15].

Functional electrical stimulation (FES) may also be viewed as an adjunct to therapeutic exercise. It has not been shown to improve function in hemiplegic patients, although Cozean reports an improvement in velocity of gait when FES is used with biofeedback [16].

FES may have a role in the rehabilitation of patients with spinal cord injury. One factor limiting its use with hemiplegic patients is the discomfort of the electrical stimulus. It may be better tolerated by patients with sensory deficits due to spinal cord injury, although further study of its physiological and functional effects is needed.

SUMMARY AND DISCUSSION

Each of the therapeutic strategies discussed here has its proponents and, indeed, zealous advocates. However, none of these nor any other approach has been proven more effective than the others in any of the published comparisons [13,17–20].

Stern and McDowell [17] compared conventional therapy with techniques based on PNF and Brunnstrom. The study is a partly randomized, unblinded comparison of 2 groups of 31 patients with hemispheric infarcts, treated for 8–9 weeks. Dickstein et al. [18] compared conventional treatment, PNF, and NDT. They assigned subjects to one of the three treatment groups by "administrative procedures of the hospital," and thus considered them essentially randomized. The study is not blinded since function was assessed by the physical therapist treating the patient. Of 196 consecutive hemiplegic patients, 131 completed the 6 week treatment program. Neither study found any significant difference between groups.

Basmajian et al. [13] performed a blinded study comparing a program including EMG biofeedback with NDT. Twenty-nine outpatients meeting strict criteria, including an infarct in the middle cerebral artery territory, were randomized and treated for 5 weeks. Only upper extremity function was studied, and again no significant difference was found.

Ernst reviewed the relevant literature through 1989 [19]. He concluded that "stroke rehabilitation is preferable to spontaneous recovery," but the optimal type of therapy had not yet been determined. One subsequent study deserves comment here. Wagenaar and colleagues considered that different stroke types and other variables among patients might confound the effects of an intervention. They studied seven patients using a single case experimental design [20]. Each patient served as his own control, alternating NDT and Brunnstrom methods every 5 weeks for a total of 20 weeks. The authors report that one patient showed more progress in walking speed with Brunnstrom's methods. There was no difference in functional improvement as measured by the Barthel index. The other six patients experienced no difference in recovery during the different treatment periods.

It may be argued that none of the studies conducted to date is ideally designed. It is now clear that a simple clinical classification of strokes results in predictable differences in outcome, and perhaps what is needed is a case-matched, controlled study utilizing this classification [21,22].

In the absence of such a study, the approach used in most centers depends upon the preference of the individual therapist. An integrated approach, in which the therapist may draw from any or all of the different philosophies, is perhaps the most common. It is supported by the rationale that this approach allows an individualized program for each patient. Furthermore, application of any of these strategies in the pure form would require the cooperation of at least the occupational as well as the physical therapists, and ideally the nursing staff as well. Each of the philosophies discussed above addresses therapeutic approaches and exercises for the upper extremity. In many centers, rehabilitation of the upper extremity and related functional skills, such as activities of daily living, is primarily the role of the occupational therapist.

Perhaps medical factors should be considered by the therapist, and by the physician, in resolving the problem of which therapeutic approach to take. The risk of venous thromboembolism can be significantly reduced by early ambulation. A 12-fold reduction in risk has been demonstrated in patients who are ambulating when compared to patients who are at mat level or pregait activities. This reduction occurred irrespective of the amount of assistance provided by the therapist, the use of assistive devices, and the use of bracing [23].

Thus, in the absence of any data demonstrating the superiority of any single approach over the others, early ambulation, with whatever assistance is necessary, can be considered a reasonable approach.

REFERENCES

1. M. Knott and D.E. Voss, *Proprioceptive Neuromuscular Facilitation: Patterns and Techniques*, Harper & Row, New York (1956).
2. B. Bobath, *Adult Hemiplegia: Evaluation and Treatment*, William Heinemann Medical Books, London (1970).
3. S. Brunnstrom, *Movement Therapy in Hemiplegia: A Neurophysiological Approach*, Harper & Row, Philadelphia (1970).
4. P.E. Sullivan, P.D. Markos, and M.A.D. Minor, *An Integrated Approach to Therapeutic Exercise*, Reston Publishing Company, Reston, CA (1982).
5. J.H. Carr and R.B. Shepherd, *A Motor Relearning Programme for Stroke*, William Heinemann Medical Books, London (1982).
6. B. Bobath, *Adult Hemiplegia: Evaluation and Treatment*, William Heinemann Medical Books, London (1978).
7. T.E. Twitchell, *Brain*, 74:443–480 (1951).
8. J.H. Carr and R.B. Shepherd, *A Motor Relearning Programme for Stroke*, William Heinemann Medical Books, London (1987).
9. C. Weiller, F. Chollet, K.J. Friston, R.J.S. Wise, and R.S.J. Frackowiak, *Ann. Neurol.*, 31:463–472 (1992).
10. J.V. Basmajian, *Arch. Phys. Med. Rehab.*, 62:469–475 (1981).

11. P. Bach-y-Rita and R. Balliet, *Motor Deficits Following Stroke* (P.W. Duncan and M.B. Badke, eds.), Year Book Publishers, New York, pp. 79–107 (1987).
12. P.M. Marzuk, *Ann. Intern. Med.*, *102*:854–858 (1985).
13. J.V. Basmajian, C.A. Gowland, A.J. Finlayson, A.L. Hall, L.R. Swanson, P.W. Stratford, J.E. Trotter, and M.E. Branstater, *Arch. Phys. Med. Rehab.*, *68*:267–272 (1987).
14. S.A. Binder, C.B. Moll, and S.L. Wolf, *Phys. Ther.*, *61*:886–891 (1981).
15. J. Inglis, M.W. Donald, T.N. Monga, M. Sproule, and M.J. Young, *Arch. Phys. Med. Rehab.*, *65*:755–759 (1984).
16. C.D. Cozean, W.S. Pease, and S.L. Hubbell, *Arch. Phys. Med. Rehab.*, *69*:401–405 (1988).
17. H.P. Stern, F. McDowell, J.M. Miller, and M. Robinson, *Arch. Phys. Med. Rehab.*, *51*:526–531 (1970).
18. R. Dickstein, S. Hocherman, T. Pillar, and R. Shaham, *Phys. Ther.*, *66*:1233–1238 (1986).
19. E. Ernst, *Stroke*, *21*:1081–1085 (1990).
20. R.C. Wagenaar, O.G. Meijer, P.C.W. van Wieringen, D.J. Kuik, G.J. Hazenberg, J. Lindeboom, F. Wichers, and H. Rijswijk, *Scand. J. Rehab. Med.*, *22*:1–8 (1990).
21. M.J. Reding and E. Potes, *Stroke*, *19*:1354–1358 (1988).
22. M.J. Reding, *Stroke*, *21*(suppl. II):II-35–37 (1990).
23. E.B. Bromfield and M.J. Reding, *J. Neuro Rehab.*, *2*:51–57 (1988).

10
Treatment of Spasticity

Peter W. Rossi

Rehabilitation Hospital of South Texas
Corpus Christi, and
University of Texas at San Antonio Health Science Center
San Antonio, Texas

INTRODUCTION AND TREATMENT GOALS

Spasticity is one of the most common problems faced by the specialist in neurological rehabilitation. It is the hallmark of disease in upper motor pathways and thus a prominent clinical manifestation of a variety of illnesses affecting the neuraxis: stroke, traumatic brain injury, multiple sclerosis, spinal cord injury, and cerebral palsy, among others. These illnesses vary widely in their pathological nature and anatomical predilection and are often nonselective by damaging both ascending and descending pathways as well as cell bodies [1]. Accordingly, a strict physiological definition of spasticity may not encompass all that the bedside clinician recognizes as spasticity.

Spasticity has been defined as "a motor disorder characterized by a velocity dependent increase in tonic stretch reflexes (muscle tone) with exaggerated tendon jerks, resulting from hyperexcitability of the stretch reflex, as one component of the upper motor neuron syndrome" [2]. In clinical parlance, spasticity is synonymous with "the upper motor neuron syndrome." This syndrome is characterized by symptoms termed "negative" because they represent a decrease in motor performance or "positive" in that they produce an increase in abnormal motor function. Negative symptoms include weakness, fatigability, decreased dexterity, and a lack of isolated movement in an extremity. Examples of positive symptoms are hypertonicity, heightened deep tendon and cutaneous reflexes, dystonic rigidity, and flexor spasms [1]. Flexor spasms are a particular concern because they are painful, forceful contractions at several joints in an extremity that can be precipitated by noxious stimuli including bowel or bladder distention, urinary tract infection, and bed sores.

It is important to differentiate spasticity from other conditions that alter the resistance of muscles to stretch [3]. Contracture, fibrosis, and ankylosis of joints represent fixed limitations in movement. Primary dystonias may cause alterations in muscle tone unaccompanied by hyperexcitability of the stretch reflex and are treated differently. Parkinsonian rigidity is recognized by the other clinical accompaniments of this disorder including cogwheel resistance to passive movement, which is not present in spasticity. Muscle cramps and spasms may be present in normal individuals or may represent manifestations of metabolic, neuropathic, or myopathic disorders.

In general, the negative symptoms of weakness and fatigability are not directly treatable and there is little evidence that patients develop increased strength or dexterity when heightened muscle tone and excitability of muscle reflexes are reduced [4]. Therapy for spasticity usually addresses the positive symptoms of abnormal posturing or discomfort induced by spasm, clonus, and muscle stiffness. Treatment goals must consider how an individual's spasticity affects his or her lifestyle, daily function, comfort, and appearance. For example, spasticity may interfere with positioning, transfers, and a patient's mobility in bed. Spasticity may make the daily tasks of dressing, bathing, and toileting extremely difficult. Left untreated, spasticity may lead to secondary complications of falls, fractures, bed sores, and interrupted sleep.

Spasticity may occasionally be beneficial to the functional needs of individual patients. For example, the paraplegic may rely upon his or her spasticity for proper positioning of the lower extremities or as an aid in withdrawing the lower extremities from noxious stimuli. Flexor spasms in the lower extremity may assist circulation and decrease the risk of thrombophlebitis. Spasticity may also help maintain muscle bulk and prevent bone demineralization. For the patient with hemiplegia, a spastic lower extremity may be needed for weight bearing during stance and ambulation. In the quadriplegic patient, intercostal spasticity may help to reduce paradoxical breathing [5].

A detailed history is therefore essential before one undertakes the treatment of spasticity. During the interview, questions should explore how a patient's spasticity interferes with his or her daily life. It is important to ascertain the precipitating factors for flexor or extensor spasms, their frequency, and diurnal variation. Examination should address the degree of hypertonicity and the resistance of an extremity to passive manipulation. The Ashworth scale is a simple and reproducible numerical scale that can help

Table 1 Ashworth Scale [6]

Score	Findings
0	No increase in tone
1	Slight increase in tone giving a "catch" when the limb was moved in flexion or extension
2	More marked increase in tone, but limb easily flexed
3	Considerable increase in tone: passive movement difficult
4	Limb rigid in flexion or extension

quantify spasticity for comparison with previous examinations [6] (see Table 1). Examination of the motor system also includes determination of muscle strength, dexterity, and fatigability, a search for hyperexcitable deep tendon reflexes and clonus, and the detection of abnormal cutaneous reflexes and flexor spasms. The patient should be observed during functional tasks such as rolling or turning in bed, transferring, attempting to stand and ambulate to determine how spasticity interferes with these tasks. Treatment goals should be directed to the functional needs of the patient, not simply to the physiological manifestations of spasticity.

PATHOPHYSIOLOGY OF SPASTICITY

The hallmark of clinical spasticity is increased resistance to passive flexion or extension of an extremity in patients with upper motor neuron lesions [7]. This increased resistance to passive movement is due to activation of muscle stretch reflexes that exist in a state of heightened central excitability due to a decrease in descending suprasegmental inhibitory influences. This was first postulated by Landau and Clare in 1964 and it continues to be supported by experimental findings [8].

Two types of stretch reflexes are identified: phasic and tonic. Phasic stretch reflexes are responsible for the heightened deep tendon reflexes, clonus, and "clasp knife" phenomenon commonly associated with spasticity. They are produced by rapid changes in muscle length and they quickly extinguish. Phasic stretch reflexes are both dependent on both velocity and length. In contrast, tonic stretch reflexes are represented clinically by heightened muscle tone and can be produced by both rapid and slow movements. Tonic stretch reflexes produce an increased resistance to movement that is sustained as long as muscle stretch persists [3,5]. Also, spasticity is associated with heightened cutaneous muscular reflexes that present clinically as flexor spasms: involuntary, forceful contractions of flexor muscle groups present most commonly in patients with spinal cord injuries [9]. They can be precipitated by a variety of noxious stimuli and may be accompanied by bowel and bladder evacuation [10]. Flexor spasms are often disturbing to the patient and may be major obstacles to reaching rehabilitation goals.

Familiarity with the anatomy and synaptic pharmacology of the spinal cord is essential to an understanding of most therapeutic strategies for spasticity. The alpha motor neuron and its peripheral extensions to muscle represent the "final common pathway" for motor control, as first suggested by Sherrington. Each alpha motor neuron receives a variety of inhibitory and excitatory influences from both segmental and suprasegmental levels. The balance and temporal summation of these influences act to determine the level of alpha motor neuron membrane polarization and, ultimately, whether the neuron discharges. Each neuronal discharge travels through the cell axon, and produces contraction of muscle fibers through chemical transmission across the neuromuscular junction. At high rates of neuronal discharge (20–30 Hz), muscle contraction increases and eventually becomes tetanic. The interplay of descending voluntary control and reflex segmental and suprasegmental influences determines the rich variety of movement possible in the normal individual. Abnormalities in one or several of these influences can result in alpha motor neuron excitability and clinical spasticity. Information from a suprasegmental level is conveyed in four main tracts. The corticospinal tract is responsible for voluntary control of movement and allows for finely coordinated movements in the extremities. In addition, it provides inhibitory influences to antigravity muscles of the trunk and limb girdles. The rubrospinal tract is similar in function to the cortical spinal tract but is vestigial in humans. The pontine reticulospinal tract provides descending excitatory influence on the alpha motor neuron, whereas the medullary reticulospinal tract is inhibitory to muscle tone. The vestibulospinal tract is responsible for the maintenance of tone in antigravity musculature. All tracts synapse directly on the alpha motor neuron and indirectly through spinal interneurons of the internuncial pool [10–12].

The alpha motor neuron receives information from the periphery as well as from central levels. This information originates from tiny muscle spindles distributed throughout muscle tissue. Muscle spindles respond to changes in muscle length and rate of stretch. Impulses are generated that are conveyed to the upper motor neuron in the ventral horn of the spinal cord by rapidly conducting large myelinated fibers, group Ia and II afferent fibers [10,13] (see Figure 1). Group Ia afferents synapse directly on the upper motor neuron after entering the cord via the dorsal roots. When muscle is stretched, as in percussion of the muscle tendon, group Ia afferents discharge and excite alpha motor neurons causing them to fire and produce reflex muscle contraction. Collateral branches of the Ia afferent travel to the dorsal horn to synapse

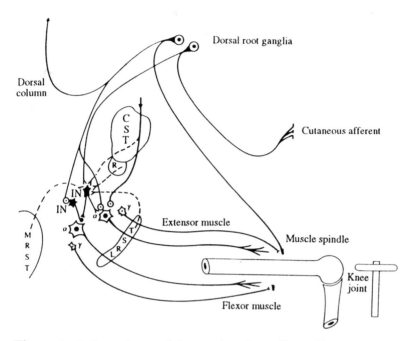

Figure 1 Reflex pathways of the spinal cord. Ia afferent fibers arising in muscle spindles of extensor muscles are activated by tendon tap. The excitatory Ia synapse (open circle) excites the extensor motor neuron (α), which fires reflexly, contracting the muscle. Simultaneously, the Ia fiber excites an interneuron (IN: black) with inhibitory synapses (filled circles) on antagonist flexor motor neurons. Interneurons of the internuncial pool mediate polysynaptic effects of descending tracts, including presynaptic inhibition (filled triangles). Other abbreviations are γ: gamma motor neuron; CST: corticospinal tract; R: rubrospinal tract; LRST: lateral reticulospinal tract; MRST: medial reticulospinal tract (including the vestibulospinal tract) (reprinted with permission from [10]).

on inhibitory neurons, which, in turn synapse on the alpha motor neuron of antagonist muscles and inhibit their contraction. This mechanism is responsible for phasic stretch reflexes.

Group II spindle afferents respond to static muscle length. They synapse on spinal interneurons. The "clasp knife" phenomenon most likely is mediated by group II afferents, which discharge at a critical degree of muscle stretch and provide sudden inhibition of alpha motor neuron output and a sudden loss of resistance [14]. Tonic stretch reflexes result from polysynaptic reflex pathways in the spinal cord generated by group II afferent fibers [10].

Muscle spindles respond to changes in muscle strength by adjusting their tension through the action of gamma motor neurons that synapse on muscle spindle fibers. The degree of muscle spindle tension is thereby adjusted to the level of muscle stretch at any given moment. This provides a regulatory gain on the motor system. These reflex pathways constitute a neuronal system designed to maintain the length of muscle and provide certain stereotyped motor behaviors.

The motor system utilizes a variety of substances for neurotransmission. Motor neurons release acetylcholine at neuromuscular synaptic terminals, producing membrane depolarization, calcium release, and muscle contraction. In the central nervous system both excitatory and inhibitory substances mediate neuronal transmission. Excitatory neurotransmitters include glutamate, aspartate, and substance P. Glutamate is the neurotransmitter utilized by the descending corticospinal tract. Aspartate provides excitatory influences between spinal interneuronal networks. Substance P is localized in small afferent fibers that mediate pain. Inhibitory neurotransmitters within the spinal cord include gamma aminobutyric acid (GABA) and glycine. Spinal interneurons and inhibitory descending motor systems utilize both GABA and glycine to provide hyperpolarization of the alpha motor neuron membrane. In particular, GABA is the neurotransmitter responsible for synaptic inhibition of the Ia afferents by spinal interneurons [15]. Although at first it was tempting to conclude that enhanced muscle spindle afferent activity was responsible for the clinical aspects of spasticity, this is not the case. Microneurographic recordings have failed to reveal muscle spindle hyperactivity [16]. Instead, it appears that heightened central excitability and, in particular, diminished presynaptic inhibition of Ia afferents by GABA, is responsible for spasticity. No evidence exists that decreased recurrent Renshaw inhibition or inhibition from group Ib or II afferents is present in spastic patients [17].

TREATMENT OF SPASTICITY: GENERAL PRINCIPLES

The clinician should have specific goals in mind when deciding to treat spasticity. Therapeutic goals may include improving functional abilities, avoiding complications such as bed sores or contractures, or improving hygiene or cosmesis. Weakness, an invariate and disabling feature of the upper motor neuron syndrome, is not improved by the treatment of spasticity. This important clinical point is sometimes forgotten. Indeed, some treatments for spasticity, such as utilization of dantrolene or nerve blocks, will increase weakness.

Therapy for spasticity should begin with treatments that are conservative, noninvasive, and specific for the muscle groups in question. Only when these are proven ineffective should more aggressive therapies be undertaken that may be irreversible or carry a high risk of morbidity. As always, informed consent should be obtained from the patient and family before one begins a spasticity treatment program. Patients should understand what benefit is hoped from a particular therapy and how to recognize complications that may arise.

For our discussion, the treatment of spasticity is classified into the following categories: general nursing management and physiotherapy; pharmacological treatment; nerve blocks and motor point blocks; surgical treatment of spasticity; and experimental therapies.

Nursing Management and Physiotherapy

The initial management of all patients with spasticity should involve the reduction of painful stimuli that may worsen spasticity and the institution of a daily stretching program that can help maintain joint, muscle, and tendon pliability and range of motion. The reduction of pain is essential to reducing spasticity and may, by itself, be adequate treatment for many patients. When confronted with a spinal cord injured patient with excessive flexor or extensor spasms, the clinician should undertake a prompt search for pressure sores, bowel or bladder distention, urinary tract infection, fractures, deep venous thrombosis, acute abdomen, or other medical conditions. Measures taken to prevent these complications should be considered in all spastic patients.

Physiotherapeutic techniques to reduce spasticity are universally accepted but their efficacy is not well documented, nor are the relative benefits of one modality over another. In particular, research has been hindered by a difficulty in providing objective and reproducible measurements of motor performance and tone [17]. In the particular case of infants with spastic diplegia, a carefully controlled study by Palmer et al. demonstrated no advantage for patients receiving routine physical therapy when motor skills such as walking were objectively measured [18].

Nevertheless, most clinicians involved with the direct care of spastic patients note that daily stretching exercises are essential to maintain and increase joint range of motion, reduce spasticity, and avoid contractures [19]. Improvement in hypertonicity may be noted for several hours when end-of-arc stretching is performed in a slow and steady fashion [20]. It is unclear whether the beneficial effects of stretching occur through changes in muscle and soft tissue, or through changes in neuronal activity within the spinal cord, or both.

Positioning the patient may also alter muscle tone. Certain postures are termed "reflex inhibiting" because of their ability to reduce tone in certain muscle groups. Detailed descriptions of tone-inhibiting postures may be found in texts by Bobath [21] or Brunnstrom [22]. The physiotherapist is able to use these postures to obtain short-term relief from hypertonicity. For example, the upright posture enhances extensor tone and reduces flexor tone in the lower extremities through labyrinthine reflexes and is important in early gait training for the hemiplegic patient [23].

Contractures can be prevented or corrected by casts or splints. The use of short-term bracing appears to offer little advantage to the spastic patient [24]. However, longer-term use of casts or splints frequently will reduce tone and increase joint range of motion [25–28]. There may be an advantage to customized adjustable braces or dynamic splints, which allow slow but changing stretch on spastic limbs. Reports documenting such beneficial effects, however, are often hampered by small sample size and lack of controls [29,30].

The topical application of cold has been used for many years to provide temporary relief from spasticity [31,32]. Cold must be applied for 20 min or more before maximal reduction in tone is noted. The initial application of cold may paradoxically increase hypertonicity [35]. The reduction in tone induced by the application of cold may last only 1–2 hr. Thus, topical application of cold may be useful as an adjunctive therapy during range-of-motion and stretching exercises but should not be considered definitive therapy for spasticity. The mechanism of action for cold and topical anesthetics is unclear but may relate to a reduction in the sensitivity of cutaneous receptors and decreased velocity of nerve conduction.

Reports of transcutaneous electrical stimulation of nerve (TENS) or muscle and its effect upon spasticity have been variable. One study using a TENS unit reported improved spasticity in only three of six spinal cord injured patients [36]. However, in contrast, another study reported dramatic reductions in spasticity in hemiplegic patients during electrical stimulation, with carryover reduction in spasticity after several treatments [37].

Pharmacological Management of Spasticity

Current pharmacological treatment of spasticity in the United States consists of the use of three principal agents: dantrolene, diazepam, and baclofen. Dantrolene differs from the others in that the site of action is muscle, whereas diazepam and baclofen act directly within the spinal cord. None of these agents is effective in reducing tonic stretch reflexes and all have a variable effect on the dystonic postures of spastic patients [38]. All may exert an effect in a nonselective fashion on both healthy and spastic muscles. These agents principally affect the positive symptoms of spasticity by reducing hypertonicity. They do not improve strength or coordination of movement and one agent in particular, dantrolene sodium, may increase muscle weakness. Adverse effects may target many organ systems and may limit their usefulness.

In general, baclofen and diazepam are used primarily to treat spasticity of spinal origin and are less effective for spasticity due to cerebral injury.

Dantrolene sodium has been used for both spinal and cerebral spasticity because of its direct effect on muscle.

These agents are most effective in reducing the spontaneous flexor spasms of patients with multiple sclerosis or spinal cord injury. They improve patient comfort and can allow more effective, safe transfers. They improve bed positioning and can improve patient hygiene. Dosage is titrated with a target symptom or functional goal in mind and is limited by the development of side effects.

Within these guidelines, the choice of agent for a particular patient remains primarily empirical and is often based on the risk profile for each particular agent and patient. In the future, a more rational selection of pharmacological agents may be based on the electrophysiological profile of spasticity in an individual patient. For example, Delwaide has been able to demonstrate that diazepam but not baclofen enhances vibratory inhibition of tendon reflexes, a normal phenomenon that is reduced in spasticity, whereas baclofen alone was able to modify abnormal recovery curves of Hoffman's reflex at the ankle. Matching the individual antispasticity agents to the pathophysiological profile determined electrophysiologically may lead to better treatment of spasticity in the future [39,40].

Dantrolene Sodium

Dantrolene interferes with the depolarization-induced release of calcium from the sarcoplasmic reticulum within skeletal muscle [41,42]. It has little or no effect on cardiac or smooth muscle [43]. By interfering with the excitation–coupling reaction, it reduces the force generated within skeletal muscle by the interaction of actin and myosin fibers. Its effect is not limited solely to spastic muscle. It produces weakness in all skeletal muscle [44].

Dantrolene appears to be more effective on "fast" muscle fibers that generate a rapid increase in tension, sustained for brief periods. It is less effective on "slow" fibers that contract in a sustained fashion and are resistant to fatigue [45]. It is effective in reducing muscle stiffness and reducing the frequency of flexor spasms. It also decreases hyperactivity of tendon reflexes [46]. When the dosage is increased slowly and blood levels are monitored, it is as effective as diazepam in reducing spasticity over long periods of time [47].

It is the only agent effective for spasticity from spinal or cerebral origin, or both [48]. Unlike baclofen or diazepam, it may be useful in patients with stroke whose spasticity limits rehabilitation [49]. Adverse effects are common and include weakness, dizziness, lethargy, headache, nausea, and vomiting. A gradual increase in the dosage of dantrolene sodium may reduce the incidence of these adverse effects. When dantrolene is used in this fashion, side effects require its withdrawal in only 2.5% of patients [43].

Of particular concern is a 0.2% incidence of fatal hepatitis observed in patients who have taken dantrolene for 60 days or longer. In these cases dantrolene sodium appears to precipitate direct hepatocellular injury. The risk of hepatitis is greater in women, in patients taking estrogens, and in patients older than 35 years [45]. Transient elevation of serum glutamic oxaloacetic transaminase levels (SGOT) occurs in approximately 10% of patients receiving dantrolene [50].

Dantrolene has been noted to exacerbate seizures in children with cerebral palsy [43] and rare pleuropericardial reactions have been reported [51].

Dantrolene sodium is metabolized in the liver and excreted in the urine. Its half-life in adults is approximately 8 hr. One-third of an oral dose is absorbed from the gastrointestinal tract and peak levels are reached in approximately 5 hr. Therapeutic blood levels vary widely from 100 to 600 ng/ml. Dosage is begun with one 25 mg tablet daily and may be increased twice weekly up to 100 mg three or four times a day. However, one report suggests that optimal effect was obtained at the daily divided dosage of 100 mg, and no benefit could be observed at dosages over 200 mg daily [47]. Dantrolene is contraindicated in patients with hepatic disease, and hepatic function should be monitored closely during dantrolene administration. Dosage is often limited by generalized weakness or diarrhea. The drug should be stopped if no benefit is observed within 6 weeks. Since the risk of fatal hepatitis has been observed in patients who have taken the drug for more than 60 days, its long-term use cannot be recommended. In addition, dantrolene is contraindicated in patients with compromised bulbar or respiratory function and, in particular, those patients with motor neuron disease. It should not be used in patients who rely upon their spasticity for functional goals such as upright stance or assistance in transfers. Bedridden quadriplegic or paraplegic patients often benefit from the improved passive mobility and improved hygiene that dantrolene allows.

Diazepam

Diazepam facilitates GABA-mediated postsynaptic inhibition in the spinal cord. This results from the interaction of diazepam with an allosteric protein regulator of GABA receptors producing enhanced affinity of these receptors for endogenous GABA. When activated, GABA receptors provide increased chloride conductance across neuronal membranes, resulting in pre- and postsynaptic inhibition [52]. Diazepam inhibits polysynaptic spinal reflex interactions and increases both pre- and postsynaptic inhibition [53,54]. Because it is effective in patients with spinal transection, diazepam is thought to exert its antispastic affect on the spinal cord. Diazepam reduces the tonic stretch reflex and has little effect on the phasic stretch reflex or the force of contraction in voluntary muscle [55].

Diazepam is very useful in reducing the frequency and severity of lower extremity flexor spasms in patients with multiple sclerosis or spinal cord injury [56]. Some observers have noted that diazepam may not be as efficient as baclofen in reducing such spasms and neither agent is useful for the treatment of spasticity of cerebral origin [52].

Diazepam's principal limitation is sedation. Other side effects include incoordination, fatigue, vertigo, and mild hypotension. Diazepam acts synergistically with other central nervous system (CNS) depressants including alcohol. It may produce psychological or physiological dependence and abrupt withdrawal has been associated with life-threatening seizures. On occasion it may produce paradoxical agitation and hostility, especially in the elderly. Such agitation should not be treated by an increase in diazepam dosage. Diazepam is contraindicated in patients with narrow-angle glaucoma and should be avoided in patients with liver, kidney, or hematological disorders.

Dosage is begun with one 2 mg tablet, two or three times daily. With gradual increases, patients may tolerate up to 20 mg four times daily without excessive sedation. Only rarely are higher dosages required. Diazepam is well absorbed from the gastrointestinal tract and therapeutic levels are reached in plasma within 30 min. Peak levels are achieved in 2–3 hr and the plasma half-life is approximately 8 hr. Diazepam is metabolized in the liver and excreted principally in urine and feces as glucuronide metabolites.

Baclofen

Baclofen (beta-4-chlorophenol-gamma aminobutyric acid) is a GABA analog and an agonist at $GABA_B$ receptors [57]. GABA is an inhibitory neurotransmitter throughout the CNS, which acts presynaptically to reduce the release of excitatory neurotransmitters. Two types of GABA receptors have been identified: those whose actions are antagonized by the agent bicuculline $(GABA_A)$ and those insensitive to bicuculline $(GABA_B)$. Baclofen exerts its actions at $GABA_B$ receptors by a reduction in the release of excitatory neurotransmitter mediated by calcium-induced depolarization of neuronal axonal projections [58,59]. At higher concentrations, baclofen also directly antagonizes the effects of excitatory neurotransmitters postsynaptically [60]. As with diazepam, baclofen is effective in patients with complete cord transection, which identifies its site of action within the spinal cord [61].

Baclofen is effective in reducing muscle hypertonus and decreasing flexor spasms [56,62]. It is also useful in treating tonic flexor dystonias in patients with multiple sclerosis or spinal cord injury [52]. In selected patients, baclofen may allow improved self-care, transfers, patient comfort, and more restful sleep. In some patients, baclofen reduces tendon reflex hyperexcitability, but this effect is variable [63]. In general, baclofen does not improve muscular strength, gait, or manual dexterity [63,64]. It also does not improve abnormal patterns of movement that involve cocontraction of agonist and antagonist muscles [65]. Baclofen does not produce weakness, unlike dantrolene. It reduces spasticity comparably to diazepam without excessive sedation. It is rarely useful for treating spasticity of cerebral origin [52,66].

Baclofen is remarkable for its low incidence of side effects, which differentiates it from other agents. The most common side effect is drowsiness, which usually can be prevented by a gradual increase in dosage. Other side effects include ataxia, respiratory and cardiac depression, and the precipitation of seizures in epileptic patients [52]. Baclofen may interfere with reflex actions in spinal cord injured patients. Some elderly stroke patients given baclofen have experienced confusion or hallucinations.

Baclofen is administered with an initial dosage of 5 mg twice daily. It may be increased up to 30 mg four times daily. Usual therapeutic dosages are 10–20 mg three to four times daily. Although higher dosages are sometimes used with clinical success, some observers have noted that dosages exceeding optimal levels may provide less relief from flexor spasms [52]. Baclofen is completely absorbed from the gastrointestinal tract. Therapeutic blood levels vary widely between individual patients. Most commonly, therapeutic serum baclofen levels are between 80 and 400 ng/ml. The serum half-life of baclofen is 3–4 hr. Peak levels are reached within 2–3 hr after a 40 mg dose in healthy subjects, and levels are sustained over 200 ng/ml for 8 hr. Thirty percent of baclofen is bound to serum protein. Eighty percent of baclofen is excreted unchanged in the urine, while 15% is excreted by the liver, and the rest in feces [52].

Other Agents

A variety of other drugs are described in the literature as useful for the treatment of spasticity. These include tizanidine, chlorpromazine, diphenylhydantoin, progabide, glycine, thiamine, and clonidine.

Although not available in the United States, tizanidine is an imidazoline derivative that facilitates the action of glycine. It has a short half-life that requires frequent administration, but it has been shown to decrease spasticity in an equivalent fashion to baclofen. Side effects include weakness, dry mouth, and mild hypotension [67,68].

Phenothiazines, especially those with alpha-adrenergic-blocking action, may be effective against spasticity, but their excessive sedation and the risk of tardive dyskinesia usually outweigh their effectiveness. However, one study demonstrated that chlorpromazine and diphenylhydantoin given together are effective in reducing spasticity [69].

Progabide has been studied in Europe for the treatment of spasticity. Like baclofen, it is a GABA derivative that is well tolerated and effectively reduces spasticity [70]. Progabide binds to both $GABA_A$ and $GABA_B$ receptors. Unlike baclofen it has been shown to decrease both tonic and phasic stretch reflexes [71].

Glycine supplementation or the use of the glycine precursor thiamine has demonstrated favorable results when used in spinal cord injured patients in two trials [72,73]. In addition, the antihypertensive agent clonidine has been shown to benefit up to 56% of spinal cord injured patients when used in conjunction with baclofen [74].

Chemical Neurolysis

Nerve roots, peripheral nerves, or terminal branches to muscle (motor points) may be blocked by either phenol or ethyl alcohol. Injection of these agents results in a chemical neurolysis and can be very effective in reducing spasticity in selected patients [75–81]. Two to 6% aqueous phenol is used most commonly, although ethyl alcohol in a 45–50% solution is also effective. The effects of these agents last generally from 6 to 12 months [75–78]. Preliminary injection with a local anesthetic may be useful in predicting the outcome from a longer-term block with phenol or ethanol. These blocks are more effective in reducing clonus than in decreasing the frequency of flexor spasms. Because of the blocking of antagonist muscles, some patients may demonstrate increased voluntary contraction after nerve or motor point block [82].

Infiltration of nerve trunks or peripheral nerves with these agents is nonselective and affects both motor and sensory fibers. It is associated with a 10–30% risk of painful dyesthesias [79,83,84]. Although these sensory disturbances diminish with time and may be treated with oral steroids or repeat phenol injection [85], they limit patients' acceptance of this procedure. The development of dyesthesias may be avoided by open injection of only motor branches of a particular nerve or by infiltration of motor points within muscle. Both procedures are technically more difficult and time consuming. Because of the vast number of motor points within a particular muscle, adequate infiltration of a sufficient number to reduce spasticity may be difficult. Motor point injection is performed with a Teflon-coated cathode hypodermic needle that allows one to identify motor points before injection. Other uncommon complications include venous thrombosis [86].

Musculocutaneous and median nerve blocks in the upper extremities may reduce elbow flexion contracture or improve range of motion in severely flexed wrist or fingers [76–78,80]. Nerve block of the obturator nerve in the lower extremity may reduce scissoring gait and allow proper perineal care [87]. Excessive ankle plantar flexion or equinovarus tone can be treated by injection of the posterior tibial nerve [79]. Injection of the paravertebral lumbar spinal nerves may be helpful in reducing excessive hip flexion in spastic patients [88]. These injections exacerbate weakness, and are usually used in bedridden or nonambulatory patients whose loss in strength is not functionally significant.

Intrathecal or epidural injection of phenol or alcohol has been reported for patients with severe lower extremity spasticity. This is an extremely risky procedure; precise positioning of the patient is required to prevent migration of the injected material cephalad. Complications include urinary and fecal incontinence, paresis, loss of sexual function, muscle atrophy, and even death. Complications have been reported in 1–10% of patients receiving intrathecal or epidural injections [89–92].

Surgical Treatment

In certain patients the results of physiotherapeutic or pharmacological treatment of spasticity may be insufficient. In these patients surgical procedures may be required to reduce spasticity adequately. In general, surgical approaches have been limited to orthopedic procedures that section, lengthen, or transfer muscle tendons and neurosurgical procedures that attempt to alter central or peripheral reflex pathways. Again, it is important for both the patient and clinician to have clearly defined functional goals before surgical therapy is undertaken.

Orthopedic procedures are principally used to improve patient function or nursing care, correct deformities, or improve cosmesis. Orthopedic procedures in the lower extremity are used to improve ambulation in stroke or head-injured patients or in children with cerebral palsy [93,94], or to improve hygiene and cosmesis in spinal cord injured patients for whom the resumption of gait is unrealistic. To relieve severe adductor spasms in the spinal cord injured patient, adductor tendon sectioning or obturator neurectomy may be performed. Hip flexion contracture or frequent flexor spasms at the hip may be treated with iliopsoas tendon sectioning. Sectioning of the hamstring tendon or insertion or transfer of its insertion proximally may correct excessive knee flexion in selected patients [95]. At the ankle, Achilles tendon sectioning or lengthening can correct plantar flexion contracture. Varus posturing at the ankle may be treated with tibialis posterior tendon transfer. In other patients who require balance and support at the ankle during gait, subtalar fusion or triple arthrodesis may be undertaken. In certain head-injured patients or those with stroke, excessive toe flexion may make walking difficult or painful and tenotomies may relieve these claw foot deformities [96].

Neurosurgical procedures designed to relieve spasticity are generally reserved for the most severe or refractory cases, since these procedures often reduce voluntary function and may be associated with profound denervation muscle atrophy, predisposing the patient to bed sores.

Neurectomies, like phenol nerve blocks, interfere with peripheral reflex pathways that contribute to spasticity. Neurectomies produce permanent and profound muscle atrophy. Dorsal rhizotomies may preclude atrophy and are performed as either open or percutaneous procedures. Open dorsal rhizotomies allow selective sectioning of fibers that contribute to spasticity by intraoperative electrophysiological study and may spare some sensation. Recurrence of spasticity may occur in 5% of patients who undergo this procedure [97,98]. Percutaneous radiofrequency rhizotomy has also been reported to reduce spasticity in more than 90% of spinal cord injured patients and recurrence of spasticity was successfully treated by repetition of this procedure [99,100].

Neurosurgical interventions to treat spasticity in the central nervous system include myelotomy of the lumbosacral cord in the longitudinal plane. This procedure may reduce spasticity while preserving some descending voluntary function in bowel and bladder control. Again, spasticity may recur. Both myelotomy and rhizotomy do not reduce the portion of hypertonicity that depends on suprasegmental reflexes [101,102].

Experimental Treatments

New approaches to the treatment of severe spasticity include intrathecal administration of baclofen or morphine, botulin injection into spastic muscles, and electrical stimulation of spinal cord or cerebellum.

The recent development of implantable intrathecal continuous-flow pumps offers the ability to administer pharmacological agents for spasticity directly to their principal site of action: the spinal cord. Reports have centered around two agents: morphine and baclofen. In 1985, Erickson et al. reported three patients with severe pain and spasticity who were treated with intrathecal injections of 1–2 mg morphine. Pain and spasticity were dramatically relieved and, with implantation of a continuous-flow pump, all three patients achieved prolonged control of their spasticity. A follow-up report 4 years later reported an additional 12 patients who had relief of spasticity within 1–4 hr after morphine injection, lasting from 12 to 36 hr. Only 1 of the 12 patients was noted to develop drug tolerance. The majority of these patients had spinal cord trauma or multiple sclerosis and their conditions had been refractory to conventional medical management. Side effects were uncommon, with the exception of nausea and vomiting at the initiation of therapy, which persisted in only one patient. Although these effects were generally favorable, a rebound effect was noted in which spasticity increased above its baseline levels with sudden discontinuation of intrathecal morphine [104]. Morphine is a receptor-specific agent and primarily affects multisynaptic reflexes in the spinal cord mediated by A-delta or C-fibers. It has little effect on the monosynaptic reflex arc [103].

In 1987, Richard Penn and Jeffrey Kroin reported seven patients with severe intractable spinal cord spasticity who received intrathecal baclofen by implantation of a drug delivery system [105]. Patients were evaluated for 2 years and demonstrated sustained reduction in hypertonicity and decreased frequency of flexor spasms. In addition, most patients reported improved functional abilities and were less awakened by painful spasms during sleep. Voluntary motor function was not improved, however. Drug dosage varied widely between patients, from 16 to 650 μg/day. During the initial 4 months of therapy it was often necessary to increase the dosage of baclofen to maintain its effectiveness, which raises the question of whether drug tolerance develops. Most complications were related to the implantable pump system that required revision, and in two patients the pump malfunctioned and produced an overdose of baclofen. A subsequent report suggested that intravenous physostigmine may reverse the respiratory depression and coma induced by intrathecal baclofen overdose [106].

These same researchers later reported a randomized double-blind crossover study of 20 patients with spinal spasticity. All patients achieved a decrease in muscle tone and spasms were improved in 18 of 19 patients who had spasms [107]. Drowsiness or confusion was not observed and pump failure was noted in only one case. Infection was not observed. The high therapeutic index of intrathecal baclofen appears to be due to its higher concentrations in the cerebral spinal fluid and its concentration within the lumbar area. Although these studies concentrated on patients with spinal spasticity, one study reported the beneficial effect of intrathecal baclofen in children with cerebral palsy [108]. Spastic patients who received intrathecal baclofen may also note improved bowel and bladder management [109,110].

Intramuscular injection of small amounts of *Clostridium botulinum* exotoxin has been reported to be beneficial in patients with a variety of movement disorders. Botulin exotoxin is produced by the bacterium *Clostridium botulinum*. When ingested, this toxin produces presynaptic neuromuscular block by preventing the release of acetylcholine from synaptic terminals at the neuromuscular junction. The clinical syndrome that results is characterized by flaccid paralysis, termed botulism. When this toxin is injected in skeletal muscle in small dosages, it can produce a dosage-dependent weakness of individual muscles [111].

Das and Park [112] have reported the beneficial effect of botulin toxin in six hemiplegic patients. Snow et al. [113] reported similar success rates in nine patients with chronic stable multiple sclerosis. Neither investigation noted adverse effects, and injections of the toxins were well tolerated by all subjects. Beneficial effects included a significant reduction in spasticity and improvement in functional scores.

Chronic cerebellar stimulation was begun by Cooper in 1972 [114] based on animal experiments in spastic cats and monkeys demonstrating a reduction in motor tone when the anterior cerebellum was stimulated electrically. Although several large uncontrolled studies have been reported, cerebellar stimulation produces only a modest reduction in spasticity and gain in function [115–117]. Double-blind studies involving smaller number of patients have generally failed to demonstrate significant improvement convincingly, although anecdotal reports of excellent results with individual patients are recorded [118–120]. Complications of this therapy include headache, hydrocephalus, death from intracranial hemorrhage, and the necessity for re-exploration and revision of electrical leads and implantable units. As such, the use of cerebellar stimulation for spasticity remains investigational and limited only to specialized centers.

Electrical stimulation of the spinal cord has also been used since the early 1970s to treat spasticity. Electrodes are placed in the epidural space over the posterior columns in the cervical or thoracic region. Electrical stimulation is performed either percutaneously or through the use of an external radiofrequency transmitter to an implanted receiver. Recent reports demonstrate only variable success. Sillis et al. evaluated 19 patients with multiple sclerosis in an uncontrolled fashion and reported "worthwhile" clinical response in only 10 [121]. Gottlieb evaluated seven patients with spinal spasticity who had appeared to have a beneficial effect from spinal cord stimulation. Gottlieb re-examined them in blinded fashion using joint compliance, stretch reflexes, and neurological examination as outcome variables. Examiners were unable to determine whether spinal cord stimulation was being administered [122]. Other investigators have reported reduction in spasticity for hemiplegic patients using spinal cord stimulation, but these studies are also hampered by small numbers of patients and uncontrolled methods [123,124].

SUMMARY

The treatment of spasticity must be tailored to an individual's needs. In some patients spasticity provides functional advantage or is inconsequential during the performance of daily activities. In these cases spasticity should not be treated. In others, treatment should be undertaken with specific functional goals in mind. Progress toward these functional goals allows the clinician to titrate the type, intensity, and duration of a particular treatment modality. All spastic patients appear to benefit from the avoidance of noxious stimuli and an active program of joint manipulation that maintains mobility and avoids secondary complications of spasticity. The decision to engage in further therapy should be undertaken in a stepwise fashion, beginning with therapies that are the least invasive and most specific and only later progressing to more aggressive measures as needed. Used judiciously, drug therapy of spasticity can benefit many patients. For the unusual patient whose severity of spasticity and its refractoriness to conventional treatment require more aggressive measures, referral to centers specializing in experimental measures may be considered.

REFERENCES

1. R.R. Young, *Neurol. Clin.*, 5(4):529–530 (1987).
2. J.W. Lance, *Spasticity and Disordered Motor Control* (R.G. Feldman and R.R. Young, eds.), Year Book, Chicago, pp. 485–494 (1980).
3. R.R. Young and P.J. Delwaide, *N. Engl. J. Med.*, 304(1):28 (1981).
4. R.R. Young, *N. Engl. J. Med.*, 320(23):1553 (1989).
5. J.W. Little and J.L. Merritt, *Rehabilitation Medicine Principles and Practice* (J.A. DeLisa, D.M. Coric, B.M. Gans, P.F. Gatens, Jr., J.A. Leonard, Jr., and M.C. McPhee, eds.), J.B. Lippincott, Philadelphia, pp. 430–432 (1988).
6. B. Ashworth, *Practitioner*, 192:540–542 (1964).
7. J.W. Lance, *Neurology*, 30:1308 (1980).
8. W.M. Landau and M.H. Clare, *Arch. Neurol.*, 10:128–134 (1964).
9. V.T. Shahani and R.R. Young, *New Developments in Electromyography and Clinical Neurophysiology* (J.E. Desmedt, ed.), Karger, Basel, pp. 734–743 (1973).
10. J.M. Cedarbaum, *Int. Med.*, 4;4:11 (1984).
11. C. Clemente, *Neurology*, 28:40–45 (1978).
12. H.G.J.M. Kuypers, *Handbook of Physiology*, Section I, Vol. II, Part I, American Physiological Society, Bethesda, MD. pp. 567–666 (1981).
13. E.R. Kandel and J.H. Schwartz, *Principles of Neuroscience*, Elsevier-North Holland, New York, pp. 269–358 (1981).
14. K. Krnjevic, *Handbook of Physiology*, Section I, Vol. II, Part I, American Physiological Society, Bethesda, MD, pp. 107–155 (1981).
15. J.C. Barber and R.A. Nicholl, *Science*, 176:1043–1045 (1972).
16. K.E. Hagbarth, G. Wallin, and L. Lofstedt, *Scand. J. Rehab. Med.*, 5:156–159 (1973).
17. R.R. Young, *Neurol. Clin.*, 5(4):535–536 (1987).
18. F.B. Palmer, B.K. Shapiro, R.C. Wachtel, M.C. Allen, J.E. Hiller, and A.J. Harryman, *N. Engl. J. Med.*, 318(13):803–808 (1988).
19. R.T. Shapiro, *Rehab. Rep.*, 3:1 (1987).
20. I. Odeen, *Scand. J. Rehab. Med.*, 13:93–99 (1981).
21. B. Bobath, *Adult Hemiplegia Evaluation and Treatment*, Heinemann Medical Books, London (1970).
22. S. Brunnstrom, *Movement Therapy in Hemiplegia*, Harper & Row, New York (1970).
23. L. Stejskal, *Am. J. Phys.*, 58:1–25 (1979).
24. J.C. Otis, L. Root, and M.A. Kroll, *J. Pediatr. Orthop.*, 5:682–686 (1985).
25. N. Kaplan, *Arch. Phys. Med. Rehab.*, 43:565–569 (1962).
26. J. Snook, *Am. J. Occup. Ther.*, 33:648–651 (1979).

27. B.J. Booth, M. Doyle, and J. Montgomery, *Phys. Ther.*, 63:1960–1966 (1983).
28. T. King, *Am. J. Occup. Ther.*, 36:671–673 (1982).
29. K. Collins, P. Oswald, G. Burger, and G. Nolden, *Arch. Phys. Med. Rehab.*, 66: 397–398 (1985).
30. J.J. McPherson, A.H. Becker, and N. Franszczak, *Arch. Phys. Med. Rehab.*, 66: 249–252 (1985).
31. K. Hartviksen, *Acta Neurol. Scand.*, *(Suppl. 3)* 79:84 (1962).
32. M.G. Levine, H. Kabat, M. Knott, and P.E. Voss, *Arch. Phys. Med. Rehab.*, 35:214–223 (1954).
33. W.J. Mills and R.S. Pozos, *Electroencephalogr. Clin. Neurophysiol.*, 61:509–518 (1985).
34. M.A. Sabbahi, C.J. De Luca, and W.R. Powers, *Arch. Phys. Med. Rehab.*, 62: 310–314 (1981).
35. C.W.Y. Chan, *Physio. Ther. Can.*, 38:85–89 (1986).
36. T. Bajd, M. Gregoric, L. Vodovmik, and H. Benko, *Arch. Phys. Med. Rehab.*, 66:515–517 (1985).
37. V. Alfieri, *Scand. J. Rehab. Med.*, 14:177–182 (1982).
38. R.R. Young, *Neurol. Clin.*, 5(4):538 (1987).
39. P.J. Delwaide, P. Martinelli, and P. Crenna, *Spasticity: Disordered Motor Control* (A.G. Feldman, R.R. Young, and W.P. Koella, eds.), Yearbook, Chicago, pp. 345–371 (1980).
40. P. Delwaide, *Ann. Neurol.*, 17:90–95 (1985).
41. W.B. Van Winkle, *Science*, 193:1130–1131 (1976).
42. J.E. Desmedt and K. Hainaut, *Biochem. Pharmacol.*, 28:957–964 (1979).
43. R.M. Pinder, T.M. Brogden, T.M. Speight, and G.S. Avery, *Drugs*, 13:4–23 (1977).
44. S.V. Chayette, J.H. Birdsong, and B.A. Bergman, *South. Med. J.*, 64:180–185 (1971).
45. R.R. Young and P.J. Delwaide, *N. Engl. J. Med.*, 304(1):31 (1981).
46. A. Glass and A. Hannah, *Paraplegia*, 12:170–174 (1974).
47. W.J. Meyler, J. Bakker, J.J. Kok, S. Agoston, and H. Wessling, *J. Neurol. Neurosurg. Psychiatry*, 44:344–349 (1981).
48. F.U. Stenberg and K.L. Ferguson, *J. Am. Geriatr. Soc.*, 23:70–73 (1975).
49. W.B. Ketel and M.E. Kolb, 9(3):161–169 (1984).
50. R. Utili, J.K. Boitnott, and H.J. Zimmerman, *Gastroenterology*, 72:610–616 (1977).
51. M.L. Petusersky, L.J. Faling, and R.E. Rocklin, *JAMA*, 242:2772–2774 (1979).
52. R.R. Young, *N. Engl. J. Med.*, 304(2):96–98 (1981).
53. R.L. MacDonald and J.C. Barker, *Nature*, 267:721 (1978).
54. W.P. Stratten and C.D. Barnes, *Neuropharmacology*, 10:685–696 (1971).
55. J.B. Cook and P.W. Nathan, *J. Neurol. Sci.*, 5:33–37 (1967).
56. N.E.F. Cartlidge, P. Hudson, and D. Weightman, *J. Neurol. Sci.*, 23:17–24 (1974).
57. A.S. Hwang and G.L. Wilcox, *J. Pharmacol. Exp. Ther.*, 248:1026–1033 (1989).
58. R.A. Davidoff and E.S. Sears, *Neurology*, 24:957–963 (1974).

59. N.G. Bowdry, D.R. Hill, A.L. Hudson, A. Doblie, D.N. Middlemiss, J. Shaw, and M. Turnbull, *Nature*, 283:92–94 (1980).

60. T.J. Blaxter and P.L. Carlen, *Brain Res.*, 341:195–199 (1985).

61. E. Pedersen, P. Arlien-Soborg, and J. Mai, *Acta Neurol. Scand.*, 50:665–680 (1974).

62. D. Burke, C.J. Andrews, and L. Knowles, *J. Neurol. Sci.*, 14:199–208 (1971).

63. G.W. Duncan, B.T. Shahani, and R.R. Young, *Neurology*, 26:441–446 (1976).

64. A. From and A. Heltberg, *Acta Neurol. Scand.*, 51:158–166 (1975).

65. R.G. Feldman, M. Kelley-Hayes, J.P. Conomy, and J.M. Foley, *Neurology*, 28: 1094–1098 (1978).

66. E. Knutsson, V. Lindblom, and A. Martensson, *J. Neurol. Sci.*, 23:473–484 (1974).

67. O.L. Hennies, *J. Int. Med. Res.*, 9:62–68 (1981).

68. C. Smolenski, S. Muff, and S. Smolenski-Kart, *Curr. Med. Res. Opin.*, 7:374–383 (1981).

69. S.L. Cohan, A. Raines, J. Panagakos, and P. Armitage, *Arch. Neurol.*, 37:360–364 (1980).

70. K. Mondrup and E. Pedersen, *Acta Neurol. Scand.*, 69:200–206 (1984).

71. K. Mondrup and E. Pedersen, *Acta Neurol. Scand.*, 69:191–199 (1984).

72. A. Barbeau, *Neurology*, 24:392 (1974).

73. A. Barbeau, M. Roy, and C. Chiuzu, *Can. J. Neurol. Sci.*, 9:141–145 (1982).

74. W.H. Donovan, R.E. Carter, C.D. Rossi, and M.A. Wilkerson, *Arch. Phys. Med. Rehab.*, 69:193–194 (1988).

75. R.T. Katz, *Am. J. Phys. Med. Rehab.*, :111–112 (1988).

76. A.A. Khalili, M. Harmel, S. Forster, and J.G. Benton, *Arch. Phys. Med. Rehab.*, 45:513–519 (1964).

77. J.K.M. Easton, T. Ozel, and D. Halpern, *Arch. Phys. Med. Rehab.*, 60:155–158 (1979).

78. D. Halpern and F.E. Meelhuysen, *Arch. Phys. Med. Rehab.*, 45:513–519 (1966).

79. C.R. Petrillo, D.S. Chu, and S.W. Davis, *Orthopedics*, 3:871–874 (1980).

80. D.E. Garland, M. Lilling, and M.A. Keenan, *Arch. Phys. Med. Rehab.*, 65: 243–245 (1984).

81. S.F. Wainaple, D. Haigney, and K. Labib, *Arch. Phys. Med. Rehab.*, 65:786–787 (1984).

82. J.W. Little and J.L. Merritt, *Rehabilitation Medicine: Principles and Practice* (J.A. DeLisa, D.M. Currie, B.M. Gans, P.F. Gatens, Jr., J.A. Leonard, Jr., and M.C. McPhee, eds.), J.B. Lippincott, Philadelphia, pp. 442 (1988).

83. M. Brattstrom, V. Moritz, and G. Srantesson, *Scand. J. Rehab. Med.*, 2:17–22 (1970).

84. A.A. Khalili and H.B. Betts, *JAMA*, 200:1155–1157 (1967).

85. M.B. Glenn, *J. Head Trauma Rehab.*, 1:72–74 (1986).

86. Medical News, *JAMA*, 249:1807 (1983).

87. E.A. Awad, *Arch. Phys. Med. Rehab.*, 53:554–557 (1972).

88.   F.E. Meelhuysen, D. Halpern, and J. Quast, *Arch. Phys. Med. Rehab.*, 49:717–722 (1968).
89.   H.D. Cain, *Paraplegia*, 3:75–76 (1965).
90.   R.E. Kelley and P.C. Gautier-Smith, *Lancet*, 2:1102–1105 (1959).
91.   P.W. Nathan, *Lancet*, 2:1099–1102 (1959).
92.   C.H. Sheldan and E. Bors, *J. Neurosurg.*, 5:385–391 (1948).
93.   G.W.N. Eggens and E.B. Evans, *J. Bone Joint Surg.*, 45:1275–1305 (1963).
94.   J.A. Fixsen, *J. R. Soc. Med.*, 72:761–765 (1979).
95.   R.L. Ray and M.G. Ehrlich, *J. Bone Joint Surg.*, 61:719–723 (1979).
96.   W.J. Treanor, *Scand. J. Rehab. Med.*, 13:123–135 (1981).
97.   V.A. Fasano, G. Broggi, G. Barolat-Romana, and A. Squazzi, *Childs Brain*, 4:289–305 (1978).
98.   W.L. Oppenheim, *Clin. Orthop. Rel. Res.*, 253:20–29 (1990).
99.   D.A. Herz, K.C. Parsans, and L.P. Pearl, *Spine*, 8(7):729–732 (1983).
100. D.L. Kasdon and E.S. Lathi, *Neurosurgery*, 15(4):526–529 (1989).
101. L. Lartinen and E. Singounas, *J. Neurosurg.*, 35:536–540 (1971).
102. P.D. Moyes, *J. Neurosurg.*, 31:615–619 (1969).
103. D.L. Erickson, J.B. Blacklock, M. Michaelson, K.B. Sperling, and J.N. Lo, *Neurosurgery*, 16(2):215–217 (1985).
104. D.L. Erickson, J.N. Lo, and M. Michaelson, *Neurosurgery*, 24(2):236–238 (1989).
105. R.D. Penn and J.S. Kroin, *J. Neurosurg.*, 66:181–185 (1987).
106. G. Muller-Schwefe and R.D. Penn, *J. Neurosurg.*, 71:273–275 (1989).
107. R.D. Penn, S.M. Savoy, D. Corcos, M. Latash, G. Gottlieb, B. Parke, and J.S. Kroin, *N. Engl. J. Med.*, 320(23):1517–1521 (1989).
108. A.L. Albright, A. Cervi, and J. Singletary, *JAMA*, 265(11):1418–1422 (1991).
109. F. Frost, J. Nanninga, R. Penn, S. Savoy, and Y. Wu, *Am. J. Phys. Med. Rehab.*, 68(3):112–115 (1989).
110. J.B. Nanninga, F. Frost, and R. Penn, *J. Urol.*, 142:101–105 (1989).
111. A.B. Scott, *Ophthalmology*, 87:1044–1049 (1980).
112. T.K. Das and D.M. Park, *Postgrad. Med. J.*, 65:208–210 (1989).
113. B.J. Snow, J.K.C. Tsui, M.H. Bhatt, M. Varelas, S.A. Hashimoto, and D.B. Calne, *Ann. Neurol.*, 28(4):512–515 (1990).
114. I.S. Cooper, *Lancet*, 1:1321 (1973).
115. I.S. Cooper, M. Riklan, I. Amin, J.M. Waltz, and M.A. Cullihan, *Neurology*, 16:744–753 (1976).
116. I.S. Cooper, M. Riklan, K. Tabaddor, T. Cullihan, I. Amin, and E.S. Walkins, *Cerebellar Stimulation In Man* (I.S. Cooper, ed.), Raven Press, New York, pp. 59–99 (1978).
117. R. Davis, Barolat-Romana, and H. Engle, *Acta Neurochi. Suppl.*, 30:317–332 (1980).
118. N.H. Gahm, B.S. Russman, R.L. Cerciello, M.R. Fiorentino, and D.M. McGrathm, *Neurology*, 31:87–90 (1981).
119. R.D. Penn, B.M. Myklebust, G.L. Gottlieb, G.C. Agarwal, and M.E. Etzel, *J. Neurosurg.*, 53:160–165 (1980).

120. C.K. Whittaker, *J. Neurosurg.*, *52*:648–653 (1980).
121. L. Sillis, E.M. Sedgewick, and R.C. Tallis, *J. Neurol. Neurosurg. Psychiatry*, *43*:1–14 (1980).
122. G.L. Gottlieb, B.M. Myklebust, D. Stefoski, K. Groth, J. Kroin, and R.D. Penn, *Neurology*, *35*:699–704 (1985).
123. S. Nakamura and T. Tsubokawa, *Neurosurgery*, *17*(2):253–259 (1985).
124. B. Cioni, M. Meglio, A. Prezioso, G. Talamonti, and M. Tirendi, *PACE Pacing Clin. Electrophysiol.*, *12*:739–742 (1989).

11

Speech Therapy and Communicative Disorders in Neurological Rehabilitation

Richard B. Lazar

*Schwab Rehabilitation Hospital and Care Network and
Northwestern University Medical School
Chicago, Illinois*

Susan M. Rubin

*Northwestern University Medical School
Chicago, Illinois*

The modern era of rehabilitation has been propelled by advances in neuroscience and technology that will have a major impact on diagnostic and treatment strategies in the communication sciences for years to come. Neural imaging by computed tomography, magnetic resonance imaging, and positron emission tomography have enhanced the understanding of language processing, articulation, phonation, and deglutition. Modern, pathophysiologically based treatment strategies are not far behind. Where restitution of function is not possible, technological advances in microcomputer science have brought alternative and augmentative devices within the reach of many.

This chapter will focus on the aphasias and their rehabilitative management; disorders of articulation, phonation, and deglutition; and special devices to augment or supplement communicative function.

APHASIA

Aphasia is the absence or impairment of the ability to communicate through speech, writing, or signs, due to a dysfunction of brain centers [1]. A more encompassing concept of aphasia must include impairment in utilizing symbols either to understand or convey meaning. In its most simple, yet global, terms, aphasia is a deficit in the ability to process symbolic materials, which exists in all stimulus modalities (auditory, visual, tactile) and in all response modalities (speaking, writing, gesturing) [2]. All language modalities and levels of communication must be considered. The rehabilitation clinician may encounter individuals with difficulties with stimulus modalities, response modalities, or both. The careful delineation of language processing disorders will help to define the type of aphasia and the nature and severity of the underlying neuropathology.

Understanding aphasia requires some familiarity with contemporary models proposed to explain speech and language organization in the brain. In right-handers, the left hemisphere subserves verbal, speech, and language functions, while the right hemisphere controls nonverbal, visual and spatial function. Hemispheric dominance is determined by the ability of the hemisphere to control speech and language function. The left hemisphere is dominant for language in right-handed individuals and is usually dominant in left-handers. Disorders that affect the left hemisphere will usually cause aphasia. The specific modality affected will be determined by the location of the lesion in that hemisphere. Aphasia is occasionally a consequence of right brain lesions in patients with anomalous dominance. In the conventional Wernicke-Geschwind model, comprehension of spoken language is processed in the temporal lobe, while motor speech is integrated in the inferior third frontal convolution [3]. These important language processing areas are connected by fibers of the arcuate fasciculus.

Aphasia is a symptom of many neurological disorders. Because of the variety of causes, there are no comprehensive estimates of the prevalence of aphasia. Approximately 85,000 new cases of aphasia occur in the United States each year from stroke alone, and approximately 100,000 cases from closed head injury [4]. With the population aging, there is good reason to expect that the number of patients with aphasia will rise substantially as the 21st century approaches.

Classification

The classification of aphasia has evolved over the years since Head first described the dichotomy of expressive and receptive aphasia in 1926 [5]. He postulated that patients with difficulty in producing language had lesions in the frontal lobe involving Broca's area. Comprehension disorders were thought to result from lesions near Wernicke's area in the temporal lobe. Geschwind expanded this concept in the late 1960s to describe better the verbal output expected of patients with lesions in these areas [6]. He classified aphasia into fluent and nonfluent types based on the amount of verbalization noted. Nonfluent aphasia was characterized by sparse, effortful output with decreased grammatical structure, originating from Broca's or surrounding areas or the anterior portions of the dominant hemisphere.

Fluent aphasia was characterized by long, effortless discourse, grammatically intact but lacking appropriate language content, originating posteriorly at or near Wernicke's area. Although these classifications helped to localize some of the different characteristics seen in patients with language disorders, they did not adequately explain all of the different patterns that occurred, including aphasia noted in patients with subcortical and nondominant hemisphere lesions.

More recently, a more specific categorization of fluent and nonfluent aphasias has emphasized a clustering of impaired speech and language characteristics [7]. The terms *cortical* and *subcortical* aphasia emphasize anatomical as well as language characteristics of speech. The advent of improved imaging techniques such as computed tomography, magnetic resonance imaging, and positron emission tomography has greatly improved our ability to correlate language deficits with anatomical lesions. Recent use of metabolic imaging studies in subjects with focal brain lesions has suggested an alternative, but not necessarily mutually exclusive, model of language processing. Lexical processing invokes the theory that the representation of language in the brain has as much to do with how words are used, such as nouns or verbs, as through which modality they are processed [8].

The most common scheme for organizing aphasia subtypes utilizes fluency and repetition disturbances for classifying clinical syndromes (Table 1). Broca's aphasia is characterized by nonfluent, aggrammatical output with effortful speech, but well-preserved auditory and reading comprehension. Repetition is usually impaired. Written language parallels spoken language in its content, if not completely impaired by hemiparesis.

Wernicke's aphasia is characterized by fluent speech output with poor comprehension, naming, and repetition. Speech is effortless and well articulated but frequently contains word or sound substitutions (paraphasias). Reading comprehension is frequently also impaired, while written output parallels verbal output.

Conduction aphasia is characterized by repetition difficulties out of proportion to the degree of output impairment [9]. Speech is relatively fluent, with occasional word substitutions or word-finding problems, and comprehension is mildly to moderately impaired. Repetition, however, is profoundly impaired, with limited ability to repeat words, phrases, or sentences despite evidence of comprehension of the task and meaning.

Anomic aphasia is characterized by the inability to generate word names in confrontational tasks and in spontaneous speech. Although this can be seen in patients with other forms of aphasia, especially other fluent aphasias, it may be the predominant deficit noted on testing and therefore should be considered a category in its own right. Patients with a true anomic aphasia have good comprehension and verbal output but a loss of content words and evidence of circumlocutory speech to describe words they cannot retrieve.

Table 1 The Aphasias: Classification of Subtypes

Function	Broca's	Transcortical Motor	Transcortical Mixed	Global
Spontaneous speech	Nonfluent	Nonfluent	Nonfluent	Nonfluent
Verbal output	Impaired	Impaired	Impaired	Impaired
Auditory comprehension	Normal	Normal	Impaired	Impaired
Naming	Normal	Normal	Impaired	Impaired
Reading	Normal	Normal	Impaired	Impaired
Writing	Impaired	Impaired	Impaired	Impaired
Repetition	Impaired	Normal	Normal	Impaired

Transcortical motor aphasia is characterized by decreased spontaneous verbal output and agrammatical speech with relative preservation of repetition, oral reading, and comprehension. The verbal output is less effortful than that seen in patients with Broca's aphasia, but there is a greater decrease in spontaneity.

Transcortical sensory aphasia is characterized by marked impairment of auditory and reading comprehension with preservation of repetition. Language output parallels the output seen in patients with Wernicke's aphasia, but repetition is strikingly preserved.

Global aphasia is characterized by global dysfunction of comprehension and spoken language, reading, and writing, Despite profound disturbances in patients' language function, retention of social skills, automatisms, self-care ability, and nonverbal communication is common.

The association of aphasia types with specific anatomical lesions is, for the most part, consistent. Broca's aphasia is associated with inferomedial frontal lobe, and Wernicke's aphasia with posterotemporal lobe lesions. Conduction aphasia usually originates from lesions near the angular or supramarginal gyrus involving the arcuate fasciculus. Anomic aphasia is believed to originate from relatively focal lesions in the second temporal gyrus or, more commonly, the angular gyrus. Global aphasia is nearly always a consequence of larger lesions involving frontal, temporal, and parietal cortex. Finally, transcortical motor and sensory aphasias have been localized to lesions surrounding but not involving Broca's and Wernicke's areas, respectively, but also can be seen with subcortical lesions.

Neurodiagnostic imaging technology has greatly improved our understanding of the relationship between subcortical lesions and aphasia. Subcortical aphasia has been described with lesions involving the thalamus, putamen, and anterior limb of the internal capsule [10]. Thalamic aphasia is

Anomic	Wernicke's	Transcortical Sensory	Thalamic	Conduction
Fluent	Fluent or hyperfluent	Fluent or hyperfluent	Fluent	Fluent or impaired
Normal	Normal	Normal to impaired	Normal to impaired	Normal
Normal	Impaired	Impaired	Normal to impaired	Impaired
Impaired	Impaired	Impaired	Normal	Normal
Normal	Impaired	Impaired	Normal	Normal
Normal	Impaired	Impaired	Normal	Normal
Normal	Impaired	Normal	Normal	Impaired

characterized by fluent speech output with occasional paraphasias and dysfluencies, mild to moderate impairment in comprehension and word retrieval, and perseveration and fluctuating attention on specific topics and words [11]. The pulvinar of the thalamus is the structure usually affected [12]. Lesions involving the putamen and the anterior limb of the internal capsule cause an aphasia similar to transcortical motor aphasia, with limited verbal output, intact repetition, and good comprehension. Depending on the extent of the lesion, mutism, articulation deficits, impairment in comprehension, or word retrieval may become apparent.

Lesions involving the nondominant hemisphere cause deficits involving nonverbal language and personality traits. Speech is usually described as copious and incessant, although it is grammatically correct and without errors. Attention span and judgment are usually impaired. Prosody (the emotional content of speech) is also impaired, so that changes in the intonation of language do not accurately reflect mood or meaning. Recognition and appreciation of the intonation patterns of others, such as sarcasm or humor, are also affected. The impact of aprosody, inattentiveness, poor judgment, or disorientation to time and space on social skills can be devastating.

Language deficits are not static and change with recovery or progression of the lesion over time [13]. Even complete global aphasia may evolve substantially over time to other forms of aphasia. The nature and extent of evolution of aphasic disorders depend on underlying pathological process affecting the central nervous system.

Diagnostic Techniques

Language assessment should always proceed from informal to formal evaluation tools. The first indication of aphasia can come from the bedside examination. Early in the history-taking process, one should get evidence of a language deficit. Even in severe aphasia, retention of social skills, nodding, smiling, gesturing, and simple automatic responses are common. Use of simple close-ended questions may not uncover limitations in comprehension or verbal output. Open-ended questions and descriptive responses should be encouraged. Naming, repetition, and comprehension of spoken language must be assessed using language of increasing complexity. Reading and writing must also be tested. Thorough assessment of reading and writing ability may be required in order to differentiate severe dysarthria or hearing loss from aphasia. As a rule of thumb, the aphasic patient will have reading deficits equivalent to his or her comprehension deficits and writing problems should parallel output problems. Formal aphasia evaluation with standardized testing instruments may be required.

Standardized language testing has greatly expanded during the past 20 years. Multiple aphasia batteries are available to quantitate and qualify language processing and functional language ability. No standardized language test is available to assess the impact of aphasia on quality of life, interpersonal skills, or family and social integration.

The Boston Diagnostic Aphasia Examination (BDAE), developed by Goodglass and Kaplan, was designed to meet three important goals of testing: (a) identification of the specific type of aphasia, which might also infer localization of the lesion; (b) provide objective measurements of performance that can be followed over time; and (c) provide assessment of strengths and weaknesses that can be used for planning therapeutic intervention [14]. Like other test batteries, the BDAE evaluates fluency, word retrieval, repetition, seriatic speech, grammar and syntax, auditory comprehension, reading comprehension, writing, and conversational speech. A number of other more cognitively weighted tasks including calculation, finger identification, right–left discrimination, time, and three-dimensional block design attributed to dominant parietal and occipital lobe function are also included.

Other aphasia batteries, such as the Porch Index of Communicative Ability (PICA) [15], the Western Aphasia Battery (WAB) [16], and the Neurosensory Center Comprehensive Examination of Aphasia (NCCEA) [17] differ in the stimulus used, ability to differentiate aphasia types (BDAE and WAB), quantitative capability (PICA and NCCEA), and sensitivity for recognizing mild aphasia. Formal tests designed to assess intensively one specific language function, such as auditory comprehension, in depth are also available.

Aphasia diagnosis is not complete without a full neurological, behavioral, and neuropsychiatric assessment. Physical and cognitive deficits are important in preparing an appropriate treatment plan. Visual field defects, for example, may limit functioning within certain language modalities and require compensatory strategies for effective communication. Hemiplegia may interfere with writing, making an alternative communication system necessary (see below). The patient's premorbid cognitive ability, language skills, literacy, and education level must be known before one can evaluate aphasia fully and set realistic treatment goals.

Therapy

The scope of the speech pathologist's duties in aphasia rehabilitation includes not only diagnostic testing but also therapy and education of the patient and family. Therapy at first should center on providing a means for the patient to communicate basic wants and needs. By addressing personal issues first, frustration is reduced and motivation for improvement enhanced. Therapy tasks should be practical and shared with family members and staff in order to promote total re-enforcement of therapy goals. The speech pathologist must insist that all caretakers are aware of the patient's limitations and best mode of communication.

Specific therapy methods are as variable as the types of aphasia. Aphasias frequently evolve, and therefore treatment strategies must be individualized. Eight general principles of effective aphasia therapy have been emphasized [2]: (a) structuring tasks at a level of difficulty that is challenging; (b) keeping stimulus material simple and relevant; (c) eliciting a large number of responses from the patient; (d) always beginning each session with a familiar task; (e) trying to introduce new tasks as an extension of familiar material; (f) providing feedback to the patient; (g) showing the patient his or her progress; and (h) directing treatment towards general abilities rather than specific responses. Some therapists have focused on tasks that stimulate fluent versus nonfluent aphasias, while others suggest tasks based on the severity of the deficits.

Specific therapy techniques have been developed to address specific language deficits. Melodic intonation therapy has been developed to encourage verbal output in patients with expressive aphasia [18]. It utilizes the concept that melodic function is contained in the right hemisphere and that aphasic patients may be able to sing even when they are unable to speak due to left hemisphere damage. Speech is facilitated by using melodies and rhythmic tapping to intone phrases and improve language output. Another technique for encouraging verbal output in aphasic patients is the use of sign language. Amer-Ind (American Indian Sign Language) and Ameslan (combining Amer-Ind and American Sign Language) have both been used effectively in patients with expressive aphasia. Sign language allows the patient a visual representation for language that is easier to produce and takes the pressure off the patient to communicate verbally. Fewer programs have been developed to treat patients with receptive aphasias and are more patient specific.

Utilizing the Token Test, aphasic subjects can be trained to follow increasingly complex commands [19]. Other workers have developed programs utilizing the neurolinguistic theory to allow patients to progress from simple comprehension tasks to more complex sentences [20]. Global aphasic patients, who are limited in both comprehension and expression, have been trained to communicate through alternative communication systems. Blissymbols, developed by Bliss in 1965, provide a visual representation of language. Visual action therapy utilizes pantomime to train patients to use gestures to communicate [21].

Pharmacological therapy has a limited but promising role in aphasia therapy. Bromocriptine, a dopamine agonist, has been found to be effective in treating patients with transcortical motor aphasia, most likely by enhancing the initiation of speech production [22]. Acupuncture has also been shown to be useful in patients in aphasia secondary to stroke [23]. The use of ganglionic blockade in aphasia therapy has recently been proposed [24].

There is extensive literature on aphasia diagnosis and treatment, but still controversy regarding the effectiveness of therapy. The effects of treatment beyond spontaneous recovery remain unclear to date. For ethical reasons, a control group randomized under a protocol for formal investigation has been nearly impossible to achieve. To date, the benefits of treatment in improving the processing of language, and the optimum duration and intensity of therapy, have not been adequately delineated.

In one comparison study of speech therapists and volunteers treating aphasic patients, there was no difference in recovery [25]. In a comparison of conventional therapy with informal counseling sessions over a 10 month trial period, there was no difference in outcome measures between treated and untreated individuals, using the Porch index of communicative ability [26]. When aphasic patients were randomized to clinic, home, or deferred treatment groups and evaluated over 24 weeks, there was no significant difference in outcome [27]. In a study of 31 patients with severe aphasia following cerebral infarction, no appreciable differences in verbal behavior could be detected between those who received programmed instruction, nonprogrammed instruction, and no treatment [28].

Two randomized studies comparing speech therapy with no treatment have concluded that those who receive speech therapy after stroke make greater gains than those receiving no treatment [29,30]. Although statistical computation favors treatment, the advantage of treatment may have been scored differences, rather than real. Whether or not formal speech and language therapy can accelerate spontaneous recovery, the provision of compensatory strategies for permanent deficits and patient and family education is useful and necessary. The medical community may rightfully argue about the efficacy of therapy for years to come, but attention to developing new techniques and improving those in current use may prove wise in the long run [31].

DYSPHAGIA

Dysphagia is disordered swallowing from any cause, with or without symptoms. Any disorder of oropharyngeal or esophageal anatomy or function may lead to dysphagia. Dysphagia as a symptom of neurological disease is prevalent across a wide variety of disorders throughout the central and peripheral nervous system.

Normal Deglutition

Normal deglutition consists of four phases: oral preparatory, oral, pharyngeal, and esophageal. During the oral preparatory phase, food is manipulated in the mouth and masticated, if necessary. Mastication involves a repeated cyclical pattern of rotary lateral movement of the labial and mandibular musculature. Once broken down into particles, food is collected into a bolus and held anterolaterally by the tongue against the palate. The motor control of the oral cavity required for appropriate bolus size and consistency requires complex sensory input, such as taste, touch, temperature, and proprioception [32].

During the oral phase, the tongue propels food posteriorly until the swallowing reflex is triggered in the area of the anterior faucial arch. A labial seal is maintained to prevent food or liquid from leaking from the mouth. Tension of the buccal musculature prevents food from falling into the lateral sulcus between the mandible and cheek. The tongue propels the food bolus posteriorly with an action described by Logemann as sequential elevation of the tongue from anterior to posterior [33].

During the pharyngeal phase, the pharyngeal swallow is triggered, and the resultant neuromuscular actions move the bolus through the pharynx. Triggering of the pharyngeal swallow occurs primarily at the anterior faucial arch [34] so that posterior movement of the bolus is not interrupted [35].

Triggering of the pharyngeal swallow results in the rapid succession of a number of physiological activities in the pharynx that are crucial to successful swallowing. The velum is elevated and retracted, and the velopharyngeal port is completely closed to prevent material from entering the nasal cavity. Pharyngeal peristalsis picks up the bolus as it passes the anterior faucial arch and carries it, by sequential peristaltic action of the pharyngeal constrictors, into and through the pharynx to the cricopharyngeal sphincter at the top of the esophagus. The larynx is elevated and closed at the true vocal cords, false vocal cords, and epiglottis and aryepiglottic folds to prevent material from entering the airway. The cricopharyngeal region then opens to allow material to pass from the pharynx into the esophagus. Laryngeal elevation and anterior movement of the larynx are thought to contribute significantly to cricopharyngeal opening by stretching the cricopharyngeal region.

During the esophageal phase, peristalsis moves the food into the stomach. The peristaltic wave, which begins in the pharynx when the pharyngeal swallow triggers, continues in sequential fashion caudally through the esophagus.

The organization of the swallowing motor sequence depends on the activity of a neuronal network, known as the swallowing center. The swallowing center is organized into three levels (the afferent, efferent, and organizing level) that correspond to the interneuronal network that programs the motor sequence of swallowing [36].

The afferent level consists of sensory receptors of the faucial arches, tonsils, soft palate, base of the tongue, and posterior pharyngeal wall that transmit neural impulses to the swallowing center through cranial nerves VII, IX, and X [37]. The fibers of the glossopharyngeal nerve (IX), contained chiefly in the superior laryngeal nerve, carry impulses to the swallowing center through the solitary tract of the medulla [38].

The efferent level consists of the motor neurons involved in swallowing, contained chiefly in cranial nerves IX, X, and XII. The trigeminal nerve (V) and facial (VII) nerves have been considered by some to have a small role in the efferent arc of deglutition [39]. More recent evidence suggests an important efferent contribution to the physiology of deglutition by the trigeminal (V) and hypoglossal (XII) nuclei, and the nucleus ambiguous [40].

The organizing level is postulated to be localized within the pontine reticular formation. In animal models, stimulation of the solitary tract or its nucleus and the adjacent reticular formation elicits swallowing [41]. These findings have been confirmed in sheep models using retrograde horseradish peroxidase and autoradiographic tracing [42]. Swallowing neurons appear to be located in two regions. A dorsal region includes the nucleus of the solitary tract and the adjacent reticular formation, and a ventral region includes the lateral reticular formation above the nucleus ambiguous [40]. The dorsal swallowing center appears to initiate and organize the swallowing motor sequence, while the ventral region distributes the motor impulses of deglutition to motor neurons directly involved in swallowing.

In addition to the medullary swallowing center, a cortical swallowing center just anterior to the orbital gyrus of the frontal lobe receives information from contralateral oropharyngeal and laryngeal receptors [35]. In animals, single-pulse stimulation of the cortical center causes a rhythmic activation of the ipsilateral nucleus of the solitary tract, but the frequency of deglutition decreases rapidly. The cortical swallowing center may have important functions in both the initiation of the motor sequence of swallowing and repeated swallowing.

Neurogenic Dysphagia

Pathological disruption of the medullary or cortical swallowing centers and its pathways in the central nervous system occurs under a variety of circumstances, leading to dysphagia as a symptom of neurological disease. Neurogenic dysphagia is well-recognized to occur in a variety of neurological diseases in all parts of the central and peripheral nervous systems (Table 2).

Under most circumstances, dysphagia can be considered oropharyngeal or esophageal in origin. In oropharyngeal dysphagia, the primary symptom complex often includes coughing, choking, or regurgitation of food or liquids. Complaints of food sticking or getting trapped in transit are more common in patients with esophageal dysphagia.

With either dominant or nondominant hemisphere cerebral involvement, reductions in labial and lingual strength, range of motion, sensation, pharyngeal swallow, and pharyngeal peristalsis have all been clearly demonstrated [43]. With brainstem involvement, reductions in lingual, labial, and buccal strength, range of motion, sensation, pharyngeal swallow, pharyngeal peristalsis, laryngeal adduction and elevation, and cricopharyngeal function have been shown clinically and radiologically [44].

Aspiration pneumonia is the feared complication of unrecognized, clinically significant neurogenic dysphagia. Broadly considered, aspiration in patients with neurological disease should be defined as entry of secretions or oral feedings below the true vocal cords. In neurogenic dysphagia, aspiration is often considered as either audible or silent aspiration [45]. How much aspiration is tolerated by individuals with neurologically disabling illness

Table 2   Neurological Causes of Oropharyngeal Dysphagia

Central Nervous System	Peripheral Nervous System	Neuromuscular Junction	Muscle
Stroke	Botulism	Myasthenia	Muscular dystrophies
Parkinson's disease	Diphtheria	gravis	Myositis
Wilson's disease	Rabies	Lambert	Metabolic myopathies
Multiple sclerosis	Diabetes	Eaton	Amyloidosis
Motor neuron	Guillain-Barré		Lupus erythematosus
disease/polio	syndrome		
Brainstem neoplasm			
Tabes dorsalis			

before leading to clinically significant aspiration pneumonia is uncertain at this time. Concerns about "silent" aspiration and its consequences arise because even the most experienced clinicians performing a bedside evaluation fail to identify a large number of patients who aspirate.

Diagnostic Techniques

The bedside swallowing evaluation should include a history of the patient's disorder, assessment of nutritional and respiratory status, oral anatomy, labial and lingual control, laryngeal control, food positioning in the oral cavity, and symptoms during attempts to swallow a variety of food and liquid types. The most prevalent signs include abnormal lingual function, abnormal gag reflex, impaired oral sensation, and abnormal cough reflex [46]. Risk factors for dysphagia in patients with neurological disease include impaired level of consciousness, gaze paresis, and sensory inattention [47].

Further clinical analysis of clinical dysphagia often requires videofluoroscopic examination under a standard protocol. This simple examination can measure prepharyngeal response time, oral motility, pharyngeal response time, pharyngeal motility patterns, and aspiration [48]. Clinical factors associated with videofluoroscopic aspiration include abnormal gag reflex and abnormal voluntary cough [49]. Wet or hoarse vocal quality is also a reliable predictor of laryngeal penetration [50]. When clinical and radiologically proven aspiration pneumonia is the endpoint, the false-positive and -negative rates for screening by videofluoroscopic examination have never been determined [51].

The technique by which videofluoroscopic evaluation of swallowing is performed may vary with different neurological diseases [52]. There is no deductive reason why the radiological examination of a dysphagic patient with myasthenia gravis should be the same as a patient with a stroke. Videofluoroscopic evaluation of a myasthenic patient requires repeated efforts during the swallowing study to look for decremental response. In patients with movement disorders, such as spasmodic torticollis, delayed reflex and pharyngeal residue may be more prevalent than other components of disordered swallow physiology [53].

Although videofluoroscopic techniques have been standardized, the effects of bolus size, viscosity, and temperature on swallowing function are poorly understood. Validation of interobserver consistency in videofluoroscopic evaluation of swallowing function has recently been established [54].

Diagnostic ultrasound is a noninvasive technique for evaluating dysphagia that has a particular advantage in the oral phases of swallowing [55]. Oropharyngeal abnormalities, such as cricopharyngeal incoordination, are extremely difficult to detect [56]. Real-time ultrasound may be used to monitor motions of the tongue, hyoid bone, and larynx [57].

Therapy

The goal of management is to return the patient with neurogenic dysphagia to as normal a diet as possible, and prevent aspiration pneumonia. Even individuals with dysphagia who are receiving nothing by mouth have a significant incidence of aspiration, due to an inability to protect the airway from intrinsic body secretions.

Bolus management should be the first consideration, with a lower incidence of aspiration pneumonia in individuals fed a soft mechanical diet with thickened liquids than those fed a pureed diet with thin liquids [58]. The optimal bolus size and consistency for oral feeding have not been determined. Oral exercises and postural facilitation may be useful before, during, or after the swallow [59]. A delayed swallowing reflex may be improved by thermal stimulation techniques, but the carryover to normal eating has not been established [60]. Simple postural compensatory strategies may improve pharyngoesophageal dysphagia by eliminating a flaccid pharyngeal wall from the bolus path and reducing upper esophageal sphincter tone [61]. In dysphagia caused by Parkinson's disease, swallowing abnormalities are improved by pharmacological management of the underlying disorder with levodopa [62].

Despite the initial severity of the patient's neurological insult, an aggressive multidisciplinary dysphagia program may be beneficial in the long term, and allow the vast majority of individuals to resume oral feeding [63]. Cognitive variables, such as arousal, behavior, judgment, and neglect, are equally important in making a final determination [64].

DISORDERS OF ARTICULATION

Definition and Diagnosis

Dysarthria is a neurogenic motor speech impairment characterized by slow, weak, imprecise, or uncoordinated movements of the speech musculature [65]. It differs from aphasia in that it encompasses difficulties in the production of speech, not the symbolic content of language. Difficulties are not with understanding, reading, writing, or choosing words to communicate. Communication difficulties are secondary to deficits in muscular control that can involve any or all of the basic processes of speech, respiration, phonation, resonance, articulation, and prosody [66].

Dysarthria must be differentiated from apraxia of speech. Apraxia is a disorder of motor programming that affects voluntary motor actions but not automatic or involuntary tasks. Difficulties in planning the actual positioning of the articulators, islands of fluent speech, and precise oral motor movements for nonspeech tasks are associated with apraxia [65]. Dysarthric individuals are unable to produce precise articulation or nonspeech motor movements due to weakness despite abilities in motor programming.

The incidence of dysarthria has been difficult to assess because of its multiple causes and variable presentations. Congenital dysarthria occurs in 31–88% of patients with cerebral palsy. Nearly 30% of patients with traumatic brain injury initially have dysarthria, with residual deficits in 15% of patients. Degenerative diseases have a high incidence of dysarthria due to their effect on the speech musculature. Studies on the incidence in the population of patients with stroke are confounded by the coincidence of aphasia and apraxia with dysarthria limiting epidemiological studies [65].

Classification

Dysarthrias have been classified using a variety of schemata. Age at onset, causes, neurophysiological and neuroanatomical classifications have all been considered. Neuroanatomical systems classify dysarthria into pyramidal, extrapyramidal, cerebellar, and peripheral nervous system disorders, associated with specific speech characteristics [67,68]. Understanding of the essential physiological components in the production of speech, including respiration, articulation, resonance, and prosody, has led to focused therapy directed at specific deficits, regardless of cause.

A framework for describing dysarthrias based on neuroanatomical as well as perceptual characteristics is commonly used today [65]. Six major categories are described (Table 3). Spastic dysarthria is characterized by slow, labored, harsh speech with consistently imprecise articulations and low, monotonous pitch. Speech is usually hyponasal and strained in quality.

Flaccid dysarthria, due to lower motor neuron lesions, is characterized by breathy speech in short phrases. There is air wastage and significant hypernasality. Articulation is imprecise secondary to weakness of the musculature and inability to develop sufficient intraoral pressure.

Mixed dysarthria is characterized by slow rate, low pitch, hoarse and

Table 3   The Dysarthrias: Classification and Prototypes

Classification	Prototype	Examples
Spastic	Pseudobulbar palsy	Cerebral palsy, stroke, head trauma, neoplasia
Flaccid	Bulbar palsy	Myasthenia gravis, poliomyelitis, Guillain-Barré syndrome
Ataxic	Cerebellar lesions	Spinocerebellar degenerations
Mixed	Abiotrophies	Motor neuron disease
Hypokinetic	Extrapyramidal	Parkinson's disease
Hyperkinetic	Dystonias, dyskinesias	Huntington's chorea, Gilles de la Tourette's syndrome

strained quality, highly defective articulation, and marked hypernasality. In the early stages either flaccid or spastic dysarthria may predominate.

Ataxic dysarthria is characterized by either intermittent disintegration of articulation with dysrhythmia and irregularity of pitch and loudness or altered prosody with prolongation of sounds, equalization of syllabic stress, and prolongation of intervals between syllables and words.

Hypokinetic dysarthria can be recognized by reduced vocal emphasis, monotonous quality, and short rushes of speech separated by illogically placed pauses. Articulation is impaired as muscles fail to go through their complete excursion.

Hyperkinetic dysarthria is characterized by unpredictable voice stoppages, disintegration of articulation, excessive variations of loudness, and distortion of vowels. Attempts at compensation lead to slow rates and inappropriate pauses.

Diagnostic Techniques

Motor speech assessment relies on the evaluation of the anatomy and physiology of its production. Muscle strength, speed of movement, range of excursion, accuracy of movements, steadiness of contraction, and musculature tone are all neuromuscular functions essential to speech production [66]. A thorough neurological exam is essential to understanding the causes of the deficits and the expected natural history of the disorder. Assessment should focus on respiration, phonation, resonance, articulation, and prosody.

The motor speech examination is classified into two parts: (a) muscular strength and coordination testing during nonspeech activities and (b) analysis of speech function for description and correlation with the remainder of the neurological findings [66]. Facial musculature, tongue movement, palatopharyngeal competency, and laryngeal control all are systematically assessed. Apraxia must also be ruled out by testing voluntary movement in comparison to automatic movements. Standardized paragraphs using phonetically balanced sentences should be utilized to evaluate contextual speech.

Additional evaluation techniques include assessment of respiratory parameters through pulmonary function tests and respiratory inductive plethysmography [69]. Indirect or direct laryngoscopy can help to assess laryngeal function, while the maximum sustained phonation time can be calculated to determine laryngeal efficiency [70]. A dysphagia evaluation reveals information about nonspeech motor competence and velopharyngeal movement.

Therapy

In light of the multiple causes of dysarthria and the variability of types, therapy must be individualized. However, basic principles underlying therapy have been proposed [66]. Therapy should be designed to encourage compensation for lost function and develop awareness of how to produce speech purposely and of self-monitoring skills. The earlier these skills are developed and the more motivated the patient, the more effective therapy will be. Specific therapy techniques should be chosen based on the natural history of the disease, with therapy goals being reassessed as the disease process changes [65].

Specific therapy techniques are designed to address specific components of speech. Respiration deficits cause inadequate breath group lengths for speech and limited volume. Therapy is designed to establish adequate and consistent subglottal air pressure. With the use of commercial or homemade water manometers, air pressure can be visualized and measured, with training designed to increase and maintain volumes for longer periods of time. A goal of 5 cm of water to 5 sec has been recommended [71]. Repositioning and postural training can also improve respiratory function [72]. Finally, respiratory pattern marking can help patients to identify more natural breath groups to normalize speech patterns.

Laryngeal disorders vary depending on the type of dysarthria. Speech may be breathy, hoarse, or harsh, with decreased volume or monotonous pitch. In extreme cases there may be an absence of phonation. Voluntary phonation can be encouraged with the use of Valsalva maneuvers, and voice quality can be improved with modification of the fundamental frequency, head rotation, or utilization of higher lung volumes [73].

Velopharyngeal function controls nasality and affects respiratory support by allowing air to escape through the nasal cavity, decreasing the intraoral air pressure needed for consonant production. Although some behavioral approaches have been suggested, management of velopharyngeal insufficiency has been primarily with prosthetic or surgical intervention.

Articulatory disorders, due to muscular weakness, respiratory, laryngeal, or velopharyngeal insufficiency may compound speech difficulty, and have a major impact on overall speech intelligibility. The goals of therapy are to improve muscular strength and coordination and to provide compensatory techniques to improve communicative function. Biofeedback has been found to be useful in both reducing tone and increasing strength [65]. Intelligibility drills and contrastive production tasks modify speech production. Rate control can improve intelligibility even without correcting articulatory errors. Pacing boards [74] and delayed auditory feedback [75] help patients to monitor their rate more effectively, slowing speech and increasing intelligibility.

Specific disorders associated with dysarthria have specific treatments. Many disorders associated with dysarthria can be medically managed (Parkinson's disease, myasthenia gravis), while in others spontaneous recovery leads to improvement (cerebral infarcts, multiple sclerosis). Degenerative diseases may benefit from early intervention to maximize speech production and delay progression and later will require compensatory techniques and ultimately augmentative communication systems (motor neuron disease). Protheses, Teflon injections, and surgical reconstruction are useful in patients with disorders involving the peripheral nervous system. Regardless of the techniques used, the role of the speech pathologist is to provide a treatment program that improves intelligibility and, ultimately, communication [66].

AUGMENTATIVE AND ALTERNATIVE COMMUNICATION

The predicament of the nonspeaking patient poses a major challenge for the rehabilitation specialist. Technological advances in microprocessing and rehabilitation engineering offer many options for those who need communicative augmentation and/or alternative speech modalities. A range of neurological disorders, from cerebral palsy to stroke, may lend themselves to special technology in order for patients to achieve functional communication [76].

Augmentative communication science is the use of aids or techniques that supplement existing vocal or verbal skills. For the individual with no vocal ability, alternative communication methods may add considerably to family, community, and environmental adaptation [77].

In general, interdisciplinary evaluation and management for patients with special communication needs are required. A team led by a rehabilitation physician with knowledge of the natural history and clinical course of the underlying disorder is essential. A physician needs to establish the prognosis for recovery or deterioration of a given neurological disorder before a costly and time-consuming commitment to a communications prosthesis is made [78]. The assistance of speech, occupational, and physical therapists is usually required. A rehabilitation engineer, although not essential in the majority of circumstances, may be extremely useful for the most effective integration of a communications device with mobility and other technical aids. No guidelines for selection of candidates for these rehabilitative interventions can be reasonably offered without considering the potential impact on quality of life in a cost-effective way [79].

Cognitive evaluation for an alternative communication device should include an assessment of alertness, level of arousal, limb function, and tone. No standardized tests are currently available for evaluation of the patient in need of a communications prosthesis, and as a result, nonstandardized testing has been accepted practice [80].

Physical evaluation by the rehabilitation engineer, occupational and physical therapist should include visuomotor and perceptual ability, gross and fine motor function, and seating and positioning needs for those who are wheelchair dependent. The overall goal of seating and positioning evaluation is to ensure maximal function and comfort. Re-evaluation periodically will be required, depending on the patient's level of physical function [81].

As a rule, differentiation should be made between temporary and permanent users of such devices. The temporary need for an alternative or augmentative communication device usually occurs early after the onset of illness. A simple picture, letter, or symbol board may be useful during the early recovery phase of patients with Broca's aphasia after stroke until functional communication is restored. When spontaneous recovery has abated, and functional gains in speech are diminished, a permanent system is recommended, such as a handheld pocket communicator with artificial speech or printout capability.

For most systems, symbols can be considered to be either dynamic (subject to change) or static (permanent). Selection techniques may be by direct choice or scanning. Dynamic symbols are usually used in electronic communications systems, while static symbols are more common in simple communication boards. In general, direct selection of symbols is the fastest selection method available. A functional body part (hand, foot, or chin) is often utilized to select items. However, a pointer, straw, or even laser activator may be required to activate selections. Scanning using a multi-dimensional matrix system may be more practical in some instances, but requires a communications partner. Linear scanning is by far the simplest method, using a sequential cursor technique for symbol selection. For more complex communication systems, row–column scanning, page–item scanning, and directed matrix scanning may be less tedious.

System selection can be organized into three categories: simple communication boards, devices with a predesignated function, and multipurpose systems [82]. A simple communication board incorporates symbols, pictures, words, or letters to establish communication. Communication devices with predesignated function, such as a call for help or bathroom assistance, are readily available and can be utilized to print or create artificial speech, respectively. Multipurpose systems are now available to combine communicative function and environmental control to promote total independence. Successful integration of a communications prosthesis into everyday living will require weeks or even months of training.

Electronic communication devices commonly use either synthesized or digitized speech output. Synthesized speech utilizes principles of mathematical modeling to produce a reproduction of the human voice. Digitized speech is produced by reformulation of acoustically processed information stored digitally in computer memory that is resynthesized upon command as human speech. Digitized human speech is more intelligible than synthesized

speech, but considerable memory is required to retain a functionally significant vocabulary.

Visual output for electronic communication devices utilizes a light-
emitting diode or a liquid crystal display. In general, the quality of visual
output in light-emitting diodes is superior, but energy requirements are
substantial. Liquid crystal displays are more energy efficient, but considerably more difficult to read.

For patients with severe dysarthria and functional quadriplegia, such as
in cerebral palsy, a viewpoint optical indicator may be utilized. An optical
light is worn on the patient's forehead, secured by an elastic band. By the
patient simply turning his or her head, using a battery-operated light indicator, a word, letter, or number can be selected from a linguistic unit on a
communication board to formulate a message. This prosthesis is best utilized
by individuals with adequate head control, but severe motor deficits in the
upper extremities.

A simple handheld communications prosthesis that generates printed
messages can be utilized by the patient with severe verbal fluency disorders
or dysarthria. This simple device is the size of a handheld pocket calculator,
and requires sufficient fine motor control in at least one upper extremity to
operate a simple key pad to generate a printed message. This device is
lightweight and portable, a distinct advantage for an ambulatory individual.

For a severely physically disabled nonspeaking patient who is able to
activate a switch and point to individual pictures, words, or characters
displayed on an overlay, the prism communication device is recommended.
This expanded augmentative communication prosthesis is designed to increase user independence and display space. It provides the user with
independent access to three sides of nine internally mounted removable
prisms, allowing a total of 540 ⅞-inch-square spaces for characters, words,
pictures, or symbols. When one depresses an externally mounted switch, the
prism set is sequenced 120 degrees. The prism communicator can be
mounted on a wheelchair lap tray, and is easily modified to meet the
functional needs of the patient.

Simple devices for patients with severe dysarthria or expressive aphasia
that utilize a touch-based system are now available commercially. A low-cost
communication prosthesis uses squares on a simple board to speak out stored
words, phrases, or sentences.

A more elaborate portable communications prosthesis using a touch-
based system consists of a liquid crystal diode display, a 128 location display,
and built-in speech synthesizer. The main program in the software for this
special prosthesis allows the user to retrieve the stored contents rapidly as
well as spell out novel words or messages. For patients with associated visual

deficits, auditory scanning software programs are now available that can be activated by a single switch. Using a built-in speech synthesizer, it scans auditory contexts, then branches to categories, cues words, and phrases. The custom display contains squares, each containing pictures, numbers, or letters that are used to compose a message that, in turn, is spoken out by the speech synthesizer. Wheelchair mountings are not necessary, but often useful, and are readily available.

Special communications prostheses with male or female real voices are available for those with severe dysarthria or expressive aphasia who have relatively good upper extremity gross and fine motor control. A portable microcomputer-based device with regular typewriter keyboard, light crystal display screen, built-in printer, and microcassette drive for vocabulary and message memory back-up purposes is currently available. An abbreviation expansion feature allows the user to type one to three letters, press a talk key, and produce a stored functional word, phrase, or message. A built-in speech synthesizer then generates a stored or novel message produced by the user. Vocabulary or message items can be easily stored, altered, or deleted. An exception table stores words that require phonetic spelling for proper pronunciation by the speech synthesizer.

REFERENCES

1. *Taber's Cyclopedic Medical Dictionary*, F.A. Davis Company, Philadelphia, pp. 106–107 (1981).
2. R.H. Brookshire, *Introduction to Aphasia*, Minneapolis, p. 18 (1978).
3. N. Geschwind, *Science*, 170:940–944 (1970).
4. M.L. Albert and N. Helm-Eastabrooks, *JAMA*, 259(8):1043–1047 (1988).
5. H. Head, *Aphasia and Kindred Disorders of Speech*, Macmillan Publishing, New York (1926).
6. N. Geschwind, *N. Engl. J. Med.*, 284:654–656 (1971).
7. H. Goodglass and E. Kaplan, *The Assessment of Aphasia and Related Disorders*, Lea & Febiger, Philadelphia (1976).
8. A. Caramazza and A.E. Heller, *Nature*, 346:267 (1990).
9. D.F. Benson, *Arch. Neurol.*, 23:339 (1973).
10. A.R. Damasio, H. Damasio, M. Rizzo, et al., *Arch. Neurol.*, 39:15–20 (1982).
11. M.H. Tuszynynksi and C. Petito, *Neurology*, 38:800–802 (1988).
12. C.W. Wallesch, H.H. Kornhuber, R.J. Brunner, et al., *Brain Language*, 20:286–304 (1983).
13. A. Kertesz and P. McCabe, *Brain*, 100:1–18 (1977).
14. H. Goodglass and E. Kaplan, *Boston Diagnostic Aphasia Examination*, Lea & Febiger, Philadelphia (1972).
15. B.E. Porch, *Porch Index of Communicative Ability*, Consulting Psychologists Press, Palo Alto, CA (1971).

16. A. Kertesz, *Western Aphasia Battery*, Grune & Stratton, New York (1982).
17. O. Spreen and A. Benton. *Neurosensory Center Comprehensive Examination for Aphasia*, University of Victoria Press, Victoria, British Columbia (1969).
18. M.L. Albert, R. Sparks, and N. Helm, *Arch. Neurol.*, 29:130–131 (1973).
19. J.A. West, *Arch. Phys. Med. Rehab.*, 54:78–86 (1973).
20. M. Naeser, *Arch. Phys. Med. Rehab.*, 67:393–399 (1986).
21. N. Helm-Estabrooks, P.F. Fitzpatrick, and B.A. Benson, *J. Speech Hearing Dis.*, 47:385–389 (1982).
22. M.L. Albert, D.L. Bachman, A. Morgan, and N. Helm-Estabrooks, *Neurology*, 38:877–879 (1988).
23. Z.J. Zhang, *J. Tradit. Chin. Med.*, 9:87–89 (1989).
24. J.B. Floyd, *Hosp. Pract.*, 24:18 (1989).
25. R. David, P. Enderby, and D. Bainton, *J. Neurol. Neurosurg. Psychiatry*, 45: 957–961 (1982).
26. J. Hartman and W.M. Landau, *Arch. Neurol.*, 44:646– 649 (1987).
27. R.T. Wertz, D.G. Weiss, J.L. Aten, R.H. Brookshire, et al., *Arch. Neurol.*, 43: 653–658 (1986).
28. M.T. Sarno, M. Silverman, and E. Sands, *J. Speech Hearing Res.*, 13:607–623 (1970).
29. A. Basso, E. Capitani, and L. Vignolo, *Arch. Neurol.*, 36:190–196 (1979).
30. C. Shewan and A. Kertesz, *Brain Lang.*, 23:272–299 (1984).
31. D.F. Benson, *Arch. Neurol.*, 36:187–189 (1979).
32. R.W. Doty, *Handbook of Physiology*, Section 6, Alimentary Canal, Volume IV, Motility, American Physiological society, Washington, D.C., pp. 1861–1902 (1968).
33. J.A. Logemann, *Evaluation and Treatment of Swallowing Disorders*, College-Hill Press, San Diego, CA (1983).
34. M. Lederman, *Clin. Radiol.*, 28:1–14 (1977).
35. A. Jean and A. Car, *Brain Res.*, 179:567–572 (1979).
36. R.W. Doty, *Handbook of Physiology*, Section 6, Alimentary Canal, Volume IV, Motility, American Physiological Society, Washington, D.C., pp. 1861–1902 (1968).
37. M.W. Donner, *Semin. Roentgenol.*, 9(4):273–282 (1974).
38. A.J. Miller, *Exp. Neurol.*, 34:210–222 (1972).
39. J. Hellemans, H.O. Agg, W. Pelemans, and G. Vantrappen, *Med. Clin. North Am.*, 65(6):1149–1171 (1981).
40. A. Jean, *Brain Behav. Evol.*, 25:109–116 (1984).
41. J.P. Kessler and A. Jean, *Exp. Brain Res.*, 57:256–263 (1985).
42. G. Holstege, G. Graveland, C. Bijker-Biemond, et al., *Brain Behav. Evol.*, 23: 47–62 (1983).
43. N.A. Leopold and M.C. Kagel, *Arch. Phys. Med. Rehab.*, 64:371–373 (1983).
44. S.L. Veis and J.A. Logemann, *Arch. Phys. Med. Rehab.*, 66(6):372–375 (1985).
45. J. Horner, *Neurology*, 38:317–319 (1988).
46. S.L. Gresham, *Med. J. Aust.*, 153:397–399 (1990).
47. D.H. Barer, *J. Neurol. Neurosurg. Psychiatry*, 52:236–241 (1989).

48. J. Robbins and R.L. Levine, *Dysphagia*, 3:11–17 (1988).
49. J. Horner, E.W. Massey, and S. Brazer, *Neurology*, 40:1686–1688 (1990).
50. P. Linden and A.A. Siebens, *Arch. Phys. Med. Rehab.*, 64:281–284 (1983).
51. M.L. Splaingard, B. Hutchins, L.D. Sulton, and G. Chaudhuri, *Arch. Phys. Med. Rehab.*, 69:637–640 (1988).
52. B. Jones and M.W. Donner, *Radiology*, 167:319–326 (1988).
53. J.E. Riski, J. Horner, and B.S. Nashold, *Neurology*, 40:1443–1445 (1990).
54. O. Ekberg, G. Nylander, F.-T. Fork, S. Sjoberg, et al., *Dysphagia*, 3:46–48 (1988).
55. S.H. Shawker, B. Sonies, M. Stone, and B.J. Baum, *J. Clin. Ultrasound*, 11:485–490 (1983).
56. T.H. Shawker, B.C. Sonies, and M. Stone, *Ultrasound Annu.*, 237–260 (1984).
57. T.H. Shawker, B. Sonies, T.E. Hall, and B.F. Baum, *Invest. Radiol.*, 19:82–86 (1984).
58. M.E. Groher, *Dysphagia*, 1:215–216 (1987).
59. J.A. Logemann, *Dysphagia*, 1(1):34–38 (1986).
60. G. de L. Lazzara, C. Lazarus, and J.A. Logemann, *Dysphagia*, 1:73–77 (1986).
61. J.A. Logemann, P.J. Kahrilas, M. Kobara, and N.B. Vakil, *Arch. Phys. Med. Rehab.*, 70:767–771 (1989).
62. M. Bushmann, S.M. Dobmeyer, L. Leeker, and J.S. Perlmutter, *Neurology*, 39:1309–1314 (1989).
63. J. Horner, F.G. Buoyer, M.J. Alberts, and M. Helms, *Arch. Neurol.*, 48:1170–1173 (1991).
64. J.A. Logemann, *Dysphagia*, 4(4):202–208 (1990).
65. K.M. Yorkston, D.R. Beukelman, and K.R. Bell, *Clinical Management of Dysarthric Speakers*, College-Hill Publishers, Boston (1988).
66. F.L. Darley, A.E. Aronson, and J.R. Brown, *Motor Speech Disorders*, W.B. Saunders, Philadelphia (1975).
67. E. Froeschel, *J. Speech Hearing Disord.*, 8:301–321 (1943).
68. R. Luchsinger and G.E. Arnold. *Voice-Speech-Language: Clinical Communicology—Its Physiology and Pathology*, Wadsworth Publishing Co., Belmont, CA (1965).
69. C. Hunter, D. Bliss, and G. Weismer, Paper presented at the American Speech–Language–Hearing Association, Los Angeles (1981).
70. R.J. Prator and R.W. Swift, *Manual of Voice Therapy*, Little, Brown, Boston (1984).
71. R. Netsell and T.J. Hixon, *J. Speech Hearing Disord.*, 43:326–330 (1978).
72. A. Putnam and T.J. Hixon, *The Dysarthrias* (M. McNeil, J. Rosenbek, and A. Aronson, eds.), College Hill Press, San Diego, CA (1984).
73. J. Smitheran and T.J. Hixon, *J. Speech Hearing Disord.*, 46:138–146 (1981).
74. N.A. Helm, *J. Speech Hearing Disord.*, 44:350–353 (1979).
75. W. Hanson and E. Metter, *J. Speech Hearing Disord.*, 45:268–276 (1980).
76. D.R. Beukelman and K.L. Garrett, *Augment. Alternate Commun.*, 4:104–121 (1988).
77. T. Mustonen, P. Locke, J. Reichle, et al., *Implementing Augmentative and*

Alternate Communication (J. Reichle, J. York, and J. Sigfoos, eds.), Paul H. Brooks, Baltimore (1991).

78. F. DeRuyter and M.R. Becker, *J. Head Trauma Rehab.*, 3:35–44 (1988).
79. D.R. Beukelman, K.M. Yorkston, and K. Smith, *Augment. Alternate Commun.*, 1:5–9 (1985).
80. G.C. Vanderheiden and K. Grilley, *Non-Vocal Communication Techniques and Aids for the Severely Physically Handicapped*, University Park Press, Baltimore (1976).
81. L.J. Bray, F. Carlson, R. Humphrey, J.P. Mastrilli, and A.S. Valko, *Community Re-Entry for Head Injured Adults* (M. Ylvisaker and Gobble, eds.), College-Hill Press, Boston (1987).
82. F. DeRuyter, L.M. Lafontaine, and M.R. Becker, *Decision Making in Speech–Language Pathology* (D.E. Yoder and R.D. Kent, eds.), Decker, Ontario (1988).

12

Rehabilitation of Cognitive Impairments

Sarah A. Raskin and Catherine A. Mateer

Good Samaritan Hospital
Puyallup, Washington

Cognitive and behavioral deficits often produce the major impairments
following a traumatic brain injury [1]. These deficits can impair the individual's ability to return to work or maintain social activities [2]. They can also
have an impact on the individual's participation in traditional rehabilitation
therapies. Therefore, professionals working with individuals who have brain
injuries would benefit from understanding these deficits and their effects on
functions such as compliance, effort, and tolerance [3]. Furthermore, a basic
understanding of the principles of cognitive rehabilitation and a knowledge of
which individuals can benefit will facilitate appropriate treatment planning
and ensure that the maximum gains are made in all therapies.

Cognitive rehabilitation has been most fully documented with individuals who have had stroke [4,5] or traumatic brain injury [6]. However, success
has been documented in a large variety of cases, including those with
Korsakoff's disease [7], age-related memory loss [8], and neurotoxin exposure [9].

In general, early intervention during more acute phases of recovery has
been shown to lead to the most profound gains following cognitive rehabilitation, and there are those who believe that rehabilitation is primarily useful in
promoting spontaneous recovery. However, it is also clear that rehabilitation
can be successful even when initiated many years after the injury, beyond the
period of spontaneous recovery [10].

MODELS OF COGNITIVE REHABILITATION

Cognitive rehabilitation is a form of intervention in which a series of procedures are applied by a trained practitioner to retrain or alleviate problems a person with brain injury encounters due to deficits in underlying cognitive functions [11,12]. Overall, any cognitive rehabilitation procedure must be based on solid, scientific knowledge of brain–behavior relationships and designed to meet specifically defined treatment goals.

There are many models of cognitive rehabilitation currently in practice [3,12–14]. However, these models can be grossly classified into two approaches, which have been termed functional skills training and process-oriented rehabilitation.

Functional skills training involves retraining specific skills of daily life, most often in a particular living or work environment. This is commonly accomplished via task analysis, followed by environmental manipulation, and development of external compensatory strategies. The skill to be retrained is broken down into its component skill parts; however, the underlying cognitive requirements of the skill or task are not examined [15]. Generalization to other skills or contexts is not expected nor considered a goal of treatment. Although the targeting of specific tasks encountered in the individual's daily life can appear to have considerable ecological validity, the narrow focus and restricted generalizability can limit the potential for recovery. Practical limitations on the number of skills that can be targeted and trained make this approach less practical.

The process approach, in contrast, involves the targeted remediation of deficits in specific cognitive areas. The separate cognitive areas most frequently identified for remediation include attention/concentration, motor planning, visual–spatial processing, learning and memory, and executive functions such as planning, reasoning, and problem solving. Each of these areas is known to be related to specific brain regions and each can be analyzed into its component parts. The process approach proceeds through one or more of these cognitive areas in a hierarchical fashion using techniques based on the cognitive, experimental, and rehabilitation psychology literature. Individualized training programs are generally based on the specific patient's pattern of cognitive impairment and his or her ultimate independent living or vocational goals. Therapy exercises are performed repeatedly until predetermined goals in each cognitive area are met.

Within the process approach, two separate methods have been utilized, both of which have been shown to be efficacious. The first involves retraining efforts focused on the restoration or improvement of specific cognitive functions; the second involves training in the use of specific compensations to assist the person in working around or in spite of cognitive limitations.

Retraining was conceptualized by Luria [16,17] as facilitating recovery of cognitive functions after brain injury through promotion of new learned connections at the level of the nervous system. He emphasized the need to focus retraining on the areas of functioning that had been disrupted, in order to facilitate new neuronal organization, including reorganization within the damaged area and transfer of function to the opposite hemisphere. This concept is based, in part, on the idea of redundancy within the brain [18].

Retraining typically begins by breaking the lost or disrupted cognitive function into its component parts. These components are arranged in a hierarchy of difficulty based on levels of cognitive involvement (e.g., auditory attention would precede auditory encoding). Then, beginning with the simplest level in the hierarchy, each step is practiced until it can be completed successfully. After each level is mastered, the person begins to practice at the next level of difficulty, until the cognitive function of focus can once again be performed. The increase in level of difficulty may be accomplished through the removal of cues or through use of more complex stimuli or more demanding tasks.

Compensation training, on the other hand, is based on the idea that some underlying cognitive functions cannot be regained once they are lost following a brain injury. Instead, the individual is taught to work around the lost function. For example, Luria [19] described a case in which tactile input was used to bypass the individual's visual–spatial deficits. In this case, the visual–spatial functions are not recovered, but a different modality is used to process the same information. Compensation training also involves the use of external aids (e.g., a watch with an alarm). This technique has most commonly been used with individuals who have memory deficits. This technique does not attempt to recover the memory functions. Instead, success in a variety of functional settings has been obtained using memory notebooks in which critical information is written down in a systematic fashion [12].

One particular method within the process approach has been referred to as the noetic approach [13]. This approach focuses on increasing awareness and on directly training the individual's capacity to recognize and regulate her or his own behavior. This approach has been used primarily with individuals with dysfunction of frontal cortical systems. Through a procedure of diminished cuing, often beginning with some external monitoring by the therapist, the individual learns through practice to internalize specific skills or behaviors and apply them to a variety of situations [20,21]. In individuals whose other cognitive functions are adequate so that this technique can be used, the greatest level of generalization can be expected.

Many specific techniques within the process approach can be useful for recovery of functional activity, whether based on retraining or development of compensation strategies, if the technique is tailored to the individual's strengths and weaknesses, as well as his or her goals. Treatment goals must be determined by the individual, based on that person's interests, needs, and social milieu. Thus, regardless of technique, the most important aspect of cognitive remediation is generalization to the individual's daily life.

The issue of generalization has been described by many authors as the most critical aspect of evaluating the effectiveness of cognitive rehabilitation [22,23]. However, the operational definition of generalization is often very different from study to study. Some studies define generalization only in terms of return to work [24], while others focus on the ability to improve performance on neuropsychological tests [25]. Generalization has been described by Gordon [23] as consisting of three levels. The first level is that the gains from remediation should hold true on the same materials on separate occasions. The second level is that improvement on the training tasks is also observed on a similar but not identical set of tasks. The third level of generalization is that the functions gained in training are shown to transfer to functions in day-to-day living.

It is perhaps uninteresting to note improvement at level I. Many studies, on the other hand, have used improvement at level II as a gross measure of generalization. For example, Sohlberg and Mateer [10] have demonstrated success in using attention training techniques by noting improvement on standardized neuropsychological measures, as presented in Table 1.

The most common method for evaluating generalization is return to work. When this is performed within a structured setting that allows for specific vocational counseling, success has been demonstrated. For example, Good Samaritan Hospital Centers for Cognitive Rehabilitation discharged a

Table 1 Average Pre- and Posttreatment Scores

PASAT[a]	Pre	S.D.	Post	S.D.	Paired t-Test
Trial 1[b]	37.2	10.4	45.5	11.6	$p < 0.01$
Trial 2	33.6	9.7	38.4	11.2	$p < 0.01$
Trial 3	28.2	9.8	33.4	13.0	$p < 0.05$
Trial 4	20.8	7.5	26.9	11.0	$p < 0.01$

Treatment consisted of attention process training, as described in text.
[a]Paced Auditory Serial Addition Test: A test of sustained auditory attention. Scores indicate number correct.
[b]Trial refers to each part of a single administration of the test. Each trial requires successively faster response.

total of 63 participants in 1987–1991. See Figure 1 for a description of the vocational status of participants before and after treatment. As can be seen in the figure, 91% of participants were unemployed at program entry, 3% were in competitive employment, and 6% were in a supported work situation or employed by a family member. At discharge, however, only 17% were unemployed, 29% were in competitive employment, 25% were in a supported work situation, 22% were in school or training, and 6% were active in some productive activity such as volunteer work. Furthermore, these gains were maintained after discharge. Thus, at 1 year after discharge 27% were unemployed, 44% were in competitive employment, 9% were in a supported work situation, 16% were in training, and 4% were involved in a productive activity.

Vocational counseling at this program takes into account an analysis of cognitive skills, premorbid vocational interests, and personal goals. Counseling involves analyzing a current job and counseling patients regarding returning to that job or finding another. Some focus is on identifying and utilizing the often considerable preserved and transferable skills. Participants are involved in a series of monitored job stations. Two months before program completion, intensive job search and placement efforts are begun. A follow-up plan for job maintenance is instituted when the patient is discharged from the program.

Although return to work is important in many ways, many aspects of finding employment are not directly under the control of the individual, such as current economic conditions. Individuals with mild cognitive deficits and excellent skills can have difficulty returning to work, especially if the employer is put off by the stigma of brain injury or if the type of work depends solely on extremely high level cognitive skills.

Of course, the definition of generalization must, like treatment, be identified on an individual basis. Meltzer [26] suggests using common activities, whether social, recreational, or occupational, that are important to the individual as the focus of treatment. Two case examples in the Appendix illustrate this point.

BASIC METHOD OF COGNITIVE REHABILITATION

The first step in developing a cognitive rehabilitation plan generally involves a comprehensive neuropsychological evaluation to determine the areas of cognitive deficits, as well as areas of cognitive strengths that can be used, especially for compensation techniques. This evaluation would also include an evaluation of mood and personality factors known to interact with cognitive functioning. Finally, the person's level of insight or awareness will be determined, since this is a critical factor in the success of rehabilitation.

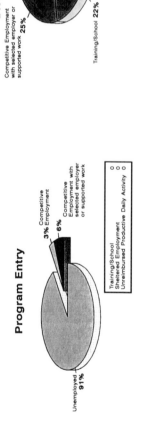

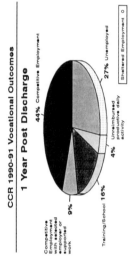

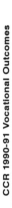

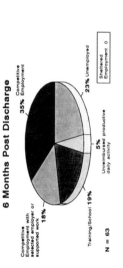

Figure 1   Vocational outcomes of participants in center for cognitive rehabilitation (CCR).

In conjunction with the neuropsychological evaluation it is essential that the individual be interviewed with regard to particular goals and specific losses in everyday functioning that he or she finds most distressing. It is helpful to use a questionnaire of everyday functioning, such as the Everyday Memory Questionnaire [27]. However, it is also important to be sure that all domains of functioning are explored. It is useful to determine how the person spends his or her time currently, so that activities that are pleasurable and productive can be increased and other activities added. For this purpose, it is helpful to use activity pattern indicators. Within these indicators, times when the individual had difficulty can also be recorded (e.g., forgetting the name of someone at work) so that an accurate account of the impact of the cognitive deficits on the person's daily life can be developed. It may be helpful to have a family member or friend help with this if such a person is available.

Next, the person's major complaints and goals must be analyzed within the context of neuropsychological performance. An example of this would be determining whether a person's difficulty with shifting mental set was because of mental rigidity, impulsivity, and/or a concentration deficit. Once a hypothesis is formed as to the neuropsychological cause of the disability, a treatment plan can be devised. If any compensation strategies are to be used, an analysis of the spared functions to be utilized must be done. Then the function to be remediated must be broken down into logical, sequential steps based on theories of cognition.

Before treatment is initiated, a measure of outcome must also be determined. This is necessary so that a criterion measure can be developed and so that a re-evaluation can be performed using the measure of outcome. Only in this way is it possible to determine if the treatment is meeting with success or should be terminated. This outcome measure may have to be created for a particular case or a standard measure may suffice. This must be determined on a case-by-case basis.

Once treatment criteria are reached, the re-evaluation should include measures of generalization as well as measures of functions that were not the focus of rehabilitation. The general finding that cognitive rehabilitation improves the functions treated and not other functions lends support to the argument that the remediation itself was responsible for the improvement, rather than a general factor related to the structure and support of coming to treatment sessions regularly.

Within the cognitive rehabilitation program, of course, psychological factors such as coping skills and degree of insight must be addressed. Prigatano [28] describes a four-step process that involves compensation training, substitution, and cognitive retraining. The first step is to reduce generalized confusion by systematically improving attentional skills. The second step is counseling to help the individual gain awareness of strengths as well as deficits. Then, the need for compensatory behaviors is demonstrated. Finally, cognitive deficits are addressed in the broader context of how they affect interpersonal skills.

Some of the complicating factors in determining the effectiveness of a cognitive rehabilitation program include specifying the effects of spontaneous recovery, individual differences in brain organization, degree of awareness of deficits, disturbance in mood, premorbid personality, and the premorbid pattern of cognitive strengths and weaknesses.

Attention Retraining

Attentional skills are disrupted by a wide variety of causes and attention is a critical underlying component of many cognitive functions. Without intact attentional skills, many other skills, including learning, communication, and problem-solving, become difficult or impossible [29]. Furthermore, attention deficits can be mistaken for memory deficits when memory functions are, in fact, intact. Moreover, disruption of the physiological systems critical to the regulation of attention may occur as the result of seemingly minor, as well as severe, neurological damage. Therefore, retraining attention skills is often the first step in a cognitive rehabilitation program [30].

Sohlberg and Mateer [10] have demonstrated the usefulness of a method for the rehabilitation of attention processes based on the experimental attention literature, clinical observation, and patients' subjective complaints. Attention is considered to be a multidimensional cognitive capacity critical to memory, new learning, and all other aspects of cognition. These authors defined attention as the capacity to focus on particular stimuli over time and to manipulate the information flexibly. This is based grossly on Broadbent's [31] model of attention as a selectivity phenomenon by means of which target stimuli receive priority processing over concurrent nontarget stimuli. Sohlberg and Mateer then expand on this model to include Baddeley's [32] concept of the central executive, which allows information to be held in short-term storage while attention is temporarily shifted to other stimuli.

These authors then developed a multilevel conceptualization of attention. The five levels identified are:

Focused attention: The ability to respond discretely to specific visual, auditory, or tactile stimuli

Sustained attention: The ability to maintain a consistent behavioral response during continuous or repetitive activity

Selective attention: The ability to maintain a cognitive set that requires activation and inhibition of responses dependent upon discrimination of stimuli

Alternating attention: The capacity for mental flexibility that allows one to move between tasks having different cognitive requirements

Divided attention: The ability to respond simultaneously to multiple tasks.

Hierarchies of treatment tasks were then developed for each of these five levels of attention, which are described below. Therapy was conducted using tasks and treatment materials specifically designed or selected for each level of attention. A multiple baseline across cognitive areas was used to assess the effectiveness of this training program in brain-injured subjects [10,33]. The Paced Auditory Serial Addition Task (PASAT) [34] was used as the outcome measure, since it presupposes the existence of focused attention and depends on the adequacy of sustained and selective attention.

Focused Attention

Although this is often disrupted early in the recovery process, none of the subjects who participated in this study had difficulty at this basic level.

Sustained Attention

Sustained attention tasks require consistent responding to either aurally or visually presented information. Visually based exercises include a variety of cancellation tasks in which the individual scans an array of stimuli and crosses out particular target(s). After each level of successful acquisition, the task is then made more difficult. This can be accomplished either through altering the stimuli (e.g., making the targets smaller, less organized, or embedded in text) or by altering the task demands (e.g., begin with canceling a single target, then two different targets simultaneously, then one target only if followed immediately by another, etc.) [14].

The Attention Process Training (APT) [10,33] also uses auditory stimuli. There are 16 audio cassette tapes and individuals respond to targets by pushing a buzzer. At higher levels of sustained attention training, there are greater demands on mental control and information processing. Subjects may be asked to respond to sequences of ascending or descending numbers or letters, then days of the week or months of the year (i.e., respond when you hear 2 months of the year that are in the correct order).

In one case, a 32-year-old male corrections officer was struck by an oncoming vehicle while driving. He apparently hit his head on the steering wheel or windshield. His wife reported that he lost consciousness momentarily and appeared dazed. No medical attention was sought until the following day, when he saw his family physician because of a severe headache. Several months later, he was referred for a neuropsychological evaluation, upon his own insistence. He had experienced difficulties returning to work and had been placed on medical leave.

The task presented to him was to repeat, in alphabetical order, five words presented in a sentence. Initial performance in trial 1 indicated a total time of 370 sec with three errors on a set of 10 sentences. On this basis, a target time goal of 295 sec (20% decrease) was set. An accuracy goal was set at 90%. The criterion for task mastery required meeting the time and accuracy goals on 2 of 3 consecutive sets of 10 sentences. This was achieved after 10 total trials utilizing the task.

Selective Attention

Training at this level involves the incorporation of distracting or irrelevant information during task performance. For visual cancellation tasks, plastic overlays with distracting designs have been found to be useful. For auditory tests, the same attention tapes are used with the addition of background distracting noise. This may be in the form of a news broadcast, a sports commentary, cafeteria noise, or conversation. Some individuals are more disrupted by internal than external distraction, that is, worry, rumination, or preoccupation with personal concerns or agendas. With these individuals, focusing on reducing these distractions may be primary. Techniques such as writing things down and then setting the paper aside before beginning a task may be helpful.

Alternating Attention

Problems at this level are evident in the individual who has difficulty changing treatment tasks once a "set" has been established and who needs extra cuing to pick up and initiate new task requirements. Training requires flexible redirection and reallocation of attention. Effective tasks require repeated changes in task demands. The patient might, for example, be asked to respond first to ascending numbers and then, on cue, to descending numbers. Training tasks often involve material that can be treated, or responded to, in different ways. Requirements are for frequent and repeated changes in cognitive or response set. In the final stages of such training, the person can be asked to generate real-life situations that are problematic (e.g., listening to a lecture and taking notes at the same time). This can then be used as the treatment material [30].

Divided Attention

This level of attention is required whenever an individual is performing multiple simultaneous tasks (e.g., driving a car while holding a conversation). Training in this area involves the use of tasks in which multiple information must be attended to simultaneously, for example, combining an auditory and a visual vigilance task.

Training Use of Compensatory Memory Devices

Individuals with profound memory loss provide a particular challenge for specialists in cognitive remediation. It is now accepted that mnemonics do not, in general, aid those with amnesia [35]. Instead, many researchers have been investigating external memory aids [36]. One type of external memory aid that has been used recently with success in persons with amnesia is a memory log book for recording information in a systematic fashion that would have otherwise been stored in memory [12,37]. These authors used a three-stage training procedure for learning use of a memory notebook based in both learning and neuropsychological theory. Effective memory book use requires that the person consistently and correctly record and refer to information in the book. These rule-based actions must be acquired and made automatic through structured, sequenced training and repetition.

In implementing a compensatory memory system the clinician must first evaluate the person's current and future needs relative to living and work environments. This provides the necessary information to determine what the notebook should contain for it to be of use. For example, some people may require orientation information with pertinent autobiographical data while others may instead need only information relevant to their work. Possible notebook sections are listed below.

Orientation: Narrative autobiographical information concerning personal data and/or information surrounding the brain injury.

Memory log: Information recorded about the activities that have been performed each hour of the day.

Calendar: A calendar with dates and times so that appointments and future activities can be scheduled.

Things to Do: A list of things that need to be performed, with space for a due date and a completion date.

Transportation: Maps and/or bus information to frequently visited places.

Feelings log: A place to chart feelings relative to specific incidents or times.

Names: A place to record names and identifying information about new people.

Today at Work: A section tailored to the specific work environment to allow the individual to record necessary information pertinent to job duties.

Things I Forgot: A dated list of times when a memory failure was evident, so that any pattern of such difficulties can be analyzed and solutions developed. This also allows one to track any decrease in such difficulties with time.

Consistent with learning theory [38], three phases of learning are implemented in memory notebook training: acquisition, application, and adaptation. Each phase imposes different demands on the learner and requires adjustment in instructional strategies.

The acquisition phase refers to learning how to perform the new skill. The person needs to become familiar with the purpose and use of each different section in the notebook. This familiarization training is achieved through repetitive administration of questions regarding notebook contents and use specific to the individual's notebook.

The second stage, application, refers to learning when and where to utilize the new skill. Role-playing has been successful. Specific home- or work-related events are role-played and the use of the notebook in those situations is demonstrated.

The final stage, adaptation, refers to the process of generalization in which the individual is able to adapt and modify the skill use to novel situations. This can be trained by accompanying the individual to a variety of naturalistic settings and monitoring performance on notebook use.

Important in each of these stages is that the use of the notebook is repeated consistently until the individual has mastered that stage before moving on to the next stage. Thus, the technique is based on exploiting procedural memory skills, which are generally intact in individuals with even severe amnesia, and utilizing repetition to facilitate learning a new skill.

CONCLUSIONS

The practice of cognitive rehabilitation for individuals with brain injury will vary substantially for each individual, depending on his or her background, personality, neuropsychological deficits, and personal goals, and thus must be individually tailored. Because there are organically based physical, cognitive, and emotional/behavioral changes following such an injury, the individual can experience a cycle of negative emotional responses that reinforces chronicity and disability. Thus, cognitive and emotional changes serve to increase stress, anxiety, and depression, which have a further impact on cognitive and emotional functioning. Early provision of realistic information and follow-up during the first few months after injury is strongly encouraged to help to avoid this cycle. Even for patients seen months or years following injury, data have been presented that support the potential for excellent cognitive and psychosocial gains and return to full-time competitive employment. Treatment of attentional, memory, and organizational skills must be systematically presented, coupled with tasks designed to generalize learned skills to everyday activities, and with effective psychosocial and vocational intervention.

APPENDIX

Case 1

Subject

A 38-year-old right-handed man had completed high school and 2 years of a chef training school. He worked as a chef in a Chinese restaurant. While at work, he fell, striking his head on the left side, and then a heavy box fell and hit the right side of his head. He lost consciousness for several hours and is unable to recall any events of the day of the accident or several days afterwards. He was taken to a nearby medical center where computed tomographic (CT) and electroencephalographic (EEG) results were normal. He complained of memory difficulties, difficulty with initiation, and difficulty doing two things at once. Interview with his wife corroborated that he was having trouble remembering events since the injury. He has also been unable to cook, even with recipes.

Neuropsychological assessment 9 months after the accident revealed that he had an above-average level of intellectual functioning, average visual attention and visual–perceptual skills, above average problem-solving and planning abilities, and average linguistic skills with some mild dysnomia. However, he exhibited severe deficits in auditory attention (divided attention in particular), verbal and visual memory, and in shifting mental set.

Given his cognitive profile, it was agreed that attention processes would be the first phase of treatment. It was also agreed that the final goal of the treatment would be for him to be able to cook successfully, since this had been a major source of pleasure for him and could lead potentially to a return to work. Since this was the goal, he was required, with his wife's help, to keep a daily log book. This served two purposes. First, given his memory difficulties, the book helped him to keep track of the events in his daily life. Second, he was to make particular note of the number of attempts and successful completions of meals. Since he was able to utilize the notebook immediately, no specific training was required for him to do this.

Materials and Procedures

Phase I (sessions twice per week for 1 hr; duration: 6 months; total sessions: 40). A hierarchy of divided attention tasks was employed. The first level of difficulty in the hierarchy involved relatively simple tasks of visual sustained attention (e.g., searching a page for a particular target) and relatively simple tasks of auditory sustained attention (e.g., listening on an audiotape for a particular target). The tasks were gradually made more difficult by moving to those requiring more mental concentration (e.g., searching a page for two numbers in a row in ascending order while listening on an audiotape for a particular sound). At each level, he was required to perform the task within the session, and to perform the task at home, under the supervision of his wife. The criterion for completing this phase of training was for him to be able to perform with two errors or fewer on each task for two consecutive sessions.

Phase II (sessions twice per week for 1 hr; duration: 1 month; total sessions: eight). Once he was able to perform two tasks simultaneously, representing improvement in divided attention, his ability to shift his attention became the focus of treatment. Thus, he was required to perform a series of tasks that involved switching between two sets (e.g., marking a "1" next to even numbers and a "2" next to odd numbers on a sheet with both even and odd numbers randomly distributed on a page). Again, the criterion was for him to perform with two errors or fewer on two consecutive sessions.

Phase III (sessions once per week for 1 hr; duration: 2 months; total sessions: eight). In the final phase, his interest in returning to work as a chef was addressed. In this phase, he was required to plan a meal in advance of the session. The meal was required to have at least three separate dishes (e.g., a main course and two side dishes). He was then supervised preparing the meal, with note taken of his ability to divide and shift his attention between the tasks at hand. After each session, his performance was evaluated and feedback given to him. Between sessions, he continued to perform tasks of shifting mental set to help maintain this skill.

Results

Level I generalization was measured in terms of his ability to demonstrate consistently improvement on the tasks given. Careful recording of his number of errors during each phase of the training was then subjected to a time series analysis. This analysis, compared to a double baseline, revealed that he had significantly improved at each phase ($p < 0.01$).

As a measure of Level III generalization, the log book he and his wife had been using was analyzed. The number of meals he successfully prepared in a week was counted and also subjected to a time series analysis. During the first week of training he was unable to complete any meals successfully. This increased only to one meal per week at the initiation of phase III. However, over the last 3 weeks of phase III, he was cooking an average of 10.2 meals per week.

Case 2

Subject

A 37-year-old left-handed woman had completed college with a degree in environmental science. She worked at various jobs and had recently set up her own business at the time of the accident. Since the accident she had begun a postgraduate academic program. She was the driver of an automobile hit broadside by another car. She believes she lost consciousness briefly and bystanders described her as disoriented. She had a laceration of her left forehead. Seven months later, due to continued complaints of difficulty concentrating, she underwent brain CT, which showed normal results.

Neuropsychological assessment 2 years after the accident revealed an average level of intellectual functioning, average linguistic skills, and gross visual perception. However, she exhibited deficits in auditory and visual attention that affected her learning and memory. She also had difficulty with constructional ability and organization.

Since she is currently in a high-pressure academic environment, and having difficulty taking notes in class, being able to follow class lectures and to comprehend material she read would be the final goal of treatment. These abilities were judged to be impaired due to her attention deficits, which were primarily in visual sustained attention and in selective attention.

Phase I (sessions once per week for 1 hr; duration: 3 months; total sessions: 11). In this phase her basic visual sustained attention was the focus of training. She was presented with a hierarchy of increasingly more difficult visual attention tasks. The criterion for each task was to make two or fewer errors of omission on two consecutive days.

Phase II (sessions once per week for 1 hr; duration: 1 month; total sessions: 4). At this time she was required to read written material and then be able to answer questions about what she had read. The initial session involved material of two or three sentences. The length of the passages was progressively increased until, by the end of this phase, the passages were 10 pages in length. She was also required to read passages and answer questions for homework.

Phase III (sessions once per week for 1 hr; duration: 4 months; total sessions: 16). In this phase she was presented with audiotapes with short paragraphs of information presented on them. Initially, the audiotapes had only white noise as distraction, and she was required to take notes and answer questions on what she had heard. The distraction became progressively more difficult, using classical music, then popular music, and finally two stories read by different speakers; she was required to follow only one of them. The criterion was to be able to listen to the stories and then correctly answer 10 questions about each one before proceeding to the next level of difficulty.

Results

Level I generalization was demonstrated by her ability to improve consistently on the training materials. Level II generalization was measured by her ability to perform tests of reading comprehension. On the Iowa level 2 test of reading comprehension, she scored at the 9th percentile for her age and level of education prior to the training. Following treatment she was given the Iowa level 3 test of reading comprehension and scored at the 60th percentile for her age and level of education. For level III generalization, her performance in classes before and after treatment was used. Prior to treatment, she was carrying only one class, and received a D in that class. The semester following treatment, she carried four classes and received one A and three Bs.

REFERENCES

1. J. Cole, N. Cope, and L. Cervelli, *Arch. Phys. Med. Rehab.*, 66:38–40 (1985).
2. N. Brooks, L. Campsie, C. Symington, A. Beattie, J. Bryden, and W. McKinlay, *Head Trauma Rehab.*, 2(3):1–13 (1987).
3. R.L. Wood and I. Fussey, *Cognitive Rehabilitation in Perspective*, Taylor & Francis, Bristol, PA (1990).
4. W. Gordon, M.R. Hibbard, S. Egelko, L. Diller, P. Shaver, A. Lieberman, and K. Ragnarsson, *Arch. Phys. Med. Rehab.*, 66:353–359 (1985).
5. B.A. Wilson, *Cortex*, 18:581–594 (1982).
6. C.A. Mateer and M.M. Sohlberg, *Neuropsychological Studies of Nonfocal Brain Damage: Dementia and Trauma* (H. Whitaker, ed.), Springer-Verlag, New York, pp. 204–219 (1988).
7. L.S. Cermak, *Cortex*, 11:163–169 (1975).
8. R. Jutagir, *Neurorehabilitation*, 2(3):55–61 (1992).
9. S.A. Raskin and W.A. Gordon, *J. Clin. Exp. Neuropsychol.*, 14(3) (abstract) (1992).
10. M.M. Sohlberg and C.A. Mateer, *J. Clin. Exp. Neuropsychol.*, 9:117–130 (1987).
11. W.A. Gordon and M.R. Hibbard, *Cognitive Rehabilitation for Persons with Traumatic Brain Injury* (J. Kreutzer and P. Wehman, eds.), Paul Brooks, Baltimore (1991).
12. M.M. Sohlberg and C.A. Mateer, *Introduction to Cognitive Rehabilitation: Theory and Practice*, Guilford Press, New York (1989).
13. K. Cicerone and D. Tupper, (1991).
14. L. Diller and W.A. Gordon, *J. Consult. Clin. Psychol.*, 49:822–834 (1981).
15. N.H. Mayer, D.J. Keating, and D. Rapp, *Clinical Neuropsychology of Intervention* (B. Uzzel and Y. Gross, eds.), Martinus Nijhoff, Boston (1986).
16. A.R. Luria, V.L. Naydin, L.S. Tsvetkova, and E.N. Vinarskaya, *Handbook of Clinical Neurology* (P.J. Vinkin and G.W. Bruyn, eds.), John Wiley & Sons, New York (1969).
17. A. Luria, *The Working Brain*, Basic Books, New York (1973).
18. S. Finger and D.G. Stein, *Brain Damage and Recovery*, Academic Press, New York (1982).
19. A.R. Luria, *Restoration of Function after Brain Injury*, Macmillan, New York (1963).
20. K.D. Cicerone and J. Wood, *Arch. Phys. Med. Rehab.*, 68:111–115 (1987).
21. M.M. Sohlberg, H. Sprunk, and K. Metzelaar, *Cognit. Rehab.*, 6:36–41 (1988).
22. I. Fussey, *Cognitive Rehabilitation in Perspective* (R.L. Wood and I. Fussey, eds.), Taylor and Francis, Bristol, PA (1990).
23. W.A. Gordon, *Neuropsychological Rehabilitation* (M. Meir, A.L. Benton, and L. Diller, eds.), Churchill Livingstone, London (1987).
24. G.P. Prigatano, D.J. Fordyce, H.K. Zeiner, J.R. Rouche, M. Pepping, and B.C. Wood, *Neuropsychological Rehabilitation After Brain Injury* (G. Prigatano, ed.), Johns Hopkins University Press, Baltimore (1986).
25. R.M. Ruff, C.A. Baser, J.W. Johnson, L.F. Marshall, A.K. Klauber, M.R. Klauber, and M. Mateer, *J. Head Trauma Rehab.*, 4(3):26–36 (1989).

26. M. Meltzer, *J. Clin. Psychol.*, 39:3–11 (1983).
27. M.M. Sohlberg and C.A. Mateer, *Community Integration Following Traumatic Brain Injury* (J.S. Kreutzer and P. Lehman, eds.), Paul H. Brookes, Baltimore (1990).
28. G. Prigatano, *Neuropsychological Rehabilitation After Brain Injury*, Johns Hopkins University Press, Baltimore (1986).
29. R.Ll. Wood, *Neuro-Behavioural Sequelae of Traumatic Brain Injury*, Taylor & Francis, Bristol, PA (1990).
30. S.A. Raskin and W.A. Gordon, *Neurorehabilitation*, 2(3):38–45 (1992).
31. D.E. Broadbent, *Perception and Communication*, Pergamon, London (1958).
32. A.D. Baddeley, *Cognition*, 10:17–20 (1981).
33. C.A. Mateer, M.M. Sohlberg, and P.K. Youngman, *Cognitive Rehabilitation in Perspective* (R.L. Wood and I. Fussey, eds.), Taylor & Francis, London (1990).
34. D. Gronwall, *Percept. Mot. Skills*, 44a:367–373 (1971).
35. M. O'Conner and L.S. Cermack, *Neuropsychological Rehabilitation* (M. Meier, L. Diller, and A. Benton, eds.), Guilford Press, New York (1986).
36. J. Harris, *Practical Aspects of Memory* (M. Gruneberg, P. Morris, and R. Sykes, eds.), Academic Press, London (1978).
37. A. Finset and S. Andresen, *Cognitive Rehabilitation in Perspective* (R.L. Wood and I. Fussey, eds.), Taylor & Francis, Bristol (1990).
38. K. Liberty, H. Haring, and O. White, *Methods of Instruction for Severely Handicapped Students* (W. Sailor, B. Wilcox, and L. Brown, eds.), Paul Brooks, Baltimore (1980).

13

Orthotic Treatment of Neurological Deficits

John W. Michael

Otto Bock U.S.A.
Minneapolis, Minnesota

Recent advances in the medical and surgical treatment of neurological conditions have significantly reduced, but not eliminated, the long-term sequelae.
As a result, more and more people are surviving with mild to moderate
physical disabilities that are amenable to orthotic management. For example,
as the result of aggressive and effective management of cerebral vascular
accidents (CVA), many survive with hemiplegic gait anomalies that respond
very well to orthotic intervention [1].

The active interest of the neurologist and neurosurgeon in orthotic
management is a recent development. The certified orthotist has much to
learn from, and to share with, this group of physicians. Based on the
experience from many decades of close collaboration, initially with orthoped-
ists and later with physiatrists as well, the development of multidisciplinary
clinic teams interested in specific problems is a proven method of making
clinical advances in the effective orthotic management of patients with
neurological deficits.

The most productive approach has been to combine the expertise of
physician and orthotist, with each contributing for the patient's benefit.
Usually the physician has the best understanding of the patient, the pathological condition, and prognosis. The orthotist contributes a practical knowledge
of functional biomechanics, the available orthotic options, and current opinion regarding the clinical effectiveness of particular designs.

Whenever the clinical picture is complex or unclear, the prescription

"Evaluate for orthosis to . . .; please call with recommendations" is appropriate. General requests such as ". . . to enhance gait" are not as helpful as specific requests such as ". . . to reduce knee flexion." There is no value in specifying a particular orthosis when it is not clear that one type is preferable. "Evaluate for orthosis to reduce knee flexion in stance" could bring a recommendation for a knee orthosis (KO), a knee–ankle–foot orthosis (KAFO), or an ankle–foot orthosis (AFO), depending on technical considerations and other clinical factors. "Evaluate for KAFO to reduce knee flexion" will generate far fewer options.

Orthotic management of various disorders has progressed significantly in recent decades, for several reasons:

1. Modern plastics have allowed the development of lighter, more acceptable, and more effective designs [2], making the cumbersome metal bracing of yesterday increasingly uncommon except in selected cases.
2. Continued upgrading of the requirements to become a certified orthotist (CO) or certified prosthetist orthotist (CPO) has resulted in a more knowledgeable and versatile clinician than the "brace technician" of the past [3].
3. Long-term collaboration between physicians and orthotists sharing an interest in a specific pathological disorder (e.g., scoliosis) has resulted in continued improvement in our understanding and management of specific problems.

Due to recent technical advances in orthotic design, literature based on experiences prior to the 1980s must be evaluated critically. Many of the cherished aphorisms of previous decades (e.g., "No plastic if spastic") have simply proven incorrect [4], and must be discarded.

Nowhere is this more apparent than in the orthotic management of individuals with a neurological deficit. This chapter will highlight and review some of the more common and effective orthoses that have proven value for this patient population.

OVERVIEW

The simplest definition of an orthosis is "An external device that applies biomechanical forces to the body." Many devices meet this definition, including plaster or synthetic casts, simple off-the-shelf supports, modular devices assembled from prefabricated modules, and custom-molded thermoplastic designs formed over a rectified positive model of the affected body part. Although today's certified orthotist is particularly proficient at providing the more complex custom-molded devices, this level of care is not always required. Particularly for short-term conditions (e.g., the dropfoot that results from a minor peroneal nerve contusion), a custom-fitted modular device or off-the-shelf item may suffice. How is the physician to select wisely from the array of choices available?

Anatomical Nomenclature

There is now widespread agreement that the most effective principle to guide orthotic prescription is the biomechanical function required. This approach was originally proposed by a joint committee of orthotists, prosthetists, engineers, and surgeons in the early 1970s [5], and avoids much of the confusion engendered when devices were formerly described by eponyms that honored the inventor or promoter but added little to our clinical understanding.

Proper descriptive terminology is now based on the segment of the body encompassed by the orthosis, often abbreviated by the acronym formed by the first letter of the body segment. Figure 1 summarizes the accepted nomenclature [6]. This has greatly simplified and clarified the description of specific orthoses and has been adopted by most English-speaking countries throughout the world. Whether in England, Australia, Canada, or the United States, a device that supports the ankle by encompassing the foot and calf region is termed an ankle–foot orthosis, usually abbreviated to an AFO.

Control of Motion

The second basic concept of the nomenclature is to describe the orthosis in terms of its control of anatomical joint motion [7]. Only five types of biomechanical control are possible, listed below from the least to most restrictive:

1. Free: unrestricted motion in the stated plane
2. Assist: application of external force to increase the range, velocity, or force of the desired motion
3. Resist: the opposite of (2), indicating application of external force to decrease the range, velocity, or force of the undesirable motion
4. Stop: completely eliminates motion in one specified direction
5. Hold: immobilizes the body segment in all planes

An orthosis to prevent the paralyzed foot from contacting the floor during swing phase could be described as an AFO with dorsiflexion assist to prevent foot drop, giving both orthotist and physician a clear image of the function desired. Note that a variety of devices could be selected to fill this prescription, based on more detailed examination of the patient and other technical considerations.

For example, if grossly fluctuating edema prevents the use of an intimately fitted plastic device, the aluminum and leather AFO with a spring-

Name_____ Date:_____

Diagnosis:

UPPER LIMB		FLEX	EXT	ABD	ADD	ROTATION Int.	ROTATION Ext.	AXIAL LOAD
SEWHO	Shoulder							
EWHO	Humerus							
	Elbow							
	Forearm					(Pron.)	(Sup.)	
WHO	Wrist			(RD)	(UD)			
HO	Hand							
	Fingers 2-5 { MP							
	PIP							
	DIP							
	Thumb { CM					(Opposition)		
	MP							
	IP							

SPINE		FLEX	EXT	LATERAL FLEXION R	LATERAL FLEXION L	ROTATION R	ROTATION L	
CTLSO	Cervical							
TLSO	Thoracic							
LSO	Lumbar							
	(Lumbo-sacral)							
SIO	Sacroiliac							

LOWER LIMB		FLEX	EXT	ABD	ADD	ROTATION Int.	ROTATION Ext.
HKAO	Hip						
KAO	Thigh						
	Knee						
AFO	Leg						
	Ankle	(Dorsi)	(Plantar)				
FO	Foot { Subtalar					(Inver.)	(Ever.)
	Midtarsal						
	Met.-phal.						

REMARKS:

KEY: Use the following symbols to indicate desired control of designated function:

F = FREE — Free motion.

A = ASSIST — Application of an external force for the purpose of increasing the range, velocity, or force of a motion.

R = RESIST — Application of an external force for the purpose of decreasing the velocity or force of a motion.

S = STOP — Inclusion of a static unit to deter an undesired motion in one direction.

v = Variable — A unit that can be adjusted without making a structural change.

H = HOLD — Elimination of all motion in prescribed plane (verify position).

L = LOCK — Device includes an optional lock.

Figure 1 Prescription chart illustrates basic terminology guidelines. Orthotic devices are described by the body segment covered and functional control desired.

loaded ankle may be the best choice. Conversely, if additional weight is a major concern and there is no edema, a lightweight, flexible plastic AFO that fits inside conventional footwear may be preferable. In the future, when miniature electronic stimulators for the peroneal nerve become commercially practical, an electronic AFO may be the best alternative. Figure 2 illustrates examples of different orthoses that would all provide the specified function.

Functional Description

Specifying the function desired allows the orthotist the latitude to select specific components, designs, and materials that best meet the patient's needs, taking into account such technical details as durability, availability, and cost-effectiveness. This approach also readily incorporates new orthoses, as they are developed, that provide appropriate biomechanical results. The physician should be as specific in the prescription as is necessary to communicate clearly: plastic AFO with plantarflexion stop to prevent toe drag ensures that neither metal alloy nor electrical stimulation would be considered, and clearly indicates that plantar flexion beyond neutral is prohibited. Figure 3 illustrates one example of a device that meets these specifications.

Four additional descriptions are used, when appropriate, to define further the function of the orthosis:

1. Lock: self-explanatory, and describes a "removable hold" such as at the knee joint
2. Degree: can be used to indicate the desired position of a stop, as in stop dorsiflexion at 5 degrees

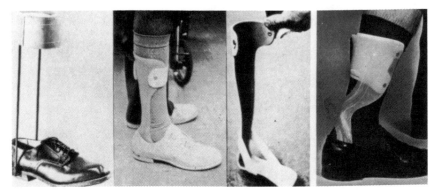

Figure 2   Four different but functionally equivalent orthoses to prevent foot drop. The orthotist selects the preferred design based on the patient's characteristics and technical considerations.

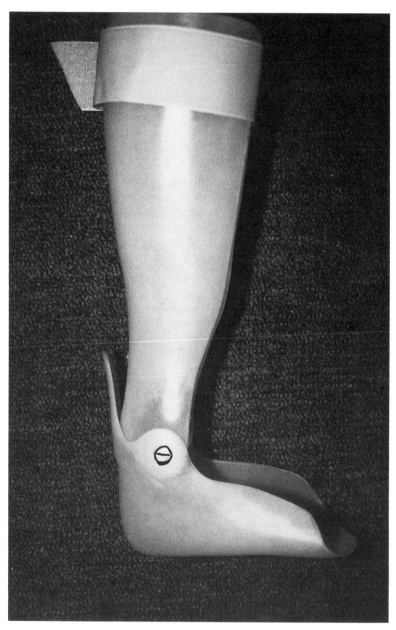

Figure 3 One AFO design in thermoplastic that allows free dorsiflexion via hinge at the ankle. Small plastic tab in Achilles tendon area of foot plate contacts the calf shell and stops excessive plantar flexion.

3. Variable: specifies an adjustable stop such as knee flexion stop adjustable from 0 to 90 degrees
4. Axial unloading: the special circumstance in which distal unweighting is desired

The advantage of this system is that it allows the physician to concentrate on the patient and his or her needs, by specifying the biomechanical assistance desired. The orthotist is then responsible for filling the prescription effectively, after taking into account the many technical factors that affect the clinical outcome. This approach combines the expertise of both orthotist and doctor, on the patient's behalf, and is far more practical than expecting the busy physician to master thoroughly the field of orthotics in addition to that of medicine. Figure 1 illustrates an orthotic prescription form developed by the American Academy of Orthopedic Surgeons that incorporates these principles [6].

Indications for Orthotic Intervention

Orthotic practice remains as much an art as a science, while advancements in materials, design, and our understanding of the biomechanical principles underlying specific disabilities are increasing at a brisk pace. As a result, it is often difficult to predict with precision when orthotic intervention will aid a particular patient. Close collaboration and frequent interaction between the prescribing physician and the certified orthotist are fundamental to developing the most effective approach. Retrospective review has demonstrated that successful orthotic devices fulfill one or more of these fundamental indications [7]:

1. Control of Motion
   a. Prevent motion (immobilize)
   b. Limit motion (to normal range or a portion of the normal range)
   c. Delay or prevent deformity (either development or recurrence)
2. Correction of deformity
3. Compensation for weakness

Correction of deformity is appropriate primarily for orthopedic problems and will not be discussed in this chapter. Compensation for weakness could be considered as a special case of motion control; it is effective primarily in non-weight-bearing situations and in the absence of spasticity.

The prescribing physician should ascertain that the recommended device can be expected to fulfill one of these indications. Use of the appropriate anatomical nomenclature along with accurate description of the motion control desired as well as the functional result intended will result in a clear, concise, and effective recommendation to the treating orthotist.

UPPER LIMB ORTHOSES

Today, the majority of upper limb orthoses are provided in a hospital setting by the occupational therapist [8]. Most are intended for short-term (often postoperative) use and require frequent modifications since the patient's condition is rapidly changing. Low-temperature plastics that can be easily softened in hot water and remolded are commonly used. The interested reader is referred to the therapy literature for a more complete discussion of these devices. The certified orthotist traditionally concentrates on patients with complex or long-term disabilities, using more durable but significantly more expensive materials.

Although this discussion will be subdivided into representative pathological conditions for convenience, it must be emphasized that there is no diagnosis-specific orthosis. The concept of a "cerebral palsy brace" or a "polio splint" is obsolete. Modern orthoses are prescribed and provided based on the biomechanical function desired, and an identical device may be used for patients with various pathological conditions, as long as the functional deficits are comparable.

Spinal Cord Injury

One common neurological problem presenting with a chronic upper limb deficit is the high-level spinal cord injury. Treatment is individualized according to the remaining functional musculature. One of the most significant deficits that may follow cervical cord injury is loss of hand function.

The three prerequisites for functional grasp may be summarized as proximal stability, hand placement, and grasp and release [7].

The primary requisite for hand function is torso stability. In patients with spinal cord injury, it is usually provided by careful positioning within the wheelchair, often supplemented by custom-molded seating systems and various restraining straps [9].

Once proximal stability is achieved, placement of the hand in space becomes the next hurdle. Many individuals with spinal cord injuries do retain limited shoulder and elbow function; however, many cannot overcome the force of gravity. One effective device to reduce the effects of gravity is the balanced forearm orthosis (BFO), illustrated in Figure 4 [7]. A series of ball bearings and fulcrums can be adjusted to counterbalance the weight of the paralyzed arm and hand, allowing the patient to use trace muscles and "body English" to move the arms voluntarily.

There are a number of effective orthotic approaches to restoring grasp and release, depending on the degree of deficit. One of the most straightforward is a simple hand orthosis (HO), fastened with Velcro, which passively attaches an implement to the paralyzed hand. Sometimes called a "utensil

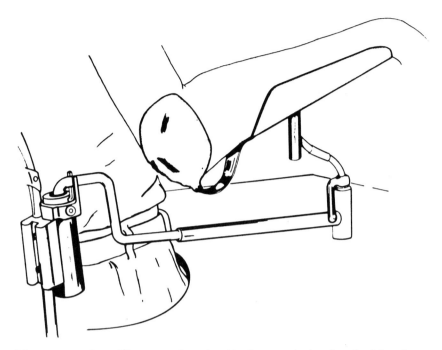

Figure 4   Balanced forearm orthosis (BFO), when attached to the wheelchair frame, counterbalances the weight of the paralyzed arm and allows even trace musculature to control arm position.

cuff," such a device is often used for shaving and similar tasks. Figure 5 illustrates examples of this orthosis [7]. The simplicity of this approach accounts for its good rate of clinical acceptance.

In many cases, significant voluntary motion is available in only one direction, and a custom-made wrist–hand orthosis (WHO) can be designed to provide both grasp and release. In the typical circumstance, good wrist extension remains without either wrist flexion or any voluntary finger motion. A WHO to provide tenodesis function links the fingers to the wrist position while stabilizing the thumb. Figure 6 shows one such design [7]. Active wrist extension drives the fingers closed; relaxation allows gravity to flex the wrist and the fingers open.

When shoulder and elbow strength is sufficient to move the arm but active wrist and finger motion is lacking, a slightly different orthosis can be beneficial. The WHO with ratchet function fixes the wrist and hand in a functional position. When the patient wishes to grasp an object, he or she pushes on the tops of the finger pieces and the orthosis passively closes them;

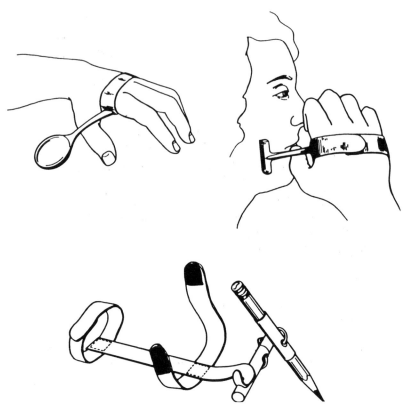

Figure 5   Utensil cuff is one of the most basic hand orthoses, yet allows the quadriplegic to grasp a variety of useful items.

a one-way ratchet prevents the grip from loosening. To release, the patient nudges a small button with the opposite arm and the ratchet opens.

The most difficult situation arises when no distal motor power is available at all even though the person can move one arm with the assistance of a balanced forearm orthosis. When body power is unavailable, external power in the form of battery-operated motorized devices is sometimes used. The externally powered WHO to provide grasp substitutes the force of a miniature motor for the absent muscle function. A mechanical switch activated by residual shoulder elevation is one common control method.

Experimental work during the past few years has demonstrated the potential for restoration of grasp by direct electrical stimulation of the denervated muscles. One control strategy being developed uses comput-

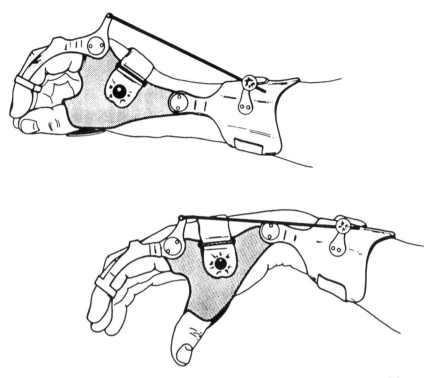

Figure 6 Tenodesis WHO converts residual wrist extension into useful grasp despite complete finger paralysis.

erized voice recognition to command the stimulator [10]. Although this device is not yet available, it seems likely that such technology will eventually allow the quadriplegic wearing an electronic orthosis simply to tell his or her hand to "grasp firmly" in order to pick up a glass of water.

Brachial Plexus Injury

Persons with brachial plexus injuries (BPI) comprise another population with varied and sometimes profound neurological deficits that can be treated orthotically [11]. As was the case with spinal cord injuries (SCI), orthotic management is based on the specific functional deficit remaining regardless of the type of lesion [12].

One pattern results in a functioning hand and wrist attached to a flail arm. This offers a high likelihood of long-term success since the functioning hand provides not only grasp but also, and even more importantly, sensation.

The literature contains a number of reports on successful application of an elbow orthosis to provide flexion/extension [13]. When shoulder strength is good, glenohumeral motion can be harnessed to provide active elbow movement using an adaptation of prosthetic arm technology. If endurance is limited, hinges with a locking mechanism can be added resulting in an EO with elbow flexion–extension lock; one such device is shown in Figure 7. For patients whose shoulder stability is limited or absent, the device must extend onto the torso to stabilize the arm; this is termed a shoulder–elbow orthosis (SEO). Although locking shoulder joints are available, experience has shown that these are difficult for many patients to operate consistently. For that reason, the most common configuration is an SEO with friction shoulder and locking elbow flexion–extension.

One of the most challenging, as well as most controversial to treat, conditions is the totally flail and insensate arm. Figure 8 shows a modular orthotic system that has been used in England for many years and has recently become available in the United States. One British surgeon has reported long-term follow-up of several hundred cases, indicating that 70% of his patients with flail arms fitted with such an orthosis continue to use it regularly for vocational or avocational tasks. The Stanmore approach is to use an SEWHO with friction shoulder, locking elbow, and prosthetic hook for grasp.

It is also possible to create an externally powered orthosis, similar to the type used for patients with quadriplegia, but adapted for ambulatory individuals. Figure 9 shows one type of SEWHO with friction shoulder, locking elbow, and electronic grasp and release. In this case, the grasp is triggered by small scapular motions that trip a hidden microswitch [12].

Cerebral Vascular Accident

Cerebral vascular accidents (CVAs) result in a significant percentage of permanent upper limb disability [14]. However, the presence of significant spasticity prevents functional use of the hand and arm with or without an orthosis. As a result, most orthoses for this population are simple devices designed to prevent fixed contractures or shoulder subluxation; few are worn on a long-term basis.

A wide variety of sling devices have been utilized immediately following the CVA to reduce shoulder subluxation until proximal control has returned. Figure 10 illustrates one variant that allows functional use of the hand without encumbering the arm, as the traditional sling and swathe would.

In patients whose marked hand spasticity persists, there is a significant risk of fixed contractures developing and hygiene can be troublesome. Figure 11 shows a WHFO with variable wrist and finger extension force plus

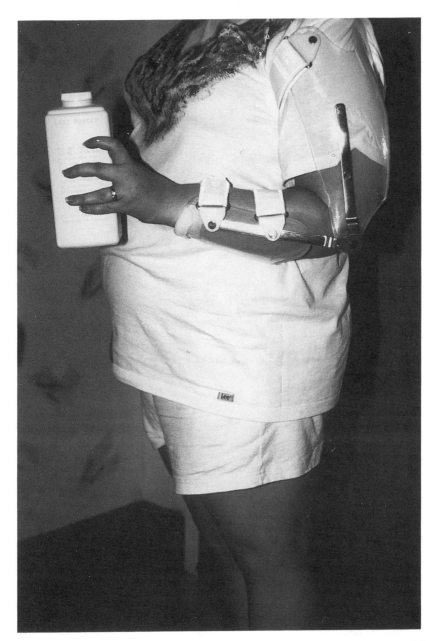

Figure 7   Elbow orthosis with ratchet elbow lock allows passive positioning of the flail elbow so that the hand can perform functional tasks.

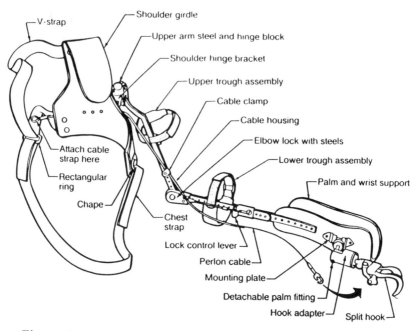

Figure 8 Stanmore modular SEWO can allow even those with complete arm paralysis a measure of useful function. Orthotic mechanisms stabilize the shoulder, lock the elbow, and replace grasp with a prosthetic hook.

hyperextension stops to reduce flexion contractures, which has been reported in the literature recently. This device has been used for selected cases, to reduce or prevent fixed contractures, with encouraging results.

Peripheral Nerve Palsy

A great variety of hand orthoses (HO) are available to treat the numerous peripheral nerve palsies. Most are either commercial designs that are premanufactured and sometimes dispensed in the physician's office or low-temperature devices molded by the therapist. Both work well for short-term applications. Many orthotists can provide such devices as well.

Traumatic Brain Injury

Long-term applications for static positioning orthoses are uncommon. Figure 12 illustrates a clear plastic WHFO to hold the wrist and hand in a functional position that was used to resist marked spasticity and maintain a functional

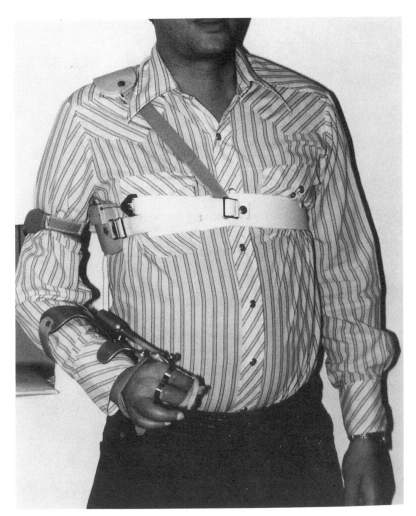

Figure 9 Sophisticated electronic arm orthosis uses a miniature motor, triggered by almost imperceptible shoulder motions, to restore grasp in a flail arm.

position following a head injury. Low-temperature devices proved too fragile and were often removed by the child, who was prone to acting out behavior. After careful consultation with the physician, parents, and school therapists, this orthosis was designed to fasten with three machine screws so it could only be applied or removed by an adult caretaker.

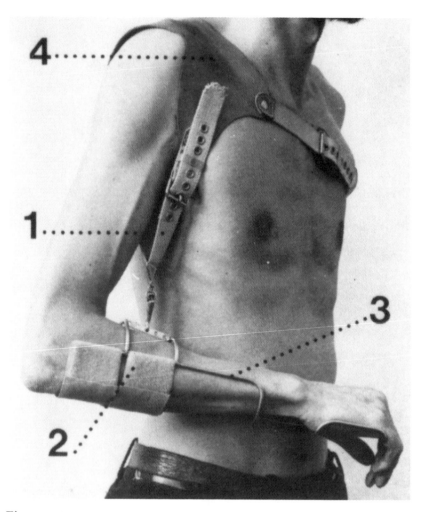

Figure 10 SEWHO from the Netherlands counterbalances the weight of the forearm and allows use of the functional thumb and fingers. Forearm support (3) is balanced by fulcrum (2); weight is transmitted through strap (1) to shoulder saddle (4) which reduces shoulder subluxation.

CERVICAL ORTHOSES

Due to the high frequency of serious cervical injuries, as well as the significant risk of progressive neurological deficit, the principles of cervical orthoses have been studied in detail. The plethora of orthotic devices available can be readily classified into less than a dozen functional groups according to the degree of biomechanical control provided.

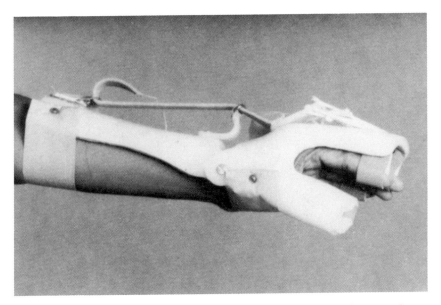

Figure 11 This device uses elastics to apply gentle traction to the fingers and wrist. Over a period of weeks, it may reduce contractures due to spastic musculature.

All orthoses, and particularly cervical orthoses, are effective only if the patient is cognizant and cooperative. It is impossible to design a device that will reliably protect the suicidal, incoherent, or uncooperative individual from him- or herself. The effectiveness of spinal orthoses is also reduced in the presence of paralysis, since the ability to function as a corrective stimulus is lost.

The head and cervical spine can be likened to a watermelon balanced on a stack of checkers. Lucas has reviewed the stability of a column according to the degree of fixation of its base and top [15]. Figure 13 demonstrates that when the top is free to displace, as is the case for most orthoses that fit between the jaw and the torso, it can support far less than if both are constrained. Since even a precisely fitted custom-molded orthosis of this type would provide only mild to moderate biomechanical control, the majority of cervical orthoses are prefabricated commercial items. Custom-made devices are typically reserved for those with anomalous anatomical structure who could not use a symmetrical premade design.

Cervical Orthoses

As a group, cervical orthoses (CO) are the least effective biomechanically. Their widespread clinical use reflects the fact that they are usually well

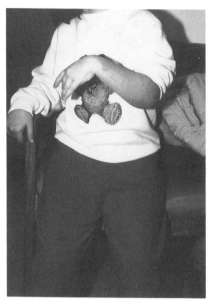

(A)

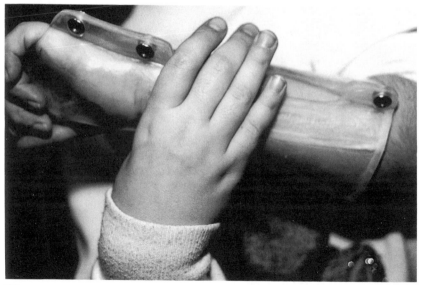

(B)

Figure 12 A, Child with closed brain injury could not use her fingers due to chronic spastic posturing of the wrist. B, Clear plastic orthosis stabilized the wrist in a functional position and allowed some grasp.

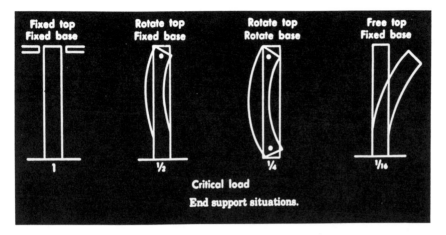

Figure 13 Lucas's research showed the inherent ligamentous stability of cadaveric spines, which is dependent upon whether the base, or top, or both are constrained. The more effectively a cervical orthosis immobilizes the head (top) or thorax (base), the greater the resulting cervical spine stability.

tolerated by patients. Table 1 summarizes the biomechanical control afforded by various cervical devices. In particular, the soft collar CO provides little more than a gentle reminder. The semirigid collar CO, such as the Philadelphia type, is significantly more effective in restricting sagittal plane motion and is also well tolerated. Although the rigid collar CO made from hard plastic provides slightly better control, it is not as frequently prescribed,

Table 1 Motion Allowed from the Occiput to the First Thoracic Vertebra with Various Orthoses

Test situation	No. of subjects	Mean age (yr)	Flexion- extension	Rotation	Lateral bending
Normal unrestricted (all subjects)	44	25.8	100	100	100
Soft collar	20	26.2	74.2	82.6	92.3
Philadelphia collar	17	25.8	28.9	43.7	66.4
Four-poster brace	27	25.9	20.6	27.1	45.9
Cervicothoracic brace	27	25.9	12.8	18.2	50.5
Halo with plastic body vest	7	40.0	4	1	4

The mean of normal motion allowed fell in the range ± 10% of indicated values.
Source: Adapted from ref. [16].

primarily because it is uncomfortable to wear and often is removed by the patient. Figure 14 illustrates examples of these COs.

Cervical Thoracic Orthoses

Orthoses that cover more of the torso provide increasingly more rigid control. Two variations are commonly used clinically. The post-type CTO may have

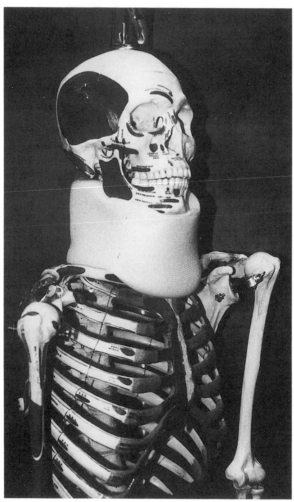

(A)

Figure 14   Common cervical orthoses, in ascending order of biomechanical control; A, soft collar; B, semirigid collar; C, rigid collar.

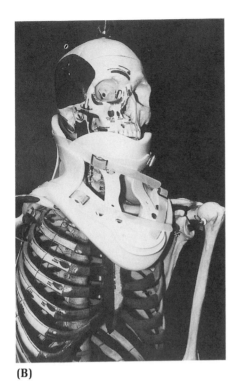

(B)

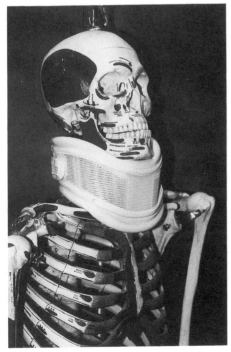

(C)

two or four rigid uprights connecting the head and thorax pieces. Although this device is somewhat difficult to tolerate, a well-fitted post type orthosis significantly restricts both extension and flexion. One commercially available variant, designed by a certified orthotist, warrants special mention because it can be fitted to the supine patient and is better tolerated in the supine position than other designs. The sternal occipital mandibular immobilizer is usually ordered by its acronym: SOMI. The CTO SOMI type has been shown to provide nearly as much immobilization as the post-type devices (Figure 15).

Cervical Thoracic Lumbosacral Orthoses

It is increasingly common to encounter posttraumatic patients with multiple spinal compression fractures as well as cervical injuries. They are sometimes managed with a removable CTLSO to stabilize the neck and thoracic spine, as shown in Figure 16. Most devices are custom-made to ensure proper torso support, but prefabricated versions are also available for use when thoracic support is less critical. One distinct advantage over plastic jackets or Minerva casts is that the anterior and posterior portions of the orthoses can be removed for hygiene or wound inspection.

The most effective orthoses to stabilize the cervical spine are the various halo apparatuses, which are by definition CTLSO devices [16]. Since the cranial attachment is relatively secure, the key difference between similar halo devices is the stability of the thoracolumbar portion. The original halo/pelvic design still provides the ultimate in stability, when metal rods are surgically inserted through the pelvis to connect the superstructure to the head ring. Fortunately, this is rarely necessary. Most patients are managed with a CTLSO halo vest (Figure 17), which has been shown to reduce most cervical motions by more than 95%. It is important to realize, however, that no orthosis can provide complete immobilization. Particularly when the patient is leaning forward, the neck can translate or "snake" even in a well-fitted halo orthosis [17].

Careful selection and fitting of the vest portion significantly enhance cervical stability in the device. Since the shoulder girdle is highly mobile, designs that contact that region are of dubious value. A properly fitted vest transmits forces to the upper chest and thorax while leaving the arms free to move. Although most traumatic cases can be managed with a prefabricated vest, unusual body contours such as kyphosis or marked scoliosis may require a custom TLSO portion for proper stability and comfort. The smallest children and adults weighing more than 300 pounds may also require a custom-molded jacket or a synthetic body cast as the foundation for the halo and superstructure.

Numerous complications have been reported from improper use of the halo ring and skull pins [18] and have become a significant source of orthotic

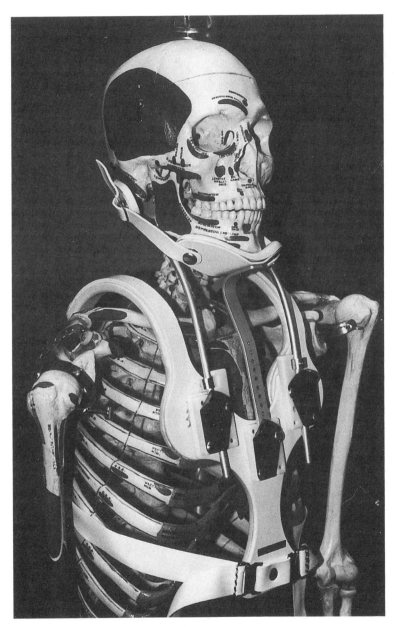

Figure 15 Sternal occipital mandibular immobilizer (SOMI) is a reasonably effective CTO that most patients tolerate well. Dual anterior posts provide head control.

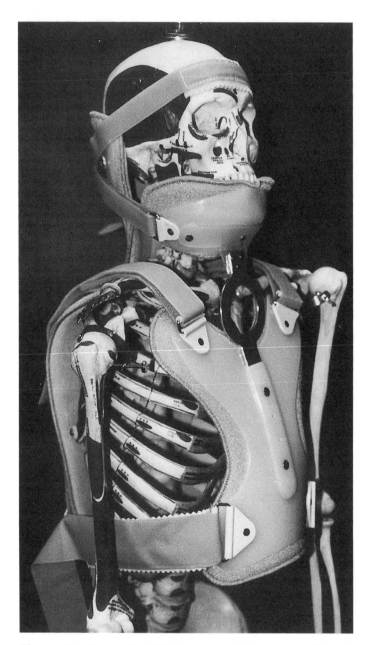

Figure 16 Removable CTLSO can provide better control than less encumbering devices, but is more difficult for patients to tolerate.

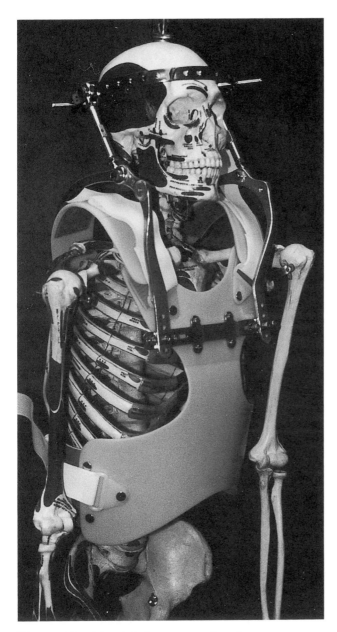

Figure 17 CTLSO halo-vest provides the greatest measure of cervical spine stability because the head (top of column) is rigidly fixed by metal pins that penetrate the outer layer of the skull.

malpractice claims. Meticulous hygiene, careful application of the pins in accordance with the manufacturer's guidelines, and regular follow-up will prevent most problems. Some manufacturers have produced excellent instructional videotapes demonstrating proper application of these devices [19].

The widespread availability of new materials that are compatible with magnetic resonance imaging (MRI) has allowed earlier application of the halo device without fear of interfering with diagnostic studies. Many are now applied in the emergency room as soon as the patient is medically stable. Muscle atrophy about the neck is a normal sequel to many months of halo use. Patients who have worn the device for extended periods of time may complain of marked neck instability when the device is removed. It is useful to provide a semirigid CO (Philadelphia collar) to be worn for a week or so after halo removal to help ease the transition to voluntary control of the head.

SPINAL ORTHOSES

The spine can be considered as a semiflexible rod, but it is impossible to design an external orthosis to apply pressure directly upon it. Indirect pressure can be applied via the torso, but this is complicated by changes in trunk contour secondary to breathing, eating, and muscle tone. The net result is that no orthosis can stabilize an unstable spinal fracture [7]; the proper function for a spinal device is to augment some degree of internal stability.

Many spinal orthoses are used for orthopedic problems such as idiopathic scoliosis or progressive juvenile kyphosis. The interested reader is referred to the orthopedic literature for discussion of these applications.

Soft Corsets

The most commonly prescribed spinal device in the United States is the lumbosacral corset [20]. This cloth garment, reinforced with both flexible and rigid metal stays, is generally well tolerated. The LSO corset with stays is often used as short-term treatment for idiopathic low back pain, and many patients report significant relief from their symptoms when wearing the orthosis. It is believed to provide three primary functions:

1. Increasing intracavitary pressure by firmly compressing the abdominal contents, which has been shown experimentally to unload the lumbar spine significantly [21]
2. Kinesthetic reminder to withdraw, which encourages the patient to maintain an upright posture since other positions are more uncomfortable
3. Psychological reassurance that "something" is being done for the patient

Although the majority are prefabricated items, it is commonly necessary to tailor the garment by sewing darts at the waist or hips for uniform support, particularly for female patients. This step is frequently omitted when the corset is provided by someone other than a certified orthotist. The first two functions are only possible if the corset is well fitted and made of a canvas or similar cloth material. Elastic devices, although they may look very similar, can only provide the third function.

A longer version of the corset with shoulder straps is termed a TLSO corset with stays and adds an additional reminder not to bend or rotate the thorax. This is sometimes useful postoperatively or as a palliative measure. Such devices provide little additional support beyond the LSO corset and are therefore much less commonly prescribed. Figure 18 contrasts these two corset types.

General consensus is emerging that spinal orthoses should not be worn indefinitely, since the abdominal muscles weaken from disuse, making it difficult to abandon the device. Bunch and Keagy have stated: "Never prescribe a support for the neck, midspine, or lumbosacral region without a plan to eliminate it" [7].

Rigid Metal Orthoses

This caveat also applies to the more rigid metal devices, which are much less commonly prescribed than in the past. Although a variety of metal designs are possible, the majority have a canvas anterior portion with a rigid posterior section, constructed from various combinations of the following common elements: thoracic band, pelvic band, paraspinal bars, lateral bars.

These devices can described succinctly by the body segments covered and the control desired. For example, an LSO with extension–lateral control indicates a device that terminates at the xiphoid and permits trunk flexion while limiting extension and lateral bending. This orthosis is sometimes prescribed to reduce excessive lumbar lordosis.

A TLSO with flexion–extension–lateral–rotary control is a much more restrictive device, as illustrated in Figure 19. Most other metal spinal orthoses are formed by hybrid combinations of these elements, providing levels of control intermediate between these two examples.

Figure 20 shows a spinal orthosis frequently prescribed after traumatic spinal compression fractures to reduce the risk of progressive deformity during the healing phase of stable lesions. Although the structure is somewhat different from the previous examples, it can be readily described in the same manner as all other devices. This is an example of a TLSO with flexion control.

Indications for rigid metal spinal orthoses remain controversial; many physicians rarely find occasion to prescribe them. One promising development has been reported by Willner of Sweden [22]. He has developed an apparatus that simulates the control provided by various spinal orthoses. He

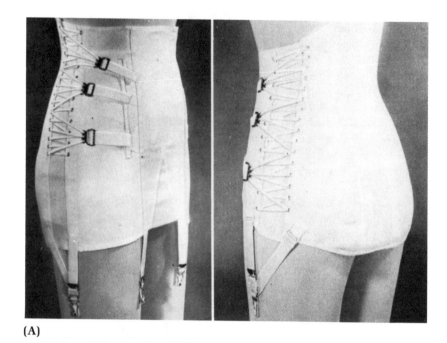

(A)

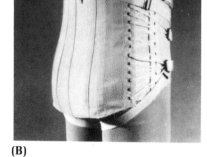

(B)

Figure 18   Cloth corsets are generally well tolerated, limit gross motion, and often reduce acute spinal pain. A, lumbosacral corset; B, thoracolumbar corset.

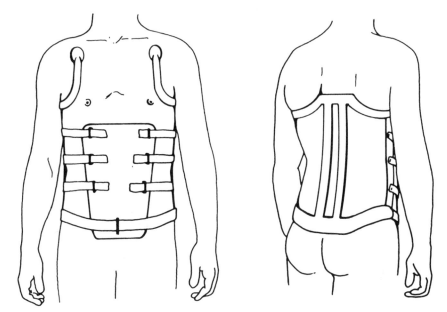

Figure 19   This metal spinal orthosis provides control of anterior, posterior, lateral, and rotary motions. It can be described as a metal TLSO with APLR control.

advocates trial wear by patients to determine functional effectiveness before a definitive device is prescribed. Clinical trials of this approach are now being conducted in the United States.

Molded Plastic Orthoses

There is widespread consensus in one area of spinal orthotics: the custom-molded plastic body jacket provides the most effective spinal control yet devised [23]. Both LSO and TLSO plastic jackets have been well accepted clinically; the latter is reserved for patients with higher-level lesions. Commonly used postoperatively or to resist progressive deformities, these devices are lightweight, easily cleaned, and usually well tolerated by patients. Most are custom-molded from a plaster impression of the torso, although a prefabricated module can be custom-fitted if the trunk contours are symmetrical.

Figure 21 illustrates one example of a TLSO body jacket with flexion–extension–lateral–rotary (FELR) control. The position of the opening can be varied according to the patients' needs; this can be specified in the prescription when desired. The most common designs are the one-piece anterior opening or posterior opening, and the two-piece bivalved or clamshell designs. Biomechanical control is similar for all styles; the primary difference is the ease and method of donning the device. For example, many postopera-

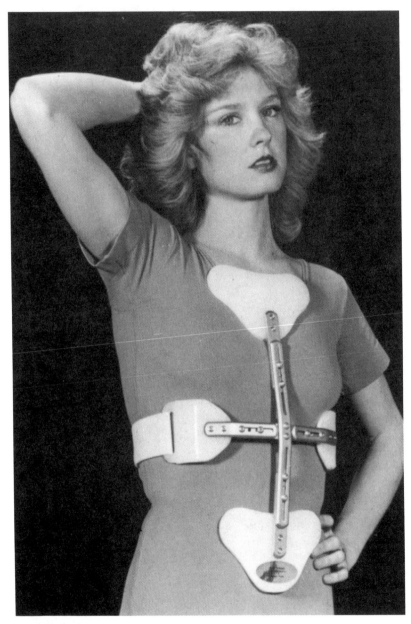

Figure 20 This simple orthosis prevents anterior bending and protects stable compression fractures during the acute healing phase.

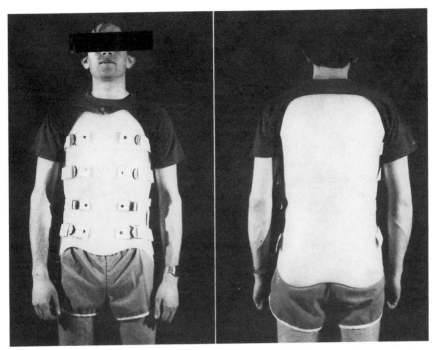

Figure 21   All-plastic TLSO body jacket provides good control of motion in all planes, is generally well tolerated by patients, and can be readily camouflaged by loose-fitting clothing.

tive devices use the bivalved style since one-half can be applied first, and the patient log-rolled in bed, before the other half is applied. The one-piece designs are easier to apply when the patient is standing and so are more commonly prescribed for ambulatory individuals.

Thanks to the availability of plastic rivets and screws, it is now possible to create a custom body jacket that is not only radiolucent but also MRI compatible. When this is desirable, it should be explicitly noted in the prescription, since most fasteners are made of ferrous materials. MRI-compatible clamshell TLSO body jacket with F–E–L–R control describes a two-piece device, extending from the sternal notch to the pubis, containing no ferrous materials.

One caveat is in order: all orthoses are less effective at their margins and are most effective at their midpoint. Norton and Brown's classic paper documented that rigid spinal orthoses may actually *increase* motion at the lumbosacral junction, since that is the first level at which any motion can occur [24]. Immobilization at this level requires a rigid extension onto the thigh by a device analogous to a hip spica cast. By the same token, very high thoracic lesions cannot be treated biomechanically with an orthosis that terminates at that level, and a CTO or CTLSO may be necessary.

LOWER LIMB ORTHOSES

Advances in lower limb orthotics have paralleled those in other areas: many effective new designs have emerged in the past two decades rendering the metal systems of yesteryear less and less common. Walking is a repetitive task [25], and for that reason is more amenable to orthotic management than more complex motions such as grasp. This may explain why the majority of orthoses prescribed are for patients with lower limb deficits.

The vast majority of lower limb orthoses provide control of motion, most frequently motion at the ankle. This discussion will therefore begin by focusing on ankle–foot orthoses (AFOs); more proximal control will be discussed subsequently.

Metal Alloy Orthoses

Even though metal alloy braces are increasingly uncommon, they provide an excellent conceptual foundation for the types of ankle control that an AFO can provide. A schematic diagram of the double-action ankle joint can be found in Figure 22. The foot is more or less constrained by the shoe, which is connected to the brace by a riveted steel "stirrup." The stirrup articulates with the ankle joints, which in turn are connected to bilateral alloy bars that terminate at a rigid calf band fastened around the leg with Velcro closures.

In the device's simplest configuration, the channels in the ankle joint are left empty and free motion is allowed in the sagittal plane. This can be described as an AFO with inversion–eversion (IE) hold, in neutral. Since all articulated AFOs prevent inversion–eversion to some degree, this control is sometimes taken for granted and the prescription is abbreviated by specifying only the sagittal plane control: free motion AFO. (A truly "free motion" AFO is logically absurd, since it would have no function!)

Imagine that the orthotist places a spring inside the posterior channel and adjusts it with the set screw to be under compression whenever the ankle is plantar flexed. This configuration substitutes the spring return for weak or missing anterior tibial muscles, allows full range of sagittal motion, yet ensures adequate toe clearance in swing phase. This is termed a dorsiflexion assist AFO; a more complete description would note with E–I hold as well.

Now consider what happens when the orthotist adds a steel pin in the anterior channel and adjusts it with the setscrew to restrain forward tibial motion beyond midstance. The device now becomes a "Dorsiflexion assist

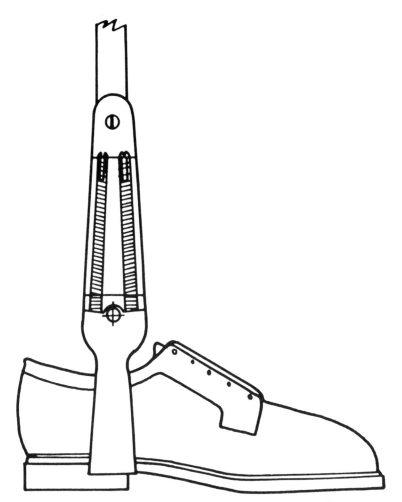

Figure 22 Schematic diagram of double-action ankle joint illustrates anterior and posterior channels. Inserting a spring or metal rod into one or both channels resists or eliminates motion at the ankle.

AFO with 5 degree dorsiflexion STOP (with I–E hold)." This is a common design to manage the flail ankle, since it allows normal sagittal motions but blocks abnormal ones.

Consider the case in which the orthotist places steel pins in both channels and eliminates all motion by tightening the set screws. It is often useful to hold the foot in such a rigid position for the higher-level paraplegic,

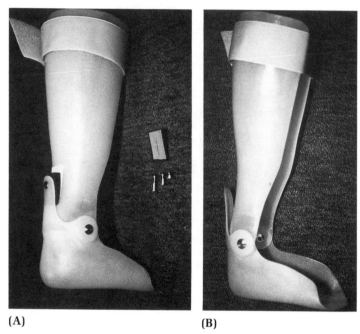

(A)   **(B)**

Figure 23   Progressive neurophysiological AFO can be modified to provide less control as the patient's neuromuscular control increases. A, solid ankle design at initial fitting; B, plantar flexion stop once spasticity begins to subside; C, plantar flexion resist once volitional control improves; D, inversion–eversion control only for residual swing-phase gait deficit.

since this provides a predictable and stable base for crutch-assisted ambulation. This is described as an AFO with I–E and F–E hold at neutral, sometimes abbreviated to solid ankle AFO in neutral. Since the angle of the ankle can be adjusted by raising one pin and simultaneously lowering its mate, it is sometimes useful to vary the position clinically until the best gait is obtained. To emphasize the adjustability, it could be termed an AFO with I–E hold and variable F–E hold, set in neutral, frequently abbreviated to adjustable solid ankle AFO.

    The versatility of the metal AFO with adjustable ankle joints remains one of its greatest advantages. As mentioned in the Overview to this chapter, it is also the preferred design to accommodate fluctuating edema since only the calf band contacts the leg. It also offers the greatest rigidity of any AFO, often making it the preferred solid ankle design for persons who body weight exceeds 300 pounds or whose work requires regular lifting of heavy weights.

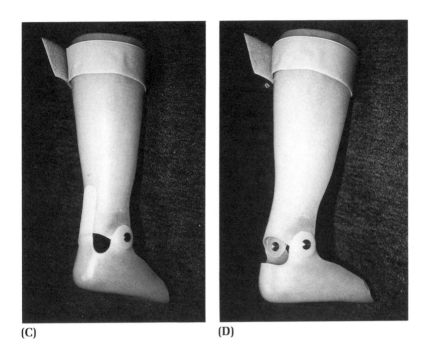

(C)   (D)

Molded Plastic Orthoses

Many articles in the literature claim that the adjustable metal AFO is the
orthosis of choice for patients with such dynamically changing conditions as
stroke [26]. Although its versatility makes it very convenient when the gait
pattern is expected to change, many modern plastic analogs can provide
similar results. Figure 23 demonstrates a very clever plastic orthosis that can
be readily modified by the orthotist to provide progressively less ankle
control as the patient's volitional control improves. Clinical experience has
proven its applicability for patients with a variety of neurological conditions
that cause hemiparesis, including CVA, traumatic brain injury (TBI), and
cranial tumors. As stated previously, orthoses are prescribed not by pathological condition but by the functional goals desired.

   Current thinking suggests that the great majority of patients with
neurological problems, with the few exceptions already noted, can be managed using thermoplastic orthoses. A number of studies comparing plastic
braces to metal equivalents have documented similar biomechanical control
but with less weight and better aesthetic appearance [27]. As a general rule,
patients accept plastic orthoses much more readily than the metal type.

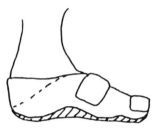

Maximum control DFO

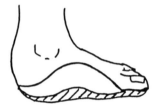

Standard moderate control DFO

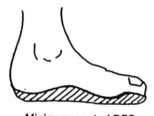

Minimum control DFO

(A)

Figure 24 (A) Lower limb orthoses can be designed with a variety of trimlines.
(B) As a general rule, the more pronounced the spasticity or deficit, the more proximal
the trimlines of the orthosis.

Cerebral Palsy

One area of significant recent advances has been in the orthotic management
of children with cerebral palsy (CP). Although the precise mechanisms
remain debated and controversial [28], a large body of clinical evidence
suggests that carefully fitted ankle–foot orthoses can significantly improve
both static standing and ambulation for many with CP [29]. Convincing proof
of efficacy is lacking, but many leading proponents advocate fitting orthoses as

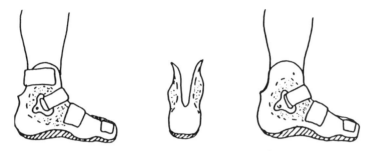

Standard DAFO with free plantar dorsiflexion

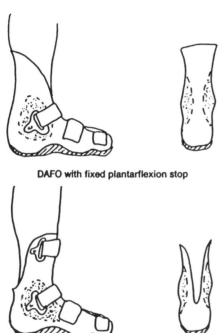

DAFO with fixed plantarflexion stop

Short Floor - Reaction DAFO

(B)

soon as the child attempts to walk, before fixed deformities have developed, in the hope of forestalling the need for corrective surgery later [30].

Figure 24 illustrates some of the varied degrees of orthotic control that have been useful for this pediatric population. The ankle-high devices provide excellent foot control while allowing free ankle motion. The general guideline is to provide the minimum amount of external control required for a normal developmental progression from standing to ambulating with assistance to walking independently. Orthotists, therapists, and physicians who work regularly with these patients often formulate the prescription collaboratively, since even minor differences in the wall thickness of the finished device can have a dramatic effect on the motion allowed.

Figure 25 demonstrates the degree of passive correction in bony alignment that an intimately fitted orthosis can achieve while allowing significant range of motion at the ankle. The orthosis used for this child was less than 1 mm ($\frac{1}{32}$″) thick; the control occurred due to specialized internal contours and a "total contact" fit against the foot.

Articulated AFOs are being prescribed for these patients more frequently, typically with a posterior stop to prevent spastic plantar flexion while allowing free dorsiflexion and good I–E control. Specialized fabrication techniques allow the orthotist to create a device whose margins become progressively thinner than the body of the device. The resulting flexible flanges, extending over much of the dorsum of the foot, significantly improve control of the foot and ankle alignment even in the face of significant spasticity. The more pronounced the spasticity, the more extensive the flanges required. Figure 26 shows one design; in this case, the child requested bright blue thermoplastic to give her brace a "sporty" appearance in combination with her pink shoes and green laces. Such individualized design is increasingly common and helps reduce the stigma associated with wearing a brace.

One specialized AFO that deserves mention for selected patients with CP is the floor reaction design, a special case within the solid ankle AFO family. Originally designed in Israel by an orthotist to manage his own postpolio paralysis, this device is characterized by a padded pretibial shell connected to a solid ankle AFO. Figure 27 illustrates an example. When uncontrolled collapse of the tibia during stance phase is the primary concern, this AFO can be of particular value. From midstance to heel-off, the pretibial shell presses back against the shin from the floor reaction forces at the anterior margin of the footplate. The net effect is much the same as a hand pushing gently just below the knee; this helps to stabilize the knee in extension. Because solid-ankle designs eliminate all ankle movement, they may make such activities as arising from a chair or from the ground more difficult. For that reason, an orthosis permitting some ankle motion is always preferable, when feasible.

Cerebral Vascular Accident

There is general agreement in North America that the patient with CVA and potential to walk can often benefit from use of an orthosis, although the particular type utilized may vary from region to region. Such patients formerly received a metal AFO with adjustable ankle attached to orthopedic shoes. Initially, the brace was locked in slight dorsiflexion to resist the spasticity,

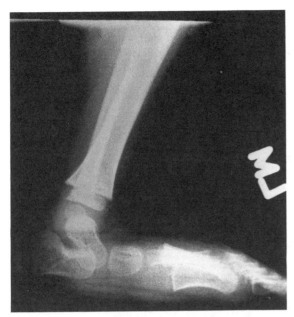

(A)

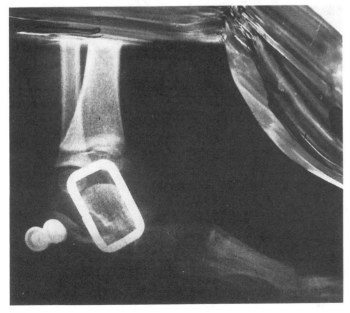

(B)

Figure 25 A, Radiograph clearly demonstrates valgus collapse of foot secondary to cerebral palsy. B, Same foot demonstrates improved anatomical alignment while patient is wearing flexible supramalleolar AFO formed from ¹⁄₃₂″ plastic.

299

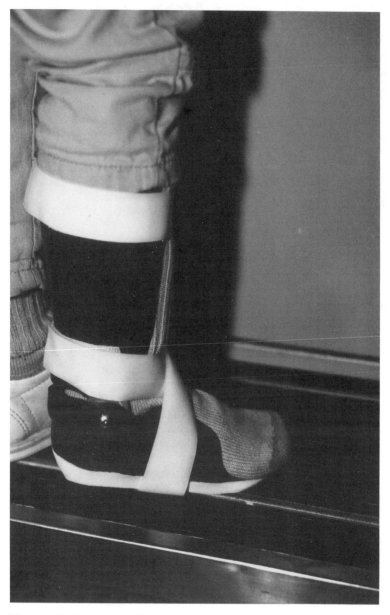

Figure 26   Moderate ankle spasticity requires extension of flexible plastic margins well up onto the forefoot and anterior tibia. Velcro strapping, combined with laced shoes, will stabilize the foot and ankle within the orthosis despite spastic plantar flexors.

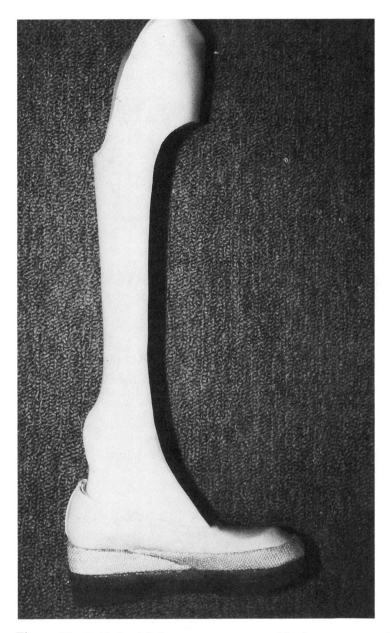

Figure 27   Padded, solid plastic anterior portion of the floor reaction AFO presses against the proximal tibia during late stance phase and encourages knee extension.

stabilize the limb, and discourage knee recurvatum. As the patient's condition improved, the degree of orthotic control was diminished until only a free-motion design with I–E control remained. Figure 24 has illustrated how this same control can be accomplished with a thermoplastic design. Although both types are clinically effective, the plastic design is significantly lighter.

A complex articulated design is not necessary for many patients with CVA, especially if spasticity is not severe. Figure 28 shows one nonarticulated design for patients with CVA. This solid ankle AFO to control spastic equinovarus demonstrates typical modifications for the hemiplegic. Note the extended lateral flanges to improve ankle varus control as well as the Velcro calf and ankle closures for one-handed function. As the patient's volitional control improves, the plastic near the ankle can be trimmed away to allow less restriction of movement. In many cases, what began as a solid ankle AFO can be ultimately trimmed back into a dorsiflexion assist design.

Knee–ankle–foot orthoses are very rarely recommended for use following CVA. If a locked knee is necessary for ambulation, the patient with CVA typically lacks sufficient hip control to advance the leg and probably to balance. Wheelchair mobility is then the safer and more practical alternative. The only exception would be if pre-existing conditions such as marked genu recurvatum required the protection of a KAFO with hyperextension stop. It is *not* necessary to lock the knee to control recurvatum; in fact, knee flexion is desirable. Such a KAFO would permit normal swing phase flexion and therefore not disrupt gait as much as one with a locked knee.

Traumatic Brain Injury

Patients with TBI and certain brain tumors often present a picture similar to that of patients with CVA. Orthotic management is therefore similar. The primary difference is that the spasticity and cognitive impairment are sometimes quite pronounced, complicating the treatment. Much has been written about the theoretical "neurophysiological principles" to reduce spasticity [31], despite the fact there is only equivocal evidence for such mechanisms. From a clinical standpoint, they are certainly harmless and since they might improve the effectiveness of the orthosis, they can be incorporated into the proven biomechanical designs.

A common observation is that clonus can often be reduced or eliminated by gently manually hyperextending the toes. When this response is noted following TBI, CVA, or similar conditions, the toes may be held in this position during the plaster-molding procedure. The AFO produced from this mold will duplicate this attitude and hold the toes in the desired extended position. Pressure on the metatarsal heads likewise often stimulates a plantar flexion spasm. Building a relief into the footplate of the orthosis will reduce pressure over the metatarsal heads and reduce this tendency [31].

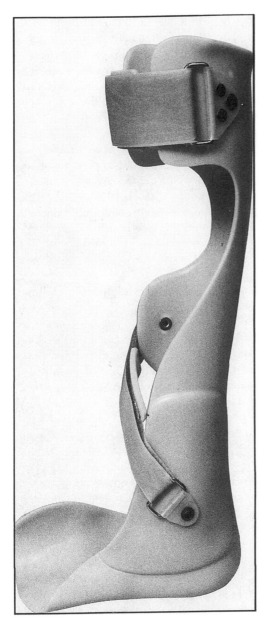

Figure 28 Solid ankle AFO to control hemiplegic gait has extended mediolateral flanges for varus/valgus control of the ankle. Velcro closure allows the patient to put it on with one hand.

One factor that seems to be important for all orthoses designed to manage spastic conditions is to maintain the hindfoot in neutral, with the talus and calcaneus centered under the tibia [32]. Why this is important is unknown. Some speculate that such "normal" alignment creates a sense of being "stable," while others argue that this position "inhibits" spasticity. Based on clinical observation, when it is impossible to hold the hindfoot securely in neutral during weightbearing, the orthosis is likely to be intolerable for the patient with spasticity.

One common-sense way to approximate the function of an orthosis is to stabilize the foot and ankle manually while the patient applies full body weight and simulates taking a step with the opposite side. This will provide a good subjective "feel" for the forces that must be exerted by an orthosis to control the leg. As a general rule, if the examiner cannot comfortably stabilize the leg with moderate hand pressure, it is unlikely an orthosis will succeed for this patient.

Multiple Sclerosis

Ankle–foot orthoses are occasionally useful for the adult with multiple sclerosis (MS). Due to the highly variable progression of the disease and resultant weakness, it is difficult to generalize beyond a few basic points.

The most important caveat is to anticipate the effect of an orthosis on more proximal joints. This is crucial when a patient has generalized weakness, since orthotic control of one joint may inadvertently affect the ability to compensate by using more distant musculature. Many with MS have learned to use "trick" motions to compensate for their condition; for example, by hyperextending the knee to compensate for weak quadriceps. If a knee orthosis with extension stop at zero degrees is prescribed to control the genu recurvatum, the likely result will be that the patient will fall when fatigued. Although this new problem could then be handled by changing the prescription to a KO with knee lock at neutral, this would disrupt swing phase by requiring circumduction or hip hiking to clear the toe. The long-term result would be more fatigue and less ability to ambulate than without bracing.

One should be cautious about using lower limb orthoses in patients with MS, particularly since most patients will not tolerate much additional superincumbent weight. Orthoses that are clinically useful tend to be very lightweight, usually flexible, and are prescribed for a specific problem such as recurrent mediolateral ankle instability. Consultation with a knowledgeable and experienced certified orthotist is often useful; occasionally a brief evaluation with a borrowed off-the-shelf leg splint will help to clarify the prescription. As a general rule, the least encumbering orthosis is the best. Few with MS will tolerate the awkwardness of a KAFO, so an AFO or even less restrictive device is most likely to succeed.

Muscular Dystrophy

Patients with the muscular dystrophies (MD) present a similar clinical picture to those with MS, but the progression is often more predictable. Timing of orthotic management remains controversial; some authorities advocate aggressive orthotic intervention to preserve upright stance and limited ambulation as long as possible [33,34], while others accept powered wheelchair mobility at an earlier age.

As with patients with MS, the emphasis is on lightweight and simple orthoses. Plastic AFOs can delay the development of plantar flexion contractures if used faithfully; sometimes use while sleeping is sufficient to maintain ankle range of motion. The AFOs should be progressively more rigid as the weakness progresses. Floor reaction designs are not commonly used because proximal hip weakness tends to make knee control tenuous.

Extremely lightweight plastic knee–ankle–foot orthoses (KAFOs) with knee locks are usually necessary as the time for ambulation nears an end. Many children will need some assistance from a caretaker to apply and remove the devices. Figure 29 illustrates one type of lightweight KAFO with locking knee mechanism; this variant accommodates a fixed knee flexion contracture. Even if little ambulation occurs, bilateral KAFOs may make transfers from the wheelchair both safer and easier at this stage.

It appears that scoliosis rarely progresses in this population until ambulation has ceased. Most authorities now believe that progressive paralytic scoliosis is inevitable for many children with MD and that surgical stabilization is unavoidable [35]. A molded TLSO body jacket or specially contoured seating system is sometimes utilized in an effort to retard the progression, but no proof exists that this is effective for these children [36].

Charcot-Marie-Tooth disease typically results in much more distal muscle weakness, and many patients remain ambulatory in the community. A common complaint is tripping when the toe fails to clear a minor obstacle in the environment, especially when the patient is fatigued. This can usually be managed with a very flexible plastic dorsiflexion assist AFO. Too stiff an orthosis will result in a tendency for the knee to buckle in early stance, if the foot is prevented from descending to the floor quickly.

Myelodysplasia

Myelodysplasia is one of the most complicated neuromuscular deficits amenable to orthotic management. For optimal results, most cases are managed in specialized multispecialty clinics with practitioners in neurology, urology, orthopedics, orthotics, and therapy in attendance.

The interested reader is referred to the extensive literature on the management of children and adults with myelomeningocele and similar conditions. Due to space constraints, this discussion will simply highlight a

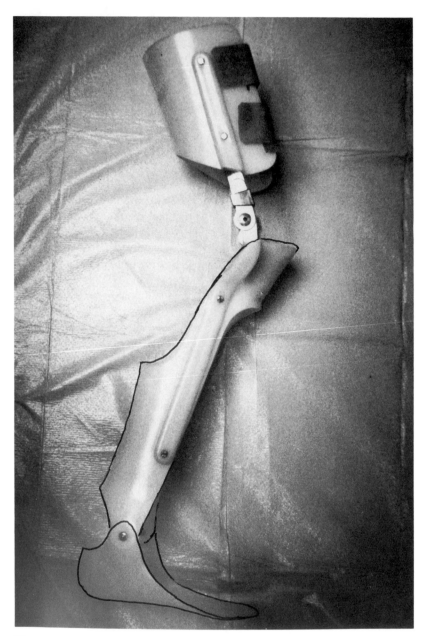

Figure 29   Thermoplastic KAFO with locking metal knee joints provides excellent biomechanical control without adding unnecessary weight. This one also accommodates a fixed knee flexion contracture of 40 degrees.

typical progression of orthotic care for a child with this disorder, without explaining the specific rationale in detail.

Positional orthoses can be useful to prevent development of fixed deformities, and may be initiated in infancy. One example is the a hip orthosis to limit extension and abduction commonly referred to as a Pavlik harness. Usually fitted in the neonatal nursery, this webbing harness keeps the femoral head contained within the acetabulum and reduces the deformity that can result from hip dysplasia. Even infants can be fitted with plastic AFOs, in an effort to hold the feet and ankles in a corrected position. Miniature solid ankle AFOs can also provide sufficient distal stability to permit the child to learn to stand and walk, for those with lower-level lesions.

Most patients with higher thoracic lesions require the use of a special TLSHKAFO standing frame, which is shown in Figure 30. This permits the small child to manipulate objects at tabletop or desktop level, encouraging both hand dexterity as well as a more normal psychosocial developmental sequence.

Once the child has mastered the static standing frame, ambulatory orthoses can be considered. As always, the least restrictive devices are the most appropriate. In the case of incomplete lesions, there will be asymmetrical loss and an AFO–KAFO combination is commonly used. Lower-level lesions will use one or two AFO's; most higher lesions will require at least the support of bilateral KAFOs.

Figure 31 shows a special type of hip–knee–ankle–foot orthosis (HKAFO) with solid ankles, locked knees, and variable hip motion that links flexion of one hip to extension of the opposite hip via a cable mechanism. This orthosis allows the patient with only one voluntary hip movement (in myelodysplasia, typically hip flexion only) to move the legs in a reciprocating step-over-step fashion. It is often abbreviated as a reciprocating gait orthosis (RGO). A significant body of information now documents that children with myelodysplasia who are fitted with this orthosis can walk further, and with less effort, than those fitted with less sophisticated alternatives [37]. Figure 32 shows one of the most complicated lower limb orthoses: a TLSHKAFO. Patients with high-level paralytic lesions often require this degree of external support if ambulation is to be attempted. In the case shown, the TLSO body jacket is intended to delay progression of a paralytic scoliosis and provide sufficient trunk stability to permit successful ambulation with the RGO type of HKAFO. Children do surprisingly well with this degree of bracing, and many can learn to ambulate for several blocks with the assistance of a rolling walker or forearm crutches.

Long-term experience shows, however, that almost all patients with thoracic-level lesions gradually become less ambulatory as they grow taller and heavier, and the majority choose wheelchair mobility as an adult. The

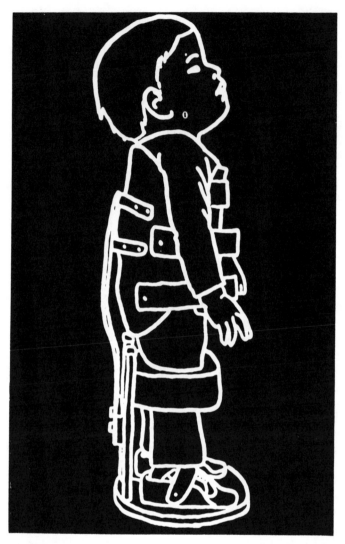

Figure 30   Standing frame supports children with thoracic level paraplegia and facilitates tabletop activities.

lower the lesion, the greater the likelihood of independent ambulation as an adult: virtually all with sacral lesions are lifetime community ambulators [38].

Spinal Cord Injury

Following the successful use of RGOs by children with paraplegia secondary to traumatic SCI, these orthoses have now been successfully utilized by adult

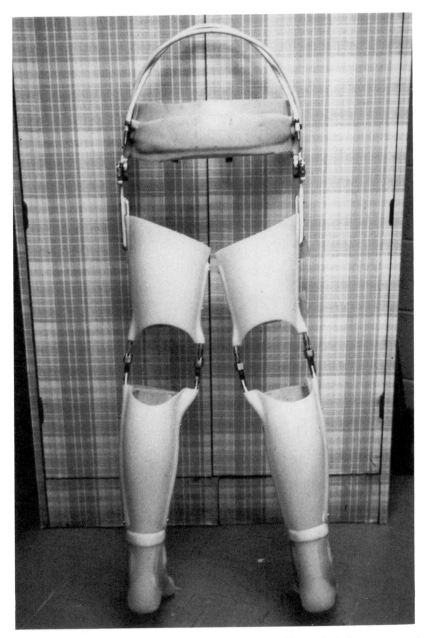

Figure 31 Reciprocating gait orthosis uses wire cables to link flexion at one hip with extension of the other. This orthosis permits some paraplegic patients to walk in a foot-over-foot manner.

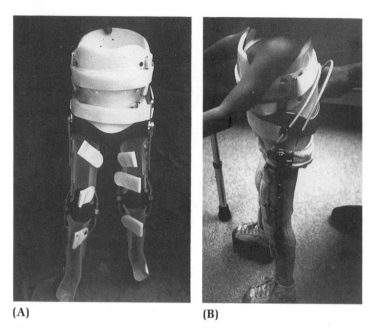

(A)   (B)

Figure 32   A, An RGO can be used in combination with a thermoplastic TLSO to control paralytic scoliosis as well as permit ambulation. B, Many small children do well with this degree of bracing, which might be overwhelming for the average adult.

paraplegics as well, if their residual spasticity is minimal to mild. A specialized design for the adult has recently been developed that combines the reciprocal motion at the hips with a gas-filled cylinder along the thighs that helps to extend the knees when the patient rises from a chair. Early results have been favorable, suggesting that a higher percentage of adult paraplegics may remain ambulatory with this design. Previous studies have shown that the overwhelming majority of adult paraplegics abandon ambulation with full-length leg braces within 2 years of discharge from a rehabilitation setting [39]. The prognosis for long-term use is significantly better when at least one of the orthoses is an AFO, presumably because this indicates better muscle function with an incomplete or lower lesion.

Several centers around the world are experimenting with the combination of RGO bracing and functional electrical stimulation (FES) to assist the paraplegic patient in walking. Although this method is not yet clinically practical, preliminary studies suggest that this combination of orthoses plus muscle stimulation can significantly reduce the effort required to cover a given distance [40].

INDIRECT ORTHOTIC INFLUENCES

Most physicians understand the direct effect a given orthosis has on a particular anatomical joint; for example, a solid ankle AFO can effectively immobilize the ankle. The indirect effect of the orthosis on adjacent joints is less obvious but often is equally important clinically. The certified orthotist is specifically trained to anticipate the influence of orthotic designs on the rest of the body and takes these factors into account when recommending a particular approach.

In addition to immobilizing the ankle, the solid ankle AFO significantly increases the knee flexion moment at heel strike since it eliminates plantar flexion motion [41]. If the patient also has an unrecognized quadriceps weakness, the AFO intended to reduce ankle motion and pain may also inadvertently increase the tendency for the knee to collapse. This is a classic example of the indirect influence that an orthosis can exert on an adjacent joint.

The solid ankle AFO likewise creates a knee extension moment at heel-off, as depicted in Figure 33 [42]. If knee collapse in late stance is a concern, this indirect effect is desirable and therapeutic; if genu recurvatum is present, the same effect may be detrimental. The key is to anticipate the indirect actions of each orthosis in order to be certain, prior to the fitting, that such influences will be desirable or at least manageable.

Although space will not permit a detailed review of all available shoe modifications, such techniques can mitigate or enhance the effects of an orthosis. The interested reader is referred to the pedorthic literature for a more detailed discussion. Here again, the certified orthotist is trained to consider the possibility of shoe modifications and to suggest them when the overall result would be improved. For example, use of a solid ankle AFO may be necessary to shield an injured ankle from motion-induced pain. Figure 34 illustrates that altering the heel of the shoe can dramatically reduce the knee flexion forces at heel strike without allowing additional ankle motion. In some cases, the orthotist may recommend a particular type of footwear (e.g., crepe sole) to improve the function without the need for other modifications. Figure 35 demonstrates the effect that altering heel height has on the forces generated at the knee by a solid ankle AFO. The orthotist will often combine the effects of such indirect influences [43] to enhance the overall result of orthotic management for a specific case.

CONCLUSION

It is hoped that this brief overview and survey of common orthotic designs will intrigue the reader and stimulate further involvement in this area.

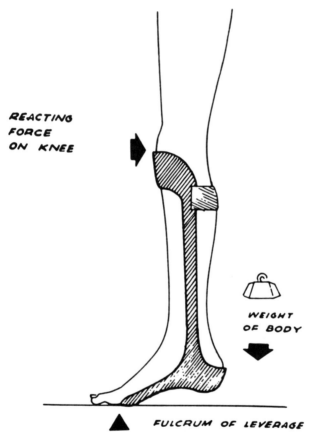

REACTING FORCE ON KNEE

WEIGHT OF BODY

FULCRUM OF LEVERAGE

Figure 33   When knee collapse is a concern, a solid ankle AFO can be used to create a knee extension force during late stance phase.

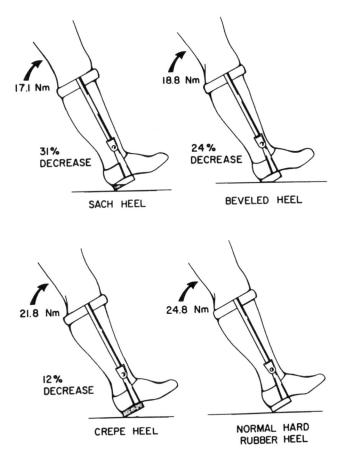

Figure 34 Softening, beveling, or cushioning the heel of the shoe reduces the knee flexion moment at heel strike induced by a solid ankle AFO.

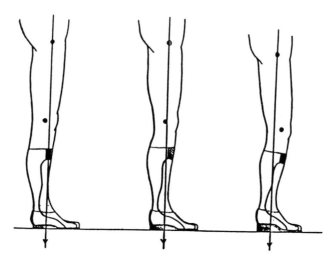

Figure 35   When a patient is wearing a solid ankle AFO, lowering the heel of the shoe tends to extend the knee during stance; raising the heel has the opposite effect. The orthotist is trained to anticipate and manage such indirect influences of orthotic design.

Orthotic treatment of neurological deficits is undoubtedly in its infancy. Continuing collaboration between interested physicians and orthotists is the key to advancing the state of the art; our patients will be the ultimate beneficiaries of such interdisciplinary efforts.

REFERENCES

1. P.W. Duncan and M.B. Badke, *Stroke Rehabilitation: The Recovery of Motor Control.* Year Book Medical Publishers, Chicago, pp. 252–271 (1987).
2. S. Fishman, N. Berger, J. Edelstein, and W. Springer. *Atlas of Orthotics: Biomechanical Principles and Application.* C.V. Mosby, St. Louis, p. 199 (1985).
3. *Orthotics Prosthetics*, *42(1)*:20–23 (1988).
4. E.A. Middleton, G.R.B. Hurley, and J.S. McIlwain, *Orthotics Prosthetics Int.*, *12*:129–135 (1988).
5. N.C. McCollough, C.M. Fryer, and J. Glancy, *Artif. Limbs*, *14(2)*:68–80 (1970).
6. E.E. Harris, *Orthotics Prosthetics*, *27(2)*:6–19 (1973).
7. W.H. Bunch, and R.D. Keagy, *Principles of Orthotic Treatment.* C.V. Mosby, St. Louis (1975).
8. M. Lohman, *Orthotics Prosthetics*, *36(2)*:42–48 (1982).
9. A.F. Bergan, J. Presperin, and T.T. Tallman *Positioning for Function: Wheelchairs and Other Assistive Technologies.* Valhalla Rehabilitation Publications, New York (1990).
10. R.H. Nathan, *Med. Biol. Eng. Comput.*, *27*:549–556 (1989).

11. C.B. Wynn Parry, *Br. J. Hosp. Med.*, 32:130–139 (1984).
12. J.A. Nunley, and J.W. Michael, *Atlas of Limb Prosthetics*, 2nd ed. (J.H. Bowker and J.W. Michael, eds.), C.V. Mosby, St. Louis (1992).
13. R.D. Leffert, *Brachial Plexus Injuries*. Churchill Livingstone, New York (1985).
14. T.P. Anderson, *Krusen's Handbook of Physical Medicine and Rehabilitation*. W.B. Saunders, Philadelphia (1990).
15. D.B. Lucas, and B. Bresler, *Report No. 40, Biomechanics Laboratory*. University of California, San Francisco.
16. R.M. Johnson, D.L. Hart, E.F. Simmons, et al. *J. Bone Joint Surg. Am.*, 59:332 (1977).
17. A.M. Johnson, J.R. Owen, D.L. Hart, and R.A. Callahan, *Clin. Orthop. Rel. Res.*, 154:34–45 (1981).
18. J.A. Baum, E.N. Hanley, and J. Pullekines, *Spine*, 14:251–252 (1989).
19. Halo-Vest Application Using the Duke Positioner (videotape). Durr-Fillauer Orthopedic, Chattanooga, TN (1980).
20. J. Perry, *J. Bone Joint Surg. Am.*, 52:1440 (1970).
21. J.M. Morris, D.B. Lucas, and B. Bresler, *J. Bone Joint Surg. Am.*, 43:327 (1961).
22. S.W. Willner, *Prosthetics Orthotics Int.*, 14:22–26 (1990).
23. M.W. Fielder, and C.M.T. Plasmans, *J. Bone Joint Surg. Am.*, 65:943–947 (1983).
24. P.L. Norton, and T. Brown, *J. Bone Joint Surg. Am.*, 39:111–138 (1957).
25. V.T. Inman, H.J. Ralston, and F. Todd, *Human Walking*. Williams & Wilkins, Baltimore (1981).
26. R.L. Waters, and J. Montgomery, *Clin. Orthop. Rel. Res.*, 102:133–143 (1974).
27. A.E. Smith, M. Quigley, and R. Waters, *Orthotics Prosthetics*, 36(2):49–55 (1982).
28. N.M. Hylton, *J. Prosthetics Orthotics*, 2(1):54–53 (1989).
29. R.S. Lin, and J.R. Gage, *J. Prosthetics Orthotics*, 2(1):1–13 (1989).
30. B. Cusick, *Phys. Ther.*, 68(12):1903–1912 (1988).
31. J.K. Shamp, *J. Prosthetics Orthotics*, 2(1):14–32 (1989).
32. M.L. Root, *Arch. Podiatr. Med. Surg.*, 1:44–46 (1973).
33. I.M. Siegel, *Arch. Phys. Med. Rehab.*, 56:322 (1975).
34. E.B. Rodilla, E. Fernandez-Bermejo, J.Z. Heckmatt, et al., *J. Child Neurol.*, 3: 269–274 (1988).
35. W. Cambridge, and J.C. Drennen, *J. Pediatr. Orthop.*, 7:436–440 (1987).
36. J.D. Hsu, *Spine*, 4:161–172 (1990).
37. F. Flandry, S. Burke, J.M. Roberts, S. Hall, A. Douilhet, G. Davis, and S. Cook, *J. Pediatr. Orthop.*, 6:661–665 (1986).
38. M.M. Hoffer, E. Fiewell, R. Perry, J. Perry, and C. Bonnet, *J. Bone Joint Surg. Am.*, 55:137–148 (1973).
39. C. Hong, E.B. San Luis, and S. Chung, *Paraplegia*, 28:172–177 (1990).
40. S. Hirokawa, M. Grimm, T. Le, M. Solmonow, R.V. Baratta, H. Shoji, and R.D. D'Ambrosia, *Arch. Phys. Med. Rehab.*, 71:687–694 (1990).
41. D.R. Wiest, R.L. Waters, E.L. Bontrager, and M.J. Quigley, *Orthotics Prosthetics*, 33(4):3–10 (1979).
42. J. Saltiel, *Orthotics Prosthetics*, 23:7 (1969).
43. T.M. Cook, and B. Cozzens, *Orthotics Prosthetics*, 30(4):43–46 (1976).

14

Adaptive Equipment

Laurie Laven

National Rehabilitation Hospital
Washington, D.C.

The effectiveness of a program of rehabilitation for a patient with neurological impairment is often measured by functional outcome. Important activities include mobility, eating, dressing, hygiene, and toileting. Adaptive equipment, wheelchairs, and home adaptations may play a major role in increasing an impaired patient's functional abilities. Therefore, it is important that all rehabilitation professionals have a basic understanding of commercially available equipment. In today's health care environment, cost is important. Prices quoted (catalog averages as of February, 1993) are for selected items.

ASSISTIVE DEVICES FOR AMBULATION

The three major indications for assistive devices are weakness of the trunk or lower extremities, poor balance in the upright posture, and decreased weightbearing on the lower extremities due to skeletal damage. Assistive devices make walking safer by increasing the base of support, by redistributing weight from the legs to the arms and the device, and by allowing a larger area within which the center of gravity can shift without the patient losing balance. Although physicians frequently write prescriptions for assistive devices without ordering a physical therapy evaluation, the cost of the evaluation is well justified by the assurance that the patient will learn safe use of the proper, well-fit device. In a survey of 124 walking aids used by 114 elderly patients referred to a physical therapy department, two-thirds of the aids were inappropriate, defective, or improperly fitted. The incidence of falls among with those with suitable aids was lower than among those with unsuitable aids, and physical therapists had issued 85% of the correct devices [1]. Selection of a device for an individual is determined by the patient's cognitive status, strength, stability, and coordination. Cardiovascular status is also considered, since oxygen consumption and heart-rate may rise significantly when the patient's trunk and arms bear weight over a paretic leg. Maximum stability and support are provided by a walker, followed by axillary crutches, forearm (Lofstrand) crutches, two canes, and one cane. However, more coordination is required to use crutches than to use a walker. Platforms can be attached to walkers or crutches for patients with a weak grip or for those unable to bear weight through their hand and wrist, such as amputees or those with severe arthritis (Figure 1).

Canes

A standard J-shaped cane has a very small base of support and the point of support is in front of the hand. Bent canes are designed to bear weight straight down the shaft, providing more support. These canes are used only for patients with minimal weakness who require more stability. Quad canes provide greater support, but are more cumbersome. Since the laterally projecting legs should be turned away from the body to avoid injury, the patient must have the cognitive ability to use the quad cane safely. The walker cane provides still greater support, is lighter and more versatile than a walker, and folds for convenience (Figure 2). The height of any cane should be the height of the wrist crease with the patient upright, arm extended.

Crutches

Axillary crutches are rarely used for patients with neurological disorders. Forearm, or Lofstrand, crutches are less stable, but are more easily maneuvered and allow free use of the hands without releasing the crutches. Lofstrand crutches are best suited for paraparetic patients with good coordination, balance, and upper limb strength who will require crutches for extended periods. Heart rate increases by as much as 48% and oxygen consumption may double during crutch walking compared to normal gait [2,3]. Crutching acts as an upper extremity cardiovascular stress test similar to a hand-cranked ergometer [4].

Walkers

A standard walker provides the greatest stability for walking, but is difficult to maneuver on stairs or in crowded areas and markedly slows gait. Most walkers

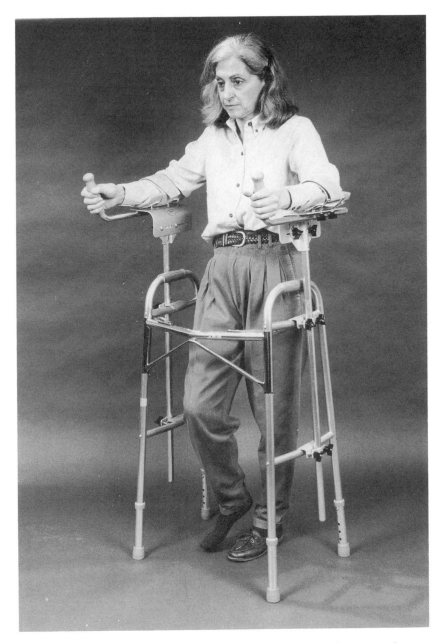

Figure 1 Platform walker can be used for amputees, those with severe arthritis, or others with weak grip unable to use a standard walker.

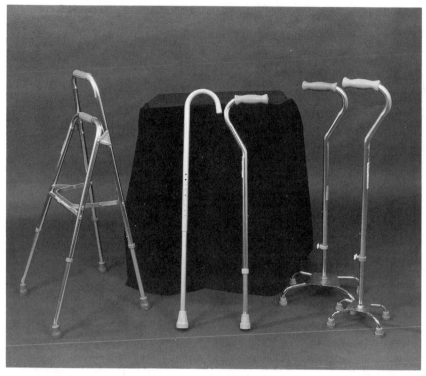

Figure 2   Left to right: walker-cane, J cane, bent cane, wide- and narrow-based quad canes.

fold for easy storage and transportation. A rolling walker is indicated for patients who are too weak to pick up the walker, do not have the cognitive ability to learn proper sequencing, or who need to improve balance by keeping their weight forward. Patients who tend to fall forward and cannot use a pick-up walker, for instance a parkinsonian patient with dementia, may benefit from an auto-stop on the rolling casters of the walker that stops forward motion when weight is borne over the front legs. Another rarely used adaptation is a walker with the hand-grip on the center cross-bar, allowing pick-up with one hand. For patients with paraparesis and inadequate upper body strength to use Lofstrand crutches, a reciprocal walker is often used. This allows one side of the walker to be advanced while full weight is supported by the stationary side (Figure 3). A walker, like a cane, should be the height of the patient's wrist crease.

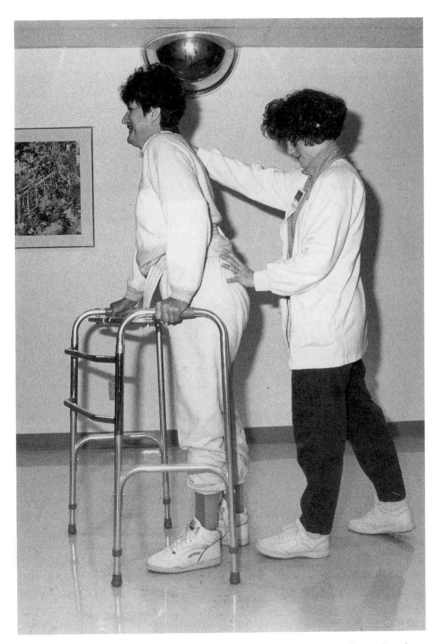

Figure 3   Reciprocal walker used by a T12 paraparetic patient. Full weight is borne on the left while the right side of the walker is advanced.

WHEELCHAIRS

There are currently 8,000–10,000 production models of wheelchairs on the market, with a wide variety of weights, sizes, and custom features. Many institutions now have wheelchair clinics for patients requiring individualized prescriptions. Every physician prescribing wheelchairs should be familiar with standard models and cushions available and recognize when evaluation for a customized wheelchair is appropriate.

Any wheelchair must be durable, easy to propel, portable, comfortable, and meet cost constraints. The patient's needs must be carefully considered. For example, a patient who is a household ambulator but lacks endurance may be homebound because a carelessly prescribed chair is too difficult to load into a car.

For patients who use wheelchairs, the proper chair and cushion are important components of self-image. The seating system must maximize user independence, enhance posture, and minimize pressure.

Size

The standard adult chair has a sling back and sling seat and folds easily. This design was introduced to allow the chair to be stored in the original invalid carriage [5]. The chair weighs 45–50 pounds without cushion and with front rigging. The seat is 19–20 inches from the floor, 18 inches wide, and 16 inches deep. A narrow adult chair is similar, except that it has a seat width of 16 inches. A tall adult chair has a seat width of 18 inches and a depth of 17 inches; a wide adult chair has a width of 20–22 inches; and a hemichair has a seat height of 17½–18 inches. The availability and cost of other sizes vary according to the manufacture. Any of these chairs is available in a lightweight version weighing 25–35 pounds. Most patients who spend little time in their chairs, like most stroke patients or elderly patients with poor endurance, can use standard lightweight chairs, which cost from $500 to $1000. Active wheelchair users, such as paraplegics or quadriplegics, often require chairs with more options to meet their individualized needs. These chairs also have a more esthetic appearance but cost $1200–$2000 or more, so cost may dictate the final choice. Ultralight sports chairs, characterized by very low backs and steeply angled seats, are not used for routine sitting and will not be discussed here. For information on seating children, the excellent text by Letts is recommended [6]. Seating for the severely disabled is also detailed by Hobson [7].

Although seat cushions and other components will be discussed later, it is crucial that the entire system—chair, cushion, and other components—be fitted at the same time.

Propulsion

Most wheelchairs are propelled with both hands. For patients with weak grasp, vertical or oblique projections on the hand rims or plasticized rims improve propulsion. Some patients also benefit from using gloves to improve traction.

The hemichair has a lower seat height and detachable footplate to enable the hemiparetic patient to propel the chair with the strong arm and leg. One-wheel drive chairs are needed only for triplegic patients with a single strong arm.

A motorized chair is appropriate for a quadraparetic patient incapable of manual propulsion. Cost is $4,000 and up, depending on the degree of mechanization needed. Normal cognition and good control of the propulsion device are mandatory. The patient and/or family must be responsible for routine maintenance of the chair (such as recharging batteries), must have a home large enough to accommodate the chair, and have means to transport the chair for repairs and outings. A back-up manual chair is provided for all power-chair users. Patients who are known to consume large quantities of alcohol or drugs, those with cognitive impairment, severe neglect, or hemianopia, are not candidates for a powered chair.

Battery-powered three- and four-wheeled scooters are marketed directly to the public. They are primarily used by household ambulators who require powered mobility for longer distances. Nonambulatory patients with good postural control and coordination who can transfer independently and are at low risk for pressure sores may also increase independence with use of these scooters. Again, cognitive impairment, neglect, or hemianopia is a contraindication to use of the powered device. Insurance coverage is variable, with costs $1,500 and up.

Safety

All wheelchairs have brakes on the larger rear wheels. Brake extenders are added for patients who cannot reach the standard-length toggle. Caster locks on the smaller front wheels are occasionally needed for quadriparetic patients who require maximum chair stability to perform independent transfers. Bilateral lower-extremity amputees have a higher center of gravity and require a chair with more posteriorly placed wheels for stability. Hand bars projecting from the upper back of the chair not only serve as grips for pushing the chair but also provide protection for the patient's head and neck should the chair tip backwards [8]. Antitip bars projecting from the lower rear of the chairs are used on lightweight chairs and for patients using a lot of ramps (Figure 4). Special brakelike devices are options on most chairs to

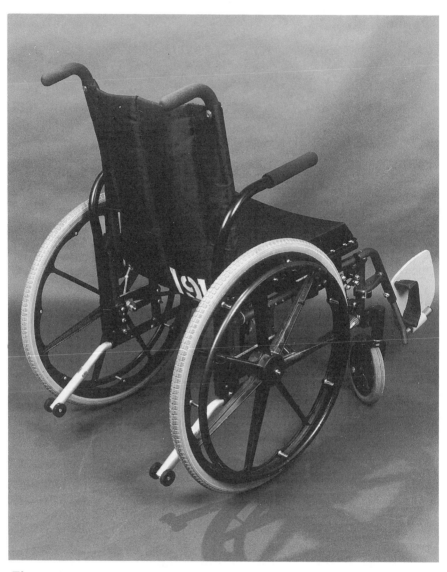

Figure 4 Antitip bars are used on lightweight chairs and for patients who frequently use ramps.

prevent backward movement while wheeling uphill. Seat belts prevent the patient from sliding or falling from the chair and should be placed at a 45 degree angle if also needed to position the pelvis. Chest straps may provide further safety and truncal support for patients with truncal weakness.

Armrests

Armrest style is determined by the patient's individual use of the arm supports and his or her transfer technique. Full-length arms provide maximum support at the front of the chair. Desk arm cutouts at the front enable the user to get closer to desks and tables and are available with adjustable height. The armrest should be 1 inch higher than the olecranon of the elbow with the arms comfortably extended, usually 9–9½ inches. If the armrests are too high, the shoulders are pushed up, causing discomfort and fatigue. If the armrests are too low, the patient may slump to keep the arms supported. The slumped posture may lead to skeletal deformity, poor balance, respiratory difficulty, and fatigue. Adjustable-height armrests are also available, and may improve standing ability, posture, and influence the difficulty of pressure-relief push-ups. Arm troughs or lap trays may be attached to position a plegic arm safely. Space-saver arms mount behind the back upholstery to decrease the width of the chair but may push on the obese patient. Clothing guards (arm panels) are standard on all but sports chairs to protect clothing from the wheel. Detachable armrests are needed for lateral transfers.

Seats

Back

For a patient with good trunk control, seat back height is measured from ½ inch below the inferior border of the scapula to the top of the seat cushion, usually 16–17 inches. The seatback must be higher or headrests added for patients with poor trunk and neck control. Too high a back restricts shoulder mobility. Too low a back decreases lateral and fore–aft stability, increasing the potential for scoliosis, kyphosis, and lordosis.

Added back height and head extension are provided for patients with truncal and neck weakness. Reclining backs compensate for truncal weakness by increasing back stability. This feature is also needed for patients with orthostatic hypotension, patients unable to perform independent weight shifts while upright, and for patients with certain leg and body casts. Some patients with severe respiratory involvement due to cervical and thoracic weakness require tilted backs to improve diaphragmatic efficiency. With the patient upright, the diaphragm is pulled down by gravity due to visceral attachments. With some gravitational force eliminated, the diaphragm returns to a more normal resting position and can move through a greater arc within the thoracic cavity [8]. Abdominal binders may be used for the same reason.

Width

Two inches of clearance is added to the widest distance between the hips and/or thigh. A seat that is too narrow will increase pressure on soft tissues. Too wide a seat may cause lateral instability, with the potential for scoliosis.

Depth

With the patient seated with his or her back firmly against the seatback, there should be 2 inch clearance between the popliteal crease and the edge of the seat. A seat that is too short will increase the pressure on the feet (heels) and the buttocks (ischial tuberosities), increasing the risk of pressure sores. A seat that is too long places increased pressure on the popliteal area, with the potential for reducing circulation and increasing thrombosis.

Height and Footrests

The distance from the back of the knee to the bottom of the heel with the foot at 90 degrees represents the minimum seat height. Footrests must have two inch clearance from the ground and should be adjusted to keep the thigh horizontal but raised slightly off the front edge of the seat. Further adjustments may be needed to allow approximately 120 degrees of elbow flexion when the handrim is held at its highest point. Varying seat height/footrest combinations may be needed to optimize comfort, pressure relief, and ease of propulsion. The potential complications of seat height and footrest combinations that are too short or too long are the same as those from improper seat depth.

Patients with dependent edema or inability to flex the knee need leg elevators. Toe and heel loops may be used to keep the feet properly positioned. Some patients with severe flexor spasms or hamstring spasticity whose feet ride over heel loops require H-straps instead (Figure 5).

Detachable footplates and armrests are needed for lateral transfers and are often requested to decrease the weight of the chair and minimize space for storage.

Angle

A seat angle of 1–3 degrees above the horizontal for the front of the seat is built in by manufacturers but is adjustable on sports chairs. Too shallow an angle may allow sliding forward, which can cause poor posture, spinal deformity, and increase the risk of pressure sores. Too steep an angle increases the pressure on the buttocks (ischial tuberosities) and may strain the hamstrings.

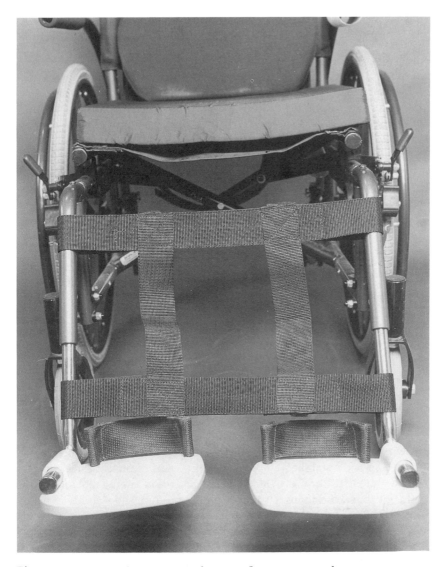

Figure 5 H-straps for patients with severe flexor spasms or hamstring spasticity.

Tires

The rear wheels are usually 24 inches in diameter and 1⅜ inches width. Some hemichairs have 22-inch tires. Pneumatic tires provide a more cushioned ride than solid rubber tries, but require frequent inflation and may make propulsion over soft surfaces, such as carpets, more difficult. Treaded tires are more durable and have better grip than smooth tires, but pick up more dirt outside that is tracked inside. Patients with weak grip who propel the chair by pushing the tires instead of the handrim find treaded tires easier to push than smooth tires. Air-free inserts are hoselike hard, rubber inserts that prevent the tire from ever becoming flat and require no air. These are more expensive than pneumatic tires. Solid rear tires, usually 1 inch wide, are most durable but provide the least shock absorption.

The small front caster wheels are eight inches in diameter. Five inch casters for a smaller turning radius may be used in sports chairs or occasionally for patients with space limitations at home. The casters may be ordered as solid hard 1 inch rubber for light indoor or pavement use; as 1½ inch semipneumatic rubber that require no air or inserts, useful on very irregular surfaces; or as 1¼ inch pneumatic tires for heaviest outdoor use on uneven surfaces, with or without airless inserts.

Mag wheels are more durable and require less maintenance than spokes, but spokes may be chosen for less air resistance in sports chairs. The types of tires provided at no additional cost vary among manufacturers. Pattern of individual use and overall cost must be considered for each patient.

Cushions

Wheelchair cushions serve many roles: they provide an effective platform from which the user performs a maximum number of tasks, reduce tissue pressure, provide stability, improve posture, absorb shock, and improve comfort. Patients with severe skeletal deformities and limited mobility benefit from customized seat inserts to control the position and stability of head, trunk, and hips. Research continues to develop specialized seating systems to meet an individual user's needs [9,10]. It is again emphasized that the cushion should be prescribed simultaneously with the wheelchair.

Pressure Reduction

Many wheelchair clinics use a pressure-monitoring device to determine the best cushion for an individual's use. Although these monitors measure surface interface pressures that are only relative indicators of deep tissue stresses, Ferguson-Pell and the researchers at Helen Hayes Hospital have developed a pragmatic scoring system for maximum acceptable pressures (see Table 1) [11]. Since no available system reduces pressure below the capillary pressure

Table 1 Recommended Maximum Acceptable Pressure (mmHg)

Level of Risk	Ischial Tuberosities	Trochanters	Sacrum	Coccyx
High: no sensation; history of sores at site of measurement	40	60	<20	<20
Moderate: no sensation; no history of tissue breakdown	60	80	40	40
Low: partial or full sensation; no history of tissue breakdown	80	80	40	40

These maximum recommended pressures assume a normal clinical status, push-ups performed every 15 min, and no other factors that would increase the risk of breakdown. Prolonged sitting (>10 hrs) and infrequent pressure relief are weighted by reducing each of the maximum allowable pressures by 10 mmHg per factor. If risk is already high, sitting time and/or pressure relief frequency must be brought to normal levels.
Source: From ref. [9].

of 30 mmHg necessary for tissue perfusion, the user with decreased sensation must be trained to perform pressure-relief techniques regularly ("push-ups"). How long an individual can withstand elevated pressure without tissue breakdown cannot be predicted, so spinal cord injured patients should be taught to perform push-ups every 15 min. The interval can be gradually increased as tolerated. Patients at highest risk for pressure sores are those with flaccid gluteals [12], poor compliance, absent sensation, previous sores, bony asymmetry, or excessive heat and moisture accumulation.

Moisture and Heat Accumulation and Loss

Spinal cord injured patients often have uncontrolled sweating. Air exchange cushion covers and cotton underwear help to reduce moisture accumulation. Air exchange is an added incentive to perform push-ups, even for those at low risk of pressure sores.

Foam cushions prevent the body from losing heat in the buttocks. Gel and fluid-filled cushions drain heat from the body. In cold environments, these cushions may make additional metabolic demands on the patient [11]. Gel cushions also have the potential to produce cold thermal injuries if not properly stored in a warm environment [13].

Posture and Positioning

Pelvic obliquity from the wheelchair sling seat results in asymmetrical pressure and can lead to scoliosis (Figure 6). A rigid seat base prevents this problem. Posterior pelvic tilt (Figure 7) places increased pressure on the coccyx. Proper positioning and restoration of lumbar lordosis can be achieved

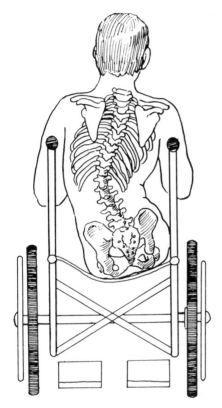

Figure 6   Hammock effect of sling seats results in asymmetrical pressures and can lead to scoliosis.

with the use of a lumbar support, a tight pelvic belt, a 10–15 degree backrest angle, and a 3–10 degree seat angle (see Figure 8). The use of armrests and the 15 degree backrest angle can also reduce ischial pressures by 25–30% [14]. Seatboards and backboards improve pelvic tilt and thoracic kyphosis in hemiplegic patients, although the seating deviations return if the supports are removed after 5–10 weeks of use [15] (Figure 9).

Commercially Available Cushions

Cushions are made of foam, gel, foam–gel combinations, air, or fluid-filled bladders. Since the Roho and Jay cushions are prescribed for 78–95% of spinal-cord-injured patients [16,17], only these cushions will be described in detail here. Other cushions for spinal-cord-injured patients are described by Ferguson-Pell [12] and Edberg and Adkins [18]. Specialized seating systems for the severely disabled are described by Letts [6]. Patients at low risk for

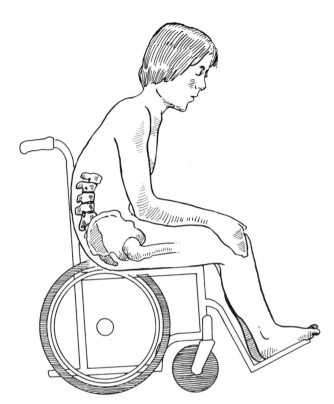

Figure 7   Posterior pelvic tilt increases pressure on the coccyx.

pressure sores may be issued seat and backboards as described above or foam cushions for comfort.

Roho cushions ($350) are made of interconnected air cells. When a localized force is applied, air is forced into neighboring cells, while air circulates freely between the cells. The cushions are available with 1, 2, or 4 inch high cells. Customized cushions may feature multiple pneumatic compartments, varying cell sizes, increased cell spacing, or deleted cells. The cushions require careful air pressure monitoring, and tend to be more sensitive to underinflation when heavily loaded cells may bottom out (Figure 10).

The Jay cushion ($325) consists of a washable molded urethane foam base covered by a wax- and oil-filled pad. A standard stretch cover, an Airexchanger cover, and an incontinent cover are available. Accessors such as adductor wedges, pelvic obliquity pads, and hip guides are available. Jay also makes a Protector that fits in a sling to wear when sitting out of the chair. Any Jay cushion can be used with a solid seat insert (Figure 11).

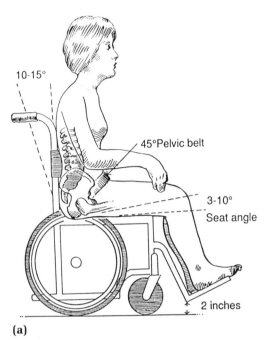

(a)

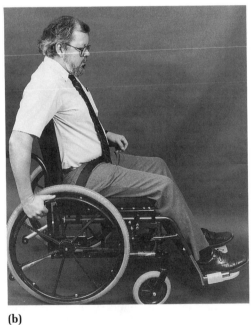

(b)

Figure 8 (a) Schematic view of proper positioning and restoration of lumbar lordosis. (b) Good patient posture in wheelchair with lumbar support, tight pelvic belt, 10 degree backrest angle, and 5 degree seat angle.

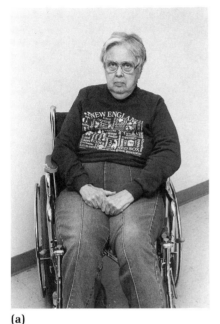 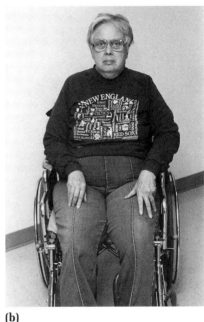

(a)   (b)

Figure 9   (a) Poor posture in patient with left hemiparesis seated in wheelchair with sling seat and back. (b) Correction of seating deviations with use of solid seat and backboard.

Some believe that the Roho provides the best protection against pressure sores, but the Jay provides better stability [16,17]. Both Roho and Jay also make back support systems.

Regardless of the cushion prescribed, patients, family, and attendants must be educated about the cushion's use and maintenance. Pressure sores can result from improper placement of the cushion [18] and no cushion alleviates the need for push-ups. Patients should be monitored regularly to ensure that the cushion is meeting their needs.

ADAPTIVE EQUIPMENT FOR ACTIVITIES OF DAILY LIVING

An overwhelming number of pieces of adaptive equipment are available to increase the self-care abilities of patients with neurological impairment. The full spectrum is best appreciated by reviewing the catalogs available in any occupational therapy (OT) department, and will not be reviewed here. This section will briefly discuss equipment frequently issued for feeding, dressing,

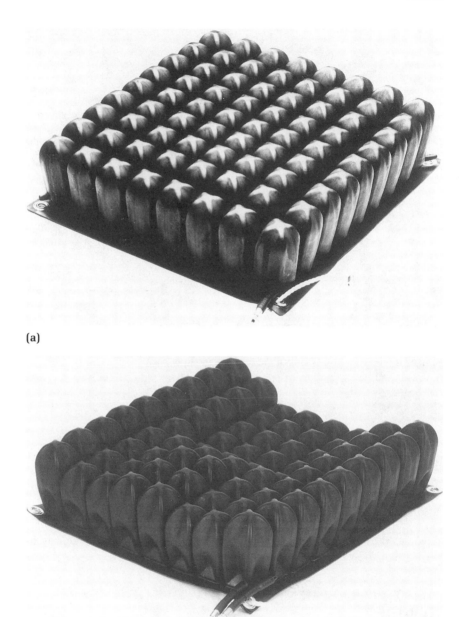

(a)

(b)

Figure 10   Roho cushions: (a) high profile; (b) enhancer (courtesy of Roho, Inc.).

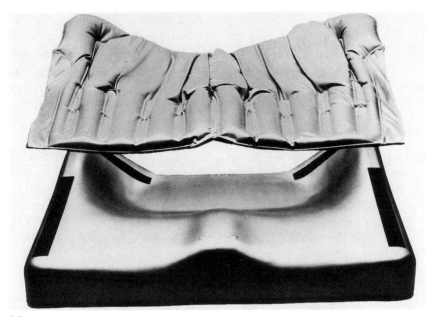

(a)

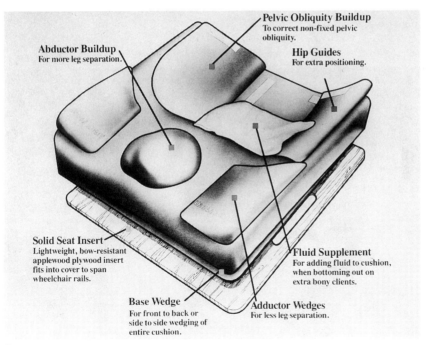

Pelvic Obliquity Buildup
To correct non-fixed pelvic obliquity.

Abductor Buildup
For more leg separation.

Hip Guides
For extra positioning.

Solid Seat Insert
Lightweight, bow-resistant applewood plywood insert fits into cover to span wheelchair rails.

Fluid Supplement
For adding fluid to cushion, when bottoming out on extra bony clients.

Base Wedge
For front to back or side to side wedging of entire cushion.

Adductor Wedges
For less leg separation.

(b)

Figure 11 (a) Jay cushion; (b) Adaptations available for Jay cushion (courtesy of Jay Medical).

and hygiene. Adaptive techniques are always stressed to minimize needed equipment. The patient must play an active role in choosing the equipment, to minimize the purchase of devices that will be quickly discarded at home. A more detailed discussion will follow on equipment for bathing and toileting.

Feeding

Several styles of built-up handles for utensils are available, as are antitip or covered cups. Weighted utensils may decrease intention tremor. Antitip spoons keep the bowl of the spoon parallel to the floor. Pizza cutters ($4) or rocker knives ($9–$15) cut meat easily without requiring fine hand dexterity or good strength. Plate guards ($18) or scoop dishes make one-handed feeding easier. Dycem or Poseygrip ($6) placed under a dish will keep it from sliding on the table (Figure 12).

Dressing

Long-handled reachers ($28) and shoe horns, dressing hooks ($6), button hooks ($4), and sock aids ($14) are often used. Clothing can be adapted with Velcro closures, elastic shoelaces, dressing loops to pull up pants, and large rings on zippers.

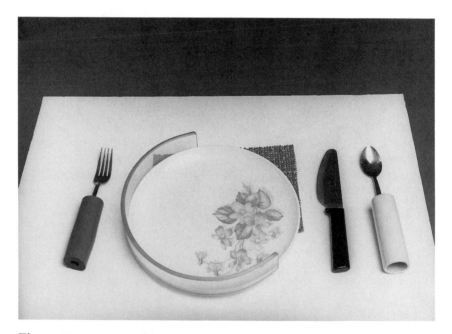

Figure 12   Common adaptive equipment for eating include foam utensil handles, plate guard, rocker knife, and Poseygrip.

Hygiene

Most stroke patients require at least a denture brush ($11) and long-handled bathing brush ($4). Patients with bilateral hand weakness but intact proximal control use equipment adapted to a universal cuff ($14), a wrist-driven flexor hinge orthosis, or powered orthosis described in Chapter 13. Dressing and feeding equipment is similarly adapted. Creative therapists custom-design equipment to fit each patient's needs, as illustrated by the device enabling a C-5 quadriplegic to apply her eye make-up (Figure 13).

Toileting

A toilet riser ($20–$25) is used for patients with good balance and control who need some assistance for sit-to-stand transfer. Grab bars may also be needed. If bars cannot be attached to a wall, a three-in-one commode provides more stability than attaching bars to the rear of the toilet. The three-in-one commode, the most commonly issued ($100), can be used at bedside or over the toilet to provide arm support. Support is further enhanced when the commode is placed against the wall. The higher seat makes standing transfers easier and the front of the seat can be angled lower to ease standing. Drop-arm commodes ($215) are used for patients who perform sliding board transfers or who require moderate or maximum assist for a Bobath transfer (Figure 14). A padded seat grips a sliding board better than the standard seat and also puts less pressure on the buttocks. Extra-wide commodes are available, but many made of polyvinyl chloride pipe are unstable.

Bathing

Hand-held shower heads ($20–$50) can be attached to any shower and some brands turn on and off at the head. Bath or shower seats ($40–$60) are used for patients able to step into the tub or shower. The seats are often used with grab bars on the front wall. Tub transfer benches ($180–$200) allow the patient to sit on the bench outside the tub or shower, then transfer laterally. Benches with slat seats provide better support but make cleaning the patient's bottom more difficult. Benches with cut-outs approximately the size of a toilet seat are also available but less supportive. Either bench can be used with a seat-belt. Many shower stalls are not big enough to allow use of a transfer bench. Showers can be customized to allow a roller shower chair ($180) to be rolled directly into the stall.

HOME ADAPTATIONS

Home adaptations for the disabled can be as simple as changing hinges to allow wheelchair access or as complex as designing environmental control systems for operating household appliances. Complex modifications may be

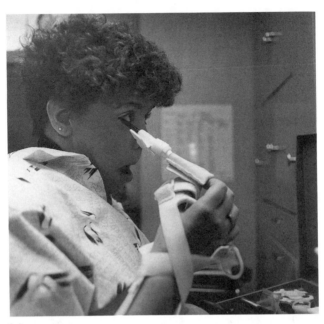

(a)

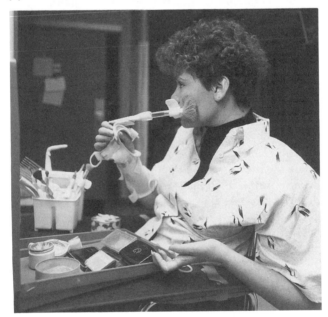

(b)

Figure 13   Custom-made devices allow a patient with C-5 quadriplegia to apply her make-up.

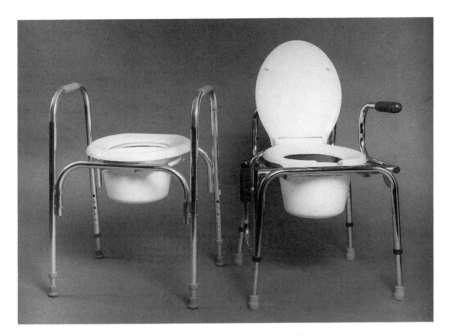

Figure 14   Three-in-one (L) and drop-arm (R) commodes.

offered by universities through homemaker rehabilitation programs or Rehabilitation Engineering Departments. Several national organizations offer plans for barrier-free homes [19,20]. This section will focus on the relatively simple, low-cost modifications most often needed.

Exterior Access

All stairs should have rails. Ready-to-install ramps or wheelchair porch lifts can be purchased [21] ($1000–$2000). Custom-made ramps of treated wood or concrete should have a minimum grade of 1 foot of ramp for 1 inch of elevation (8.3% slope). Surfaces must be nonskid. Turning points must be at least 3 × 5 feet and should be inserted at least every 25 feet of ramp. Ramp width must allow 3 inches clearance on either side of the wheelchair with a 32 inch high safety railing and 2 inches edging. The ramp must be well-lighted, with a 5 × 5 foot platform for a door opening outward or a 3 × 5 foot platform for a door opening inward.

Doors

Exterior doors are usually wide enough for wheelchairs. Offset hinges ($12) widen the entrance by the thickness of the door by allowing it to fit flush with the door frame. A wheelchair can be made 2–4 inches narrower by using a hand-cranked device, or ½–1 inches narrower by removing wheel rims. Interior doors and molding may be removed and replaced by curtains.

Thick foam door knob covers or lever-type handles ($10) may be added to or replace existing door knobs. Door locks can be moved or replaced by push-button combination lock systems that can be operated by a finger or mouth stick. This system unlocks and partially opens the door. Card-access or voice-activated systems are also available from locksmiths.

Interior Adaptation

Furniture frequently needs to be rearranged or removed to allow wheelchair mobility, or can be strategically placed to give support for ambulation. Bedrooms of patients unable to navigate stairs quickly and independently should be on a floor with an outside door (and ramp if needed) to facilitate emergency exits. Light-switch extenders can be placed at a wheelchair-accessible height. Chairs, sofas, and beds may need to be raised or lowered to ease wheelchair transfers. Wedges or solid-seat inserts may improve transfers from soft, overstuffed furniture. Grab-bars are frequently needed for bathroom transfers. Their specific location is best evaluated by a therapist on home visit, since location depends on bathroom layout, location of studs, and type of transfer. Many other adaptations can be recommended after a home visit by an occupational therapist. Often, however, health-care professionals can learn from the ingenious adaptations designed by the disabled patient or his or her family.

SUMMARY

The ultimate outcome of training for functional independence is determined by a patient's use of adaptive techniques and equipment in his or her home or other residential setting. Adaptive equipment or home adaptations should be recommended only after careful consideration of the patient's individual needs. For example, a rocker knife and dressing hook may be appropriate for a hemiparetic patient living alone but inappropriate for a hemiparetic patient whose caretaker will provide assistance rather than wait for the patient to cut his or her own food. If the patient and caretakers are consulted and educated about adaptive equipment, the amount of suitable equipment issued will be minimized and the patient's outcome maximized.

ACKNOWLEDGMENTS

The author thanks David Good, M.D., Helen Minder, P.T., Michelle Porter, P.T., Lori Edwards, O.T., and Katie Mullen, O.T., for their patience, support and recommendations; and Marilyn Tate for her assistance in preparation of the manuscript.

REFERENCES

1. C.S. Simpson, and L. Purie, *Physiotherapy*, 77:231–234 (1991).
2. C.A. Hinton, and K.E. Culle, *Phys. Ther.*, 62:813–819 (1982).
3. S.V. Fisher, and R.P. Patterson, *Arch. Phys. Med. Rehab.*, 62:250–256 (1981).
4. R. Patterson, and S.V. Fisher, *Arch. Phys. Med. Rehab.*, 62:257–260 (1981).
5. M. Harms, *Physiotherapy*, 76:266–271 (1990).
6. R.M. Letts, *Principles of Seating the Disabled*. CRC Press, Boca Raton (1991).
7. D.A. Hobson, *Rehabilitation Engineering*. CRC Press, Boca Raton (1990).
8. J. Wetzel, *Spinal Cord Injury* (H.V. Adkins, ed.), Churchill Livingstone, New York, pp. 75–98 (1985).
9. M. Ferguson-Pell, G.V.B. Cochran, V.R. Palmieri, and J.B. Brunski, *J. Rehabil. Res. Dev.*, 23:63–76 (1986).
10. S. Springle, K.C. Chung, and C.E. Brubaker, *J. Rehabil. Res. Dev.*, 27:135–140 (1990).
11. M.W. Ferguson-Pell, *J. Rehabil. Res. Dev. Clin. Suppl.*, 21:49–73 (1990).
12. S. Springle, K.C. Chung, and C.E. Brubaker, *J. Rehabil. Res. Dev.*, 27:127–134 (1990).
13. I.R. Odderson, K.M. Jaffe, C.A. Sleicher, R. Price, and R.J. Kropp, *Arch. Phys. Med. Rehabil.*, 72:1017–1020 (1991).
14. S.O. Brattgard, and K. Severinsson, *Biomechanics Vi-B: International Series on Biomechanics* (E. Asmussen and K. Jorgenson, eds.), University Park Press, Baltimore, pp. 270–273 (1978).
15. D.F. Borello-France, R.G. Burdett, and Z.L. Gee, *Phys. Ther.*, 68:67–71 (1988).
16. J.E. Latter, and E. DeHoux, *Principles of Seating the Disabled* (R.M. Letts, ed.), CRC Press, Boca Raton, pp. 237–254 (1991).
17. S.L. Garber, and L.R. Dyerly, *Am. J. Occup. Ther.*, 45:550–554 (1991).
18. E. Edberg, and H.V. Adkins, *Spinal Cord Injury* (H.V. Adkins, ed.), Churchill Livingstone, New York, pp. 177–197 (1985).
19. M.H. Malek, and B.S. Almasy, *Willard and Spackman's Occupational Therapy* (H.L. Hopkins and H.D. Smithy, eds.), J.B. Lippincott, Philadelphia, pp. 231–250 (1983).
20. V. Nixon, *Physical Therapy* (R.M. Scully and M.R. Barnes, eds.), J.B. Lippincott, Philadelphia, pp. 1073–1102 (1989).
21. J.J. Somerville, and H.M. Pendleton, *Spinal Cord Injury* (H.V. Adkins, ed.), Churchill Livingstone, New York, pp. 243–270 (1985).

15

Pharmacological Enhancement of Recovery

Larry B. Goldstein

Duke University and
Durham Department of Veterans Affairs Medical Center
Durham, North Carolina

INCIDENCE AND EXTENT OF INJURY

Stroke and traumatic brain injury are major causes of neurological disability. The prevalence of stroke is between 5 and 6:1000 population [1]. In 1986, there were over 2 million Americans alive who had survived a stroke [2]. One-third of these patients were wage earners who became unemployed because of their disabilities. In 1989, the American Heart Association estimated the annual costs of stroke-related health care to be $13.5 billion [2]. Twelve billion dollars of this was the result of lost wages, hospital expenses, and nursing home services. Traumatic brain injury affects 200–400:100,000 population in the United States and has a peak incidence in the second and third decades [3]. A second peak in incidence occurs in the sixth decade [3]. Although 5–10% of traumatic brain injuries are fatal (overall mortality rate of 25:100,000 population), most individuals have only minor injuries and do not come to medical attention [3]. Moderate head injury (Glasgow coma scale 9–12) affects 60,000–75,000 persons per year [4]. Of patients with moderate traumatic brain injury, two-thirds are moderately to severely disabled 3 months after the injury [5].

RECOVERY AFTER FOCAL BRAIN INJURY

General Clinical Features

Although many survivors of acute stroke or traumatic head injury have significant disabilities, most patients recover some degree of function. Functional improvements can occur over the first 3–6 months after stroke [6]. In some individuals, recovery can continue over a period of years [7]. However, spontaneous recovery is largely completed by 1 month after stroke [8–13].

In humans, a series of diverse biological and environmental factors may influence recovery from brain injury (Table 1). The strongest predictor of the extent of eventual recovery is the severity of the initial neurological deficit [8,14–16]. In addition, the impact of an individual's age on subsequent recovery has been long recognized as an important prognostic factor [17]. Racial differences also may affect the ultimate degree of physical impairment after stroke [18]. The size and location of the brain lesion and the presence of prior lesions are critical [17]. For example, Knopman and co-workers found that lesion volume correlated with recovery from aphasia after stroke [19]. Patients with small lesions recovered fluency whereas those with large lesions had poor outcomes. However, language recovery in patients with intermediate-sized lesions depended on lesion location. The importance of lesion location also was demonstrated in a study in which infarct size and location were determined by brain computed tomography or cerebral angiography and correlated with the motor deficit after stroke [20]. The site (subcortical versus cortical), but not the size of the lesion correlated with ultimate recovery. Nutritional status, prelesion experience, and postlesion training are also relevant to recovery [17]. Grafman and co-workers investigated the relationships of preinjury intelligence or education, brain-tissue volume loss, and lesion location on the persistence of cognitive deficits after penetrating brain wounds [21]. Preinjury intelligence and education were more important predictors of postinjury performance than other variables. Routine physical

Table 1 Clinical Factors Influencing Recovery

Biological factors	Environmental factors
Age	Nutritional status
Race	Preinjury experience
Lesion size	Postinjury experience
Lesion location	Social factors
Lesion mechanism	
Comorbidity	

therapy is a type of postinjury training aimed at reducing complications and improving functional outcome. The "forced use" of a paretic limb represents a novel clinical strategy designed to maximize the recovery of a specific impaired function [22,23]. The noninvolved hand of a patient is restrained so that the individual is constantly "forced to use" the paretic limb. Based on anecdotal reports, such patients have demonstrated marked functional improvement. Other potentially important covariates include medical comorbidity, the presence of mood disorders [24,25], and the availability of a caring spouse or caretaker [16,26].

Neurobiology of Recovery

The neurobiological basis of spontaneous behavioral recovery after focal brain injury is not completely understood. However, laboratory investigations provide insights into the recovery process. In analogy to the situation in humans, a variety of environmental and biological factors have an impact on the recovery process (Figure 1). For example, lesion location can be a better predictor of behavioral performance in monkeys after focal brain injury than lesion size [27,28]. In fact, some lesion loci are associated with significant improvements in a certain behavior [28]. Recovery also is influenced by the pathological sequelae to acute brain injury, the brain's adaptive responses to injury, and by a variety of neuronal rearrangements (Table 2). Laboratory studies now suggest that pharmacological management of patients during the period of recovery may be possible.

Pathological Sequelae of Acute Brain Injury

Cerebral Edema   Cerebral edema commonly accompanies brain injury and has a complex pathophysiology [29]. Brain edema due to focal ischemia begins as a cytotoxic type occurring in both grey and white matter. Cytotoxic edema involves the accumulation of intracellular fluid. This is followed by vasogenic edema that involves a leakage of proteins and fluid from damaged blood vessels (a defect of the blood–brain barrier). Edema may produce local functional depression in the area immediately surrounding the lesion. Remote functional depression can be caused by compression of normal structures distant from the site of primary injury. Clinical worsening and spontaneous improvement in patients after acute brain injury may be due, in part, to the development and subsequent resolution of edema.

Diaschisis   Diaschisis, a term originated by the German pathologist Von Monakow [30], refers to sudden functional depression of brain regions distant from the site of primary injury [31]. Reductions in blood flow and metabolism following hemispheric stroke have been demonstrated in humans by positron emission tomography in the noninjured ipsilateral cerebral hemisphere, the

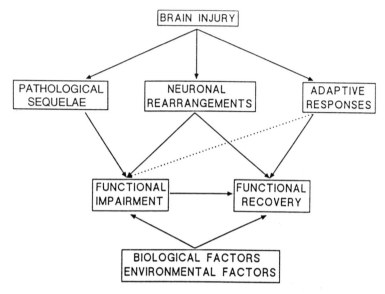

Figure 1 Brain injury results in tissue responses that are influenced by a variety of biological and environmental factors to produce functional impairment. Adaptive cellular responses and some neuronal rearrangements may then contribute to functional recovery. Other neuronal rearrangements may be maladaptive and contribute to the functional deficit. Drugs may influence these processes at many different levels (from ref. [209]).

contralateral cerebral hemisphere, and the contralateral cerebellum [32–34]. Crossed cerebellar–cortical diaschisis occurs in patients with unilateral cerebellar infarctions [35]. Capsular or thalamic stroke also can have remote effects on metabolism in the cerebral cortex and cerebellum [36].

The pathophysiological mechanism underlying diaschisis is not under-

Table 2 Neurobiology of Recovery

Pathological sequelae of acute brain injury	*Neuronal rearrangements*
Cerebral edema	Axonal rearrangements
Diaschisis	Regeneration
Denervation supersensitivity	Pruning
Adaptive responses	Collateral sprouting
Unmasking	Ingrowth
"Relearning" and long-term potentiation	Dendritic rearrangements

stood [31,37]. Depression of metabolic activity in brain regions distant from the primary site of injury might be a reflection of regional changes in cerebral blood flow. As an alternative, decreased regional cerebral blood flow may be a secondary phenomenon reflecting locally depressed cerebral metabolism. These remote areas of depressed cerebral metabolic activity could result from injury to excitatory projections from the injured region. It has also been suggested that diaschisis could result from the release of vasoactive or neuroactive substances from damaged brain [38].

Denervation Supersensitivity As in the peripheral nervous system, lesions in the central nervous system may result in enhanced responses of targets to neurotransmitters [39]. The possible relationship of this phenomenon to behavioral recovery has been extensively reviewed [17]. In brief, partial damage to the dendritic tree results in an acute decrease in the amount of neurotransmitter available at the synapse. An upregulation of postsynaptic receptors ensues. Subsequent presentation of a smaller amount of neurotransmitter then results in an exaggerated physiological response that may restore (or impair) function.

Adaptive Responses

Adaptive responses refer to the mechanisms by which uninjured brain assumes the functions previously performed by injured neurons. Several general hypotheses have been offered to explain this process.

Unmasking One hypothesis is that redundant neural networks perform functions lost due to brain injury. This hypothesis was suggested by Lashley [40] and Luria [41,42] and has also been discussed as "unmasking" [43]. More recent studies with positron emission tomography in human stroke patients demonstrate metabolic changes consistent with "unmasking." In uninjured humans, motor movement is associated with increases in regional cerebral blood flow (rCBF) in the contralateral primary sensorimotor cortex. However, in patients who had recovered from stroke that had resulted in limb paresis, movement of the previously paralyzed limb is associated with significant changes in rCBF in widespread areas of the brain including both ipsilateral and contralateral sensorimotor cortex and cerebellar hemispheres [44].

"Relearning" and Long-term Potentiation A second general hypothesis is that the cellular mechanisms that underlie behavioral recovery also may be responsible for normal learning. For example, task-specific postlesion experience can hasten recovery of locomotor abilities in rats that had motor cortex lesions [45–48]. The impact of certain drugs on the recovery process may be blocked [49–51] or diminished [52] if the animals are not given task-specific experience during the period of intoxication.

The best-understood putative cellular mechanism of learning and memory is long-term potentiation (LTP) [53–55]. LTP has been described by

Collingridge and Bliss as a "kind of activity-dependent change in synaptic efficacy that is assumed to provide the physiological basis of information storage in the brain" [56]. LTP has been best characterized in the hippocampal formation, but has also been demonstrated in several other brain regions including hypothalamus [57], visual cortex [58,59], and motor cortex [60]. In the hippocampal formation, LTP is induced by a single, transient, high-frequency stimulation of excitatory neural inputs. This produces an increase in synaptic responses that can last for prolonged periods of time [54,55]. The development of LTP is mediated, at least in part, by the N-methyl-D-aspartate (NMDA) subtype of glutamate receptor [56,61,62]. The administration of NMDA receptor antagonists block the induction of LTP and disrupt learning and memory [63–65]. Other neurotransmitters such as catecholamines [61,66–68], γ-aminobutyric acid (GABA) [69–72], and acetylcholine [73,74] can modulate the induction of LTP and have been implicated in the memory process. As discussed below, these neurotransmitters may also influence recovery after brain injury.

Neuronal Rearrangements

It is clear that a variety of neuronal rearrangements occur after many types of brain injuries [17,75–77]. Both axonal (presynaptic) and dendritic (postsynaptic) rearrangements may occur. Some of these rearrangements are beneficial while others are maladaptive and may contribute to the ultimate functional deficit (Figure 2).

Axonal Rearrangements

REGENERATION   Regeneration refers to the regrowth of an injured neuron's axon to reinnervate the denervated target [75]. Axonal regeneration would be the ideal rearrangement to restore function. Although controversial

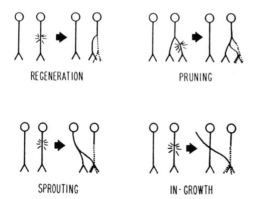

REGENERATION   PRUNING

SPROUTING   IN-GROWTH

Figure 2   Theoretical classification of axonal rearrangements (from ref [75]).

and difficult to demonstrate, functional regeneration of axons may occur in the central nervous system [78,79].

PRUNING   Pruning occurs in highly collateralized neurons (single neurons with many axons). When one axon is injured, collateral branches extend to reinnervate the target [80]. Unlike regeneration, pruning has been clearly demonstrated in the adult brain and should be a beneficial adaptive rearrangement [81–86].

COLLATERAL SPROUTING   Collateral sprouting (the most extensively studied neuronal arrangement) refers to neurite outgrowth from an uninjured neuron in response to damage to an adjacent fiber [75]. Sprouting has been demonstrated in the central nervous system [76] and can result in the formation of electrophysiologically functional synapses [87,88]. Collateral sprouting may be maladaptive because it usually results in hyperinnervation of the target.

INGROWTH   Ingrowth is the response of an uninjured nerve to a remote injury [75]. A foreign neuron grows to innervate a target in response to the loss of the target's normal innervation. The most extensively studied example of ingrowth is the expansion of sympathetic fibers from surface blood vessels into the brain parenchyma after certain lesions [89]. Sympathetic ingrowth interferes with recovery after various specific experimental lesions in laboratory animals [90,91].

DENDRITIC REARRANGEMENTS   Changes in receptor numbers following partial denervation represents a type of postsynaptic receptor plasticity (see above). A variety of other short-term synaptic changes may occur [92]. Rapid morphological changes in dendritic spines have been observed in different species under a variety of conditions [92,93] and may play a role in learning and memory [94,95]. Changes in the shape and/or number of dendritic spines can occur in association with the development of LTP [96–98]. Changes in synaptic contacts also may be induced by environmental enrichment [99]. Behavioral recoveries from lesions of the deep cerebellar nuclei in cats are associated with the formation of new synapses in the motor cortex [100].

PHARMACOLOGY OF FUNCTIONAL RECOVERY

Laboratory Studies

The preceding discussion provides a framework for considering the effects of drugs on the recovering brain (Figure 1). It is possible that a given class of drug may influence the recovery process through a variety of mechanisms. Furthermore, certain drugs may be beneficial if given soon after the acute injury, but detrimental if given later.

Steroids

Treatment with glucocorticoids reduces cerebral edema in patients with brain tumors and other mass lesions. This often results in dramatic, but transient, symptomatic improvement. Studies of the effects of glucocorticoids following cerebral infarction in laboratory animals have yielded conflicting results [29,101,102]. Injury to neurons following transient ischemia is actually potentiated by glucocorticoids and diminished or delayed by adrenalectomy in the rat [103]. Early clinical studies reported that treatment with glucocorticoids improved the outcome of patients with stroke who had clinical signs of cerebral edema [104–106]. However, these studies were anecdotal and may have included patients with other conditions. Recent clinical studies indicate that glucocorticoid treatment is ineffective after both ischemic stroke [107,108] and supratentorial intracerebral hemorrhage [109].

New treatment strategies aimed at interrupting the processes responsible for the edema following cerebral infarction and ischemia are currently being tested in animal models. The 21 aminosteroids, a new class of steroid drugs with little mineralocorticoid or glucocorticoid activity, may decrease cerebral edema by inhibiting lipid peroxidation [110]. These experimental therapies may become clinically important in the future.

Drugs that Influence Central Neurotransmitters

Drugs that influence the activities of a variety of neurotransmitter systems also affect functional recovery following focal brain injury. These drugs may be either beneficial or detrimental. They could act through a variety of potential mechanisms including enhancement or impairment of learning, hastening or slowing of recovery from diaschisis, and relieving or intensifying the effects of denervation supersensitivity. These and other potential mechanisms of action remain largely speculative.

Catecholamines Amphetamine is perhaps the most extensively studied drug with the capacity to facilitate recovery after focal brain injury. It was recognized as early as 1946 that treatment with amphetamine restored righting and other postural activity in low decerebrate cats [111]. Amphetamine treatment also reinstated long-standing absent placing responses in hemidecorticate and neodecorticate cats [112–114]. More recently, an enduring recovery of function has been demonstrated in cats subjected to bilateral visual cortex ablations [50,115]. This lesion results in a complete and permanent deficit of stereopsis. Treatment with amphetamine, when combined with visual experience, results in a recovery of binocular depth perception. Relearning of a visual discrimination task in visually decorticated rats is also facilitated by amphetamine [116].

Because motor function is a particularly important determinant of physical function and independence in activities of daily living after brain injury in humans [16], the impact of drugs on motor recovery after focal cortex injury has been the subject of extensive laboratory investigations. A sensorimotor cortex lesion in the rat does not result in a dramatic motor deficit when the animals are observed on a flat field, but becomes obvious when the animals traverse a narrow elevated beam (beam-walking ability) [117,118]. Feeney et al. devised a simple system for grading this motor deficit and found that a single dose of D-amphetamine administered 24 hr after unilateral sensorimotor cortex ablation accelerated the rate of functional recovery [49,119]. Postlesion treatment with amphetamine also enhanced motor recovery in cats with unilateral frontal cortex ablation lesions [51,113,120].

Understanding of the pharmacological mechanism of amphetamine-facilitated recovery is hampered because the drug has diverse central and peripheral effects. Systemic administration of amphetamine may produce raised blood pressure with reflex bradycardia, behavioral arousal, and hypermotility [121]. Dextroamphetamine also may induce changes in regional cerebral blood flow [122]. The behavioral and pharmacological effects of amphetamine are also dose dependent. For example, amphetamine's beneficial effect on beam-walking recovery occurs over a narrow range of dosages (Figure 3). The dose–effect curve forms an inverted U, with a decline in response at higher dosages [123]. This decline is likely to be due to amphetamine-induced stereotypies. The levels of norepinephrine in rat brain are decreased when amphetamine is administered in relatively high dosage. This effect is most likely caused by depletion of granular amine stores combined with an inhibition of the reuptake mechanism [124]. However, acute pharmacological effects of the drug may be related to the release of extragranular accumulations catecholamines [124]. In addition, amphetamine may induce a disaggregation of brain polysomes through a dopaminergic mechanism, thereby interfering with protein synthesis [125].

Amphetamine's central actions may be mediated through noradrenergic, dopaminergic, or serotonergic neurons [124]. A dopaminergic mechanism for amphetamine's action is suggested by the observations that coadministration of haloperidol blocks amphetamine-promoted recovery [49,126], that haloperidol impairs motor recovery when given alone [49], and that the administration of haloperidol reinstates motor deficits in recovered animals [127]. However, in addition to its action as a dopamine receptor antagonist, haloperidol has antagonist effects at noradrenergic receptors [128]. Other coincident lines of evidence suggest that amphetamine-promoted recovery of function is mediated through noradrenergic neurons. Intraventricular [129] or cerebellar [130] infusions of NE facilitate recovery. Apomorphine has no effect. Treatment with a centrally acting α_1-adrenergic receptor 'antagonist (i.e., prazosin) interferes with motor recovery [131,132]. Postlesion systemic administration of an α_2-adrenergic receptor antagonist (i.e., yohimbine,

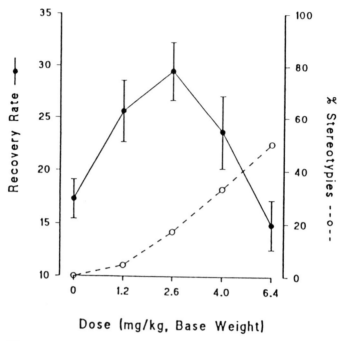

Dose (mg/kg, Base Weight)

Figure 3   Dose–effect relationship for amphetamine-facilitated recovery of beam-walking in the rat following a unilateral suction–ablation lesion of the sensorimotor cortex. Amphetamine was given as a single dose the day after cortex lesion. Recovery rate for each rat is calculated from the area under the time–effect curve when beam-walking scores are plotted against time after drug administration (see [46] and [135] for methodological details). Mean recovery rate (± S.E.M.) for each dosage of amphetamine is shown. The maximally effective dosage is between 1.2 and 4.0 mg/kg. The percentage of animals at each dosage that exhibited stereotypies is also shown. These data were presented at the 17th Princeton Conference on Cerebrovascular Diseases [133] (from ref. [123]).

idazoxan) enhances motor recovery [131–134] while administration of α_2-adrenergic receptor agonist clonidine impairs motor recovery (Figure 4) [135] and reinstates beam-walking deficits in recovered rats [131,132,136]. Furthermore, pretreatment with the neurotoxin DSP-4, a drug that selectively depletes central norepinephrine (NE), slows beam-walking recovery (Figure 5) [137,138].

   Taken together, these data suggest that amphetamine influences recovery indirectly through its effects on central norepinephrine. Although this work was largely carried out in rats with suction lesions of the cerebral cortex,

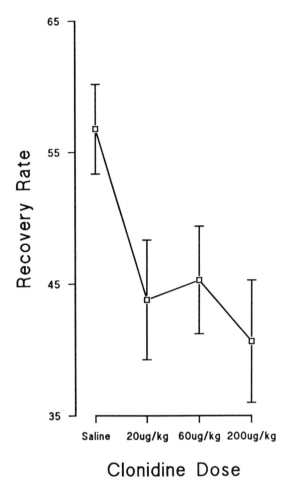

Clonidine Dose

Figure 4 The relationship between a single dose of saline or clonidine administered 24 hr after unilateral sensorimotor cortex suction–ablation injury in rats and the "rate" of beam-walking recovery over the next 12 days. Mean overall "recovery rates" (lower panel) were calculated from the areas under the time–effect curves when each rat's beam-walking scores were plotted as a function of time after surgery (see [46] and [135] for methodological details). The error bars indicate ±1 S.E.M. A single dose of clonidine as low as 20 μg/kg significantly impairs subsequent recovery (from ref. [135]).

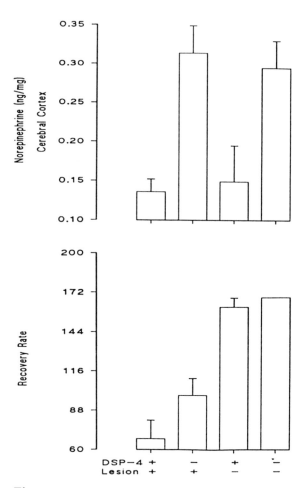

Figure 5 Half of the rats in this experiment received the neurotoxin DSP-4 and half received saline. DSP-4 selectively depletes central norepinephrine. Two weeks later, half of the DSP-4 treated and half of the saline-treated rats underwent right sensori-motor cortex suction–ablation. The remainder of the rats underwent sham operation. Motor recovery was measured over the next 12 days. The upper panel shows the mean cerebral cortical norepinephrine values for each group of rats. Mean overall "recovery rates" (lower panel) were calculated from the areas under the time–effect curves when each rat's beam-walking scores were plotted as a function of time after surgery (see [46] and [135] for methodological details). The error bars indicate ±1 S.E.M. +, The group of animals received that treatment (injection of DSP-4 or unilateral right cortex suction-ablation). Rats pretreated with DSP-4 that underwent subsequent cortex abla-tion had poorer recoveries than lesioned rats pretreated with saline. Although DSP-4 pretreatment had similar effects on lowering central norepinephrine in sham operated controls, these rats did not have a beam-walking deficit. These data suggest that central norepinephrine depletion impairs subsequent motor recovery (from ref. [137]).

the effect of noradrenergic agents on recovery is similar for traumatic cerebral contusion and infarction injury models [139–142].

The mechanism of the amphetamine effect remains speculative, but consistent with a variety of hypotheses. For example, the size and location of the cortical receptive field responding to a specific peripheral stimulus can be mapped with 2-deoxyglucose autoradiography. This receptive field is increased by treatment with amphetamine [142]. Thus, the administration of amphetamine could facilitate recovery by promoting the "unmasking" of alternative neural pathways. It also has been proposed that drugs such as amphetamine may act to accelerate the resolution of diaschisis and thereby facilitate the functional recovery [31,143]. The effect of treatment with amphetamine on the induction of LTP is particularly intriguing in view of the hypothesis that recovery after brain injury entails a type of "relearning." Administration of amphetamine facilitates the development of LTP in a dose-dependent manner [144] and enhances memory retrieval [145,146]. In addition to these effects, even a single dose of amphetamine can cause increases in the numbers of dendritic spines in certain brain regions [147].

GABA　Intracortical infusion of the inhibitory neurotransmitter GABA increases the hemiparesis produced by a small motor cortex lesion in rats [148]. Even short-term intracortical infusion of a GABA agonist can produce long-term impairment of behavioral recovery [149]. The deleterious effect of GABA is increased by the systemic administration of phenytoin [150], which may act through a GABA-mediated mechanism [151]. The administration of diazepam, a benzodiazepine that acts as an indirect GABA agonist, impedes recovery from the sensory asymmetry caused by anterior–medial neocortex damage in the rat [152]. Coadministration of the benzodiazepine antagonist Ro 15-1788 blocks this detrimental effect [153]. The diazepam effect is mimicked by infusion of the GABA agonist, muscimol, into the sensorimotor cortex adjacent to the lesion [154]. Thus, GABA or GABA agonists interfere with the recovery process whereas GABA antagonists may be beneficial.

GABA influences the induction of LTP and learning and memory. Stimulation of inhibitory GABAergic inputs to the hippocampal formation [70,71], as well as the administration of indirect GABA agonists (e.g., benzo-diazepines) [155,156], suppresses the induction of LTP. The administration of benzodiazepines impairs learning and memory [157,158]. In contrast, GABA antagonists facilitate hippocampal LTP [69] and may enhance learning and memory [159]. Because GABA is an inhibitory neurotransmitter, it also may act to slow the resolution of diaschisis. It is interesting to note recent evidence suggesting that amphetamine administration also may influence the activity of GABAergic neurons, leading to lower extracellular GABA concentrations [160].

Acetylcholine　Much of the data concerning the impact of cholinergic drugs on recovery of function are old and inadequate when evaluated against current standards. As early as 1942, Ward and Kennard reported that cholinergic agonists increased the rate of motor recovery after motor cortex lesions in monkeys [161]. The beneficial effects of cholinergic agonists were blocked by administration of phenytoin [162]. Recent data suggest that the anticholinergic drug scopolamine interferes with motor recovery following cortex infarction in rats [163]. As reviewed by Feeney and Sutton, acetylcholine administration appears to enhance recovery of function [164].

Acetylcholine would be expected to facilitate the induction of LTP by suppressing voltage-activated potassium conductance [56]. Activation of the muscarinic cholinergic receptor facilitates the induction of LTP in the rat dentate gyrus [165]. Anticholinergics are potent amnestic agents. However, the putative effects of cholinergic drugs on recovery also may be mediated by their indirect actions on noradrenergic neurons [166,167].

N-Methyl-D-Aspartate   The availability of drugs that competitively and noncompetitively block specific subtypes of the glutamate receptor has led to trials of these agents in experimental ischemia. The noncompetitive NMDA receptor antagonists MK-801 [168–170], dextromethorphan, and dextrorphan [171–174], and the competitive NMDA receptor antagonists CGS 19755 and CPP [175] have been reported to reduce brain injury following focal or global ischemia.

As discussed above, the development of LTP is mediated, at least in part, by the NMDA subtype of glutamate receptor [56,61,62]. The administration of NMDA receptor antagonists blocks the induction of LTP and disrupts learning and memory [63–65]. Thus, NMDA receptor antagonists would be hypothesized to interfere with the recovery process. In fact, administration of the NMDA receptor antagonist MK 801 reinstates sensory deficits in rats that had *recovered* from anteromedial frontal cortex injury [176]. The drug had a slightly beneficial effect if given soon after the brain injury. These results would not have been anticipated based on MK-801's mode of action (i.e., blocks induction but has no effect on maintenance of LTP [177]). MK-801 had no effect on beam-walking recovery in rats whether it was administered to the animals soon after the injury or after spontaneous recovery was complete [178]. Thus, if "relearning" is involved in motor recovery after cortex injury, the results of these two sets of experiments suggest that the process is not susceptible to permanent disruption by the early administration of an NMDA receptor antagonist.

Growth Factors/Transplants

As discussed above, a variety of neuronal rearrangements occur after many types of brain injuries. Because neuronal rearrangements may be either beneficial or detrimental, to be most clinically efficacious, a drug should selectively promote only beneficial neuronal rearrangements.

The use of growth factors to improve functional outcome following brain injury is the topic for a separate review [179]. A large number of substances can promote neuronal survival or growth [179]. Treatment with nerve growth factor (NGF), one of the first of these substances identified, improves spatial learning following nucleus basalis magnocellularis lesions in rats [180] and prevents neuronal death after brain trauma [181].

Although originally considered a neuronotrophic factor, GM1 ganglioside may have several mechanisms of action [182]. Several laboratory studies suggest that postlesion administration of gangliosides may improve functional outcome [183–185].

An extensive literature is available that provides evidence for successful structural and functional grafts of homotypic fetal brain tissue (see [186]). For example, fetal neurons grafted to the brains of adult rats with ischemic lesions of the hippocampus become structurally incorporated and establish connections with the host brain [186]. Intracerebral chromaffin cell autografts accelerate functional recovery in adult cats with unilateral frontal cortex ablation [187]. At this time, the use of neural grafts or transplants to facilitate recovery after brain injury in humans remains controversial.

Summary

Laboratory studies show that a variety of drugs may influence recovery after focal brain injury. The mechanisms underlying these drug effects remain speculative. One hypothesis is that the effects on recovery of drugs that influence central neurotransmitters can largely be predicted based on their effects on learning (and the induction of LTP, see Table 3). However, the effects some drugs (i.e., MK-801) cannot be predicted based solely on this hypothesis.

Clinical Studies

The use of drugs to improve recovery after brain injury in humans was attempted as early as the 1940s. More recent preliminary clinical studies indicate that many of the drugs that influence recovery in laboratory animals have similar effects on recovery in humans.

Physicians' Prescribing Patterns: Use of "Deleterious" Drugs After Stroke

To determine what drugs were currently being used in the treatment of patients with stroke, a retrospective study of physicians' prescribing patterns was carried out [188]. More than 80% of individuals were taking at least one drug at the time of the stroke. Sixty-five percent of patients were receiving multiple drugs. Antihypertensive agents such as clonidine and prazosin and sedative hypnotics including benzodiazepines were among the most commonly prescribed medications (Figure 6). As noted above, many of these drugs have deleterious effects on recovery of function in laboratory animals.

A retrospective study has recently been performed to test the hypoth-

Table 3   Effects of Some Drugs on Recovery and Induction of LTP

Transmitter/Drug	Effect on Recovery	Effect on LTP Induction
Norepinephrine	+	+
Amphetamine	+	+
Clonidine	−	−
Haloperidol	−	−
Prazosin	−	
GABA	−	−
Diazepam	−	−
Muscimol	−	−
Phenytoin	−	
Acetylcholine	+	+
Scopolamine	−	−
MK-801	−/neutral	−

Comparisons of the effects of various neurotransmitters and drugs on recovery following sensorimotor cortex injury with their effects on the induction of long-term potentiation (LTP). +, Beneficial effect on recovery and a facilitation of the induction of LTP; −, detrimental effect on recovery and a suppression of the induction of LTP. References are provided in the text. *Source:* Revised from ref. [123].

esis that drugs that interfere with recovery in laboratory animals are also detrimental in human stroke victims [189]. These potentially detrimental drugs included the antihypertensives clonidine and prazosin, neuroleptics, benzodiazepines, and phenytoin. The motor recoveries of patients with stroke who received one or a combination of these drugs were compared to the recoveries of a similar group of patients who did not receive these agents. Motor function was measured prospectively with the Fugl-Meyer assessment [190] by observers who were blind to the study hypothesis. This scale measures selective and synergistic movements and has both concurrent and predictive validity [190] and high inter- and intratester reliability [191]. The two groups of patients were similar with respect to a variety of characteristics including age, blood pressure, gender, and medical comorbidity. Although the results of this study need to be interpreted with caution, patients who received one or a combination of the hypothesized "detrimental" drugs at the time of stroke or during the subsequent hospitalization had slower motor recoveries than patients who did not receive one of these drugs (Figure 7). Additional, largely anecdotal reports indicate that treatment with haloperidol [164,192] and certain antihypertensives [193] may interfere with language recovery in patients with aphasia following stroke.

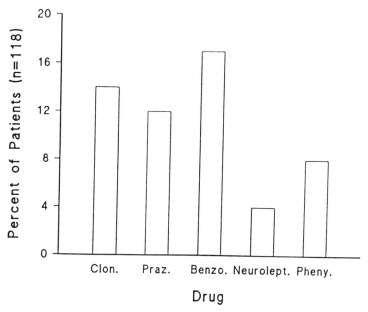

Figure 6   The drugs prescribed for patients admitted to the hospital within 48 hr of a carotid distribution ischemic stroke [188]. The percentage of patients prescribed the indicated drugs are shown (clon., clonidine; praz., prazosin; benzo., benzodiazepine; neurolept., neuroleptic; pheny., phenytoin). The results of studies in laboratory animals suggest that these drugs are harmful if given during the period of recovery from brain injury (from ref. [210]).

Amphetamine-Facilitated Recovery in Humans

Anecdotal reports indicate that treatment with amphetamine improves cognitive function in young adults with posttraumatic organic brain syndrome [194,195]. Motivation in elderly patients refractory to rehabilitation procedures also improves with amphetamine treatment [196]. These effects are likely to be due to the stimulant properties of the drug rather than a specific effect on functional recovery. However, administration of amphetamine has been reported to be of benefit in the treatment of aphasia due to stroke [197,198]. A small, prospective, double-blind study was carried out to determine whether the amphetamine's effect on motor recovery occurs in humans [199]. Motor function was measured with the Fugl-Meyer assessment [190]. A group of eight patients with stable motor deficits following ischemic stroke were randomized to receive either a single dose of amphetamine or placebo. Within 3 hr of drug administration, all of the patients underwent intensive

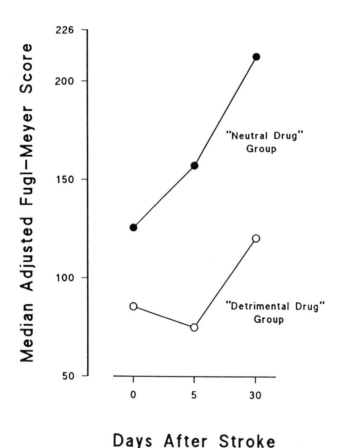

Days After Stroke

Figure 7   The motor recoveries of a cohort of patients with stroke were analyzed retrospectively. Motor function had been measured prospectively with the Fugl-Meyer Assessment [190]. The medications taken by patients at the time of stroke or during the subsequent hospitalization were determined by review of their medical records. The patients were then organized into two groups. One group ("Detrimental" drug group) had received one or a combination of the drugs hypothesized to be harmful based on laboratory animal experiments (see text). The remaining patients, all of whom had received at least one drug, were included in the "Neutral" drug group. Patients in the "Detrimental" drug group had greater initial deficits and recovered motor function more slowly than patients in the "Neutral" drug group (from ref. [189]).

physical therapy. The following day, the patients' abilities to use their affected limbs were reassessed. The amphetamine-treated patients had significant motor improvements while none of the placebo-treated patients had a significant change in performance (Figure 8). Because this study involved only a small group of highly selected patients, the results may not be applicable to patients with stroke with other types of deficits. Because only short-term motor recovery was measured, the longer-term efficacy of amphetamine treatment is unknown. Furthermore, the results must be viewed with caution because the study has not been replicated. However, the study provides some of the only controlled data showing a beneficial effect of amphetamine treatment on motor recovery in humans.

Other Drugs and Recovery in Humans

Early reports suggested that cholinergic agents might facilitate recovery following brain injury in humans [200,201]. However, much of the data

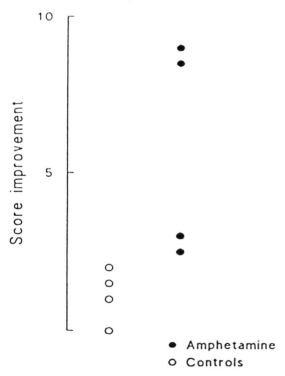

Figure 8 The differences in Fugl-Meyer scores between amphetamine-treated patients with stroke and controls is shown (modified from ref. [199]).

concerning the impact of cholinergic drugs on recovery of function are old and inadequate when evaluated against current standards. These reports have been reviewed by Feeney and Sutton [164]. Administration of cytidine-5'-diphosphocholine (CDP-choline) to rats after ischemia lessens the resultant neurological deficit [202]. Although CDP-choline accelerates phospholipid synthesis and may suppress the release of free fatty acids by ischemic neurons [202], administration of the drug may also lead to an enhancement of cholinergic function. A recent double-blind multicenter clinical trial indicates that CDP-choline may improve functional outcome in patients with ischemic stroke [203].

GM1-ganglioside has been the subject of clinical trials for the treatment of patients with a variety of neurological disorders, including a recent report of benefit in individuals with spinal cord injury [204]. Trials in patients with stroke suggest that the drug may be of some benefit [205–207]. However, the clinical significance of the reported effects in these studies is unclear and one trial failed to demonstrate any impact of the drug on recovery in stroke patients [208]. Two large clinical trials of GM1-gangliosides for the treatment of patients with acute stroke are currently in progress.

SUMMARY

The development of an understanding of the basic neurobiology underlying functional recovery after focal brain damage is leading to new strategies for the treatment of patients with stroke and traumatic brain injury. It is important to recognize that some of the drugs currently used to treat coexisting medical conditions may be harmful. In combination with new treatments designed to limit acute damage and salvage injured but not dead neurons, new strategies aimed at facilitating functional recovery offer the hope of improved outcomes for the brain-injured patient.

ACKNOWLEDGMENT

The author thanks Dr. James N. Davis for his support and helpful suggestions.

REFERENCES

1. J.F. Kurtzke, *Cerebrovascular Survey Report 1985* (F.H. McDowell and L.R. Caplan, eds.), National Institutes of Health, Bethesda, pp. 1–34 (1985).
2. American Heart Association, *1989 Stroke Facts*. American Heart Association, Dallas (1988).
3. R.F. Frankowski, J.F. Annegers, and S. Whitman, *Central Nervous System Trauma Status Report—1985*. (D.P. Becker and J.T. Povlishock, eds.), National

Institute of Neurological and Communicative Disorders and Stroke, Bethesda, pp. 33–43 (1985).

4. L.F. Marshall, and S.B. Marshall, *Central Nervous System Trauma Status Report—1985.* (D.P. Becker and J.T. Povlishock, eds.), National Institutes of Health, Bethesda, pp. 45–51 (1985).

5. R.W. Rimel, M.A. Giordani, T.J. Barth, and J.A. Jane, *Neurosurgery, 11*:344–351 (1982).

6. C.E. Skilbeck, D.T. Wade, R.L. Hewer, and V.A. Wood, *J. Neurol. Neurosurg. Psychiatry, 46*:5–8 (1983).

7. P. Bach-y-Rita, *Arch. Phys. Med. Rehabil., 62*:413–417 (1981).

8. P.W. Duncan, L.B. Goldstein, G.W. Divine, D.B. Matchar, and J. Feussner, *Stroke, 23*:1084–1089 (1992).

9. M. Newman, *Stroke, 3*:702–710 (1972).

10. D.T. Wade, H.R. Langton, V.A. Wood, C.E. Skilbeck, and H.M. Ilsmail, *J. Neurol. Neurosurg. Psychiatry, 46*:521–524 (1983).

11. S.C. Loewen, and B.A. Anderson, *Stroke, 21*:78–81 (1990).

12. D.T. Wade, V.A. Wood, and R.L. Hewer, *J. Neurol. Neurosurg. Psychiatry, 48*: 7–13 (1985).

13. G. Kinsella, and B. Ford, *Med. J. Aust., 2*:662–666 (1980).

14. L. Jongbloed, *Stroke, 17*:765–776 (1986).

15. A.W. Heinemann, E.J. Roth, K. Cichowski, and H.B. Betts, *Arch. Neurol., 44*: 1167–1172 (1989).

16. N.B. Lincoln, M. Blackburn, S. Ellis, J. Jackson, J.A. Edmans, F.M. Nouri, M.F. Walrer, and H. Haworth, *J. Neurol. Neurosurg. Psychiatry, 52*:493–496 (1989).

17. S. Finger, and D.G. Stein, *Brain Damage and Recovery.* Academic Press, New York (1982).

18. R.D. Horner, D.B. Matchar, G.W. Divine, and J.R. Feussner, *Stroke, 22*:1497–1501 (1991).

19. D.S. Knopman, O.A. Selnes, and N. Niccum, *Neurology, 33*:1170–1178 (1983).

20. J. Lundgren, K. Flodstrom, K. Sjogren, B. Liljequist, and A.R. Fugl-Meyer, *Scand. J. Rehab. Med., 14*:141–143 (1982).

21. J. Grafman, A. Salazar, and H. Weingartner, *J. Neurosci., 6*:301–307 (1986).

22. S.L. Wolf, D.E. Lecraw, L.A. Barton, and B.B. Jann, *Exp. Neurol., 104*:125–132 (1989).

23. C.G. Ostendorf, and S.L. Wolf, *Phys. Ther., 61*:1022–1028 (1981).

24. S. Finklestein, L. Benowitz, R. Baldessarini, et al., *Ann. Neurol., 12*:463–467 (1982).

25. M.J. Reding, L.A. Orto, S.W. Winter, I.M. Fortuna, P. Di Ponte, and F.H. McDowell, *Arch. Neurol., 43*:763–765 (1986).

26. S. Shah, F. Vanclay, and B. Cooper, *Stroke, 20*:766–769 (1989).

27. E. Irle, *Brain Res. Rev., 12*:307–320 (1987).

28. E. Irle, *Brain Res. Rev., 15*:181–213 (1990).

29. R. Katzman, R. Clasen, I. Klatzo, J.S. Meyer, H.M. Pappius, and A.G. Waltz, *Stroke, 8*:512–540 (1977).

30. C. von Monakow, *Die Lokalisation im Grosshirn und der Abbau der Funktion Durch Kortikale Herde*. J.F. Bergmann, Wiesbaden (1914).
31. D.M. Feeney, and J.-C. Baron, *Stroke*, *17*:817–830 (1986).
32. G.L. Lenzi, R.S.J. Frackowiak, and T. Jones, *J. Cereb. Blood Flow Metab.*, *2*: 321 (1982).
33. W.R.W. Martin, and M.E. Raichle, *Ann. Neurol.*, *14*:168–176 (1983).
34. M. Fiorelli, J. Blin, S. Bakchine, D. Laplane, and J.C. Baron, *J. Neurol. Sci.*, *104*:135–142 (1991).
35. M.I. Botez, J. Leveille, R. Lambert, and T. Boetz, *Eur. Neurol.*, *31*:405–412 (1991).
36. S. Pappata, B. Mazoyer, T. Dinh, H. Cambon, M. Levasseur, and J.C. Baron, *Stroke*, *21*:519–524 (1990).
37. Y. Castella, W.D. Dietrich, B.D. Watson, and R. Busto, *J. Cereb. Blood Flow Metab.*, *9*:329–341 (1989).
38. R. Slater, M. Reivich, H. Goldberg, R. Banka, and J. Greenberg, *Stroke*, *8*: 684–690 (1977).
39. I. Creese, D. Burt, and S. Snyder, *Science*, *197*:596–598 (1977).
40. K.S. Lashley, *Brain Mechanisms and Intelligence*. University of Chicago Press, Chicago (1929).
41. A.R. Luria, *Restoration of Function after Brain Injury*. MacMillan, New York (1963).
42. A.R. Luria, *Higher Cortical Functions in Man*. Basic Books, New York (1966).
43. P.D. Wall, *Recovery of Function: Theoretical Considerations for Brain Injury Rehabilitation* (P. Bach-y-Rita, ed.), University Park Press, Baltimore, pp. 91–105 (1978).
44. F. Chollet, V. DiPiero, R.J.S. Wise, D.J. Brooks, R.J. Dolan, and R.S.J. Frackowiak, *Ann. Neurol.*, *29*:63–71 (1991).
45. J.M. Held, J. Gordon, and A.M. Gentile, *Behav. Neurosci.*, *99*:678–690 (1985).
46. L.B. Goldstein, and J.N. Davis, *J. Neurosci. Methods*, *31*:101–107 (1990).
47. J. Stephens, *Soc. Neurosci. Abstr.*, *12*:1285 (1986).
48. J. Stephens, *Phys. Ther.*, *66*:781–780 (1986).
49. D.M. Feeney, A. Gonzalez, and W.A. Law, *Science*, *217*:855–857 (1982).
50. D.M. Feeney, and D.A. Hovda, *Brain Res.*, *342*:352–356 (1985).
51. D.A. Hovda, and D.M. Feeney, *Brain Res.*, *298*:358–361 (1984).
52. L.B. Goldstein, and J.N. Davis, *Restor. Neurol. Neurosci.*, *1*:311–314 (1990).
53. T.V.P. Bliss, and A.C. Dolphin, *T.I.N.S.*, *5*:289–290 (1982).
54. T.V.P. Bliss, and T. Lomo, *J. Physiol.*, *232*:331–356 (1973).
55. T.V.P. Bliss, and A.R. Gardner-Medwin, *J. Physiol.*, *232*:357–374 (1973).
56. G.L. Collingridge, and T.V.P. Bliss, *T.I.N.S.*, *10*:288–293 (1987).
57. D. Corbett, *Brain Res. Bull.*, *5*:637–642 (1980).
58. A. Artola, and W. Singer, *The NMDA Receptor* (G.L. Collingridge and J.C. Watkins, eds.), Oxford University Press, Oxford, pp. 153–166 (1989).
59. V.A. Aroniadou, and T.J. Teyler, *Brain Res.*, *562*:136–143 (1991).
60. A. Keller, A. Iriki, and H. Asanuma, *J. Comp. Neurol.*, *300*:47–60 (1990).

61. L.W. Swanson, T.J. Teyler, and R.F. Thompson, *Neurosci. Res. Prog. Bull.*, *20*: 601–769 (1982).

62. G.L. Wenk, C.M. Grey, D.K. Ingram, E.L. Spangler, and D.S. Olton, *Behav. Neurosci.*, *103*:688–690 (1989).

63. M.J. Benvenga, and T.C. Spaulding, *Pharmacol. Biochem. Behav.*, *30*:205–207 (1989).

64. G.E. Handelmann, P.C. Contreras, and T.L. O'Donohue, *Eur. J. Pharmacol.*, *140*:69–73 (1987).

65. R.G.M. Morris, E. Anderson, G.S. Lynch, and M. Baudry, *Nature*, *319*:774–776 (1986).

66. P.K. Stanton, and J.M. Sarvey, *Brain Res.*, *361*:276–283 (1985).

67. D. Dahl, and J.M. Sarvey, *Proc. Natl. Acad. Sci. USA*, *86*:4776–4780 (1989).

68. W.F. Hopkins, and D. Johnston, *Science*, *226*:350–352 (1984).

69. H. Wigstrom, and B. Gustafsson, *Acta Physiol. Scand.*, *125*:159–172 (1985).

70. R.M. Douglas, G.V. Goddard, and M. Riives, *Brain Res.*, *240*:259–272 (1982).

71. R.M. Douglas, B.L. McNaughton, and G.V. Goddard, *J. Comp. Neurol.*, *219*: 285–294 (1983).

72. H.R. Olpe, and G. Karlsson, *Naunyn Schmiedebergs Arch. Pharmacol.*, *342*: 194–197 (1990).

73. T. Ito, Y. Miura, and T. Kadokawa, *Can. J. Physiol. Pharmacol.*, *66*:1010–1016 (1988).

74. S. Williams, and D. Johnston, *Science*, *242*:84–87 (1988).

75. J.N. Davis, *NIH Central Nervous System Trauma Status Report—1985*. (D.P. Becker and J.T. Povlishock, eds.), National Institutes of Health, Bethesda, pp. 491–501 (1985).

76. C.W. Cotman, M. Nieto-Sampedro, and E.W. Harris, *Physiol. Rev.*, *61*:684–784 (1981).

77. R.D. Lund, *Development and Plasticity of the Brain*. Oxford University Press, New York (1978).

78. D.R. Bernstein, and D.J. Stelzner, *J. Comp. Neurol.*, *221*:382–400 (1983).

79. A.P. Foerster, *J. Comp. Neurol.*, *210*:335–356 (1982).

80. G.E. Schneider, and S.R. Jhaveri, *Plasticity and Recovery of Function in the Central Nervous System*. Academic Press, New York, pp. 65–109 (1974).

81. J.H. Haring, G.D. Miller, and J.N. Davis, *Brain Res.*, *368*:233–238 (1986).

82. J.H. Haring, and J.N. Davis, *Brain Res.*, *360*:384–388 (1985).

83. F.H. Gage, A. Bjorklund, U. Stenevi, and S.B. Dunnett, *Brain Res.*, *268*:39–47 (1983).

84. F.H. Gage, A. Bjorklund, and U. Stenevi, *Brain Res.*, *268*:27–37 (1983).

85. V.M. Pickel, H. Krebs, and F.E. Bloom, *Brain Res.*, *59*:169–179 (1973).

86. F.H. Gage, A. Bjorklund, and U. Stenevi, *Nature*, *819*:819–821 (1983).

87. O. Steward, C.W. Cotman, and G.S. Lynch, *Exp. Brain Res.*, *18*:396–414 (1973).

88. N. Tsukahara, H. Hultborn, F. Murakami, and Y. Fujito, *J. Neurophysiol.*, *38*: 1359–1372 (1975).

89. K.A. Crutcher, *Brain Res. Rev.*, *12*:203–233 (1987).
90. L.E. Harrell, T.S. Barlow, and J.N. Davis, *Exp. Neurol.*, *82*:379–390 (1983).
91. L.E. Harrell, and D.S. Parsons, *Brain Res.*, *474*:353–358 (1988).
92. R.S. Zucker, *Annu. Rev. Neurosci.*, *12*:13–31 (1989).
93. Y. Geinisman, F. Morrell, and L. De Toledo-Morrell, *Brain Res.*, *480*:326–329 (1989).
94. C.H. Bailey, and M. Chen, *J. Neurobiol.*, *20*:356–372 (1989).
95. R.N. Walsh, *Int. J. Neurosci.*, *12*:33–51 (1981).
96. F.-L.F. Chang, and W.T. Greenough, *Brain Res.*, *309*:35–46 (1984).
97. N.L. Desmond, and W.B. Levy, *Brain Res.*, *265*:21–30 (1983).
98. N.L. Desmond, and W.B. Levy, *Synapse*, 5:139–143 (1990).
99. C. Beaulieu, and M. Colonnier, *J. Comp. Neurol.*, *274*:347–356 (1988).
100. A. Keller, K. Arissian, and H. Asanuma, *Exp. Brain Res.*, *80*:23–33 (1990).
101. U. Ito, K. Ohno, Y. Suganuma, K. Suzuki, and Y. Inaba, *Stroke*, *11*:166–172 (1980).
102. A.M. Bremer, K. Yamada, and C.R. West, *Neurosurgery*, 6:149–154 (1980).
103. R.M. Sapolsky, and W.A. Pulsinelli, *Science*, 229:1397–1399 (1985).
104. B.M. Patten, J. Mendell, B. Bruun, W. Curtin, and S. Carter, *Neurology*, *22*: 377–383 (1972).
105. H.I. Russek, A.S. Russek, and B.L. Zohman, *JAMA*, *159*:102–105 (1955).
106. M.K. Rubenstein, *J. Nerv. Ment. Dis.*, *141*:291–299 (1965).
107. J.W. Norris, and V.C. Hachinski, *Br. Med. J.*, *292*:21–23 (1986).
108. R.B. Bauer, and H. Tellez, *Stroke*, 4:547–555 (1973).
109. N. Poungvarin, W. Bhopat, A. Viriyavejakul, P. Rodprasert, P. Buranasiri, S. Sukondhabhant, M.J. Hensley, and B.L. Strom, *N. Engl. J. Med.*, *316*:1229–1233 (1987).
110. W. Young, J.C. Wojak, and V. DeCrescito, *Stroke*, *19*:1013–1019 (1988).
111. H.M. Maling, and G.H. Acheson, *J. Neurophysiol.*, 9:379–386 (1946).
112. M.B. Macht, *Am. J. Physiol.*, *163*:731–732 (1950).
113. P.M. Meyer, J.A. Horel, and D.R. Meyer, *J. Comp. Physiol. Psychol.*, 56:402–404 (1963).
114. D.M. Feeney, and D.A. Hovda, *Fed. Proc.*, *39*:1095 (1980).
115. D.A. Hovda, R.L. Sutton, and D.M. Feeney, *Behav. Neurosci.*, *103*:574–584 (1989).
116. J.J. Braun, P.M. Meyer, and D.R. Meyer, *J. Comp. Physiol. Psychol.*, *61*:79–82 (1986).
117. F.J.J. Buytendijk, *Arch. Neerl. Physiol. Homme Anim.*, *17*:370–434 (1932).
118. N.R.F. Maier, *J. Comp. Neurol.*, *61*:395–405 (1935).
119. D.M. Feeney, A. Gonzalez, and W.A. Law, *Proc. West. Pharmacol. Soc.*, *24*: 15–17 (1981).
120. R.L. Sutton, D.A. Hovda, and D.M. Feeney, *Behav. Neurosci.*, *103*:837–841 (1989).
121. N. Weiner, *The Pharmacological Basis of Therapeutics* (A.G. Gilman, L.S. Goodman, T.W. Rall, and F. Murad, eds.), Macmillan, New York (1985).
122. R.J. Mathew, and W.H. Wilson, *Psychopharmacology*, *87*:298–302 (1985).

123. L.B. Goldstein, *Stroke*, *21* (Suppl III):139–142 (1990).
124. K. Fuxe, and U. Ungerstedt, *Amphetamines and Related Compounds* (E. Costa and S. Garattini, eds.), Raven Press, New York, pp. 257–288 (1970).
125. M.A. Moskowitz, B.F. Weiss, L.D. Lytle, H.N. Munro, and R.J. Wurtman, *Proc. Natl. Acad. Sci. USA*, *72*:834–836 (1975).
126. D.A. Hovda, and D.M. Feeney, *Proc. West. Pharmacol. Soc.*, *28*:209–211 (1985).
127. S. Brailowsky, and R.T. Knight, *Neurobiol. Aging*, *8*:441–447 (1987).
128. J.N. Davis, C.D. Arnett, E. Hoyler, L.P. Stalvey, J.W. Daly, and P. Skolnick, *Brain Res.*, *159*:125–135 (1978).
129. M.G. Boyeson, and D.M. Feeney, *Pharmacol. Biochem. Behav.*, *35*:497–501 (1990).
130. M.G. Boyeson, K.A. Krobert, and J.M. Hughes, *Soc. Neurosci. Abstr.*, *12*:1120 (1986).
131. R.L. Sutton, and D.M. Feeney, *Soc. Neurosci. Abstr.*, *13*:913 (1987).
132. M.S. Weaver, L.J. Farmer, and D.M. Feeney, *Soc. Neurosci. Abstr.*, *13*:477 (1987).
133. L.B. Goldstein, *Cerebrovascular Diseases. Sixteenth Research (Princeton) Conference*. (M.D. Ginsberg and W.D. Dietrich, eds.), Raven Press, New York, pp. 303–308 (1989).
134. L.B. Goldstein, H.V. Poe, and J.N. Davis, *Ann. Neurol.*, *26*:157 (1989).
135. L.B. Goldstein, and J.N. Davis, *Brain Res.*, *508*:305–309 (1990).
136. J. Stephens, G. Goldberg, and J.T. Demopoulos, *Arch. Phys. Med. Rehab.*, *67*: 666–667 (1986).
137. L.B. Goldstein, A. Coviello, G.D. Miller, and J.N. Davis, *Restor. Neurol. Neurosci.*, *3*:41–47 (1991).
138. M.G. Boyeson, and T.R. Callister, *Soc. Neurosci.*, *16*:778 (1990).
139. D.M. Feeney, and V.S. Westerberg, *Can. J. Psychol.*, *44*:233–252 (1990).
140. B.E. Hurwitz, W.D. Dietrich, P.M. McCabe, B.D. Watson, M.D. Ginsberg, and N. Schneiderman, *Soc. Neurosci. Abstr.*, *14*:1132 (1988).
141. B.E. Hurwitz, W.D. Dietrich, P.M. McCabe, B.D. Watson, M.D. Ginsberg, and N. Schneiderman, *Cerebrovascular Diseases. The Sixteenth Research (Princeton) Conference* (M.D. Ginsberg and W.D. Dietrich, eds.), Raven Press, New York, pp. 309–318 (1989).
142. W.D. Dietrich, O. Alonso, R. Busto, and M.D. Ginsberg, *Stroke*, *21* (Suppl. III):147–150 (1990).
143. D.M. Feeney, R.L. Sutton, M.G. Boyeson, D.A. Hovda, and W.G. Dail, *Physiol. Psychol.*, *13*:197–203 (1985).
144. P.E. Gold, R.L. Delanoy, and J. Merrin, *Brain Res.*, *305*:103–107 (1984).
145. H.J. Altman, and D. Quartermain, *Behav. Brain Res.*, *7*:51–63 (1983).
146. D. Quartermain, and C.Y. Botwinick, *J. Comp. Physiol. Psychol.*, *88*:386–401 (1975).
147. R.R. Dawirs, G. Teuchert-Noodt, and M. Busse, *Neuropharmacology*, *30*:275–282 (1991).
148. S. Brailowsky, R.T. Knight, and K. Blood, *Brain Res.*, *362*:322–330 (1986).
149. T.D. Hernandez, and T. Schallert, *Restor. Neurol. Neurosci.*, *1*:323–330 (1990).
150. S. Brailowsky, R.T. Knight, and R. Efron, *Brain Res.*, *376*:71–77 (1986).

151. A.Y. Chweh, E.A. Swinyard, and H.H. Wolf, *Pharmacol. Biochem. Behav.*, 24: 1301–1304 (1986).
152. T. Schallert, T.D. Hernandez, and T.M. Barth, *Brain Res.*, 379:104–111 (1986).
153. T.D. Hernandez, G.H. Jones, and T. Schallert, *Brain Res.*, 487:89–95 (1989).
154. T.D. Hernandez, T.A. Jones, and T. Schallert, *Soc. Neurosci. Abstr.*, 14:844 (1988).
155. I.P. Riches, and M.W. Brown, *Neurosci. Letts*. S42–S40 (1986).
156. M. Satoh, K. Ishihara, T. Iwama, and H. Takagi, *Neurosci. Letts.*, 68:216–220 (1986).
157. R. Lister, *Neurosci. Biobehav. Rev.*, 9:87–93 (1985).
158. T. Roth, T. Roehrs, R. Wittig, and F. Zorick, *Br. J. Clin. Pharmacol.*, 18 (Suppl.):45S–49S (1984).
159. H. Lal, B. Kumar, and M.J. Forster, *FASEB J.*, 2:2707–2711 (1988).
160. A. Bourdelais, and P.W. Kalivas, *Brain Res.*, 516:132–136 (1990).
161. A.A. Ward, Jr., and M.A. Kennard, *Yale J. Biol. Med.*, 15:189–228 (1942).
162. C.W. Watson, and M.A. Kennard, *J. Neurophysiol.*, 8:221–231 (1945).
163. M. De Ryck, H. Duytschaever, and P.A.J. Janssen, *Stroke*, 21 (Suppl. III):158–163 (1990).
164. D.M. Feeney, and R.L. Sutton, *CRC Crit. Rev. Neurobiol.*, 3:135–197 (1987).
165. E.C. Burgard, and J.M. Sarvey, *Neurosci. Letts.*, 116:34–39 (1990).
166. D.L. Cheney, H.F. LeFevre, and G. Racagni, *Neuropharmacology*, 14:801–809 (1975).
167. M.J. Kuhar, S.F. Atweh, and S.J. Bird, *Cholinergic–Monoaminergic Interaction in the Brain* (L.L. Butcher, ed.), Academic Press, New York, pp. 211 (1978).
168. A. Kochhar, J.A. Zivin, and P.D. Lyden, *Arch. Neurol.*, 45:148–153 (1988).
169. R. Gill, A.C. Foster, and G.N. Woodruff, *Neuroscience*, 25:847–855 (1988).
170. C.K. Park, D.G. Nehls, D.I. Graham, G.M. Teasdale, and J. McCulloch, *Ann. Neurol.*, 24:543–551 (1988).
171. G.K. Steinberg, J. Saleh, and D. Kunis, *Neurosci. Letts.*, 89:193–197 (1988).
172. G.K. Steinberg, J. Saleh, D. Kunis, R. DeLaPaz, and S.R. Zarnegar, *Stroke*, 20: 1247–1252 (1989).
173. G.K. Steinberg, C.P. George, R. De La Paz, D.K. Shibata, and T. Gross, *Stroke*, 19:1112–1118 (1988).
174. D.W. Choi, *Brain Res.*, 403:333–336 (1987).
175. C.A. Boast, S.C. Gerhardt, G. Pastor, J.F. Lehmann, P.E. Etienne, and J.M. Liebman, *Brain Res.*, 442:345–348 (1988).
176. T.M. Barth, M.L. Grant, and T. Schallert, *Stroke*, 21 (Suppl. III):153–157 (1990).
177. V. Heale, and C. Harley, *Pharmacol. Biochem. Behav.*, 36:145–149 (1990).
178. L.B. Goldstein, and A. Coviello, *Brain Res.*, 580:129–136 (1992).
179. S.A. Lipton, *Arch. Neurol.*, 46:1241–1248 (1989).
180. R.J. Mandel, F.H. Gage, and L.J. Thal, *Exp. Neurol.*, 104:208–217 (1989).
181. L.F. Kromer, *Science*, 235:214–216 (1987).
182. A. Carolei, C. Fieschi, R. Bruno, and G. Toffano, *Cerebrovasc. Brain Metab. Rev.*, 3:134–157 (1991).

183. B.A. Sabel, G.L. Dunbar, and D.G. Stein, *J. Neurosci. Res.*, *12*:429–443 (1984).
184. B.A. Sabel, M.D. Slavin, and D.G. Stein, *Science*, *225*:340–342 (1984).
185. A. Ortiz, J.S. MacDonall, C.G. Wakade, and S.E. Karpiak, *Pharmacol. Biochem. Behav.*, *37*:679–684 (1990).
186. N. Tonder, T. Sorensen, J. Zimmer, M.B. Jorgensen, F.F. Johansen, and N.H. Diemer, *Exp. Brain Res.*, *74*:512–526 (1989).
187. R.L. Sutton, D.A. Hovda, and D.M. Feeney, *Brain Dysfunct.*, *2*:201–210 (1989).
188. L.B. Goldstein, and J.N. Davis, *Neurology*, *38*:1806–1809 (1988).
189. L.B. Goldstein, D.B. Matchar, J.C. Morgenlander, and J.N. Davis, *J. Neurol. Rehab.*, *4*:137–144 (1990).
190. A.R. Fugl-Meyer, L. Jaasko, I. Leyman, S. Olsson, and S. Steglind, *Scand. J. Rehab. Med.*, *7*:13–31 (1975).
191. P.W. Duncan, M.A. Propst, and S.G. Nelson, *J. Am. Phys. Ther. Assoc.*, *63*: 1606–1610 (1983).
192. B. Porch, J. Wyckes, and D.M. Feeney, *Soc. Neurosci. Abstr.*, *11*:52 (1985).
193. B.E. Porch, and D.M. Feeney, *Clin. Aphasiol.*, *16*:309–314 (1986).
194. R.W. Evans, C.T. Gualtieri, and D. Patterson, *J. Nerv. Ment. Dis.*, *175*:106–110 (1987).
195. S. Lipper, and M.M. Tuchman, *J. Nerv. Ment. Dis.*, *162*:366–371 (1976).
196. A.N.G. Clark, and G.D. Mankikar, *J. Am. Geriatr. Soc.*, *27*:174–177 (1979).
197. R. Homan, J. Panksepp, J. Mcsweeny, P. Badia, E. Borroughs, L. Chapman, and R. Conner, *Soc. Neurosci.*, *16*:439 (1990).
198. D. Walker-Batson, H. Unwin, S. Curtis, E. Allen, M. Wood, P. Smith, M.D. Devous, S. Reynolds, and R.G. Greenlee, *Restor. Neurol. Neurosci.*, *4*:47–50 (1992).
199. E.A. Crisostomo, P.W. Duncan, M.A. Propst, D.B. Dawson, and J.N. Davis, *Ann. Neurol.*, *23*:94–97 (1988).
200. L.B. Perelman, *Sov. Med.*, 8–9 (1946).
201. T.C.A.M. van Woerkom, J.M. Minderhoud, T. Gottschal, and G. Nicolai, *Eur. Neurol.*, *21*:227–234 (1982).
202. M. Kakihana, N. Fukuda, and M. Suno, *Stroke*, *19*:217–222 (1988).
203. Y. Tazaki, F. Sakai, and E. Otomo, *Stroke*, *19*:211–216 (1988).
204. F.H. Geisler, F.C. Dorsey, and W.P. Coleman, *N. Engl. J. Med.*, *324*:1829–1838 (1991).
205. L. Battistin, A. Cesari, F. Galligioni, G. Marin, M. Massarotti, D. Paccagnella, A. Pellegrini, G. Testa, and P. Tonin, *Eur. Neurol.*, *24*:343–351 (1985).
206. S. Bassi, M.G. Albizzati, M. Sbacchi, L. Frattola, and M. Massarotti, *J. Neurosci. Res.*, *12*:493–498 (1984).
207. C. Argentino, M.L. Sacchetti, D. Toni, G. Savoini, E. D'Arcangelo, F. Erminio, F. Federico, F.F. Milone, V. Gallai, D. Gambi, A. Mamoli, G.A. Ottonello, O. Ponari, G. Rebucci, U. Senin, and C. Fieschi, *Stroke*, *20*:1143–1149 (1989).
208. B.I. Hoffbrand, P.J. Bingley, S.M. Oppenheimer, and C.D. Sheldon, *J. Neurol. Neurosurg. Psychiatry*, *51*:1213–1214 (1988).
209. L.B. Goldstein, and J.N. Davis, *Stroke*, *21*:1636–1640 (1990).
210. L.B. Goldstein, *J. Neurol. Rehab.*, *5*:129–140 (1991).

IV

SPECIAL MEDICAL PROBLEMS

16

Bladder Dysfunction

David A. Gelber

Southern Illinois University School of Medicine and Memorial Medical Center
Springfield, Illinois

Bladder dysfunction occurs in a variety of neurological diseases, resulting clinically in incontinence or urinary retention. Serious medical complications may ensue, including urinary tract infections, skin breakdown, injury to the upper urinary tract, and development of renal or bladder calculi. In addition, bladder dysfunction may have serious psychological and social consequences. Urinary incontinence often results in social embarrassment and a feeling of lost autonomy. The need to address excessive time to one's bodily functions is demoralizing to many patients. Furthermore, the need to learn compensatory techniques, such as self-catheterization, is burdensome to patients and caregivers. From a rehabilitation standpoint, bladder dysfunction may be a major factor in determining whether a patient will return home or require placement in a skilled care facility.

The following is a review of bladder dysfunction as it affects the rehabilitation of patients with neurological diseases. The anatomy and physiology of normal micturition will be outlined and abnormalities in voiding resulting from specific neurological conditions discussed. The evaluation of bladder dysfunction will be reviewed briefly. Treatment strategies will then be discussed in detail.

ANATOMY

Upper and Lower Urinary Tract

The urinary system can be classified anatomically into the upper urinary tract, lower urinary tract, and nervous system pathways (both peripheral and central) that control micturition. If any component of the urinary system is injured, bladder dysfunction may result.

The upper urinary tract is comprised of the kidneys and ureters. These are not primarily affected by diseases of the nervous system and will not be discussed further in this chapter.

The bladder is comprised primarily of the detrusor muscle and posteriorly situated trigonal region where the ureters enter the bladder [1]. Both of these structures are composed of intertwined smooth muscle bundles. Distally the bladder tapers into the bladder neck, which empties into the urethra [2].

The urethra is comprised of two muscular layers. The inner and outer layers are directly continuous with the inner and outer muscular layers of the detrusor [2]. In males the prostate lies between these two muscular layers in the proximal urethra [3]. The inner urethral muscle layer is surrounded in its proximal half by the outer smooth muscle layer extending from the bladder neck to the urogenital diaphragm [4]. This outer smooth muscle layer, which encircles the proximal urethra ventrally, comprises the internal urinary sphincter and allows for closure at the bladder neck and proximal urethra. The internal sphincter is under involuntary control mediated by the sympathetic nervous system [5]. The external urinary sphincter, on the other hand, is comprised of striated muscle and has two separate components. The first component is the urogenital diaphragm (pelvic floor musculature), which surrounds the urethra as a "pelvic sling" [6]. This component is under voluntary control and is innervated by the somatic nervous system [7]. The second component is intrinsic urethral striated muscle that surrounds the distal urethra [4,6]. This portion is also referred to as the intrinsic external sphincter and, in contrast to the pelvic floor muscles, receives innervation from the somatic, parasympathetic, and sympathetic nervous system (triple control) [8] (Figures 1 and 2).

During normal micturition, the detrusor muscle contracts and the internal and external urinary sphincters relax in a coordinated fashion. At rest the bladder wall is relaxed and the sphincters are tonically contracted to maintain continence.

Nervous System Control of Micturition

Bladder emptying is facilitated primarily by the parasympathetic nervous system. Parasympathetic neuronal cell bodies are located in the intermediolateral cell column in the sacral spinal cord, levels S2–4 [9]. Motor nerves exit

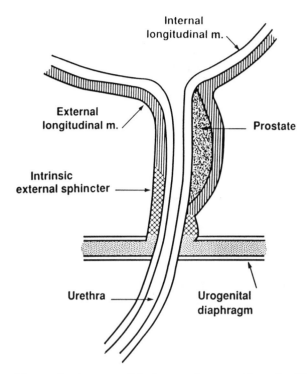

Figure 1 Anatomy of the lower urinary tract in males. The inner and outer smooth muscle layers of the bladder wall are continuous with the inner and outer muscular layers of the proximal urethra. The prostate lies between these smooth muscle layers. The external sphincter is composed of striated muscle reflected down from the pelvic floor muscles (urogenital diaphragm), and intrinsic striated muscle surrounding the distal urethra (intrinsic external sphincter) (from ref. [3]).

via the ventral roots, course in the pelvic nerves, and synapse in ganglia located in and just outside the bladder wall [10]. Postganglionic fibers end primarily in the detrusor muscle; however, there is parasympathetic innervation as well, of the proximal urethra and external sphincter [8]. Parasympathetic afferents, responsible for the sensation of bladder filling, course back to the sacral spinal cord with the pelvic nerves [10]. Activation of the parasympathetic system causes the detrusor muscle to contract and the bladder to empty.

Continence is maintained, in part, by the sympathetic nervous system. Although it has been classically taught that sympathetic neurons involved in micturition arise in the intermediolateral cell column at levels T11–L2 [10], one recent study could not precisely determine the spinal levels of origin [11]. Sympathetic preganglionic fibers synapse in the paravertebral ganglia; post-

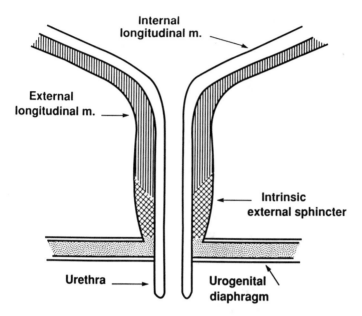

Figure 2   Anatomy of the lower urinary tract in females (from ref. [3]).

ganglionic fibers course with the hypogastric nerves and terminate on receptors in the detrusor muscle, bladder neck, and urethra [7]. In addition, sympathetic fibers also synapse on parasympathetic ganglia [10]. The sympathetic system has reciprocal function to the parasympathetic system. Activation causes relaxation of the detrusor muscle, mediated by beta-adrenergic receptors, and contraction of the bladder neck and proximal urethra (internal sphincter), mediated by the alpha-adrenergic receptors [12]. In addition, sympathetic fibers inhibit parasympathetic outflow at the parasympathetic ganglia level through presynaptic inhibition [13]. Overall, activation of the sympathetic system results in urine storage and continence (Figure 3).

The somatic nervous system is also responsible for maintaining continence through its innervation of the external urinary sphincter. The somatic (pudendal) nucleus is located in the ventral gray matter of the sacral spinal cord, levels S2–S4, and extends one segment rostral to the pelvic nucleus [7,14]. Efferents course along the wall of the pelvis in the pudendal nerve to innervate the pelvic floor musculature and striated intrinsic external sphincter. As noted above, this system is under voluntary control, in contrast to the parasympathetic and sympathetic system. Activation of the pudendal nucleus results in contraction of the pelvic floor muscles and external sphincter, which also helps to maintain continence.

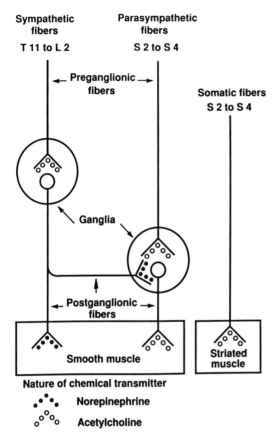

Figure 3 Neuropharmacological innervation of the bladder, urethral smooth muscle, and striated external sphincter. Parasympathetic pre- and postganglionic neurons and sympathetic preganglionic neurons are cholinergic; sympathetic postganglionic neurons are adrenergic. In addition to innervation of the bladder and proximal urethra, sympathetic postganglionic fibers also synapse on parasympathetic ganglionic cells, allowing for sympathetic inhibition of parasympathetic activity (from ref. [96]).

Thus, during micturition, the parasympathetic system is activated and sympathetic and somatic system inhibited to facilitate bladder emptying; the detrusor muscle contracts and the bladder neck, proximal urethra, and striated external sphincter relax. This is mediated via the caudal spinal cord reflex loops described above. Intersegmental reflexes are also involved to further modulate this system [10]. Other neurotransmitters, such as vasoactive intestinal peptide (VIP), leu-enkephalin, neuropeptide Y, substance P, somatostatin, calcitonin gene-related peptide (CGRP), ATP, and histamine, may also be involved as neuromodulators of the neuromicturition pathways [15–23].

The bladder and sphincter centers in the caudal spinal cord appear to be coordinated through descending neural pathways arising from a pontine micturition center [24–26]. Although this center has not been definitively

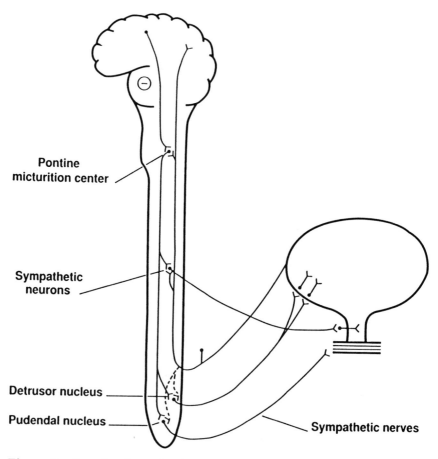

Figure 4 Central and peripheral nervous system pathways affecting micturition. The pontine micturition center coordinates bladder and sphincter activity through descending tracts projecting to the caudal spinal cord. Parasympathetic outflow from the detrusor nucleus in the sacral spinal cord is directed predominantly to the bladder wall. Sympathetic outflow from the thoracolumbar cord projects primarily to the bladder neck and proximal urethra (internal sphincter). Somatic outflow from the pudendal nucleus in the sacral spinal cord projects to the external striated sphincter (from ref. [52]).

identified in humans [27], animal studies have localized a micturition center to the nucleus lateralis dorsalis, in the pontine reticular formation rostral to the locus ceruleus [28]. Efferent fibers from this pontine micturition center course through the reticulospinal tracts to terminate on the pelvic and pudendal nuclei in the sacral spinal cord. Afferent proprioceptive input from the bladder and sphincters ascends in the cord in the posterior columns to terminate in the pontine micturition center, thus completing another reflex loop [7] (Figure 4).

In addition to afferent input from the caudal spinal cord, the pontine micturition (coordinating) center receives facilatory and inhibitory input from various cortical and subcortical structure which, in part, allows for conscious control over micturition. In animal studies, the red nucleus, midbrain tegmentum, ventrolateral nucleus of the thalamus, substantia nigra, subthalamus, pallidum, cortical regions including supermedial frontal lobe, anterior cingulate gyrus, and genu of the corpus callosum, and the fastigial nucleus of the cerebellum have been shown to inhibit micturition [7,29,30]. Stimulation of the medulla, mesencephalon, rostral hypothalamus, and septum, on the other hand, have been shown to facilitate micturition through connections to the pontine micturition center [7,31].

Summary

In summary, micturition results from reflex activity arising in the caudal spinal cord. Parasympathetic activity results in detrusor muscle contraction and subsequent bladder emptying. Conversely, the sympathetic system is responsible for maintaining continence through relaxation of the bladder wall and tonic contraction of the bladder neck and proximal urethra (internal sphincter). The somatic nervous system, under voluntary control, is also responsible for maintaining continence, through activation of the striated external sphincter. The pontine micturition center, through a reflex loop with the caudal spinal cord, acts to coordinate bladder and sphincter function. This center, in turn, is modulated by various cortical and subcortical pathways that allow for conscious control of micturition.

EVALUATION OF BLADDER DYSFUNCTION

The evaluation of bladder dysfunction should begin with a detailed history. Specific information regarding past history of childhood enuresis, genitourinary surgery, renal or bladder stones, urinary tract infections, or history of sexual dysfunction should be sought. Present history, including onset and duration of specific urological symptoms (incontinence, urinary retention, frequency, urgency, nocturia, hesitancy) should also be obtained.

Physical examination should include a thorough genitourinary and neurological examination. The integrity of the sacral micturition arc can be assessed indirectly by eliciting several cutaneous reflexes. The bulbocavernosus reflex, elicited by squeezing the glans penis or clitoris results in contraction of the external anal sphincter. The anal wink is a reflex contraction of the external anal sphincter elicited by stimulation of the perianal skin, usually with a pin. Both of these cutaneous reflexes are mediated by spinal cord segments S2–S4 and are lost with lesions affecting the sacral spinal cord or roots [32].

Laboratory studies, including measurement of blood urea nitrogen (BUN), creatinine, and urinalysis should be performed on all patients as part of a urological work-up. If further evaluation of the upper urinary tract (kidneys, ureters) is indicated, measurement of creatinine clearance or performance of an intravenous pyelogram may be necessary.

Evaluation should also include measurement of postvoid residual urine volumes (PVR), usually obtained by intermittent straight catheterization after voluntary voiding. A PVR greater than 50 ml is considered abnormal [33], indicative of impaired bladder emptying. PVR can also be measured by ultrasound technique. This method has the advantage of being noninvasive, but does require the use of a portable ultrasound unit. Ultrasound is relatively accurate in the measurement of PVR when performed by trained personnel [34–36].

The most definitive diagnostic procedure for evaluation of bladder dysfunction is a urodynamic study [37]. This consists of a cystometrogram (CMG), and external sphincter electromyogram (EMG), and often includes measurement of a urethral pressure profile (UPP), and uroflowmetry [33,38,39].

A cystometrogram graphs bladder pressure versus volume in response to bladder filling with either fluid (usually isotonic saline) or gas (carbon dioxide), instilled via a catheter directly into the bladder [36,40]. Pressures are measured by transducers located in the bladder and urethra [37]. The bladder volume at which the patient first senses filling is noted. Bladder capacity, defined as the volume at which the patient notes the urge or desire to void, or when strong uninhibited detrusor contractions are noted on the cystometrogram, is also recorded [38].

The bladder/volume pressure ratio gives a measure of bladder compliance (tone) [36,41]. A normally compliant bladder shows little change in bladder pressure with filling, due to the elastic properties of the bladder wall. A hypocompliant bladder, due to bladder wall fibrosis or scarring, generates a more rapid rise in bladder pressure at low volumes. A hypercompliant bladder, usually due to chronic overstretching of the bladder wall, shows extremely low pressures at high bladder volumes.

At the conclusion of the urodynamic study, as the catheter is being withdrawn, measurements of urethral pressure along varying points of the urethra can be obtained (urethral pressure profile) [33,38]. After the catheter is removed entirely, the patient can empty the bladder into a uroflowmeter to give a measure of urine flow rate [36]. Urine flow rate can be slowed by bladder outlet obstruction or a poorly contracting bladder.

External urethral sphincter activity is measured throughout the cystometrogram [37]. Normally the external sphincter and pelvic floor musculature is contracting during bladder filling but relaxes at the onset of a detrusor contraction in a coordinated fashion. The sphincter should remain relaxed throughout the duration of the bladder contraction [42]. Sphincter function can be measured in several ways. Direct needle electromyography of the periurethral striated muscle is preferred; however, the electrodes may be difficult to place, especially in young children [42]. Alternatives include placement of perineal surface electrodes or needle electrodes into pelvic floor muscles, or placement of needle electrodes into the external anal sphincter. Recently, an anal plug electrode has been developed. Although some have questioned the reliability of recording anal sphincter activity as a measure of urethral sphincter activity [43], recent studies have found an excellent correlation between the two [44]. In most cases, measurement of anal sphincter activity is as useful as direct placement of urethral sphincter electrodes.

PHYSIOLOGY OF MICTURITION

Normal Micturition

Normal individuals will tolerate bladder filling to approximately 400–500 ml (bladder capacity). At approximately 25% of bladder capacity (125–200 ml), one first senses bladder filling [45]. Sensation of bladder filling is mediated by bladder sensory afferents that return to the sacral cord and subsequently travel to the sensory cortex via the posterior columns [46]. If it is not a socially appropriate time to void, micturition can be consciously inhibited via descending cortical inhibitory influences on the pontine micturition center. Inhibition of the pontine micturition center results in decreased parasympathetic and increased sympathetic and somatic outflow from the caudal spinal cord. This causes detrusor relaxation, increased bladder neck and proximal urethral tone, and increased activity of the external striated sphincter, all of which serve to maintain continence.

When the bladder fills to capacity, one senses bladder fullness and the urgency to void. If it is an appropriate time to void, cortical inhibition of the pontine micturition center is removed, resulting in increased parasympathetic activity and decreased sympathetic and somatic activity. This results in detrusor contraction with coordinated relaxation of the urinary sphincters.

The urodynamic study can be organized into filling and voiding stages.

During filling there should be only minimal rise in detrusor pressure due to the elastic properties of the bladder wall (normal bladder tone or compliance). During voiding, bladder pressures typically rise to 40–80 cm H_2O, with urine flow rates of 20–25 ml/sec [45]. Urethral sphincter activity, as measured by sphincter EMG, is present during bladder filling, but ceases at the onset of voiding (Figure 5).

Bladder Dysfunction Based on Lesion Location

Bladder dysfunction can result from a lesion anywhere along the neuraxis interrupting the reflex pathways described previously (Table 1). Lesions rostral to the pontine micturition center (e.g., due to stroke, tumor, Parkinson's disease or cerebral palsy) characteristically cause detrusor hyperreflexia with sphincters that relax in a coordinated fashion during voiding [47–51].

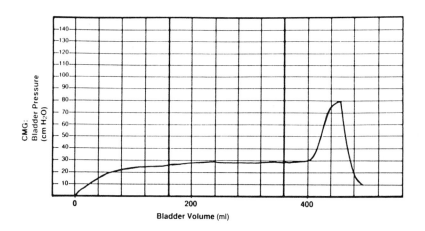

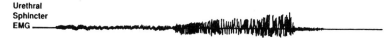

Figure 5 Appearance of a normal urodynamic study. The cystometrogram (CMG) is displayed on upper panel, and simultaneous urethral sphincter EMG on lower panel. One normally senses bladder filling at approximately 200 ml volume. At this point the external urethral sphincter is activated to help maintain continence. When voiding is consciously initiated at bladder capacity (400–500 ml), the bladder contracts, generating intravesical pressures of 40–80 cm H_2O, and the external sphincter relaxes in a coordinated fashion to allow for complete bladder emptying (courtesy J. Texter, M.D., SIU School of Medicine, Springfield, IL).

Table 1   Bladder Dysfunction Based on Lesion Location

Lesion Location	Urodynamic Study Pattern
Rostral to pons	Detrusor hyperreflexia with coordinated sphincters
Between pons and sacral spinal cord	Detrusor hyperreflexia with sphincter dyssynergia
Sacral spinal cord	Detrusor and sphincter areflexia
	Detrusor areflexia with normal sphincter function
	Normal detrusor function with areflexic sphincter
Cauda equina or peripheral nerves	Detrusor and sphincter areflexia

Patients are usually unable to inhibit micturition consciously, resulting in urge incontinence [52]. Urodynamic studies demonstrate uninhibited bladder contractions greater than 15 cm H_2O occurring during the bladder filling stage [26]. Bladder capacity may be significantly reduced. Because the urethral sphincters do relax appropriately during a detrusor contraction, bladder emptying is usually complete (Figure 6).

Lesions located between the pontine micturition center and caudal spinal cord, most commonly due to traumatic spinal cord injury, multiple sclerosis, or transverse myelitis, result in an overactive bladder with uncoordinated sphincters (detrusor hyperreflexia with sphincter dyssynergia) [52–54]. During voiding, the bladder contracts against a closed sphincter; this results clinically in urinary retention and, if untreated, can eventually cause damage to the upper urinary tract. Urodynamic studies show a significantly reduced bladder capacity with the detrusor contracting vigorously at low bladder volumes. Extremely high intravesical pressure is generated, often higher than 100 cm H_2O. Sphincter EMG shows the urethral sphincter reflexively contracting during detrusor contraction [26] (Figure 7).

Lesions affecting the peripheral nerves, cauda equina, or conus medullaris, secondary to sacral spinal cord trauma, spinal cord tumors, multiple sclerosis, myelomeningocele, spinal stenosis, or diabetic neuropathy [55–59], typically result in both an underactive bladder and sphincters. This leads to urinary retention and overflow incontinence. Urodynamic studies show a significantly increased bladder capacity. Sensory awareness of bladder filling is usually diminished [45]. By definition, if minimal, nonsustained bladder contractions are present on cystometrogram, it is termed "bladder hyporeflexia." If no bladder contractions occur with filling to bladder capacity, it is termed "bladder areflexia" [60] (Figure 8). Occasionally conus medullaris lesions can result in detrusor areflexia with normal sphincter

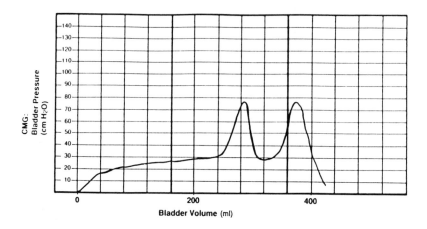

Figure 6   Urodynamic study characteristic of detrusor hyperreflexia with coordinated sphincters. As the bladder fills to approximately 200 ml, the patient senses the urge to void and is able to activate the external sphincter to maintain continence. Voiding does occur prematurely, however, at low bladder volumes because the patient is not able to continue to inhibit micturition consciously. Because the bladder and sphincter activity is coordinated, bladder pressures are usually normal and bladder emptying complete. In this figure, two uninhibited bladder contractions during filling are shown (courtesy J. Texter, M.D., SIU School of Medicine, Springfield, IL).

activity if the pudendal nucleus is spared, or normal detrusor function with an areflexic sphincter if the pelvic nucleus is spared [52].

CLASSIFICATION OF BLADDER DYSFUNCTION

Over the years, various systems to classify bladder dysfunction have been developed [52,61–63]. Because of different terminology used, this has caused confusion, particularly in the urologic literature. None of the classification schemes is perfect for all types of bladder dysfunction. Some systems are more appropriate for bladder dysfunction caused by neurological diseases, others for primary urological diseases. Several schemes are anatomically based, with bladder dysfunction classified on the basis of neurological lesion location [64–66]. Others are more functionally oriented, with urological dysfunction classified on the basis of a problem with urine storage or bladder

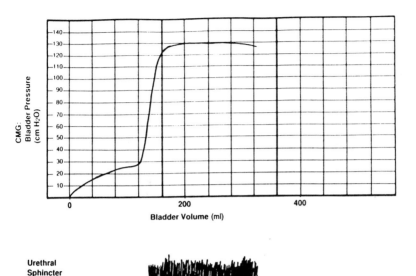

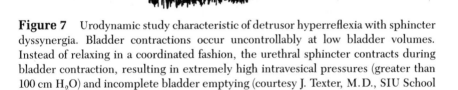

Figure 7 Urodynamic study characteristic of detrusor hyperreflexia with sphincter dyssynergia. Bladder contractions occur uncontrollably at low bladder volumes. Instead of relaxing in a coordinated fashion, the urethral sphincter contracts during bladder contraction, resulting in extremely high intravesical pressures (greater than 100 cm H_2O) and incomplete bladder emptying (courtesy J. Texter, M.D., SIU School of Medicine, Springfield, IL).

emptying [67]. Other systems are based primarily on the results of urodynamic studies [52,68].

To help standardize terminology, the International Continence Society developed a new classification system in 1981 [60]. This system classifies both detrusor and urethral function as normal, overactive, or underactive, on the basis of urodynamic study results. Detrusor function is considered "normal" if there is no significant rise in bladder pressure during filling, if there are no involuntary detrusor contractions during filling, and if normal voiding can be voluntarily initiated, sustained, and suppressed. A normal detrusor may also be referred to as "stable." Detrusor function is considered "overactive" if there are involuntary detrusor contractions during filling that cannot be voluntarily suppressed. If there is no apparent neurological cause for this, it is termed an "unstable detrusor." If there is an attributable neurological lesion present, this condition is called "detrusor hyperreflexia" [60]. It is recommended that one avoid use of the terms hypertonic, upper motor neuron,

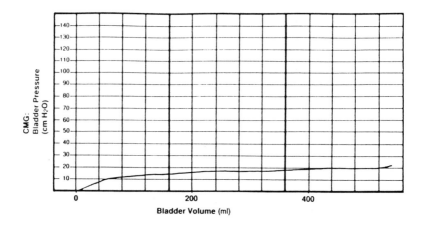

Figure 8 Urodynamic study characteristic of detrusor and urethral sphincter areflexia. Minimal or no bladder contractions are generated, even with bladder filling to high bladder volumes (greater than 500 ml). There is minimal urethral sphincter activity during bladder filling (courtesy J. Texter, M.D., SIU School of Medicine, Springfield, IL).

reflex, spastic, and uninhibited bladder, all of which have been used previously to describe an overactive bladder [50,52]. The detrusor is defined as "underactive" if there are no contractions during filling, and an absent or poorly sustained contraction occurs during voluntary attempts to void. If there is an apparent neurological lesion responsible, this disorder is termed "detrusor areflexia" [60]. Previous terminology including atonic, hypotonic, autonomic, and flaccid bladder should also be avoided.

Urethral closure is also defined as normal, overactive, or incompetent [60]. If urethral closure is "normal," there is positive urethral closure pressure during filling and a decrease in urethral pressure during micturition to allow for unobstructed flow. This can be voluntarily controlled. Urethral closure is defined as "overactive" if the urethra fails to relax or contracts involuntarily during a detrusor contraction. This can also be referred to as "detrusor–urethral" or "detrusor–sphincter dyssynergia," depending on whether the bladder neck or external striated sphincter is involved. If the urethral closure mechanism is "incompetent," there may be leakage of urine between voiding.

BLADDER DYSFUNCTION ASSOCIATED WITH NEUROLOGICAL DISEASES

Introduction

Urinary incontinence and urinary retention may occur as a result of various neurological diseases. The following is a review of bladder dysfunction associated with several of the more common chronic neurological conditions: stroke, Parkinson's disease, multiple sclerosis, and spinal cord injury.

Stroke

Urinary incontinence is a common stroke sequela, with incidence ranging from 38 to 60%, depending on the series [48,69–71]. Incontinence may result directly from injury to the micturition neural pathways causing detrusor hyperreflexia, or may be due to stroke-related physical or mental impairments.

Several studies have attempted to correlate the location of the stroke with the development of bladder dysfunction. Khan et al. performed urodynamic studies on incontinent patients following stroke. Injury to the basal ganglia or frontoparietal cortex was associated with detrusor hyperreflexia with coordinated sphincter activity [72]. Tsuchida et al. found detrusor hyperreflexia in patients with stroke involving the frontal lobe, internal capsule, and putamen. Patients retained voluntary sphincter control following putaminal stroke but not in cases of stroke involving the frontal cortex or internal capsule [73]. A subsequent study by Khan evaluated 33 patients with bladder dysfunction following stroke. 26 of whom had detrusor hyperreflexia, which correlated with lesions involving the cerebral cortex or the internal capsule [47].

Although these studies suggested that detrusor hyperreflexia results from injury to frontoparietal cortex, internal capsule, or basal ganglia, more recent prospective studies have not been able to correlate side of stroke, stroke side, or location of infarct with the development of poststroke incontinence [48,70,71]. Therefore, the precise nature of the various cortical and subcortical influences on micturition remains speculative at this time.

Studies of poststroke bladder dysfunction have also shown an association between the development of incontinence and the presence of certain neurological deficits including moderate or severe motor deficits [69], mental status deficits [69], the combination of hemiplegia, proprioceptive deficits, and visual neglect [48], and aphasia [48,69,71]. This suggests that in some individuals incontinence does not result from lesions of the micturition pathways but is due indirectly to their deficits. In a prospective study of bladder dysfunction following acute stroke, Gelber and Good found that a majority of aphasic patients with stroke actually had a normal urodynamic study [71]. In these patients incontinence was considered to be secondary to their inability to communicate the need to void.

Poststroke urinary incontinence improves with time, even without treatment. In a prospective study by Borrie et al., 151 patients with stroke were evaluated for 1 year. Of these, 60% were incontinent at 1 week post-stroke, 42% at 4 weeks, and 29% at 12 weeks. Of patients with mild incontinence at 4–6 weeks, 67% eventually regained continence without treatment while only 18% of patients with moderate or severe incontinence did [69].

Impaired bladder emptying may also develop after a stroke. Garrett et al. found that 56% of patients admitted to a rehabilitation unit after stroke had elevated post void residuals [74]. Impaired bladder emptying persisted in 33% and was associated with a higher incidence of urinary tract infection. No definitive correlation could be made between the size or location of the stroke and development of urinary retention. The cause of impaired bladder emptying after stroke remains uncertain; urodynamic studies were not performed on patients in Garrett's series.

Parkinson's Disease

Bladder dysfunction develops in 37–71% of patients with Parkinson's disease [75,76]. This is not an unexpected finding, since the basal ganglia is thought to modulate micturition pathways, as discussed earlier. This notion is supported further by studies evaluating the results of stereotactic thalamotomy on patients with Parkinson's disease. Murnaghan found that a stereotactic lesion placed in the ventrolateral thalamus caused or worsened detrusor hyper-reflexia while a lesion placed in the posterior limb of the internal capsule diminished bladder tone [75]. Porter and Bors also found that thalamotomy increased detrusor hyperreflexia [76].

The most common abnormality seen on urodynamic studies of patients with Parkinson's disease is detrusor hyperreflexia. In various studies of those with urological symptoms, the incidence of detrusor hyperreflexia ranges from 50 to 93% [26,49,77–80]. As is expected with suprapontine lesions, there is coordinated sphincter activity in most cases. In a small percentage of patients (7–18%), however, sphincter pseudodyssynergia occurs [26,80]. In contrast to true sphincter dyssynergia, in which involuntary sphincter activity occurs during bladder contraction, pseudodyssynergia is defined as voluntary contraction of the perineal muscles during bladder contraction in order to prevent leaking. Pavlakis et al. also noted external sphincter bradykinesia, defined as slow relaxation of the sphincter during bladder contraction, in 11% of patients with Parkinson's disease [80]. This finding, however, has not been reproduced in other studies [49].

Overall, urological symptoms are relatively common in patients with

Parkinson's disease, usually as a result of detrusor hyperreflexia. Results of studies on this patients population give further support to the premise that the basal ganglia exerts inhibitory influences on micturition pathways.

Multiple Sclerosis

Urinary urgency, urge incontinence, increased frequency, and urinary retention are common symptoms in patients with multiple sclerosis [81,82]. Miller et al. studied 297 patients with probable multiple sclerosis [MS]: 78% had urological symptoms at some point in their disease course, 12% as part of the initial symptom complex, and 3% as the sole presenting symptom [82]. Andersen and Bradley evaluated 52 patients with MS for 12 years; 94% eventually developed urological symptoms [81].

In several studies urodynamic studies have been performed on patients with multiple sclerosis. In 99 patients Bradley et al. studied with urological symptoms, 60% had detrusor hyperreflexia, and 40% detrusor areflexia [56]. Andersen and Bradley evaluated 52 patients and found detrusor hyperreflexia in 64% and detrusor areflexia in 33%. External sphincter EMG showed normal external sphincter function in 50%, sphincter dyssynergia in 31%, and areflexic sphincter in 15%. Overall, 96% of the patients studied had abnormalities of bladder or sphincter function [81].

Other factors may also be important in the development of bladder dysfunction in patients with MS. Schoenberg et al. found that in some patients with urinary tract infections, detrusor hyperreflexia resolved entirely after the infection was treated with antibiotics [83].

In summary, as expected, multiple sclerosis commonly results in bladder dysfunction. In fact, if evaluated long enough, almost all patients with MS will experience urological symptoms at some point during their disease course. The type of bladder dysfunction depends on the location of the MS plaques, with detrusor hyperreflexia expected from lesions in the cerebrum, detrusor–sphincter dyssynergia from lesions in the suprasacral spinal cord, and detrusor areflexia from lesions involving the sacral spinal cord.

Spinal Cord Injury

Urological dysfunction can result from spinal cord injury of any type, including trauma, tumor, or congenital anomalies [53,58,59,84–87]. The type of bladder dysfunction depends on the spinal cord levels involved and whether the lesion is complete or not.

In patients with complete suprasacral spinal cord lesions there is usually an initial period of "spinal shock" during which the bladder and sphincters are areflexic. During recovery from spinal shock the sphincters regain activity first, usually within days of the injury, while bladder reflex activity does not usually return until much later, typically 6–12 weeks following injury [88].

Ultimately, a pattern of detrusor hyperreflexia with sphincter dyssynergia will develop [53]. In patients with incomplete suprasacral spinal cord lesions, detrusor hyperreflexia also develops. However the incidence of sphincter dyssynergia is less than that for complete spinal cord lesions (44% versus 89%) [26].

Lesions of the sacral spinal cord can lead to varying patterns of urological dysfunction, depending on whether the pelvic nuclei, pudendal nuclei, or nerve roots are affected. Urodynamic patterns include detrusor and external sphincter areflexia, bladder hyperreflexia with an areflexic sphincter, or an areflexic bladder with a hyperreflexic sphincter. This latter pattern may also be seen following suprasacral spinal cord lesions where there is chronic overstretching of the bladder wall [89].

Infants born with myelomeningocele commonly have urological dysfunction. As with traumatic spinal cord injury, the bladder and sphincters may be normal, overactive, or underactive, depending on the level of the lesion [85]. There may also be an initial period of spinal shock. In one series, all infants who initially had an areflexic bladder with an active sphincter went on to develop bladder hyperreflexia [90]. Sphincter dyssynergia is common in suprasacral myelomeningocele and can be complicated by development of intrarenal reflux, renal scarring, and frequent urinary tract infections [85].

TREATMENT

Introduction

A variety of options are available to treat bladder dysfunction. Strategies include easily instituted nursing protocols, such as a regularly scheduled voiding program, medications, surgical procedures, and other modalities, including biofeedback, and electrical stimulation.

Empiric treatment of bladder dysfunction is not recommended. A patient may be incontinent, for example, because of detrusor hyperreflexia, sphincter incompetence, or unrelated factors, such as aphasia secondary to stroke. In each one of these situations the treatment strategies are different. Therefore, a urodynamic study is recommended for all patients with persistent bladder dysfunction, to define the abnormal micturition pattern and to help guide the most appropriate therapy.

The following is a review of available treatments for bladder dysfunction as defined by urodynamic study results.

Normal Urodynamic Study

Despite a normal urodynamic study, patients may be incontinent due to factors such as impaired mobility, aphasia, or cognitive impairment. In these individuals, nonpharmacological treatment is recommended. Gelber and Good found that in aphasic incontinent patients after stroke with normal urodynamic studies, the number of incontinent episodes per day dropped markedly with use of a scheduled voiding program alone [71]. This involves offering the patient a urinal or placing him or her on a bedpan or commode at regular intervals, typically every 2–4 hr, depending on the patient's voiding frequency. In persistently incontinent male patients, an external collection device (e.g., condom catheter) may also be beneficial.

Detrusor Hyperreflexia

The most common urodynamic abnormality associated with cerebral lesions is detrusor hyperreflexia with coordinated sphincter activity leading to increased urinary frequency and urge incontinence. Treatment is aimed specifically at diminishing the bladder hyperreflexia (Table 2).

Urinary tract infections (UTIs) should be treated promptly. Schoenberg et al. found that in some patients with multiple sclerosis, detrusor hyperreflexia, and a UTI, symptoms resolved entirely after treatment of the infection. No additional therapy was needed [83].

Table 2 Treatment of Bladder Dysfunction

Detrusor Hyperreflexia	Detrusor Hyporeflexia
Scheduled voiding program	Fluid restriction
Medications	Intermittent catheterization program
Propantheline	Crede or Valsalva techniques
Oxybutynin	Medications
Dicyclomine	Bethanechol
Flavoxate	Naloxone
Imipramine	Surgical procedures
Baclofen	Urinary diversion
Indomethacin	Vesicostomy
Verapamil	Electrical nerve stimulation
Surgical procedures	
Sacral rhizotomy	
Neurectomy	
Cystolysis	
Augmentation cystoplasty	
Electrical nerve stimulation	
Biofeedback	
External collection device	
Suprapubic tapping	

In patients with detrusor hyperreflexia but only occasional incontinent episodes, a scheduled voiding program, as discussed above, may be of benefit [91,92]. Biofeedback may also be helpful in selected cases [93].

For more severe cases of symptomatic detrusor hyperreflexia, pharmacological intervention is warranted. The hallmark of treatment has been the use of anticholinergic medications, including propantheline (Probanthine), which acts by cholinergic (muscarinic) receptor blockade [94]. The dosage is 15–30 mg every 4–6 hr. Response can be predicted by administering it intravenously during a cystometrogram. Its use may be limited by anticholinergic side effects (dry mouth, blurred vision, tachycardia, constipation, orthostasis, and impotence). Oxybutynin (Ditropan) has anticholinergic, antispasmodic, and local anesthetic effects. It is as effective as propantheline at dosages of 5 mg 2–4 times per day [95,96] and has fewer anticholinergic side effects, especially in the elderly [97]. Intravesical administration of oxybutynin has been shown to be beneficial in patients unable to tolerate oral administration [98].

Dicyclomine (Bentyl) has both anticholinergic and antispasmodic effects [96,99] and has been shown to be efficacious in the treatment of detrusor hyperreflexia at dosages of 20 mg three times daily [96,100]. Less effective is flavoxate (Urispas) given at dosages of 100–200 mg three or four times daily. It has weak antispasmodic and anticholinergic activity [96,101]. Imipramine is also efficacious; it has multiple sites of action including peripheral cholinergic receptor blockade, direct relaxation of bladder smooth muscle, inhibition of reuptake of norepinephrine, and central antidepressant activity [96].

Other medications may also have benefit in selected cases. Baclofen, in addition to its effect on the external striated sphincter (discussed below), also inhibits bladder contractions at dosages of 60–160 mg/day [102]. It is thought to act on spinal cord interneurons, inhibiting polysynaptic spinal cord reflexes [103]. It is most efficacious in treating detrusor hyperreflexia secondary to spinal cord lesions, especially when sphincter dyssynergia is present [104]. Baclofen may also be administered intrathecally via an implantable pump [105,106]. Alpha-adrenergic blockers (e.g., phenoxybenzamine, phentolamine, and prazosin) have their major site of activity on alpha-adrenergic receptors in the bladder neck; in the normal bladder these agents have little direct effect on the detrusor muscle. In a parasympathetically denervated hyperreflexic bladder, however, alpha-adrenergic blockers do appear to diminish detrusor hyperreflexia, possibly because the alpha-adrenergic receptors in the bladder wall proliferate or become suprasensitive. Alpha-adrenergic blockers are most often used in combination with anticholinergics, especially when there is an associated overactive bladder neck (internal sphincter) [107–109]. Indomethacin may also have limited use through action of prostaglandin inhibition [110] at dosages up to 100 mg twice daily. Intravesical administration of verapamil has also been shown to diminish detrusor hyperreflexia [111].

If pharmacological treatment does not result in significant symptomatic improvement, surgical options may be considered; these procedures involve selective lesioning of the peripheral neural pathways from spinal cord to bladder. Sacral rhizotomy at levels S2–S4 will eliminate bladder hyperreflexia but also causes loss of reflex erections in men, loss of vaginal lubrication in women [112], and impaired anal sphincter activity [113]. The posterior roots may be selectively lesioned in combination with placement of an anterior root stimulator, allowing for adequate urine storage and electrically triggered bladder emptying [112]. A nerve plexus–presacral neurectomy can be performed; this involves lesioning the sympathetic chain and dividing the presacral nerve, thus interrupting the sensory limb of the sacral micturition reflex arc [114]. Another option is cystolysis, which involves selective denervation of the bladder. This procedure has the advantage of not interfering with sphincter activity [115]. The long-term effects of this procedure are not known. Electrical nerve stimulation may be of benefit in refractory cases. Stimulation of the pelvic or pudendal nerve results in increased sphincter activity, which, in turn, diminishes detrusor hyperreflexia through inhibition of the reflex arc [116,117].

In patients with detrusor hyperreflexia and a small noncompliant bladder, adequate urine storage may be difficult to achieve, even with pharmacological or surgical denervation procedures. In these individuals an augmentation cystoplasty may be of benefit [118,119]. This procedure involves enlarging the bladder with an interposed piece of colon or small bowel.

The result of pharmacological or surgical treatment of detrusor hyperreflexia is often conversion of the bladder to a hyporeflexic state. Bladder hyporeflexia is more easily managed, especially with an intermittent catheterization program; this is discussed in detail below.

Detrusor Hyperreflexia with Sphincter Dyssynergia

This pattern usually occurs as a result of a suprasacral spinal cord lesions, often following a period of detrusor areflexia (spinal shock). Because the bladder is contracting against a closed sphincter, bladder emptying is incomplete and can lead to urinary tract infections and eventual damage to the upper urinary tract. Sphincter dyssynergia may involve the external striated sphincter, internal sphincter (bladder neck and proximal urethra), or both.

One mode of treatment is to initiate spinal reflex voiding by inducing detrusor contractions [112]. One technique that paraplegics can perform easily is light suprapubic tapping, which causes reflex initiation of bladder contractions. Heavy tapping, however, should be avoided since it will also induce sphincter cocontraction and can result in incomplete bladder emptying. The light tapping technique can be augmented with use of biofeedback. The patient, through audio or visual feedback of bladder and sphincter activity, can learn the best place to tap and the force needed to induce bladder contraction but limit sphincter cocontraction [89].

If there is significant external sphincter dyssynergia, pharmacological intervention may be necessary. Baclofen, administered either orally (average dosages are 120 mg/day) or intrathecally has been shown to decrease external sphincter activity [96,103,104,106]. Side effects at high dosages include somnolence and mild generalized weakness. Baclofen acts at the spinal cord level, inhibiting polysynaptic spinal cord reflexes. Diazepam may also be used as adjunctive therapy [96]. Dantrolene sodium (Dantrium) also reduces external sphincter activity, resulting in significant decrease in residual urines at dosages of 25–100 mg four times daily [120,121]. Its site of action is the sarcoplasmic reticulum of skeletal muscle. Unfortunately, its use is limited by side effects including dizziness, fatigue, generalized weakness, and potential hepatotoxicity.

If pharmacological management is not successful, surgical intervention can be employed. The most commonly employed procedure in men is a transurethral external sphincterotomy. This is, however, an irreversible procedure and can result in urinary incontinence [112]. Pudendal neurectomy is also effective; however, this results in loss of reflex erections in men [89,122]. Sacral rhizotomy will abolish detrusor hyperreflexia and sphincter dyssynergia but is also limited by loss of reflex bowel activity and reflex erections [113].

One newer treatment that deserves mention is use of botulin toxin. Dykstra et al. studied 11 men with detrusor–sphincter dyssynergia [123]. Injection of toxin into the external striated sphincter resulted in a significant drop in urethral pressure and postvoid residuals. An average of 3 injections was needed and the effect lasted for an average of 50 days. It remains to be seen whether use of botulin toxin will eventually replace the more invasive, irreversible surgical procedures (Table 3).

If there is significant dyssynergia of the internal sphincter (bladder neck and proximal urethra), pharmacological intervention can also be employed. Because alpha-adrenergic activity results in contraction of the bladder neck, treatment of internal sphincter dyssynergia involves use of alpha-adrenergic blockers [124]. Phenoxybenzamine can be used at dosages of 10–60 mg/day, although its use is limited by side effects including orthostasis, tachycardia, miosis, diarrhea, and retrograde ejaculation [96]. Prazosin (Minipres), a selective alpha-1 blocker, may also be used [107]. However, a recent study by Petersen et al. did not show significant improvement in bladder emptying, despite a lowering of resting urethral pressure [108]. This may be because prazosin acts peripherally, while dyssynergia is centrally (cord) mediated.

Table 3   Treatment of Sphincter Dysfunction

Overactive external sphincter	*Overactive internal sphincter*
Medications	Medications
Baclofen	Phenoxybenzamine
Diazepam	Prazosin
Dantrolene	Methyldopa
Botulin toxin injection	Clonidine
Surgical procedures	
External sphincterotomy	
Pudendal neurectomy	
Sacral rhizotomy	
Biofeedback	
Areflexic external sphincter	*Areflexic internal sphincter*
Surgical procedures	Medications
Artificial sphincter	Ephedrine
Bladder neck reconstruction	Pseudoephedrine
Fascial sling bladder suspension	Phenylpropanolamine
	Propranolol
	Conjugated estrogen

Methyldopa (Aldomet), at dosages of 1–2 g/day results in improved bladder emptying. Although its precise action is not known, it is thought to act centrally to diminish sympathetic outflow [125]. Clonidine, an alpha-2 agonist, has also been shown to decrease urethral pressure, probably also acting centrally to diminish sympathetic outflow. It may be preferred over alpha-adrenergic blockers because it has fewer side effects [126] (Table 3).

Once the dyssynergic sphincter is addressed, treatment then shifts to the hyperreflexic bladder, especially if there is persistent incontinence. Strategies are the same as outlined in the section above. Often a combination of treatments (e.g., anticholinergic plus alpha-adrenergic blocker, or anticholinergic plus external sphincterotomy) is needed. If incomplete bladder emptying persists, an intermittent catheterization program may be needed [127].

Detrusor Hyperreflexia with Sphincter Areflexia

This is a rare urodynamic pattern seen in 15% of patients with myelomeningocele and incomplete sacral spinal cord lesions [89,112]. Patients with detrusor hyperreflexia and an areflexic sphincter are constantly incontinent because of diminished resistance to urinary outflow. In the past, management consisted of use of a chronic indwelling catheter or a urinary diversion surgical procedure (placement of a sigmoid or ileal loop). It is now recommended that chronic indwelling catheters be avoided, if possible, because of the risk of urinary tract infection, bladder stone formation, and urethral stricture formation [128]. Fewer urinary diversion procedures are now performed because of frequent postsurgical complications and poor long-term results [129].

Initial management for this type of bladder dysfunction should include treatment of bladder hyperreflexia, as outlined above, in combination with a scheduled voiding program [89]. If incontinence persists, because of an incompetent sphincter, newer surgical procedures should be considered including placement of an artificial urinary sphincter, bladder neck reconstruction, or a fascial sling bladder neck suspension (in women) [112]. These may need to be combined with augmentation cystoplasty if there is significant detrusor hyperreflexia or decreased bladder compliance [118,119] (Table 3).

Detrusor Areflexia with Sphincter Areflexia

This urodynamic pattern is seen with complete conus medullaris lesions, cauda equina syndrome, severe peripheral neuropathy [112], or as part of the spinal shock phase in suprasacral spinal cord injury [88]. Bladder hypo- or areflexia usually results in impaired bladder emptying and overflow incontinence.

Initial management involves an intermittent catheterization program. Fluid restriction is also important to prevent overfilling of the bladder. Fluid intake should be restricted to 1800–2400 ml/day and catheterization performed often enough to keep residuals less than 500 ml [88,89]. Urine cultures should be checked every 3 days initially and symptomatic infections should be treated promptly. A study by Mohler et al. showed no advantage in using suppressive antibiotics, treating asymptomatic infections, or in using more than 3 days of antibiotics [130]. Again, an intermittent catheterization program is preferred over use of an indwelling catheter or urinary diversion procedure.

The use of cholinergic medications has been advocated to induce bladder contractions. Bethanechol chloride (Urecholine) is a parasympathomimetic drug that stimulates bladder postganglionic cells [131]. It may be administered subcutaneously at dosages of 2.5–10 mg every 4–6 hr or orally 50 mg every 6 hr [131,132]. It causes severe muscarinic side effects (e.g., diarrhea, vomiting, sweating, bronchospasm, and bradycardia) if given intramuscularly or intravenously [96]. Bethanechol is effective in improving bladder contractility if low-amplitude detrusor contractions are present; it is not efficacious in a completely areflexic bladder [131,133]. Cholinergic medications should be avoided if there is significant bladder outlet obstruction, because of the potential creation of a pseudodyssynergic state.

In incomplete spinal cord lesions, naloxone may also enhance the detrusor reflex [134]. Naloxone may act by potentiating spinal cord reflexes through inhibition of enkephalins.

Patients can often augment bladder emptying by using Credé or Valsalva techniques [135]. These techniques create increased intravesical pressure to allow for passive voiding. Because high pressures need to be generated to open the bladder neck, ureteral reflux can result; therefore patients must be evaluated closely for development of upper urinary tract damage [112]. Crede and Valsalva techniques should be used cautiously if there is increased sphincter activity, because these can induce sphincter dyssynergia.

Electrical stimulation has been studied as a means of facilitating bladder contraction. The sacral nerve roots can be stimulated; this does result in increased bladder emptying but causes side effects of penile erection, pelvic pain, and piloerection [136]. The pelvic nerves can also be stimulated, however this also results in pain and increased outflow resistance [117]. Transurethral intravesical electrical stimulation has also been studied but was only beneficial in patients with incomplete lesions [137] (Table 2).

If there is significant sphincter areflexia, incontinence may be persistent. Treatment of external sphincter areflexia is outlined in the section above. If the internal sphincter is incompetent there are several potential pharmacological interventions aimed at increasing bladder neck and proximal urethral tone. Use of alpha-adrenergic agonists, including ephedrine 25–50 mg four times daily, pseudoephedrine 30–60 mg four times daily, and phenylpropanolamine 50 mg three times daily increases urethral closure pressure and improves sphincteric incontinence [96]. Side effects include hypertension, anxiety, and insomnia. Beta blockers, such as propranolol also increase urethral closure pressure, possibly by unmasking the alpha receptors [96]. Conjugated estrogen (Premarin) has also been shown to improve sphincteric incontinence, although the mechanism of action is not known [96] (Table 3).

Detrusor Areflexia with Sphincter Hyperreflexia

This is a rare urodynamic pattern that results from incomplete sacral spinal cord lesions or following suprasacral lesions if the detrusor is chronically overstretched [89]. Clinically, urinary retention results.

The easiest form of treatment for this type of bladder dysfunction is an intermittent catheterization program, as described above. Again, use of chronic indwelling catheters should be avoided. One can also use Valsalva or Crede technique to augment bladder emptying. If significant outflow obstruction persists, external sphincterotomy or pudendal neurectomy can be considered.

SUMMARY

Bladder dysfunction occurs as a result of many neurological diseases, usually due to impairment of the neural pathways controlling micturition. The specific type of bladder dysfunction depends on the localization of the lesion, with lesions involving the sacral cord and roots causing bladder and sphincter areflexia, lesions between the pons and sacral cord causing bladder hyper-reflexia with sphincter dyssynergia, and suprapontine lesions causing bladder hyperreflexia with coordinated sphincters. Evaluation of bladder dysfunction should include a detailed history and physical examination, measurement of postvoid residual urine volumes, and urinalysis, but most importantly should include a urodynamic study with a cystometrogram and urinary sphincter EMG, to define the type of bladder and sphincter dysfunction and to guide appropriate therapy. Although some forms of bladder dysfunction are easily treatable or resolve spontaneously, long-term medical management or surgical intervention is often required. We are fortunate that many forms of treatment are currently available.

REFERENCES

1. E.A. Tanagho, and R.C.B. Pugh, *Br. J. Urol.*, 35:151–165 (1963).
2. E.A. Tanagho, and D.R. Smith, *Br. J. Urol.*, 38:54–71 (1966).
3. J.A. Hutch, and O.N. Rambo, Jr., *J. Urol.*, 97:696–704 (1967).
4. J.A. Hutch, *J. Urol.*, 97:705–712 (1967).
5. F.J. Kleeman, *J. Urol.*, 104:549–554 (1970).
6. T. Koyanagi, *J. Urol.*, 124:400–406 (1980).
7. W.E. Bradley, G.W. Timm, and F.B. Scott, *Urol. Clin. North. Am.*, 1:3–27 (1974).
8. A. Elbadawi, and E.A. Schenk, *J. Urol.*, 111:613–615 (1974).
9. S.A. Awad, and J.W. Downie, *Urol. Int.*, 32:192–197 (1977).
10. W.C. de Groat, and A.M. Booth, *Ann. Intern. Med.*, 93 (Part 2):312–315 (1980).
11. J. Nordling, H.H. Meyhoff, and T. Hald, *Scand. J. Urol. Nephrol.*, 15:7–19 (1981).
12. S.A. Awad, A.W. Bruce, G. Carro-Ciampi, J.W. Downie, and M. Lin, *Br. J. Pharmacol.*, 50:525–529 (1974).
13. W.C. de Groat, *Brain Res.*, 87:201–211 (1975).
14. G.L. Rockswold, W.E. Bradley, and S.N. Chou, *J. Comp. Neurol.*, 193:521–528 (1980).
15. P. Milner, R. Crowe, G. Burnstock, and J.K. Light, *J. Urol.*, 138:888–892 (1987).
16. P. Alm, J. Alumets, E. Brodin, R. Hakanson, G. Nilsson, N.-O. Sjoberg, and F. Sundler, *Neuroscience*, 3:419–425 (1978).
17. G. Burnstock, T. Cocks, R. Crowe, and L. Kasakov, *Br. J. Pharmacol.*, 63:125–138 (1978).

18. R. Crowe, H.E. Moss, C.R. Chapple, J.K. Light, and G. Burnstock, *J. Urol.*, *145*:600–604 (1991).
19. A. Dray, and R. Metsch, *Eur. J. Pharmacol.*, *104*:47–53 (1984).
20. J. Gu, M.A. Blank, W.M. Huang, K.N. Islam, G.P. McGregor, N. Christofides, J.M. Allen, S.R. Bloom, and J.M. Polak, *Urology*, *24*:353–357 (1984).
21. O.P. Khanna, G.J. DeGregorio, R.G. Sample, and R.F. McMichael, *Urology*, *10*:375–381 (1977).
22. J. Gu, M.A. Blank, W.M. Huang, K.N. Islam, G.P. McGregor, N. Christofides, J.M. Allen, S.R. Bloom, and J.M. Polak, *Urology*, *24*:353–357 (1974).
23. J. Gu, J.M. Restorick, M.A. Blank, W.M. Huang, J.M. Polak, S.R. Bloom, and A.R. Mundy, *J. Urol.*, *55*:645–647 (1983).
24. W.E. Bradley, and C.J. Conway, *Neurology*, *16*:237–249 (1966).
25. P.C. Tang, *J. Neurophysiol.*, *18*:583 (1955).
26. M.B. Sirkoy, and R.J. Krane, *J. Urol.*, *127*:953–957 (1982).
27. J.G. Blaivas, *J. Urol.*, *127*:958–963 (1982).
28. N.N. Bhatia, and W.E. Bradley, *Female Urology* (S. Raz, ed.), W.B. Saunders, Philadelphia, pp. 13–32 (1983).
29. R.J. Lewin, G.V. Dillard, and R.W. Porter, *Brain Res.*, *4*:301–307 (1967).
30. F. Andrews, and P.W. Nahtan, *Proc. R. Soc. Med.*, *58*:553–555 (1965).
31. C-A. Carlsson, *Acta Pharmacol. Toxicol.*, *43*(II):8–12 (1978).
32. E. Bors, and K.A. Blinn, *J. Urol.*, *82*:128 (1959).
33. C. Norton, *Geriatr. Nurs. Home Care*, 11–14 (1987).
34. T.L. Massagli, K.M. Jaffe, and D.D. Cardenas, *J. Reprod. Med.*, *35*:925–931 (1990).
35. J. Kjeldsen-Kragh, *Paraplegia*, *26*:192–199 (1988).
36. B.M. Churchill, R.F. Gilmour, and P. Williot, *Pediatr. Clin. North Am.*, *34*: 1133–1157 (1987).
37. R.C. Bump, *Urogynecology*, *16*:795–816 (1989).
38. A.C. Diokno, *J. Am. Geriatr. Soc.*, *38*:300–305 (1990).
39. H.A. Thiede, and F.K. Thiede, *J. Reprod. Med.*, *35*:925–931 (1990).
40. S.B. Bauer, *Controversies in Neuro-urology* (D.M. Barrett and A.J. Wein, eds.), Churchill Livingstone, New York, pp. 193–202 (1984).
41. P. Abrams, J.G. Blaivas, S.L. Stanton, and J.T. Andersen, *Int. Urogynecol. J.*, *1*: 45–58 (1990).
42. E. McGuire, *Urol. Clin. North Am.*, *6*:121–124 (1979).
43. R.L. Vereecken, and H. Verduyn, *Br. J. Urol.*, *42*:457 (1970).
44. G. Lose, and J.T. Andersen, *J. Urol.*, *137*:249–252 (1987).
45. H.M. Saxton, *Radiology*, *175*:307–316 (1990).
46. W.K. Yeates, *Bladder Control and Enuresis* (I. Kolvin, R.C. Mackeith, and S.R. Meadow, eds.), J.B. Lippincott, Philadelphia, pp. 28–36 (1973).
47. Z. Khan, P. Starer, W.C. Yang, and A. Bhola, *Urology*, *35*:265–270 (1990).
48. M.J. Reding, S.W. Winter, S.A. Hochrein, H.B. Simon, and M.M. Thompson, *J. Neurol. Rehab.*, *1*:25–30 (1987).
49. Y. Berger, J.G. Blaivas, E.R. DeLaRocha, and J.M. Salinas, *J. Urol.*, *138*:836–838 (1987).

50. M. Fall, B.L. Ohlsson, and C-A. Carlsson, *Br. J. Urol.*, *64*:368–373 (1989).
51. R.M. Decter, S.B. Bauer, S. Khoshbin, F.M. Dyro, C. Krarup, A.H. Colodny, and A.B. Retik, *J. Urol.*, *138*:1110–1112 (1987).
52. R.J. Krane, and M.B. Siroky, *Clinical Neuro-urology* (R.J. Krane and M.B. Siroky, eds.), Little, Brown, Boston, pp. 143–158 (1979).
53. J.J. Wyndaele, *Paraplegia*, *25*:10–15 (1987).
54. M.S. Weinstein, D.D. Cardenas, E.J. O'Shaughnessy, and M.L. Catanzaro, *Arch. Phys. Med. Rehab.*, *69*:923–927 (1988).
55. C. Frimodt-Moller, *Dan. Med. Bull.*, *23*:267–278 (1976).
56. W.E. Bradley, J.L. Logothetis, and G.W. Timm, *Neurology*, *23*:1131–1139 (1973).
57. R.S. Kirby, *Ann. R. Coll. Surg. Engl.*, *70*:285–289 (1988).
58. A.Y. Smith, and J.R. Woodside, *Urology*, *32*:474–477 (1988).
59. J. Snape, H.M. Duffin, and C.M. Castleden, *Br. J. Urol.*, *59*:50–52 (1987).
60. C.P. Bates, W.E. Bradley, E.S. Glen, H. Melchior, D. Rowan, A.M. Sterling, T. Sundin, D. Thomas, M. Torrens, R. Turner-Warwick, N.R. Zinner, and T. Hald, *J. Urol.*, *53*:333–335 (1981).
61. R.J. Krane, and M.B. Siroky, *Controversies in Neuro-Urology* (D.M. Barrett and A.J. Wein, eds.), Churchill Livingstone, New York, pp. 233–238 (1984).
62. D.M. Barrett, and A.J. Wein, *Controversies in Neuro-Urology* (D.M. Barrett and A.J. Wein, eds.), Churchill Livingstone, New York, pp. 239–250 (1984).
63. D.R. Staskin, *Clinical Neuro-Urology*, 2nd edition (R.J. Krane and M.B. Sirkoy, eds.), Little, Brown, Boston, pp. 411–424 (1991).
64. E. Bors, and A.E. Comarr, *Neurologic Urology*. University Park Press, Baltimore (1971).
65. W.E. Bradley, *Campbell's Urology* (P. Walsh et al., eds.), W.B. Saunders, Philadelphia, pp. 129–185 (1986).
66. T. Hald, and W.E. Bradley, *The Urinary Bladder*. Williams and Wilkins, Baltimore (1982).
67. A.J. Wein, *J. Urol.*, *125*:605 (1981).
68. J. Lapides, *JAMA*, *201*:618 (1967).
69. M.J. Borrie, A.J. Campbell, T.H. Caradoc-Davies, and G.F. Spears, *Age Ageing*, *15*:177–181 (1986).
70. J.C. Brocklehurst, K. Andrews, B. Richards, and P.J. Laycock, *J. Am. Geriatr. Soc.*, *33*:540 (1985).
71. D.A. Gelber, and D.C. Good, *Neurology*, *41*(Suppl 1):352 (1991).
72. Z. Khan, J. Hertanu, W.C. Yang, A. Melma, and E. Leite, *J. Urol.*, *126*:86–88 (1981).
73. S. Tsuchida, H. Noto, O. Yamaguchi, and M. Itoh, *Urology*, *21*:315–317 (1983).
74. V.E. Garrett, J.A. Scott, J. Costich, D.L. Aubrey, and J. Gross, *Arch. Phys. Med. Rehab.*, *70*:41–43 (1989).
75. G.F. Murnaghan, *Br. J. Urol.*, *33*:403–409 (1961).
76. R.W. Porter, and E. Bors, *J. Neurosurg.*, *34*:27–32 (1971).
77. J.T. Andersen, S. Hebjorn, C. Frimodt-Moller, S. Walter, and J. Worm-Petersen, *Acta. Neurol. Scand.*, *53*:161–170 (1976).

78. J.T. Andersen, and W.E. Bradley, *J. Urol.*, *116*:75–78 (1976).
79. M. Greenberg, H.L. Gordon, and J.J. McCutchen, *South Med. J.*, *65*:446–448 (1972).
80. A.J. Pavlakis, M.B. Siroky, I. Goldstein, and R.J. Krane, *J. Urol.*, *129*:80–83 (1983).
81. J.T. Andersen, and W.E. Bradley, *Br. J. Urol.*, *48*:193–198 (1976).
82. H. Miller, C.A. Simpson, and W.K. Yeates, *Br. Med. J.*, *1*:1265–1269 (1965).
83. H.W. Schoenberg, and J.M. Gutrich, *Urology*, *16*:444–447 (1980).
84. R.H. Hackler, M.K. Hall, and T.A. Zampieri, *J. Urol.*, *141*:1390–1393 (1989).
85. J.D. Van Gool, T.P. De Jong, and A.A. Van Wijk, *Acta. Urol. Belg.*, *57*:497–501 (1989).
86. B.E. Glahn, *Urol. Clin. North Am.*, *1*:163–173 (1974).
87. S.A. Koff, and P.A. Deridder, *J. Urol.*, *118*:87–89 (1977).
88. W.F. O'Donnell, *Crit. Care Clin.*, *3*:599–617 (1987).
89. J.L. Opitz, *Controversies in Neuro-Urology* (D.M. Barrett and A.J. Wein, eds.), Churchill Livingstone, New York, pp. 437–451 (1984).
90. L.S. Baskin, B.A. Kogan, and F. Benard, *Br. J. Urol.*, *66*:532–534 (1990).
91. B.A. Greengold, and J.G. Ouslander, *J. Gerontol. Nursing*, *12*:31–35 (1986).
92. A.W. Pengelly, and C.M. Booth, *J. Urol.*, *52*:463–466 (1980).
93. L.D. Cardozo, P.D. Abrams, S.L. Stanton, and R.C.L. Feneley, *Br. J. Urol.*, *50*: 521–523 (1978).
94. G.S. Benson, A.J. Wein, D.M. Raezer, and J.N. Corriere, Jr., *J. Urol.*, *116*:174–175 (1976).
95. C.U. Moisey, T.P. Stephenson, and C.B. Rendler, *J. Urol.*, *52*:472–475 (1980).
96. A.J. Wein, *Surgery of Female Incontinence* (S.L. Stanton and E.A. Tangho, eds.), Springer-Verlag, New York, pp. 186–199 (1980).
97. J.G. Ouslander, J. Blaustein, A. Connor, S. Orzeck, and C-L. Yong, *J. Urol.*, *140*:47–50 (1988).
98. C.B. Brendler, L. C. Radebaugh, and J.L. Mohler, *J. Urol.*, *141*:1350–1352 (1988).
99. I.M. Thompson, and R. Lauvetz, *Urology*, *8*:452–454 (1976).
100. C.P. Fischer, A. Diokno, and J. Lapides, *J. Urol.*, *120*:328–329 (1978).
101. A.E. Finkbeiner, L.T. Welch, and N.K. Bissada, *Urology*, *12*:231–235 (1978).
102. M.C. Taylor, and C.P. Bates, *J. Urol.*, *51*:504–505 (1979).
103. J.F.J. Leyson, B.F. Martin, and A. Sporer, *J. Urol.*, *124*:82–84 (1980).
104. H. Kiesswetter, and W. Schober, *Urol. Int.*, *30*:63–71 (1975).
105. F. Frost, J. Nanninga, R. Penn, S. Savoy, and Y. Wu, *Am. J. Phys. Med. Rehab.*, *68*:112–115 (1989).
106. J.B. Nanninga, F. Frost, and R. Penn, *J. Urol.*, *142*:101–105 (1989).
107. D. Jensen, Jr., *Scand J. Urol. Nephrol.*, *15*:229–233 (1981).
108. T. Petersen, S.E. Husted, and P. Sidenius, *Scand. J. Urol. Nephrol.*, *23*:189–194 (1989).
109. M.B. Scott, and J.W. Morrow, *J. Urol.*, *119*:483–484 (1978).
110. L.D. Cardozo, and S.L. Stanton, *J. Urol.*, *123*:399–401 (1980).
111. A. Mattiasson, B. Ekstrom, and K-E. Andersson, *J. Urol.*, *141*:174–177 (1989).

112. H. Madersbacher, *Paraplegia*, 28:217–229 (1990).

113. R.P. MacDonagh, M.C. Forster, and D.G. Thomas, *J. Urol.*, 66:618–622 (1990).

114. G.E. Leach, D. Goldman, and S. Raz, *Female Urology* (S. Raz, ed.), W.B. Saunders, Philadelphia, pp. 326–334 (1983).

115. F.S. Freiha, and T.A. Stamey, *J. Urol.*, 123:360–363 (1980).

116. B.L. Ohlsson, M. Fall, and S. Frankenberg-Sommar, *Br. J. Urol.*, 64:374–380 (1989).

117. E.A. Tanagho, and R.A. Schmidt, *J. Urol.*, 140:1331–1339 (1988).

118. A.A. Sidi, Y. Reinberg, and R. Gonzalez, *J. Urol.*, 138:1120–1122 (1987).

119. E.J. Kass, and S.A. Koff, *J. Urol.*, 129:553–555 (1983).

120. R.H. Hackler, B.H. Broecker, F.A. Klein, and S.M. Brady, *J. Urol.*, 124:78–81 (1980).

121. M.M. Murdock, D. Sax, and R.J. Krane, *Urology*, 8:133–137 (1976).

122. G. Stark, *Arch. Dis. Child.*, 44:698 (1969).

123. D.D. Dykstra, A.A. Sidi, A.B. Scott, J.M. Pagel, and G.D. Goldish, *J. Urol.*, 139:919–922 (1988).

124. R.J. Krane, and C.A. Olsson, *J. Urol.*, 110:650–652 (1973).

125. S. Raz, J.J. Kaufman, G.W. Ellison, and L.W. Mayers, *Urology*, 9:188–190 (1977).

126. J. Nordling, H.H. Meyhoff, and N.J. Christensen, *Invest. Radiol.*, 16:289–291 (1979).

127. E. Geraniotis, S.A. Koff, and B. Enrile, *J. Urol.*, 139:85–86 (1988).

128. B. Connolly, R.J. Fitzgerald, and E.J. Guiney, *Z. Kinderchir.*, 43(Suppl II):17–18 (1988).

129. M. Castro-Gago, I. Nov, A. Cimadevila, J. Pena, A. Rodriguez-Nunez, and A. Marques-Queimadelos, *Eur. J. Pediatr.*, 150:62–65 (1990).

130. J.L. Mohler, D.L. Cowen, and R. C. Flanigan, *J. Urol.*, 138:336–340 (1987).

131. A.C. Diokno, and R. Koppenhoefer, *Urology*, 8:455–458 (1976).

132. J. Lapides, *J. Urol.*, 91:658–659 (1964).

133. J.K. Light, and F.B. Scott, *J. Urol.*, 128:85–87 (1982).

134. S. Vaidyanathan, M.S. Rao, K.S.N. Chary, P.L. Sharma, and N. Das, *J. Urol.*, 126:500–502 (1981).

135. N.M. Resnick, and S.V. Yalla, *N. Engl. J. Med.*, 313:800–805 (1985).

136. J.H. Grimes, B.S. Nashold, and E.E. Anderson, *J. Urol.*, 113:338–340 (1975).

137. H. Madersbacher, *Paraplegia*, 28:349–352 (1990).

17

Chronic Pain Management

Russell K. Portenoy

Memorial Sloan-Kettering Cancer Center
New York, and
Cornell University Medical College
White Plains, New York

Michael J. Brennan

The Rehabilitation Center of Fairfield County
Bridgeport, Connecticut

Clinicians of every discipline encounter patients who experience persistent pain as a primary condition or potentially disabling complication of a medical disorder. The therapeutic approach to this diverse population must integrate the management of the underlying disease process, if identified, with specific interventions for the pain itself. In all cases, pain management should pursue the dual goals of enhanced comfort and restoration of physical and psychosocial function. For many patients, these goals can be substantially advanced by the efforts of a single physician, who provides continuing assessment, implements one or more interventions, and appropriately refers the patient to other clinicians for additional modalities. Refractory patients, who remain highly distressed by pain or significantly disabled despite therapy, should be evaluated by specialists in pain management. Subspecialization in this area has evolved in many disciplines, including neurology, rehabilitation, anesthesiology, and psychiatry.

This chapter discusses the general approach to the patient with chronic pain, emphasizing the assessment and management of the heterogeneous population with chronic nonmalignant pain. The comprehensive management of cancer pain is reviewed elsewhere [1–3]. Issues related to the treatment of specific disorders associated with chronic pain, such as arthritis or postherpetic neuralgia, are not discussed and may need to be reviewed by the clinician on a case-by-case basis.

DEFINITIONS

Pain has been defined by the International Association for the Study of Pain as "an unpleasant sensory and emotional experience associated with actual or potential tissue damage, or described in terms of such damage" [4]. Implicit in this definition is the observation that the relationship between tissue damage and pain is neither uniform nor predictable. This is a fundamental principle, which can be clarified by the distinctions among nociception, pain, and suffering [5].

Nociception, Pain, and Suffering

Nociception is the activity produced in the afferent nervous system by noxious mechanical, thermal, or chemical stimuli [6,7]. Pain is the perception of nociception, and like other perceptions, relates to a complex interaction between activity in the sensorineural apparatus and other processes. Pain may be absent despite extensive tissue damage, or severe in the absence of any sufficient organic explanation.

From the clinical perspective, pains that appear excessive for the degree of overt tissue injury (i.e., for the degree of nociception inferred to exist), are most problematic. Some of these syndromes, such as those with clear neuropathic mechanisms, have an unequivocal organic cause. Others will be perceived to have a likely organic cause that remains to be identified. Some patients will present positive evidence for a psychological causation, and many will be assumed to have pain that is multiply determined by organic processes and psychological influences. Given this variability, the clinician should be cautious in applying diagnostic labels. Patients with pain that is perceived to be unexplained by the degree of nociception occurring and cannot be convincingly ascribed to some other pathophysiology (organic or psychological) should receive the neutral label of "idiopathic pain" [8].

In an effort to clarify the complex phenomenology of pain and its relationship to nociception, models have been developed that postulate a hierarchy of dimensions [9]. The sensory–discriminative dimension reflects the fundamental need to identify, localize, and discriminate noxious stimuli. When related to tissue injury, this information is probably transmitted in afferent pathways that have been well characterized in animal models of nociception [6,7]. The clinician uses the description of this sensory dimension to elaborate hypotheses for the underlying organic contribution to the pain. These hypotheses may then be pursued through imaging or other evaluation techniques, the findings of which clarify the degree to which the pain can be explained by nociception or some other process.

Two other dimensions have been posited to reflect the highly variable and dynamic reactive component of the pain: the motivational–affective dimension suggests the emotional response and the cognitive–evaluative dimension suggests the individual's attempt to understand the meaning of the pain and manage it [9]. It may be conjectured that these reactions are mediated through different neural systems than those that transmit sensory information. For example, the multiple polysynaptic afferent pathways that interconnect with brainstem reticular neurons and the limbic system may subserve the motivational–affective dimension.

The construct of suffering may also illuminate the experience of chronic pain. Suffering is a more global experience, which suggests some fundamental threat to the person, the combined effect of numerous losses, or the overall impairment in quality of life. Although pain may contribute profoundly to suffering, other aversive perceptions may be equally or more salient. Symptoms other than pain, such as loss of function, familial dissolution, or financial concerns, may all contribute. Suffering may be more related to a concurrent psychiatric disorder (e.g., depression or anxiety) than to the pain with which it is associated. Evaluation of all these factors is an essential component of the comprehensive pain assessment. A clinical focus on pain to the exclusion of other factors contributing to the suffering of the patient may lead to an unsatisfactory outcome, even if comfort is enhanced.

Chronic Pain Versus Chronic Nonmalignant Pain Syndrome

The chronic pain population is extraordinarily heterogeneous. This heterogeneity, which is evident even among those with the same diagnoses, relates to variability in the characteristics of the pain itself, the physical impairments and medical disorders associated with the pain, and the prominence of psychological and behavioral comorbidity. Given the differences among patients, the appellation "chronic pain" should be viewed as a nonspecific term that indicates a temporal feature of the pain. A recent definition that encompasses many earlier ones designates a pain as chronic if it persists for a month beyond the usual course of an acute illness or a reasonable duration for an injury to heal, if it is associated with a chronic pathological process, or if it recurs at intervals for months or years [10].

Distinct from the nonspecific label of "chronic pain" are such terms as "chronic pain syndrome," "chronic nonmalignant pain syndrome," or "intractable nonmalignant pain syndrome." The latter are generally applied to patients whose chronic pain has become associated with marked affective and behavioral disturbances, that is, patients with substantial pain-related disability. Many of these patients have idiopathic pain; some fulfill criteria for a diagnosis of a defined psychiatric disorder of which pain is a component [11]. When pain is experienced in a specific region of the body, patients with a chronic nonmalignant pain syndrome may be labeled by other terms, including atypical facial pain, failed low back syndrome, chronic tension headache, or chronic pelvic pain of unknown cause.

The failure to differentiate the chronic pain syndrome from chronic pain in general has led to confusion in the medical literature. Publications originating from multidisciplinary pain clinics, for example, often describe the characteristics of patients with "chronic pain" without adequately defining the subgroup as one that contains a disproportionate number of patients with severe chronic pain syndrome. Research findings from this group, although informative, may not generalize to other large segments of the chronic pain population, who have much less pain-related disability and never present to multidisciplinary pain clinics. Clinicians who treat patients with chronic pain must recognize the diversity of this population and make no a priori assumptions about the characteristics of the pain or associated findings. All such characteristics must be defined on a patient-by-patient basis through the process of a comprehensive pain assessment.

PRINCIPLES OF PAIN ASSESSMENT

A comprehensive assessment clarifies the organic and psychological contributions to the pain and characterizes the range of problems (physical, psychological, sexual, familial, social, financial, and so on) that may also require treatment. In some patients with multiple problems, a useful way of conceptualizing the goal of this assessment is the development of a pain-oriented problem list.

The information required to develop the pain-oriented problem list derives from the history, as well as accompanying records, physical examination, laboratory tests, and imaging studies. Among other outcomes, this information may allow the clinician to define the pain syndrome and infer a predominating pain pathophysiology, both of which may be useful in planning the subsequent evaluation and organizing a therapeutic approach.

The pain history should clarify the temporal features (onset, course, and daily pattern), location, severity, quality, and factors that provoke or relieve the pain. The history of present illness should be supplemented by queries intended to elicit a past history of persistent pain, prior pain treatments, and previous use of licit drugs (including alcohol, tobacco, and both over-the-counter and prescription medicines) and illicit drugs. Pending litigation should be clarified. A psychosocial assessment should characterize premorbid psychiatric disease or personality disorder, coping styles demonstrated during earlier episodes of physical disease or psychological stress, current psychological state with particular reference to anxiety and depression, current resources (social, familial, and financial), and functional status. The patient's activities during the day should be enumerated to help clarify his or her degree of physical inactivity and social isolation.

The physical examination of patients with chronic pain should clarify the organic contributions to the pain. If further evaluation is necessary, the information obtained from the history and this examination guide the selection of appropriate laboratory and imaging procedures.

It must be emphasized that the discovery of a lesion during this comprehensive assessment does not indicate that the predominating pathogenesis for the pain is organic. A competent evaluation identifies potentially treatable organic conditions and clarifies the degree to which pain and disability can be ascribed to these factors or to other identifiable pathological conditions, including psychological disturbances.

Relevance of Pain Characteristics

The characteristics of the pain may clarify its syndrome or pathogenesis, or guide the selection of treatments.

Severity

The severity of the pain may be assessed on a verbal rating scale (none, mild, moderate, severe, or excruciating), a numerical scale (0–10 or 0–100, in which 0 is no pain and 10 or 100 is the worst pain imaginable) or a visual analog scale (a line of defined length anchored by appropriate descriptors, e.g., "no pain" and "worst possible pain"). Scaling of the pain severity through one of these simple techniques greatly facilitates the process of monitoring changes over time.

Temporal Features

Acute pain has a recent onset and is expected to be short-lived. It usually has a well-defined cause (e.g., surgical incision). There is an association between acute pain and specific pain behaviors (e.g., moaning, grimacing, and splinting of the painful part), signs of sympathetic hyperactivity (including tachycardia, hypertension, and diaphoresis), and the affect of anxiety. In contrast, these clinical concomitants are usually absent in patients with chronic pain, which is more often associated with sleep disturbance and other vegetative signs (such as lassitude and anorexia), and with depressed affect [12].

From the clinical perspective, it is important to recognize that chronic pain itself is characterized by diverse temporal profiles. Most patients have fluctuating pain with some pain-free intervals and, indeed, some patients have such discrete painful episodes that it is useful to conceptualize the problem as recurrent acute pain, rather than chronic pain. Even those with continuous pain experience large fluctuations in the intensity of pain or acute episodes of severe exacerbation that the patient perceives as distinct from the baseline pain. In a survey of patients with pain due to cancer, for example, almost two-thirds experienced transitory breakthrough pains [13].

Topographic Features

Therapeutic options vary among pains that are focal, multifocal, and generalized. Only focal pains, for example, are generally amenable to neural blockade. This feature should be noted during the pain assessment.

Recognition of pain referral patterns is likewise important, particularly when one is selecting appropriate assessment procedures. There are numerous subtypes of referred pain. For example, a lesion at any level of the neuraxis can refer pain anywhere in the cutaneous distribution innervated by the injured structure. Thus, pain in the foot may be referred from a pathological process affecting the peripheral nerves that supply this site, the appropriate nerve root, or specific spinal cord tract or brain region. Lesions affecting diverse nonneural structures, including bone, muscle, and viscera, may also refer pain to a remote site [14,15]. Shoulder pain, for example, can be referred from irritation of the ipsilateral diaphragm or from trigger points in the sternocleidomastoid muscle. Common pain referral patterns must be appreciated by the clinician, so that imaging of potentially diseased regions can proceed efficiently.

Quality

Although no verbal descriptor is specific, the quality of the pain may provide useful clues about its underlying pathogenesis. Burning or shooting pain, for example, suggests a possible neuropathic mechanism.

Pain Syndromes

Syndrome identification may delineate associated organic processes, suggest an efficient evaluation, guide the selection of treatments, and indicate prognosis. The development of criteria for syndrome identification has recently been advanced through the development of a pain taxonomy by the International Association for the Study of Pain [4].

Inferred Pathophysiology

Although it is very likely that most chronic pain is multiply determined by a complex interaction between organic factors and psychological disturbances, it is usually possible to impute a predominating mechanism based on the clinical evaluation of the patient. This inferred pathophysiology can be very useful in selecting a multimodality treatment approach for the patient.

Pains that appear clinically to have a predominating organic contribution have been termed "nociceptive" or "neuropathic." Nociceptive pain is perceived to be commensurate with the degree of continuing tissue damage from an identifiable peripheral lesion that involves either somatic or visceral structures. Nociceptive pain originating from somatic structures (somatic pain) is typically described as aching, stabbing, throbbing, or pressure-like. Visceral pain associated with obstruction of hollow viscus is usually gnawing or crampy; pain related to distention or torsion of organ capsules or other mesentery is typically aching or stabbing in quality. Designation of a pain as nociceptive has clinical implications, since this type of pain can often be ameliorated through interventions that improve the peripheral nociceptive lesion. For example, joint replacement can usually relieve refractory arthritic pain.

Neuropathic pain is related to aberrant somatosensory processes induced by an injury to the peripheral or central nervous system [16]. Major subtypes include those in which the abnormal focus of neural activity responsible for perpetuating the pain is in the peripheral nervous system (so-called peripheral neuropathic pain), those in which this focus is in the central nervous system (so-called deafferentation pain), and those in which the pain is dependent on efferent activity in the sympathetic nervous system (so-called sympathetically maintained pain). The pains are often dysesthetic (abnormal pain, unfamiliar to the patient) and disproportionate to any evident nociceptive lesion. Identification of a neuropathic mechanism is extremely important, since specific therapies may be useful for these syndromes (see below).

As discussed previously, most patients who lack the criteria to fulfill a pathophysiological diagnosis of nociceptive or neuropathic pain can be said to have an idiopathic pain syndrome. Some of these patients have pain that is believed to have a predominating psychological pathogenesis, including a subgroup who meet criteria for specific psychiatric diagnoses [11].

This concept of inferred pathophysiology has been extended in the population with chronic nonmalignant pain through the development of a multiaxial pain assessment, which attempts to integrate medical–physical, psychosocial, and behavioral dimensions of the pain [17,18]. In this approach, an empirically derived psychosocial and behavioral classification, which categorizes patients into three groups ("dysfunctional," "interpersonally distressed," and "adaptive copers"), is combined with a medical–physical classification, such as the aforementioned taxonomy of pain developed by the International Association for the Study of Pain [4]. Validation of this model in clinical practice is needed, but it demonstrates well the complexity of chronic pain patients and the need to target specific factors that contribute to the pain, or are associated with it, through a multimodality treatment plan.

MANAGEMENT OF CHRONIC PAIN

The many treatments for chronic pain may be categorized into six broad categories (Table 1). Many patients with chronic pain benefit from a multimodality approach in which each of several treatments is targeted to the specific needs of the patient. The comprehensive assessment should provide the information necessary to select and coordinate these multiple modalities of therapy. For example, the patient who experiences chronic pain without severe disability or psychological disturbance may be well managed by the single knowledgeable practitioner who can administer one or more analgesic treatments. This model of care is completely appropriate for most patients with pain due to cancer, for example. The patient with a severe chronic pain syndrome, on the contrary, may be better served by a multidisciplinary, multimodality approach that emphasizes the rehabilitation of physical, psychological, and social functioning. In this group, the latter therapies are as important as primary analgesic treatments, and should be administered by specialists familiar with the vagaries of chronic pain management.

Patients must be told explicitly that the major therapeutic goals of all chronic pain therapy are comfort and function. For those with little pain-related disability, the need to maintain function should be stressed, even if no specific rehabilitative therapies are necessary. Those with compromised function, who require a more coordinated program, must often be encouraged in the strongest terms to accept the need for nonanalgesic (rehabilitative or psychotherapeutic) initiatives. Many patients who present for management of a chronic pain syndrome believe that the only goal of therapy is relief of pain, and that comfort alone will immediately lead to better function. These patients must be taught to redefine the clinical agenda so that functional considerations become at least as important as pain relief.

The traditional multidisciplinary pain clinic may provide optimal care

Table 1   Approaches Used in the Management of
Chronic Pain

Primary therapies directed against the underlying cause
Primary analgesic therapies
   Pharmacological approaches
   Anesthetic approaches
   Surgical approaches
   Physiatric approaches
   Neurostimulatory approaches
   Psychological approaches

---

for the subpopulation of patients with substantial pain-related disability, whose physical and psychosocial function is perceived to be a major target of therapy. Although the single practitioner could possibly organize a comprehensive approach for these patients through the development of a referral network, many of these patients present such complex interactions among symptoms, physical impairments, and functional disturbances that the coordinated skills of pain specialists in several disciplines are needed to elaborate an adequate multimodal therapeutic approach. It is the responsibility of the primary clinician to perform a comprehensive pain assessment, and thereby determine the need for this approach.

Pharmacological Approaches

Analgesic drugs can be classified into three categories: nonsteroidal anti-inflammatory drugs (NSAIDs), adjuvant analgesics, and opioids. Adjuvant analgesics are a diverse group of drugs in varied classes that have primary indications other than pain but are analgesic in selected circumstances. Although all three categories of analgesic drugs may be explored in any patient with chronic pain, the customary approach continues to emphasize the use of NSAIDs and adjuvant analgesics in the management of chronic nonmalignant pain and the use of opioids for pain due to cancer.

Nonsteroidal Anti-Inflammatory Drugs

The NSAIDs inhibit the enzyme cyclo-oxygenase and may thereby produce analgesia at a peripheral level by reducing tissue concentrations of inflammatory mediators known to sensitize or activate peripheral nociceptors [19,20]. A central analgesic mechanism may also be important [21], however, and could explain the marked disproportion between anti-inflammatory effects and the analgesia observed with some of these drugs, such as acetaminophen.

NSAID analgesia is characterized by a lack of demonstrable physical dependence or tolerance, and the existence of a ceiling dose. The ceiling dose, beyond which additional increments fail to yield greater pain relief, is unknown in any individual patient and, like the minimal effective dose and the dose associated with adverse effects, may be higher or lower than the standard recommended dose.

Drug Selection Numerous NSAIDs are available commercially [22] (Table 2). Relatively few have been specifically approved as analgesics, but clinical experience suggests that any can potentially be useful for this indication.

The risk of toxicity must be considered in the selection of NSAID therapy. All NSAIDs should be used cautiously in patients with kidney disease. Although acetaminophen has the potential for renal toxicity [23], it is generally the preferred drug in this setting. Acetaminophen is also preferred

Table 2   Nonsteroidal Anti-Inflammatory Drugs

Chemical Class	Generic Name	Approximate Half-Life (hr)	Dosing Schedule	Recommended Starting Dosage (mg/Day)[a]
p-Aminophenol derivatives	Acetaminophen[b]	2–4	q 4–6 hr	1400
Naphyl-alkanone	Nabumetone	20–35	q 24 hr	1000
Salicylates	Aspirin[b]	3–12[c]	q 4–6 hr	1400
	Diflunisal[b]	8–12	q 12 hr	1000 once, then 500 q 12 hr
	Choline magnesium trisalicylate[b]	8–12	q 12 hr	1500, then 1000 q 12 hr
	Salsalate	8–12	q 12 hr	1500, then 1000 q 12 hr
Proprionic acids	Ibuprofen[b]	3–4	q 4–8 hr	1200
	Naproxen[b]	13	q 12 hr	500
	Naproxen sodium[b]	13	q 12 hr	550
	Fenoprofen	2–3	q 6 hr	800
	Ketoprofen	2–3	q 6–8 hr	150
	Flurbiprofen[b]	5–6	q 8–12 hr	100
Acetic acids	Indomethacin	4–5	q 8–12 hr	75
	Tolmetin	1	q 6–8 hr	600
	Sulindac	14	q 12 hr	300

Maximum Recommended Dosage (mg/Day)	Comment
6000	Overdosage produces hepatic toxicity. Not anti-flammatory and therefore not preferred as first-line analgesic or coanalgesic in patients with bone pain. Lack of gastrointestinal (GI) or platelet toxicity, however, may be important in some patients with cancer. At high dosages, platelet counts and liver function tests should be done monthly.
2000	Experience too limited to evaluate higher doses. Once daily doses may be advantageous in some patients.
6000	Standard for comparison. May not be tolerated as well as some of the newer NSAIDs[d]
1500	Less GI toxicity than aspirin[d]
4000	Unlike other NSAIDs, choline magnesium trisalicylate and salsalate have minimal GI toxicity and no effect on platelet aggregation, despite potent anti-flammatory effects. May therefore be particularly useful in some patients with cancer.[d]
4000	
4200	Available over-the-counter[d]
1000	Available as a suspension. Some studies show greater efficacy of higher dosages, specifically 1500 mg/day, with little to no increase in adverse effects; long-term efficacy of this dosage and safety in a medically ill population are unknown, however, and it should be used cautiously in selected patients.[d]
1100	Some studies show greater efficacy of higher dosages, specifically 1650 mg/day, with little to no increase in adverse effects; long-term efficacy of this dosage and safety in a medically ill population are unknown, however and it should be used cautiously in selected patients.[d]
3200	[d]
300	[d]
300	Experience too limited to evaluate higher dosages, although it is likely that some patients would benefit.[d]
200	Available in sustained-release and rectal formulations. Higher incidence of side effects, particularly GI and central nervous system (CNS), than proprionic acids[d]
2000	[d]
400	Less renal toxicity than other NSAIDs.[d]

Table 2   (Continued)

Chemical Class	Generic Name	Approximate Half-Life (hr)	Dosing Schedule	Recommended Starting Dosage (mg/Day)[a]
	Diclofenac	2	q 6 hr	75
	Ketorolac	4–7	q 4–6 hr	150
Oxicams	Piroxicam	45	q 24 hr	20
Fenamates	Mefenamic acid[b]	2	q 6 hr	500, then 250 q 6 hr
	Meclofenamic acid	2–4	q 6–8 hr	150
Pyrazoles	Phenylbutazone	50–100	q 6–8 hr	300

[a]Starting dosage should be one-half to two-thirds recommended dosage in the elderly, those on multiple drugs, and those with renal insufficiency. Dosage must be individualized. Low initial dosage should be titrated upward if tolerated and clinical effect is inadequate. Dosage can be increased weekly. Studies of NSAIDs in patients with cancer are meager; dosing guidelines are thus empiric.

in patients with a history of a bleeding disorder or peptic ulcer disease. If the risk of bleeding or ulcer formation is relatively small and an NSAID with stronger anti-inflammatory effects would be preferable, the most reasonable choice is a nonacetylated salicylate, either choline magnesium salicylate or salsalate. The latter are less likely to produce gastropathy than other NSAIDs, and at usual clinical dosages, do not impair platelet aggregation [24]. All NSAIDs may cause fluid retention, and must therefore be administered cautiously to patients with congestive heart failure, peripheral edema, or ascites.

Drug-specific toxic effects must also be considered. For example, the pyrazole subclass, of which only phenylbutazone is presently available in the United States, is associated with a greater risk of adverse effects than the other NSAIDs and has been supplanted by newer drugs. High dosages of acetamin-

Maximum Recommended Dosage (mg/Day)	Comment
200	d
120	Parenteral formulation available. Experience limited to the treatment of acute pain, for which the maximum first day dosage has been 150 mg and the maximum daily dosage thereafter has been 120 mg. There is no experience yet with the chronic administration of this drug and both efficacy and safety of long-term administration remain to be determined. Experience is also too limited to evaluate higher dosage.
40	Administration of 40 mg for more than 3 weeks is associated with a high incidence of peptic ulcer, particularly in the elderly.[d]
1000	Not recommended for use longer than 1 week and therefore not indicated in the treatment of pain due to cancer[d]
400	d
400	Not a first-line drug due to risk of serious bone marrow toxicity. Not preferred for treatment of pain due to cancer.

[b]Pain is approved indication.
[c]Half-life of aspirin increases with dosage.
[d]At high dosage, stool guaiac tests should be done bimonthly and liver function tests, measurement of blood urea nitrogen (BUN), creatinine, and urinalysis should be checked every 1–2 months.

ophen may likewise cause hepatopathy, and pre-existing liver disease mandates prudence in the administration of this drug.

The availability of agents that may reduce the likelihood of NSAID-induced gastropathy could potentially influence drug selection. Unfortunately, the use of prophylactic agents remains controversial. The administration of misoprostol, a prostaglandin analog, diminishes the risk of gastric ulceration [25], but a recent study questions its cost-effectiveness in the absence of significant risk factors for gastrointestinal hemorrhage [26]. A study in normal individuals suggests that cimetidine, an H_2-blocker, can reduce gastropathy [27], but controlled trials have failed to confirm this benefit in patients during long-term treatment. Sucralfate reduces gastrointestinal symptoms but does not lower the incidence of ulceration, and omeprazole, a new hydrogen–potassium ATPase pump inhibitor, blocks gastric acid production and may be protective, but has not been adequately tested.

Given current information, it is reasonable to administer misoprostol concurrent with NSAID therapy to patients who have risk factors for gastric ulceration, including patients with a history of ulcer disease or gastritis, the elderly, those receiving corticosteroids, and those with recent upper abdominal pain or gastrointestinal side effects from NSAIDs. As noted, the use of a nonacetylated salicylate is also appropriate in patients in this group. Patients at high risk who cannot tolerate misoprostol might be considered for an alternative treatment, such as a combination of sucralfate and an H_2 blocker [28] or omeprazole.

Other factors may also be relevant in the selection of an NSAID. Given the known intraindividual variability in the response to different NSAIDs, the patient's previous experience with drugs in this class should be considered when treatment is selected. A drug that produced intolerable side effects in the past should be avoided, and, conversely, a drug that yielded very favorable effects should be considered more strongly. Concern about compliance or ease of administration may also be important. Patients who might benefit from the use of an NSAID on an "as needed" basis (e.g., those with intermittent pains) may prefer a drug with a short half-life, such as aspirin or ibuprofen, whereas those who would benefit from less frequent administration should receive an NSAID with once daily (e.g., piroxicam) or twice daily dosing (e.g., choline magnesium trisalicylate, diflunisal, naproxen, and others). Finally, the cost of the different NSAIDs varies widely, and if appropriate, decisions can be made on the basis of this factor.

An injectable formulation of an NSAID, ketorolac, has recently become available in the United States. This drug has efficacy comparable to morphine in the postoperative setting [29]. It is presently recommended for short-term use, and is particularly valuable for patients predisposed to adverse effects from opioids.

Dose–Response Relationship   The standard recommended dosage of an NSAID is empirically derived from dosage-ranging studies. These dosages may or may not be appropriate for the individual patient. In most cases, therefore, it is reasonable to explore the dose–response relationship through trials of escalating dosages. This is particularly important for patients who may be predisposed to adverse effects (e.g., the elderly or those with mild renal insufficiency). Administration should be initiated at a level below the standard recommended dosage, then increased on a weekly basis or less frequently. Through this process, the minimal effective dosage and the ceiling dosage may be identified. Given the potential for dose-related toxicities, including some effects for which there may be no effective forewarning (e.g., bleeding ulcer or renal failure), this process of dosage exploration should be limited by an empirical maximum dosage; a range of 1.5–2 times the standard dosage is reasonable for this purpose. Long-term therapy at dosages above the standard should be monitored more carefully with a test for occult fecal blood, urinalysis, and serum tests of renal and hepatic function on a bimonthly basis.

Duration of Trials   Several weeks are needed to evaluate the efficacy of an NSAIDs for the treatment of a grossly inflammatory lesion, such as arthritis. Based on clinical experience, a shorter period, such as a week, may be adequate for the same purpose in patients with pain without a grossly inflammatory lesion.

Switching Drugs   It is generally accepted that failure with one of the NSAIDs should be followed by a trial with another. The order of these sequential drug trials is currently selected empirically.

Adjuvant Analgesics

The term "adjuvant analgesic" refers to a diverse group of drugs that have primary indications other than pain but are analgesic in selected circumstances. This group comprises specific drugs in varied drug classes (Table 3).

Several principles guide the selection and administration of the adjuvant analgesics. First, the optimal use of these drugs requires a comprehensive assessment of the patient. The information acquired from this assessment may allow more rational selection of a drug on the basis of specific characteristics of the pain or patient, and encourages the integration of pharmacotherapy with other pain-related interventions. Second, appropriate treatment with these agents depends on the clinician's knowledge of their pharmacology and appreciation for the differences between the use of each drug for its primary indication and its use as an analgesic. Third, dosing guidelines, as described below, must recognize the large interindividual and intraindividual variability that characterizes the response to these drugs.

Finally, polypharmacy must be recognized as a necessary approach for many patients. Although single-agent therapy is preferable, the combined use of analgesic drugs may yield enough benefit to justify the increased risk of adverse drug effects. Various combinations of an opioid, NSAID, and one or more adjuvant analgesic are commonly used. A rational approach to the institution of multiple adjuvant analgesics follows from the guidelines applied for each agent. A drug should be selected and the dosage adjusted to clarify the risk/benefit relationship. Treatment should be discontinued if the drug does not produce meaningful analgesia at a maximally safe or tolerated dosage. If such a dosage yields meaningful partial analgesia, the treatment should usually be maintained, even if the overall relief is not adequate. In the latter situation, consideration should then be given to a trial of second drug, usually from a different class. This process can potentially identify a group of

Table 3   Adjuvant Analgesics

Drug Class	Examples
Antidepressants	
Tricyclic antidepressants	Amitriptyline
	Doxepin
	Imipramine
	Nortriptyline
	Desipramine
"Newer" antidepressants	Trazodone
	Fluoxetine
	Maprotiline
	Paroxetine
Monoamine oxidase inhibitors	Phenelzine
Anticonvulsants	Carbamazepine
	Phenytoin
	Valproate
	Clonazepam
Oral local anesthetics	Mexiletine
	Tocainide
Neuroleptics	Fluphenazine
	Haloperidol
	Methotrimeprazine
	Pimozide
Muscle relaxants	Orphenadrine
	Carisoprodol
	Methocarbamol
	Chlorzoxazone
	Cyclobenzaprine
Antihistamines	Hydroxyzine
Psychostimulants	Caffeine
	Methylphenidate
	Dextroamphetamine
Corticosteroids	Dexamethasone
	Prednisone
	Methylprednisolone
Sympatholytic drugs	Prazosin
	Phenoxybenzamine
Calcium channel blockers	Nifedipine
Miscellaneous	Baclofen
	Clonidine
	Capsaicin

drugs, each of which contributes sufficient analgesia to warrant continued treatment, but none of which possesses enough efficacy to sustain therapy alone. As long as the overall benefits exceed adverse drug effects (including both side effects and potentially negative effects on function), and patients undergo assessment with periodic consideration of drug holidays or dosage reduction, this approach is acceptable.

Antidepressants   Tricyclic antidepressants (TCAs) have demonstrated analgesic effects in many chronic pain syndromes [30–33]. Analgesic effects were first believed to be related to specific antidepressant effects, but this conclusion has been negated by numerous observations, including the occurrence of analgesia earlier than mood change in patients with chronic pain and the development of analgesia in patients with chronic pain without depression [34,35]. Analgesic effects have also been demonstrated in animal models [36].

   The analgesic action of TCA drugs may be due to enhanced activity in monoamine-dependent endogenous pain-modulating pathways [6,37]. Both tertiary amine compounds (e.g., amitriptyline), whose activity is relatively greatest at serotonin synapses, and secondary amine TCAs (e.g., nortriptyline and desipramine), which have relatively selective effects at norepinephrine synapses, are analgesic. TCAs also bind to many other receptors [38,39], some of which use neurotransmitters and neuromodulators that have been implicated in the process of pain modulation [6,40]. The potential interactions of the TCAs with endogenous pain-modulating pathways are thus complex and have prevented the clear elucidation of the analgesic mechanism of these drugs.

   Many controlled trials have confirmed the analgesic efficacy of the TCAs. These studies have demonstrated that amitriptyline is analgesic in patients with diabetic neuropathy, postherpetic neuralgia, tension and migraine headache, myofascial pain, and psychogenic pain [34,35,41–43]. Imipramine was effective in patients with arthritis [44] and painful diabetic neuropathy [45], and doxepin was analgesic in those with psychogenic headache [46] and coexistent chronic pain and depression [47]. Desipramine was demonstrated to be analgesic in patients with postherpetic neuralgia and diabetic neuropathy [32], and clomipramine was efficacious in several pain syndromes [48].

   Studies of the "newer" antidepressants have yielded more equivocal results. Maprotiline was favorably compared with amitriptyline in the treatment of postherpetic neuralgia [49]. One study suggested that trazodone was effective in patients with pain due to cancer [50], but another could not confirm analgesic effects from this drug when administered to patients with pain due to traumatic myelopathy [51]. Zimelidine, which is similar to trazodone in its relative selectivity at the serotonin synapse, was analgesic in a controlled trial of patients with mixed organic and psychogenic pain syndromes [52], but was ineffective in an open-label comparison against amitriptyline in patients with postherpetic neuralgia [53]. Convincing analgesic effects were identified in a study of another selective serotonin reuptake inhibitor, paroxetine [54]. Zimelidine is not currently available in the United States. There have been no published controlled analgesic trials of fluoxetine, and clinical experience with this drug has been disappointing.

Monoamine oxidase inhibitors, which also increase the availability of central monoamines, may also be analgesic. These agents are used in the treatment of refractory migraine [55] and a controlled trial in patients demonstrated analgesia in patients with atypical facial pain [56]. Given the potential for hypertensive crisis after ingestion of tyramine-containing foodstuffs, however, the use of these drugs cannot be recommended except in the situation of severe refractory vascular headache. If a monoamine oxidase inhibitor is considered, dietary restrictions must be explained to the patient and a list provided of prescription and over-the-counter medications that may interact adversely with these drugs. It must also be recognized that meperidine is absolutely contraindicated in patients who are receiving a monoamine oxidase inhibitor due to the risk of a serious hyperpyrexic syndrome.

A trial of a TCA should be considered in virtually all patients with chronic pain. Those with neuropathic pain, who often respond poorly to other modalities, are a particularly important subgroup. Data from controlled studies suggest that diverse neuropathic pains may respond, including those characterized by continuous dysesthesias and by lancinating dysesthesias [32]. Clinical experience strongly confirms the potential efficacy of these drugs in patients with continuous dysesthesias; the response of lancinating pains is more variable, and it may be reasonable to consider the TCAs as second-line agents for these pains, most efficiently used after an anticonvulsant or two, baclofen, and perhaps an oral local anesthetic fails (see below).

Contraindications to the use of the TCAs include significant cardiac arrhythmias, symptomatic prostatic hypertrophy, and narrow-angle glaucoma. Given the supporting data from controlled studies, a tertiary amine TCA, specifically amitriptyline, doxepin, imipramine, or clomipramine, is preferred as the initial trial; the evidence for analgesic effects is greatest for amitriptyline. Patients who experience intolerable side effects from one of these agents, or are predisposed to side effects, should undergo a trial with a secondary amine TCA, specifically nortriptyline or desipramine.

Dosing guidelines for the use of TCAs as analgesics are amply supported by clinical experience. Initial dosages of the tertiary amine compounds should be low, such as 10–25 mg at night. Dosages should be increased gradually over 1–2 weeks to 50–150 mg at night; the rate of escalation should be selected based on the severity of the pain, the occurrence of early favorable responses, and the patient's ability to tolerate the side effects of the drug. If possible, the dosage should be held in this range for a week or so before upward titration is resumed. Analgesic effects usually begin 4–7 days after an effective dosage is reached. With the exception of nortriptyline, the analgesic dose range for the TCA drugs is typically 50–150 mg per night [32,34]. The usually effective dosage for nortriptyline is not known, but may be lower. Most patients can be adequately treated with a single nighttime dose, but some experience waning of analgesic effects toward evening and are better managed with twice-daily dosing.

Some studies have suggested that analgesia is a dose-dependent effect [34]. Upward titration of the dose should continue if neither analgesia nor intolerable side effects occur in the usual therapeutic range. Higher dosages may also be needed if depression is prominent. Although the plasma level associated with analgesic effects is unknown, measurement of plasma TCA concentration is useful if analgesic effects do not occur as the usual therapeutic range is approached. Relatively low plasma concentration suggests that noncompliance, poor absorption, or unusually rapid catabolism may be compromising therapy. In the absence of side effects, dosages should be increased until plasma concentration is in the antidepressant range. At the present time, there is no justification to seek analgesic effects at dosages that yield a plasma concentration higher than this. The existence of a biphasic analgesic response (loss of efficacy as the dosage is increased) during treatment with nortriptyline has been suggested in anecdotal evidence, but confirmatory data are lacking. If such an effect exists with any of the TCAs, it is unlikely to pose a clinical problem if low initial dosages and upward titration are used.

Anticonvulsants   Anticonvulsant medications (Table 3) have become widely accepted in the management of chronic neuropathic pain syndromes characterized by lancinating pains [57]. The mechanism of analgesia is unknown, but presumably relates to the mechanisms that underlie anticonvulsant effects, such as the capacity to suppress paroxysmal discharges, neuronal hyperexcitability, or spread of abnormal discharges [58]. Spontaneous and paroxysmal electrical activity can be produced by nerve injury and may be the substrate on which anticonvulsants act to reduce pain in these conditions [59–62].

Case series have suggested that phenytoin is effective in trigeminal neuralgia [3,64], and favorable effects of this drugs have been reported in patients with glossopharyngeal neuralgia, tabetic lightning pains, paroxysmal pain in postherpetic neuralgia, thalamic pain, postsympathectomy pain, and posttraumatic neuralgia [65–67]. A controlled trial has confirmed that beneficial effects are produced in patients with painful diabetic neuropathy [68]. As noted, most of the neuropathic pains in these syndromes were characterized by a prominent lancinating component.

Controlled trials have established the efficacy of carbamazepine in trigeminal neuralgia, in the lancinating (but not continuous) pains of postherpetic neuralgia, and in painful diabetic neuropathy [69–71]. Case reports have also suggested that patients with glossopharyngeal neuralgia, tabetic lightning pains, paroxysmal pain in multiple sclerosis, postsympathectomy pain, lancinating pains due to cancer, and posttraumatic neuralgia may benefit from this drug [67,72–75].

Uncontrolled clinical trials and anecdotal reports have similarly depicted favorable outcomes in patients with varied neuropathic pains following treatment with clonazepam or valproate. Clonazepam has been reported to be useful in the treatment of trigeminal neuralgia, paroxysmal postlaminectomy pain, and posttraumatic neuralgia [67,76,77], and valproate was beneficial in the management of trigeminal neuralgia, postherpetic neuralgia, and other pains [67,78].

Several agents that are not anticonvulsants have also been demonstrated to have analgesic effects in trigeminal neuralgia and are, therefore, considered with the aforementioned agents as potential treatments for patients with lancinating neuropathic pains. Baclofen, a gamma-aminobutyric acid (GABA) agonist approved for the treatment of spasticity, is a second-line agent in the treatment of trigeminal neuralgia [79]. This drug has a favorable safety profile and should be considered for the treatment of lancinating neuropathic pains of any type. The finding that an oral local anesthetic, tocainide, is effective in trigeminal neuralgia [80] likewise justifies a therapeutic trial with drugs in this class for any refractory lancinating pain. Mexiletine is widely regarded to be the safest available oral local anesthetic (see below) and is preferred for this indication. Pimozide is a neuroleptic recently demonstrated to be analgesic in trigeminal neuralgia [81]. As discussed below, the potential adverse effects of the neuroleptics during long-term administration suggest that the use of pimozide for lancinating neuropathic pains should be reserved for patients who fail to respond to other agents.

Although the clearest indication for a trial of one of the aforementioned drugs is a lancinating neuropathic pain, occasional patients with refractory continuous dysesthesias respond favorably. Hence, a therapeutic trial of one or more of these agents may be appropriate in these pain syndromes following failed attempts with TCAs and other drugs, particularly an oral local anesthetic (see below). The use of an anticonvulsant or related agent for nonneuropathic pains is not supported by available data.

In all cases, drugs are administered as they are for their primary indication. A conservative oral loading dosage of phenytoin is reasonable, but the other drugs should be initiated at low dosages, then gradually titrated upward until limiting side effects occur or the plasma concentration exceeds the therapeutic range. Patients may have markedly different analgesic responses to the various anticonvulsant drugs [67], and sequential trials should be considered in refractory cases.

Oral Local Anesthetics The potential for analgesic effects from systemically administered local anesthetics has been appreciated for many years [82] and the advent of oral formulations has opened new possibilities for analgesic therapy. As noted previously, the efficacy of tocainide has been established in trigeminal neuralgia [80]. A carefully controlled trial has also demonstrated the efficacy of mexiletine in patients with painful diabetic polyneuropathy [83]. Together, these data suggest that oral local anesthetics can be effective drugs for either lancinating or continuous dysesthesias. Mexiletine is the safest compound [84], and a trial of this drug should be considered for neuropathic pain of any type. Dosing is empiric and should mimic that applied in the treatment of cardiac arrhythmias.

Neuroleptics Numerous surveys have suggested that haloperidol, fluphenazine, perphenazine, thioridazine, chlorprothixene, and chlorpromazine can be analgesic in a variety of painful disorders, including refractory neuropathic pain syndromes [85–88]. There are, however, very few controlled confirmatory studies. The analgesic efficacy of methotrimeprazine has been established [89], and this drug, which is available in a parenteral formulation and has prominent sedative and hypotensive effects, is commonly used in the management of patients with advanced cancer. As discussed previously, pimozide has been suggested to be effective in trigeminal neuralgia [81], and can be considered a second-line agent in the management of lancinating neuropathic pains. A controlled single-dose study failed to confirm the efficacy of chlorpromazine [90].

Given the meager data supporting the analgesic efficacy of neuroleptic drugs and the risk of serious movement disorders associated with their long-term use, it is appropriate to restrict therapeutic trials to patients with intractable neuropathic pain. Clinical experience is greatest with fluphenazine and haloperidol. Dosages reported to be effective are generally low, and concerns about side effects usually limit dosage titration.

Clonidine Clonidine is an alpha-2 adrenergic agonist that has proven analgesic effects [91]. Although long-term analgesic trials of oral or transdermal clonidine have not been conducted, the drug has been used to treat chronic and recurrent pains [92,93], and clinical experience supports therapeutic trials in patients with refractory pain, including neuropathic pains.

Calcitonin A recent controlled trial has demonstrated that treatment with intravenous calcitonin can have beneficial effects in patients with phantom limb pain, at least during the early stages of this syndrome [94]. Another

controlled trial demonstrated benefit from intranasal calcitonin in patients
with sympathetically maintained pain [95]. Although the mechanism of
analgesic action in these disorders is not known and confirmatory studies are
needed, it is reasonable to consider this treatment in refractory cases of these
neuropathic pains.

Muscle Relaxants   The so-called muscle relaxant drugs, which are usually
administered in the treatment of acute musculoskeletal pains, must be
differentiated from drugs used for muscle spasm and those indicated for
spasticity. Musculoskeletal pains, which often relate to acute sprains or
strains, may or may not be associated with muscle spasm, which is a focal area
of increased muscle activity associated with tenderness and splinting of the
painful part. Spasticity, which is usually not painful, typically involves a large
region of hypertonicity and results from a lesion in the central nervous
system. Muscle relaxant drugs may be helpful in the treatment of acute
musculoskeletal pain, but are not specifically useful in relieving muscle
spasm. Drugs useful in the treatment of true spasticity, such as baclofen and
dantrolene, are not indicated for common musculoskeletal pains or spasm,
and muscle relaxant drugs are not indicated in the treatment of true spasticity. The exception to these distinctions is diazepam, which may be useful
in all three conditions.

The muscle relaxant drugs include orphenadrine, carisoprodol, chlor-
zoxazone, methocarbamol, and cyclobenzaprine (Table 3). Controlled studies
have demonstrated efficacy greater than placebo for each of these agents in
the treatment of musculoskeletal pain [96,97]. Some studies favorably compare one of these drugs to aspirin or acetaminophen, or demonstrate that the
analgesia obtained from the combination of a muscle relaxant and either
aspirin or acetaminophen is greater than that provided by the analgesic alone
[98]. There have been no long-term repeated dose studies or trials in which
the various muscle relaxant drugs were compared to each other or to different
NSAIDs, opioids, or sedative/hypnotic drugs.

The mechanism of the analgesic effects produced by the muscle relaxant
drugs is conjectural. These agents suppress polysynaptic myogenic reflexes in
experimental preparations [99], but the relevance of this phenomenon is not
known. There is no evidence that they actually reduce contraction of striated
muscle. Thus, these are clearly analgesic drugs, but the available data are
inadequate to determine whether these favorable responses are due to
nonspecific sedative effects, a primary analgesic effect, a partial lessening of
muscle tension, or some combination of these effects.

Short-term therapy with muscle relaxant drugs is commonly accepted
in the treatment of acute musculoskeletal pain, and there are sufficient data
to confirm the safety and efficacy of this approach. Both the selection of a
specific drug and dosing are empirical, and there is no evidence that upward

titration beyond usually recommended dosages produces any other effect than progressive sedation, with an unknown degree of accruing risk. There are no studies of chronic treatment, and anecdotal data originating from multidisciplinary pain programs indicate that some patients may misuse or abuse these drugs, or, at least, use them in a manner that appears to compromise rehabilitative efforts. Given these observations, long-term treatment should be undertaken cautiously, with continued assessment of efficacy and side effects.

Benzodiazepines Single-dose controlled studies in the postoperative setting have concluded that some of the benzodiazepine drugs are analgesic. In a recent open-label trial, alprazolam provided analgesia to patients with neuropathic cancer-related pain [100]. In contrast, a small controlled study of chlordiazepoxide failed to demonstrate any benefit [101].

Although benzodiazepines may have analgesic effects, concerns about adverse cognitive effects and abuse have limited their use. With the exception of diazepam, which is commonly administered for the treatment of acute musculoskeletal pain (particularly if associated with clear muscle spasm), these drugs are not usually offered for a primary pain indication. However, some patients who receive a benzodiazepine for anxiety or acute muscle spasm report very positive analgesic effects, and occasional patients appear to obtain sustained benefits, similar to the sustained anxiolytic effects sometimes observed in patients who are administered these drugs for a primary indication of anxiety. It may be reasonable to continue treatment in such circumstances, as long as the patient can be closely monitored and continued benefits without adverse pharmacological effects or abuse can be documented.

Antihistamines Numerous studies, including some controlled trials, have demonstrated the analgesic efficacy of antihistamine drugs, including orphenadrine, diphenhydramine, hydroxyzine, and others [97,98,102,103]. The mechanisms of these analgesic effects are not known, but could potentially relate to the existence of specific histamine receptors in the endogenous pathways for pain modulation [102].

Although the data from studies have been favorable, clinical experience has not confirmed the utility of antihistamines as analgesics. These drugs are used in combination products marketed as minor analgesics, usually for headache, and orphenadrine is administered as a muscle relaxant.

Drugs for Sympathetically Maintained Pain Patients with sympathetically maintained pain (reflex sympathetic dystrophy or causalgia) who are unable to tolerate nerve blocks, or have failed to benefit from these procedures, have been empirically treated with sympatholytic drugs. Case reports and clinical series have demonstrated favorable effects from phenoxybenzamine [104],

prazocin [105], oral guanethidine [106], and propranolol [107]. Corticosteroids [108] and nifedipine [109] have also been suggested to be useful in
anecdotal reports, and as noted above, calcitonin was recently reported to be
useful [95].

Psychostimulant Drugs   Psychostimulant drugs, specifically dextroamphetamine, methylphenidate, and caffeine, are analgesic [110–112]. Caffeine is
commonly added to combination products marketed as headache remedies,
and both dextroamphetamine and methylphenidate are used to reverse
opioid-induced sedation in patients with pain due to cancer.

Miscellaneous Drugs   Analgesic effects have been established for both cannabinoid drugs and L-tryptophan, but neither are in clinical use for the
indication of pain. The psychotomimetic side effects observed during trials of
cannabinoid drugs have discouraged additional analgesic studies or anecdotal
trials of these agents for a primary indication of pain. Cannabinoids are used
as antiemetics in patients with cancer. L-Tryptophan is also analgesic and was
used anecdotally until several years ago, at which time an association with a
rare systemic disease, eosinophilia–myalgia syndrome, was confirmed. The
drug has been removed from the market in the United States and can no
longer be recommended where still available.

Opioid Analgesics

The administration of opioid analgesics is strongly encouraged in the treatment of chronic cancer pain, and guidelines for use in the population with
cancer have achieved a broad consensus [1–3]. In contrast, chronic administration of opioids for nonmalignant pain has traditionally been rejected due to
persistent concerns about the potential for loss of efficacy over time (i.e., the
development of tolerance), adverse pharmacological effects, and most importantly, the development of addiction. Recently, however, the potential benefits to selected patients from this approach have been suggested in numerous
surveys [113–118]. The patients reported in these surveys were treated with
opioids for long periods, obtained sustained partial analgesia (in some cases
associated with improved functioning), and did not present untoward problems related to adverse pharmacological effects or abuse.

   This experience has led to a critical reappraisal of the concerns that have
heretofore justified the general rejection of this approach [119]. For example,
the notion that analgesic tolerance inevitably results in the gradual loss of
efficacy is contradicted by numerous surveys performed in the population
with cancer [120–122], as well as the aforementioned surveys of patients with
nonmalignant pain. For reasons that are not understood, analgesic tolerance
is rarely the "driving force" for dosage escalation in the clinical setting; in the
absence of a progressive lesion capable of increasing pain, opioid dosages

usually remain stable. Hence, the potential for tolerance should not justify the decision to withhold chronic opioid therapy.

Some of the concerns about the potential for addiction may relate to confusion in the nomenclature of drug dependence, specifically the misidentification of physical dependence as addiction. Physical dependence is a pharmacological property of opioid drugs, and other compounds, characterized solely by the potential for an abstinence syndrome following abrupt dosage reduction or administration of an antagonist drug. Extensive experience in the population with cancer strongly suggests that the phenomenon of physical dependence poses no clinical burden as long as drug dosages are tapered and antagonist drugs avoided.

Addiction may be defined as a psychological and behavioral syndrome characterized by psychological dependence, compulsive drug use, and other aberrant drug-related behaviors. Patients who become addicted to a substance demonstrate loss of control, compulsive behaviors, and continued use despite harm to themselves or others. Unlike physical dependence, the phenomenon of addiction is a serious adverse outcome that must be addressed as a potential risk during chronic opioid therapy.

Abundant data can be adduced to support the view that addiction is extraordinarily rare among patients with no prior history of substance abuse who are administered opioids for painful medical disease [119,123–125]. The concern that long-term exposure to these drugs, by itself, can lead to addiction is strongly negated by the highly favorable experience with this therapy in the population with cancer. This clinical experience, combined with research in the population of addicts indicates that addiction represents the final outcome of a complex set of determinants, some related to properties inherent in a drug and others to characteristics of the individual. Genetic, psychological, social, and situational factors are all probably involved. Mere exposure to an opioid, or any other drug that has potentially inherent reinforcing effects, is not a sufficient condition for the development of addiction.

Although studies are needed to confirm the efficacy and safety of long-term opioid therapy for patients with nonmalignant pain and define the populations most likely to benefit, current data strongly suggest that this approach is a useful alternative for a selected group of these patients. At the present time, clinical experience suggests that a prior history of substance abuse may increase the likelihood of problems during therapy and should be viewed as a relative contraindication. For the large majority of patients without this history, chronic opioid therapy might be considered as a means of providing increased comfort after other reasonable approaches have failed. Guidelines for management have been suggested (Table 4).

Table 4 Proposed Guidelines in the Management of Opioid Therapy for
Nonmalignant Pain

1. Should be considered only after all other reasonable attempts at analgesia have
failed.
2. A history of substance abuse should be viewed as a relative contraindication.
3. A single practitioner should take primary responsibility for treatment.
4. Patients should give informed consent before the start of therapy; points to be
covered include recognition of the low risk of psychological dependence as an
outcome, potential for cognitive impairment with the drug alone and in combination with sedative/hypnotics, and understanding by female patients that children
born when the mother is receiving opioid maintenance therapy will likely be
physically dependent at birth.
5. After drug selection, doses should be given on an around-the-clock basis; several
weeks should be agreed upon as the period of initial dosage titration. Although
improvement in function should be continually stressed, all should agree to at
least partial analgesia as the appropriate goal of therapy.
6. Failure to achieve at least partial analgesia at relatively low initial dosages in the
nontolerant patient raises questions about the potential treatability of the pain
syndrome with opioids.
7. Emphasis should be given to attempts to capitalize on improved analgesia by
gains in physical and social function.
8. In addition to the daily dosage determined initially, patients should be permitted
to escalate the dosage transiently on days of increased pain. Two methods are
acceptable:
    A. Prescription of an additional four to six "rescue doses" to be taken as needed
    during the month.
    B. Instruction that one or two extra doses may be taken on any day, but must be
    followed by an equal reduction of dose on subsequent days.
9. Most patients must be seen and drugs prescribed at least monthly. Patients
should be assessed during each visit for the efficacy of treatment, adverse drug
effects, and the appearance of either misuse or abuse of the drugs. The results of
the assessment should be clearly documented in the medical record.
10. Exacerbations of pain not effectively treated by transient, small increases in
dosage are best managed in the hospital, where dosage escalation, if appropriate,
can be observed closely and return to baseline dosages can be accomplished in a
controlled environment.
11. Evidence of drug hoarding, acquisition of drugs from other physicians, uncontrolled dosage escalation, or other aberrant behaviors should be followed by
tapering and discontinuation of opioid maintenance therapy.

Rehabilitation Approaches

Rehabilitation approaches epitomize the dual objectives of chronic pain management: functional restoration and comfort. Beyond comprehensive physical therapy and occupational therapy programs, physiatric approaches include the use of assistive devices and numerous physical modalities, such as electrical stimulation techniques and the application of therapeutic heat and cold. Biofeedback, trigger point injections, behavioral modification techniques, acupuncture, and newer technologies such as low-energy lasers are also applied in rehabilitation settings. Patients treated within a multidisciplinary pain management model may receive the latter therapies by various specialists on the team, under medical supervision.

The proper application of physiatric approaches should consider realistic short-term and long-term goals; guidelines for therapists, including the weight-bearing status of all limbs and any precautions that must be observed; and the frequency and duration of therapy. When physical or occupational therapists are involved, or rehabilitation approaches are integrated with treatments directed by specialists in other disciplines, the goals of therapy are facilitated by regular team meetings, which review both the medical and rehabilitation progress of the patient and ensure that adjustments can be made.

Physical Modalities

Physical modalities are widely used in the management of soft tissue, orthopedic, and neuropathic pain syndromes [126–130]. In addition to their ability to decrease pain, these techniques may have beneficial secondary effects, such as improved tissue compliance with heating or reduction of inflammation with cold [127]. In all cases, they should be selected with specific goals in mind and coordinated with other approaches based on a comprehensive assessment of the patient.

Therapeutic Heat   The application of heat to a painful body part is one of the oldest forms of analgesic intervention, dating to antiquity [126]. The potential benefits of heat include local and systemic relaxation, increase in local blood flow, increase in tissue compliance, and analgesia.

Therapeutic heat may be administered through a variety of means [127,128]. Selection of the appropriate diathermy technique in an individual case depends on the amount of heating desired, the depth and type of tissues to be heated, and where the patient will be treated (bedside or physical therapy area). Regardless of the technique chosen, several precautions apply in the administration of either superficial or deep heat. Most important is the avoidance of insensate areas, ischemic regions, and tissues adjacent to neoplasms. Patients who are unable to communicate and those with bleeding diatheses should not be treated, and paralyzed patients require close supervision during therapy.

Superficial heating of tissue (i.e., less than 1.5 cm penetration) may be readily accomplished with the use of hot packs, heating pads, radiant heat lamps, and hydrotherapy. Hot packs, which deliver heat through conduction, are simple to use and can be applied easily to most areas. Common types of hot packs include the Kenny and hydrocolator pack. Electrically powered heating pads are also useful, and may offer advantages over conventional packs because they provide heat at a relatively constant temperature for a more prolonged period. These devices must be applied cautiously, however, since prolonged periods of heat exposure may cause burning. Radiant heat may be produced by either white or infrared light, and provides heating through conversion of electromagnetic energy to heat. The amount of heat administered to the patient by these units depends on the distance from the light source, among other factors, and is somewhat more difficult to control.

Hydrotherapy also may be used as a form of superficial heat. Common devices available include the whirlpool, which is used for limb immersion, and the much larger Hubbard tank, which can accommodate the entire person. The swimming pool is another version of hydrotherapy. Hospital pools come in a wide variety of sizes and may be used to provide exercise, relaxation, or ambulation training to the patient with pain. Patients with painful soft tissue or arthritic conditions may find the use of the pool to be an effective analgesic intervention.

Ultrasound, short-wave diathermy, and microwave units are used to heat deeper tissues. The selection of the device is determined by the desired amount and depth of heat to be delivered. Ultrasound is probably the most frequently used, and may be effective in a variety of painful musculoskeletal disorders. In this technique, sound waves generated through piezoelectric crystals are directed into the patient, where their interaction with tissue interfaces that differ in sound absorption qualities leads to the production of heat. Heat generation is greatest at bone and ligament interfaces, and in joint capsules, where temperature may increase as much as 5°C.

Ultrasound may also be used to effect phonophoresis of analgesic substances. Phonophoresis is the ability of ultrasound energy to drive biologically active agents into body tissues by combining them with the conducting medium used with the device. Cortisol and lidocaine have been administered to soft tissues this way [126].

Clinical experience suggests that ultrasound may provide analgesia to patients with diverse musculoskeletal disorders, including those with joint ankylosis, contractures, muscle spasms, exacerbations of chronic low back pain, and tendinitis or bursitis; some patients with postherpetic neuralgia or sympathetically maintained pain also appear to benefit [126,128,131]. Ultrasound should not be used in proximity to fluid-filled cavities (i.e., orbit, gravid uterus), or near the heart, nerve ganglia, infections, and neoplastic tissues. Special care also should be taken to avoid the application of ultrasound over endoprosthetic implants (metal or plastic) and areas in which methylmethacrylate was used.

Cryotherapy   Therapeutic cold may diminish inflammation, decrease muscle spasm, and reduce pain [126–128,132]. The mechanisms that result in these effects are poorly understood. Theories proffered to explain the benefits of cold application have variably suggested a role for decreased receptor function, slowed conduction in nociceptive fibers, or attenuated inflammatory responses. None of these explanations has been confirmed.

Cold is most effective in patients with musculoskeletal pain. The application of cold alone has been extensively used to treat acute and chronic myofascial pain syndromes, and cold in conjunction with heat (contrast baths) has been effective in rheumatological disorders.

Cold therapy may be applied through ice massage, cold packs, or the administration of vapocoolant sprays, such as ethylchloride or fluorimethane. Contraindications include insensate tissue, ischemic regions, and a history of Raynaud's syndrome or other cold hypersensitivity.

Assistive Devices and Orthoses

Assistive devices and orthoses are frequently prescribed in the management of physical impairments. The analgesic potential in these devices is poorly appreciated. Orthoses, which may provide support, relieve stress, or supplant the function of weakened joints, may also stabilize, immobilize, or unload painful tissues. These appliances, which may be prefabricated or custom-molded, can be fitted to virtually any joint in the body [133–135]. The most frequently prescribed in the treatment of pain are spinal braces, which are appropriate for patients with back pain caused by any of a variety of causes.

The optimal back brace depends on the level of disease, amount of stabilization required, and patient tolerance [135–138]. When the spine is stable and not at risk for further injury, soft prefabricated devices, such as neck collars, corsets, or sacroiliac belts, may suffice. These devices are easily fitted and are usually well tolerated. If they do not afford adequate pain relief, a trial of a more restrictive device may be attempted. For those individuals with compromised spinal integrity in need of greater stabilization, rigid orthoses are available. The custom-molded plastic body jacket provides maximum orthotic control and immobilization of the spine.

Contraindications for the use of bracing are few. Insensate, injured, or hyperpathic tissue may preclude the use of devices that come in direct contact with skin, especially if the patient's mental status is compromised.

Patients who are obese, or rely on accessory abdominal breathing, may not tolerate the binding of the abdomen that results from corsets and other back braces. Although there have been concerns about the potential for deleterious effects from long-term bracing, including weakening of abdominal or spinal muscles and decreased calcium deposition in the spine, recent evidence has been reassuring about the safety of this approach [139]. Patients with painful musculoskeletal disorders should undergo expert evaluation to determine the potential for analgesia or functional benefits that could result from bracing of the painful site.

Assistive devices refer to crutches, canes (both straight and four-pronged), and a variety of walkers. These are used to aid in ambulation by increasing ground contact points. They lessen weight bearing by altering the distribution of mass while ambulating, and, in patients with paretic limbs, supplant lost function and thus promote independence and mobility [133, 140]. These devices may have important analgesic consequences in patients with pain on walking. For example, patients with hip pain may greatly benefit from the use of a cane in the contralateral hand while ambulating. This causes weight to be distributed between the painful leg and the assistive device, which may ameliorate pain by reducing both the weight borne by the joint and the intrinsic muscle forces that act upon this region. Weight bearing on a painful limb may be reduced up to 25% by the use of a cane, as much as 45% by use of a single arm crutch, and almost completely by double-supported ambulation from either crutches or walkers [141].

The safe and effective use of assistive devices requires a good fit and integrity of the upper extremity and shoulder girdle. Weight transfer from the lower extremities to the arm may predispose the patient to joint pain and bony injury if degenerative or metastatic disease is present. In the presence of neoplastic involvement of the arm or shoulder, a variety of adaptations can be made to the assistive device to protect the patient. Assistive devices should also be used with caution in patients with impaired mental status. Falls from improper use of leg braces, canes, or crutches can have devastating consequences, including fractures and head injury.

Comprehensive Rehabilitation Programs

In many cases, the difference between an inpatient or outpatient multidisciplinary pain treatment program and a rehabilitation program is only a matter of emphasis. Both include intensive physical therapy and physical medicine techniques, and many offer specific vocational counseling. Pain programs usually provide a stronger psychotherapy component, specifically behavioral therapy and training in cognitive techniques, and all address analgesic drug use in a systematic way. Although an approach that lacks these other components is probably not optimal for pain management, a comprehensive rehabilitation program of any type may be considered for the patient with a chronic pain syndrome who lacks access to a formal pain management program. This is particularly appropriate when pain-related disability is high. The outcome of such programs, as measured by return of the patient to premorbid levels of activity, vary [142,143], but favorable results are clearly possible [144]. It is likely that successful outcome relates to adequate patient selection, which, in turn, is based on the type of comprehensive assessment described previously.

Anesthetic Approaches

Therapies traditionally considered to be within the purview of anesthesiologists play an important role in the management of chronic pain. The most important of these techniques include neural blockade and intraspinal treatments.

Neural blockade refers to a large group of procedures that transiently or more permanently block sympathetic and/or somatic nerves [145,146]. Temporary nerve blocks, which are accomplished with local anesthetic, have been categorized as diagnostic, prognostic, or therapeutic. Diagnostic blocks help to clarify the afferent neural pathways involved in the experience of pain. Prognostic blocks are traditionally used to evaluate the utility of a subsequent neurolytic procedure. The predictive value of these blocks has not been proved, but they are commonly used clinically as an aid to patient selection. Although a favorable response to a temporary block does not predict permanent relief following neurolysis, the failure to achieve pain relief with local anesthetic suggests that neurolysis will be ineffective, and such patients are typically excluded. Finally, local anesthetic blocks can be therapeutic in chronic pain if relief outlasts the duration of the drug. For example, repeated sympathetic blocks with local anesthetic are considered a mainstay approach for sympathetically maintained neuropathic pains. Therapeutic neurolytic nerve blocks are an important modality in cancer pain management, but are only rarely considered in the population with nonmalignant pain.

Local anesthetics have recently been used to provide more prolonged neural blockade through techniques of perineural or epidural infusion. For example, epidural local anesthetic infusion, either alone or in combination with opioid drugs, has become an accepted modality in cancer pain management. Rare patients with chronic nonmalignant pain have been treated using these approaches.

Although trigger point injection is typically classified as an anesthetic approach, this simple technique is within the purview of all practitioners [132]. Trigger points in muscle are extremely common causes of pain (so-called myofascial pain syndrome), and the use of saline or local anesthetic injections may be a useful approach in patients with these pains. Injection into tender areas within other soft tissues also appears to benefit some patients. These injections may be supplemented by the application of heat or cold; transcutaneous electrical nerve stimulation over the painful region may also be useful. Following the treatment of myofascial trigger points, systematic stretching of the muscle should be performed. In some patients, these other techniques may obviate the need for injections; for example, the local application of cold using a vapocoolant, following by stretching ("spray and stretch"), is a well-known technique for the treatment of trigger points. Injections should be used cautiously in the immunocompromised patient and avoided in those with coagulopathy.

Neurostimulatory Approaches

It has been appreciated for some time that stimulation of afferent neural pathways can relieve pain. The best-known application of this principle is transcutaneous electrical nerve stimulation (TENS). Other approaches include counterirritation (systematic rubbing of the painful part), percutaneous electrical nerve stimulation, dorsal column stimulation, deep brain stimulation, and acupuncture.

TENS has been purported to be effective in numerous conditions [147,148]. Recent studies, however, have raised questions about its efficacy. For example, a controlled trial in chronic back pain demonstrated that TENS was no more effective than exercise alone [149]. Nonetheless, there is an extensive clinical experience with this approach, and it is generally accepted that some patients truly benefit for prolonged periods.

The mechanism of TENS is assumed to involve the activation of segmental and suprasegmental pain-modulating systems by stimulation of large-diameter, heavily myelinated primary afferent fibers [130]. At a segmental level, it is likely that this input stimulates inhibitory interneurons, the activity of which impedes afferent transmission mediated by lightly myelinated or unmyelinated primary afferent nociceptors. A role for suprasegmental processes is suggested by some effects, such as prolonged diminution of pain after cessation of stimulation and analgesia produced by stimulation of areas remote from the pain, that are not adequately explained by segmental mechanisms.

TENS may be administered through a variety of wave forms. These include monophasic waves, symmetrical and asymmetrical biphasic waves, and polyphasic waves. Although it is commonly observed that patients respond better to one or another waveforms, there are no established relationships between specific waveforms and analgesia, either in general or in selected conditions. Hence, optimal stimulation parameters must be found by trial and error.

It is likewise taken as axiomatic that responses can vary with electrode placement, but the optimal placement in any individual patient is not known. Most patients appear to benefit maximally when electrodes are applied to the painful area itself. Some respond better, however, when stimulation is applied to acupuncture meridians, superficial nerves or motor points, or areas remote from the painful site [126].

A therapeutic trial of TENS is warranted in most patients with chronic, well-localized pain. Although clinical observation suggests that conditions characterized by mild to moderate pain are most responsive, severe pain itself should not exclude the use of a therapeutic trial. Patients with cardiac pacemakers and those with severe dysrhythmias should not be treated, and electrodes should not be placed over the carotid sinus or on damaged skin. A therapeutic trial, if undertaken, should be performed in a manner that recognizes the great patient variability in the response to this modality. Such a trial should include repeated periods of stimulation, during which the electrode placement, waveform, stimulation intensity, and timing of stimulation are varied. This usually requires several weeks, and is generally accomplished most effectively when the patient is able to bring the unit home.

A treatment related to TENS, electrical massage, is frequently used to treat painful muscle spasms [126]. These devices produce strong, at times tetanic, contractions of muscles. In some patients, these contractions yield analgesia.

Surveys of other techniques, such as acupuncture and dorsal column stimulation, have suggested that outcome is similar to TENS: many patients will report analgesia soon after the approach is implemented, but far fewer obtain prolonged relief. There have been no comparative studies of stimulatory approaches, and factors that may predict response are unconfirmed. The ability of one technique (such as TENS) to predict the response to another (such as dorsal column stimulation or deep brain stimulation) is also unknown. Trials of the invasive techniques should be performed only by experienced practitioners, and are best reserved for patients who have failed to respond to the expert administration of other pain management techniques.

Neurosurgical Approaches

Surgical procedures designed to denervate the painful part have been developed for every level of the nervous system, from peripheral nerve to cortex [150]. These procedures are used in the management of pain due to cancer;

with few exceptions, they are very rarely appropriate for patients with nonmalignant pain. Peripheral neurectomy can be useful in patients with painful peripheral mononeuropathies, such as that caused by neuroma, and the use of the dorsal root entry zone lesion has gained acceptance in the management of patients with avulsion of neural plexus [151].

Other neurosurgical procedures, such as cingulotomy, are not antinociceptive but, instead, reduce the affective concomitants of the pain. These approaches are now performed very rarely and virtually never in those with nonmalignant pain.

Psychological Approaches

The comprehensive assessment clarifies the psychological needs of the patient and allows psychological interventions to be targeted appropriately. Specific cognitive and behavioral approaches have become widely accepted in the management of pain [152]. Cognitive approaches, which include relaxation training, distraction techniques, hypnosis, and biofeedback, may enhance the sense of personal control and potentially reduce pain. Behavior therapy may be effective in improving the functional capabilities of the patient with chronic pain. Combined with intensive physiatric therapies, these cognitive and behavioral approaches are the foundation of the multidisciplinary pain management approach preferred for patients with chronic pain associated with pain-related disability.

It is important to recognize that psychological interventions should be considered for all patients with chronic pain, including those whose affective disturbance or pain-related disability are not sufficient to warrant referral to a multidisciplinary pain program. For example, many patients can benefit from simple cognitive techniques, such as relaxation training or distraction, which may provide periods of increased comfort and bolster a sense of personal control over the pain. Other types of cognitive therapy, such as biofeedback training or hypnosis, clearly help some patients as well. There have been few comparative studies of these various techniques, and patients usually receive training in the approaches available to the clinician.

Some simple behavioral therapies can be offered as part of multimodal pain treatment organized by a single practitioner. For example, a graduated exercise program can be implemented through the use of a activity diary maintained by the patient. The patient is provided with detailed instructions about the timing and nature of the exercise (e.g., swimming, walking, stretching) and uses the diary to document adherence to the program. By referring to the diary, the clinician can identify areas in need of additional assistance and monitor the patient's progress.

CONCLUSION

The management of chronic pain evolves from a comprehensive assessment, which guides the selection and implementation of a multimodality treatment plan designed to enhance comfort and address specific pain-related disturbances in function. A subgroup of patients requires the type of intensive management provided through multidisciplinary pain treatment programs, and the assessment process should identify those in need of this referral. Many other patients can be greatly helped through the efforts of a single concerned clinician who can implement a suitable pain management program.

REFERENCES

1. K.M. Foley, N. Engl. J. Med., 313:84–95 (1985).
2. R.K. Portenoy and K.M. Foley, Handbook of Psychooncology: Psychological Care of the Patient with Cancer (J.C. Holland and J.H. Rowland, eds.), Oxford University Press, New York, p. 369 (1989).
3. World Health Organization, Cancer Pain Relief. World Health Organization, Geneva (1986).
4. H. Merskey, Pain, 3:S1–S225 (1986).
5. J.D. Loeser and K.J. Egan, Managing the Chronic Pain Patient: Theory and Practice at the University of Washington Multidisciplinary Pain Center. Raven Press, New York, pp. 3–20 (1989).
6. J.-M. Besson and A. Chaouch, Physiol. Rev., 67:67–185 (1987).
7. W.D. Willis, The Pain System: The Neural Basis of Nociceptive Transmission in the Mammalian Nervous System. Karger, Basel (1985).
8. S. Arner and B.A. Myerson, Pain, 33:11–23 (1988).
9. R. Melzack and K.L. Casey, The Psychology of Pain, 2nd ed. (R. A. Sternbach, ed.), Raven Press, New York, pp. 1–24 (1968).
10. J.J. Bonica, The Management of Pain (J. J. Bonica, ed.), Lea & Febiger, Philadelphia, pp. 18–27 (1990).
11. American Psychiatric Association, Diagnostic and Statistical Manual of Mental Disorder, 3rd ed. American Psychiatric Association, Washington, D.C. (1980).
12. J.M. Romano and J.A. Turner, Psychol. Bull., 97:18–34 (1985).
13. R.K. Portenoy and N.A. Hagen, Pain, 41:273–281 (1990).
14. J.G. Kellgren, Clin. Sci., 4:35–46 (1939).
15. H.E. Torebjork, J.L. Ochoa, and W. Schady, Pain, 18:145–156 (1984).
16. R.K. Portenoy, Towards a New Pharmacotherapy of Pain (A. Basbaum and J.-M. Besson, eds.), John Wiley & Sons, New York, pp. 393–416 (1991).
17. D.C. Turk and T.E. Rudy, Pain, 43:27–35 (1990).
18. D.C. Turk and T.E. Rudy, J. Consult. Clin. Psychol., 56:233–238 (1988).
19. G.A. Higgs and S. Moncada, Advances in Pain Research and Therapy, vol. 5 (J.J.

Bonica, U. Lindblom, and A. Iggo, eds.), Raven Press, New York, pp. 617–626 (1983).

20. J.R. Vane. *Nature New Biol.*, *231*:232–235 (1971).

21. J.-C. Willer, T. De Broucker, B. Bussel, A. Roby-Brami, and J.-M. Harrewyn, *Pain*, *38*:1–8 (1989).

22. A. Sunshine and N.Z. Olson, *Textbook of Pain*, 2nd ed. (P.D. Wall and R. Melzack, eds.), Churchill Livingstone, New York, pp. 670–685 (1989).

23. D.P. Sandler, J.C. Smith, C.R. Weinberg, V.M. Buckalew, V.W. Dennis, W.B. Blythe, and W.P. Burgess, *N. Engl. J. Med.*, *320*:1238–1243 (1989).

24. B.J.Z. Danesh, A.R. Saniabadi, R.I. Russell, and G.D.O. Lowe, *Scot. Med. J.*, *32*:167–168 (1987).

25. D.Y. Graham, N.M. Agrawal, and S.H. Roth, *Lancet*, *2*:1277–1280 (1988).

26. J.T. Edelson, A.N.A. Tosteson, and P. Sax, *J.A.M.A.*, *264*:41–47 (1990).

27. W.O. Frank, B.A. Wallin, J.M. Berkowitz, M.B. Kimmey, R.H. Palmer, F. Rockhold, and M.D. Young, *J. Rheumatol.*, *16*:1249–1252 (1989).

28. S.H. Roth, *J. Rheumatol.*, *15*:912–919 (1988).

29. D.A. O'Hara, R.J. Fragen, M. Kinzer, and D. Pemberton, *Clin. Pharmacol. Ther.*, *41*:556–561 (1987).

30. S. Butler, *Advances in Pain Research and Therapy*, vol. 7. (C.R. Benedetti, C.R. Chapman, and G. Moricca, eds.), Raven Press, New York, pp. 173–198 (1984).

31. C.J. Getto, C.A. Sorkness, and T. Howell, *J. Pain Symptom Manage.*, *2*:9–18 (1987).

32. M.B. Max, R. Kishore-Kumar, S.C. Schafer, B. Meisler, R. H. Gracely, B. Smoller, and R. Dubner, *Pain*, *45*:3–9 (1991).

33. R.K. Portenoy, *Pain Syndromes in Neurology* (H. L. Fields, ed.), Butterworths, London, pp. 257–278 (1990).

34. M.B. Max, M. Culnane, S.C. Schafer, R.H. Gracely, D.J. Walther, B. Smoller, and R. Dubner, *Neurology*, *37*:589–594 (1987).

35. J.R. Couch, D.K. Ziegler, and R. Hassanein, *Neurology*, *26*:121–127 (1976).

36. K. Spiegel, R. Kalb, and G.W. Pasternak, *Ann. Neurol.*, *13*:462–465 (1983).

37. D.L. Hammond, *Advances in Pain Research and Therapy*, vol. 9 (H.L. Fields, R. Dubner, and F. Cervero, eds.), Raven Press, New York, pp. 499–513 (1985).

38. D.S. Charney, D.B. Menkes, and F.R. Heninger, *Arch. Gen. Psychiatry*, *38*: 1160–1180 (1981).

39. E. Richelson, *Psychiatry Annu.*, *9*:186–194 (1979).

40. M. Sosnowski and T.L. Yaksh, *J. Pain Symptom Manage.*, *5*:204–213 (1990).

41. S. Diamond and B.J. Baltes, *Headache*, *11*:110–116 (1971).

42. S. Carette, S., G.A. McCain, D.A. Bell, and A.G. Fam, *Arthritis Rheum.*, *29*: 655–659 (1986).

43. I. Pilowsky, E.C. Hallet, K.L. Bassett, P.G. Thomas, and R.K. Penhall, *Pain*, *14*:169–179 (1982).

44. M.A. Gingras, *J. Int. Med. Res.*, *4*:41–49 (1976).

45. B. Kvinesdal, J. Molin, A. Froland, and L.F. Gram, *J.A.M.A.*, *251*:1727–1730 (1984).

46. A. Okasha, A.A. Ghaleb, and A. Sadek, *Br. J. Psych.*, *122*:181–183 (1973).
47. S.R. Hameroff, R.C. Cork, K. Scherer, R. Crago, C. Neuman, J.R. Womble, and T.P. Davis, *J. Clin. Psychiatry*, *43*:22–27 (1982).
48. H.D. Langohr, M. Stohr, and F. Petruch, *Eur. Neurol.*, *21*:309–317 (1982).
49. C.P.N. Watson, R.J. Evans, and V.R. Watt, Ninth Annual Scientific Meeting of the American Pain Society, St. Louis, MO, October 25–28 (1990).
50. V. Ventafridda, C. Bonezzi, A. Caraceni, F. DeConno, G. Guarise, G. Ramella, L. Saita, V. Silvani, M. Tamburini, and F. Toscani, *Ital. J. Neurol. Sci.*, *8*:579–587 (1987).
51. G. Davidoff, M. Guarracini, E. Roth, J. Sliwa, and G. Yarkony, *Pain*, *29*:151–161 (1987).
52. F. Johansson and L. Von Knorring, *Pain*, *7*:69–78 (1979).
53. C.P.N. Watson and R.J. Evans, *Pain*, *23*:387–394 (1985).
54. S.H. Sindrup, L.F. Gram, K. Brosen, O. Eshoj, and E.F. Mogensen, *Pain*, *42*:135–144 (1990).
55. M. Anthony and J.W. Lance, *Arch. Neurol.*, *21*:263–268 (1969).
56. R.G. Lascelles, *Br. J. Psychiatry*, *122*:651–659 (1966).
57. M. Swerdlow, *Clin. Neuropharmacol.*, *7*:51–82 (1984).
58. J. Weinberger, W.J. Nicklas, and S. Berl, *Neurology*, *26*:162–173 (1976).
59. D. Albe-Fessard and M.C. Lombard, *Advances in Pain Research and Therapy*, vol. 5 (J.J. Bonica, U. Lindblom, and A. Iggo, eds.), Raven Press, New York, pp. 691–700 (1982).
60. J.D. Loeser, A.A. Ward, and L.E. White, *J. Neurosurg.*, *29*:48–50 (1968)
61. B. Nystrom and K.E. Hagbarth, *Neurosci. Lett.*, *27*:211–216 (1981).
62. P.D. Wall and M. Gutnick, *Exp. Neurol.*, *43*:580–593 (1974).
63. S. Blom, *Arch. Neurol.*, *9*:285–290 (1963).
64. J. Braham and A. Saia, *Lancet*, *2*:892–893 (1960).
65. J.B. Green, *Neurology*, *11*:257–258 (1961).
66. V.S. Hatangdi, R.A. Boas, and E.G. Richards, *Advances in Pain Research and Therapy*, vol. 1 (J.J. Bonica and D. Albe-Fessard, eds.), Raven Press, New York, pp. 583–587 (1976).
67. M. Swerdlow and J.G. Cundill, *Anesthesia*, *36*:1129–1132 (1981).
68. V.S. Chadda and M.S. Mathur, *J. Assoc. Physicians India*, *26*:403–406 (1978).
69. F.G. Campbell, J.G. Graham, and K.J. Zilkha, *J. Neurol. Neurosurg. Psychiatry*, *29*:265–267 (1966).
70. J.M. Killian and G.H. Fromm, *Arch. Neurol.*, *19*:129–136 (1968).
71. B.W. Rockliff and E.H. Davis, *Arch. Neurol.*, *15*:129–136 (1966).
72. K. Ekbom, *Arch. Neurol.*, *26*:374–378 (1972).
73. F. Elliot, A. Little, and W. Milbrandt, *N. Engl. J. Med.*, *295*:678 (1976).
74. M.L.E. Espir and P. Millac, *J. Neurol. Neurosurg. Psychiatry*, *33*:528–531 (1970).
75. S. Mullan, *Surg. Clin. North Am.*, *53*:203–210 (1973).
76. M.R. Caccia, *Eur. Neurol.*, *13*:560–563 (1975).
77. G. Martin, *Ann. R. Coll. Surg. Engl.*, *63*:244–252 (1981).
78. H. Raftery, *J. Irish Med. Assoc.*, *72*:399–401 (1979).

79. G.H. Fromm, C.F. Terence, and A.S. Chatta, *Ann. Neurol.*, *15*:240–247 (1984).
80. P. Lindstrom and U. Lindblom, *Pain*, *28*:45–50 (1987).
81. F. Lechin, B. Van Der Dijs, M.E. Lechin, J. Amat, A.E. Lechin, A. Cabrera, F. Gomez, E. Acosta, L. Arocha, S. Villa, and V. Jimenez, *Arch. Neurol.*, *46*: 960–962 (1989).
82. S. Glazer and R.K. Portenoy, *J. Pain Symptom Manage.*, *6*:30–39 (1991).
83. A. Dejgard, P. Petersen, and J. Kastrup, *Lancet*, *1*:9–11 (1988).
84. W. Kreeger and S.C. Hammill, *Mayo Clin. Proc.*, *62*:1033–1050 (1987).
85. R. Kocher, *Advances in Pain Research and Therapy*, vol. 1 (J.J. Bonica and D. Albe-Fessard, eds.), Raven Press, New York, pp. 279–282 (1976).
86. L.H. Margolis and A.J. Gianascol, *Neurology*, *6*:302–304 (1956).
87. P.W. Nathan, *Pain*, *5*:367–371 (1978).
88. O. Weis, K. Sriwatanakul, and M. Weintraub, *S. Afr. Med. J.*, *62*:274–275 (1982).
89. L. Lasagna and T.J. DeKornfeld, *J.A.M.A.*, *178*:119–122 (1961).
90. R.W. Houde and S.L. Wallenstein, *Fed. Proc.*, *14*:353 (1966).
91. M.B. Max, S.C. Schafer, M. Culnane, R. Dubner, and R.H. Gracely, *Clin. Pharmacol. Ther.*, *43*(4):363–371 (1988).
92. J. Shafar, E.R. Tallett, and P.A. Knowlson, *Lancet*, *1*:403–407 (1972).
93. Y.-M. Tan, and J. Croese, *Ann. Intern. Med.*, *105*:633 (1986).
94. H. Jaeger and C. Maier, *Pain*, *48*:13–20 (1992).
95. C. Gobelet, M. Waldburger, and J.L. Meier, *Pain*, *48*:171–175 (1992).
96. N.A. Bercel, *Curr. Ther. Res.*, *22*:462–468 (1977).
97. R.H. Gold, *Curr. Ther. Res.*, *23*:271–276 (1978).
98. I.W. Birkeland and D.K. Clawson, *Clin. Pharmacol. Ther.*, *9*:639–646 (1968).
99. C.M. Smith, *Physiological Pharmacology*, vol. 2 (W.S. Root and F.G. Hoffmann, eds.), Academic Press, New York, pp. 2–96 (1965).
100. F. Fernandez, F. Adams, and V.F. Holmes, *J. Clin. Psychopharmacol.*, *7*:167–169 (1987).
101. S. Yosselson-Superstine, A.G. Lipman, and S.H. Sanders, *Israel J. Med Sci.*, *21*:113–117 (1985).
102. M.M. Rumore and D.A. Schlichting, *Pain*, *25*:7–22 (1986).
103. J.E. Stambaugh and C. Lance, *Cancer Invest.*, *1*:111–117 (1983).
104. S.Y. Ghostine, Y.G. Comair, D.M. Turner, N.F. Kassell, and C.G. Azar, *J. Neurosurg.*, *60*:1263–1268 (1984).
105. S.E. Abram and R.W. Lightfoot, *Reg. Anesth.*, *6*:79–81 (1981).
106. T. Tabira, H. Shibasaki, and Y. Kuroiwa, *Arch. Neurol.*, *40*:430–432 (1983).
107. G. Simson, *J.A.M.A.*, *227*:327 (1974).
108. F. Kozin, L.M. Ryan, G.F. Carerra, L.S. Soin, and R.L. Wortmann, *Am. J. Med.*, *70*:23–29 (1981).
109. D.S. Prough, C.H. McLeskey, G.P. Poehling, L.A. Koman, D.B. Weeks, T. Whitworth, and E.L. Semble, *Anesthesiology*, *62*:796–799 (1985).
110. E. Bruera, S. Chadwick, C. Brenneis, J. Hanson, and R.N. MacDonald, *Cancer Treat. Rep.*, *71*:67–70 (1987).

111. W.H. Forrest, B. Brown, C. Brown, R. Defalque, M. Gold, E. Gordon, K.E. James, J. Katz, D.L. Mahler, P. Schroff, and G. Teutch, *N. Engl. J. Med.*, *296*: 712–715 (1977).

112. E.M. Laska, A. Sunshine, F. Mueller, W.B. Elvers, C. Siegel, and A. Rubin, *J.A.M.A.*, *251*:1711–1718 (1984).

113. R.D. France, B.J. Urban, and F.J. Keefe, *Soc. Sci. Med.*, *19*:1379–1382 (1984).

114. R.K. Portenoy and K.M. Foley, *Pain*, *25*:171–186 (1986).

115. A. Taub, *Narcotic Analgesics in Anesthesiology* (L.M. Kitahata and D. Collins, eds.), Williams and Wilkins, Baltimore, pp. 199–208 (1982).

116. F.S. Tennant and G.F. Uelman, *Postgrad. Med.*, *73*:81–94 (1983).

117. B.J. Urban, R.D. France, E.K. Steinberger, D.L. Scott, and A.A. Maltbie, *Pain*, *24*:191–197 (1986).

118. M. Zenz, M. Strumpf, and M. Tryba, *J. Pain Symptom Manage.*, 7:69–77 (1992).

119. R.K. Portenoy, *J. Pain Symptom Manage.*, 5:S46–S62 (1990).

120. F.J. Brescia, R.K. Portenoy, M. Ryan, L. Drasnoff, and G. Gray, *J. Clin. Oncol.*, *10*:149–155 (1992).

121. R.M. Kanner and K.M. Foley, *Ann. N.Y. Acad. Sci.*, *362*:161–172 (1981).

122. R.G. Twycross, *Int. J. Clin. Pharmacol. Ther.*, 9:184–198 (1974).

123. C.R. Chapman, *Advances in Pain Research and Therapy*, vol. 11 (C.S. Hill and W.S. Fields, eds.), Raven Press, New York, pp. 339–352 (1989).

124. S. Perry and G. Heidrich, *Pain*, *13*:267–268 (1982).

125. J. Porter and H. Jick, *N. Engl. J. Med.*, *302*:123 (1980).

126. J.R. Basford, *Rehabilitation Medicine: Principles and Practice* (J.A. Delisa, ed.), J.B. Lippincott, Philadelphia, pp. 257–275 (1988).

127. J.F. Lehmann and B.F. deLateur, *Textbook of Pain*, 2nd ed. (P.D. Wall and R. Melzack, eds.), Churchill Livingstone, Edinburgh, pp. 932–941 (1989).

128. J.F. Lehmann and B.J. deLateur, *Krusen's Handbook of Physical Medicine and Rehabilitation*, 4th ed. (F.J. Kottke and J.F. Lehmann, eds.), W.B. Saunders, Philadelphia, pp. 285–367 (1982).

129. B.A. Meyerson, *Advances in Pain Research and Therapy*, vol. 5 (J.J. Bonica, U. Lindblom, A. Iggo, and C. Benedetti, eds.), Raven Press, New York, pp. 495–534 (1983).

130. C.J. Woolf, *Textbook of Pain*, 2nd ed. (P.D. Wall and R. Melzack, eds.), Churchill Livingstone, Edinburgh, pp. 884–896 (1989).

131. M.M. Portwood, J.S. Lieberman, and R.G. Taylor, *Arch. Phys. Med. Rehabil.*, 68:116–118 (1987).

132. J.G. Travell and D.G. Simons, *Myofascial Pain and Dysfunction: The Trigger Point Manual*, Williams and Wilkins, Baltimore, pp. 5–164 (1983).

133. C.W. Britell and S.R. McFarland, *Rehabilitation Medicine: Principles and Practice* (J.A. Delisa, ed.), J.B. Lippincott, Philadelphia, pp. 372–388 (1988).

134. H.R. Lehneis, *Rehabilitation Medicine* (J. Goodgold, ed.), C.V. Mosby, St. Louis, pp. 823–841 (1988).

135. K.T. Ragnarsson, *Rehabilitation Medicine: Principles and Practice* (J.A. Delisa, ed.), J.B. Lippincott, Philadelphia, pp. 307–329 (1988).

136. G.R. Cybulski, *Neurosurgery*, 25:240–252 (1989).
137. S. Fisher, *Krusen's Handbook of Physical Medicine and Rehabilitation*, 4th ed. (F.J. Kottke and J.F. Lehmann, eds.), W.B. Saunders, Philadelphia, pp. 593–601 (1990).
138. H. Flor and D.C. Turk, *Pain*, 19:105–121 (1984).
139. N.E. Walsh and R.K. Schwartz, *Am.J.Phys.Med.Rehabil.*, 69:245–250 (1990).
140. L.R. Leslie, *Krusen's Handbook of Physical Medicine and Rehabilitation*, 3rd ed. (F.J. Kottke and J.F. Lehmann, eds.), W.B. Saunders, Philadelphia, pp. 564–570 (1990).
141. M. Williams and H.R. Lissner, *Biomechanics of Human Motion*. W.B. Saunders, Philadelphia (1962).
142. J.E. Cassisi, G.W. Sypert, A. Salamon, and L. Kapel, *Neurosurgery*, 25:877–883 (1989).
143. S.L. Chapman, S.F. Brena, and L.A. Bradford, *Pain*, 11:255–268 (1981).
144. J.C. King and W.J. Kelleher, *Phys.Med. State of the Art Rev.*, 5:165–186 (1991).
145. P.P. Raj, *Neural Blockade in Clinical Anesthesia and Management of Pain*, 2nd ed. (M.J. Cousins and P.O. Bridenbaugh, eds.), J.B. Lippincott, Philadelphia, pp. 899–934 (1988).
146. M.J. Cousins, B. Dwyer, and D. Gibb, *Neural Blockade in Clinical Anesthesia and Management of Pain*, 2nd ed. (M.J. Cousins and P.O. Bridenbaugh, eds.), J.B. Lippincott, Philadelphia, pp. 1053–1084 (1988).
147. M.R. Gersh and S.L. Wolf, *Phys. Ther.*, 65:314–336 (1985).
148. G. Thorsteinsson, H.H. Stonnington, G.K. Stillwell, and L.R. Elveback, *Pain*, 5:31–41 (1978).
149. R.A. Deyo, N.E. Walsh, D.C. Martin, L.S. Schoenfeld, and S. Ramamurthy, *N. Engl.J. Med.*, 332:1627–1634 (1990).
150. J.M. Gybels and W.H. Sweet, *Neurosurgical Treatment of Persistent Pain*. Karger, Basel (1989).
151. R.F. Young, *J. Neurosurg.*, 72:715–720 (1990).
152. D.C. Turk, D. Meichenbaum, and M. Genest, *Pain and Behavioral Medicine: A Cognitive–Behavioral Perspective*. Guilford Press, New York (1983).

18
Medical Complications in the Rehabilitation Patient

James R. Couch, Jr.

The University of Oklahoma Health Sciences Center
Oklahoma City, Oklahoma

Physicians caring for patients with chronic neurological disease encounter a variety of medical conditions that can complicate rehabilitation. These medical illnesses may precede the neurological illness, or may be a consequence of it. Because of the frequency of comorbid conditions, it is imperative that physicians practicing neurorehabilitation be alert to their presence, be comfortable in treating minor medical problems, and recognize when consultation with another physician is necessary for serious conditions. Finally, rehabilitation physicians must recognize when rehabilitation programs must be altered because of concurrent medical problems.

This chapter will focus on stroke, the most frequent neurological illness requiring rehabilitation. However, many of the topics discussed apply equally to other patients with other chronic neurological conditions. Medical complications are also discussed in many of the other chapters in this book that deal with specific conditions.

In the literature on rehabilitation of stroke, there is relatively little information on medical complications in the patient with stroke. Work by Dobkin [1], Feigenson et al. [2], and Adler et al. [3] all cover aspects of this problem. Adler et al. noted that 69% of their patients had significant medical problems on admission to the rehabilitation service [3] and McClatchie found that 45% of his 174 patients developed medical problems while on the rehabilitation unit [4]. Relatively few articles provide a compendium of complications in a fashion designed to help the neurorehabilitation physician

Table 1 Categories of Medical Conditions in Patients Undergoing Stroke
Rehabilitation as Suggested by Relation to the Rehabilitation Process

Premorbid conditions that contribute to the stroke
Comorbid conditions that interfere with the rehabilitation process
Conditions that develop while the patient is on the rehabilitation ward and have an
  impact on or interfere with the rehabilitation process

in day-to-day patient care. In this chapter some of the material was taken from
articles specifically related to medical complications, some from the geriatric
literature, and some reflects the author's experience.

It is well known that the most common factor related to stroke is age. In
the Mayo Clinic study of stroke incidence [5], the incidence of stroke rose
from 6:100,000 in the group less than 55 years of age to 488:100,000 in the
seventh decade to 1129:100,000 in the eighth decade, and the incidence in the
ninth decade was 1500:100,000. With these data in mind, it is obvious that the
patient with stroke is more likely to be an elderly patient. As a consequence,
the complications seen in the patient with stroke would include those
specifically related to stroke as well as conditions commonly seen in the
elderly.

In approaching the topic of medical problems in the patient with stroke,
it is apparent that there are different categories of problems and these relate
differently to the patient. Table 1 is a suggested listing of categories into which
medical complications may be divided.

PREMORBID CONDITIONS THAT CONTRIBUTE TO STROKE

The Framingham study has identified six major risk factors for stroke [6,7].
These include hypertension, cardiac disease, lipid abnormalities, primarily
hypercholesterolemia, smoking, diabetes, and obesity. These problems are
all common in the elderly patient and all except obesity show a statistically
significant contribution to the risk of stroke. Of note, these are also major
factors in the occurrence of coronary disease, another major premorbid
condition in the patient with stroke [8].

Hypertension is a very common condition that occurs in 10 percent of
patients greater than 70 years old and 20 percent of those greater than 80
years old [9]. In general, the risk of stroke is directly related to the level of
hypertension, both systolic and diastolic [6]. In addition to cerebrovascular
disease, hypertension influences the development of cardiac disease and
renal disease and is a significant factor in cerebral hemorrhage [6,7,9]. The
most common cause of hypertension is essential hypertension [9]. Sympto-

matic hypertension may also be seen in patients with renal vascular disease in either small or large vessels and in endocrine abnormalities including hyperthyroidism, hyperaldosteronism, hyperadrenalism, Cushing's disease, and pheochromocytoma.

Hypertension was a major problem in the studies of McClatchie [4] and Dobkin [1] and was seen in 60–63% of subjects. The morbidity directly associated with hypertension was not tabulated in these studies.

Mild hypertension may have relatively few symptoms. More severe hypertension may result in malaise and increased fatigability because of the increased afterload on the heart. Essential hypertension can also be associated with cardiomyopathy, cardiac hypertrophy, and myocardial infarction. Any or all of these factors will diminish the ability of the patient to participate in and benefit from the rehabilitation program.

The second major area of stroke-related conditions is cardiac disease. The Framingham study found that cardiac disease defined by cardiac enlargement with electrocardiographic criteria, or by x-ray criteria, was significantly associated with ischemic, nonembolic stroke [6]. This may reflect in part the relation to hypertension and in part arteriosclerosis as an underlying condition predisposing to myocardial infarction, cerebrovascular disease, and renal disease as well as hypertension.

Many cardiac conditions may also lead to embolic stroke. These conditions include recent myocardial infarction, cardiac enlargement due to congestive heart failure and subsequent poor ejection fraction, noncontractile myocardial wall, and ventricular aneurysm. Atrial arrhythmias such as atrial fibrillation are strongly associated with embolic stroke [10]. This and other arrhythmias may transiently alter cardiac function. Clots may form on the inner surface of dysfunctional areas of heart wall or on dysfunctional valves, with subsequent cerebral embolization.

Because cardiac and cerebrovascular disease are so often related, it is necessary for the rehabilitation physician to evaluate the cardiac system very carefully. Arrhythmias, especially paroxysmal arrhythmias that may be related to exercise, must be recognized. If not treated appropriately, these may result in significant risks to the patient when progressive physical activity is required in the rehabilitation program [1].

Congestive heart failure is another problem of major potential importance in the patient undergoing rehabilitation [3,4]. Adler et al. found this problem in 11% of their patients [3] and McClatchie in 15% of theirs [4]. Patients with congestive heart failure will find this condition worsened by the physical activity of the rehabilitation program. At times patients who are in borderline compensation for congestive heart failure may find their heart failure becoming clinically symptomatic during the exercise program required by the rehabilitation regimen [1,4,12]. Congestive heart failure must be recognized and treated to avoid the danger of sudden cardiac decompensation while the patient is participating in the exercise programs. Recognition and treatment of congestive heart failure will help to maximize participation in the rehabilitation program.

The medications employed for treating cardiac problems and hypertension include beta-adrenergic blocking agents, alpha-2 adrenergic agonists, calcium channel blocking agents, angiotensin-converting enzyme inhibitors, diuretics, digitalis derivatives, guanidine, procainamide, and a number of other drugs. These all have side effects and many produce sedation, nausea, and hypotension. The diuretics may produce alteration of electrolyte balance and dehydration. The patient should be watched carefully for side effects [9]. If these occur the medication regimen should be re-evaluated to see if some of the drugs can be changed or their dosage altered. In some cases, these side effects may diminish the patient's motivation to participate in the program or may even slow recovery.

Diabetes mellitus (DM) is a problem of great significance in patients undergoing stroke rehabilitation. Diabetes can be classified into type I or autoimmune type (juvenile type, insulin-dependent type) [13] and type II or non-insulin-dependent type [14]. Type II DM is the most common cause of adult hyperglycemia and has an overall prevalence of 2–5% in the United States. Prevalence varies greatly among identifiable subgroups and may be up to 35% in some Native American tribes. Incidence rises with age. Prevalence of DM is 8–18% in the 65–74 year age group and over 20% at age 80.

DM was a frequent problem in the studies of patients undergoing rehabilitation. Dobkin [1], McClatchie [4], and Adler et al. all found DM in 15–20% of their patients.

Type I DM is predominantly of childhood or juvenile onset and there is a genetic predisposition. A smaller percentage of patients will develop late-onset type I DM. In some subjects the differentiation between type I and type II DM can be difficult to make.

Table 2 reviews the major complications of type I and type II DM. In the usual population undergoing rehabilitation, type II DM is relatively more common. The major complications occur in both types, and the discussion below will cover type I and type II DM as a single entity.

Hypoglycemia may appear in the diabetic patient as exercise levels increase. As the patient becomes significantly more active in the rehabilitation program, insulin requirements may decrease and the patient on insulin may become hypoglycemic. Hypoglycemia, likewise, is not infrequent when the sulfonylurea oral agents for treatment of DM are used. Use of medication such as salicylates, warfarin, monoamine oxidase inhibitors, and beta-adrenergic blocking agents may predispose to hypoglycemia. Because of an

Table 2 Complications of Diabetes and Relative Frequency in
Types I and Type II

Complications	Type I	Type II
Hypoglycemia	+++	++
Ketoacidosis	+++	rare
Nonketotic hyperosmolar coma	+	+++
Hypersensitivity to insulin	++	rare
Nephropathy	+++	+ to +++
	(up to 30%)	depending on age
Retinopathy	+++	++
Microvascular insufficiency (coronary, cerebral, renal, peripheral arterial disease)	+++	+++
Neuropathy (somatic, autonomic)	+++	+++
Dermopathy	++	+

age-related decrease in beta-adrenergic function and autonomic neuropathy, the elderly diabetic patient may not respond to early hypoglycemia and may develop severe hypoglycemia rapidly.

Hypoglycemia is a major risk for all diabetic patients and careful monitoring is needed. As activity increases, insulin requirements may decrease. The diet should be monitored carefully and times for meals and snacks maintained. Therapists should be made aware of the problem and provide sugar if the patient complains of symptoms of hypoglycemia including headache, severe hunger, tremulousness, weakness, sudden increase in irritability, disorientation, confusion, loss of consciousness, or seizure.

Hyperosmolar, hyperglycemic nonketotic coma is another major risk in the older diabetic patient [14]. This syndrome develops in relation to increased levels of stress hormones (corticosteroid and epinephrine) that may occur in acute disease processes in patients with modest glucose intolerance. Dehydration and falling renal perfusion contribute to the situation and accelerate the rising glucose level. Coma may occur rapidly and be followed by death. Treatment is directed at rehydration and lowering blood glucose by rapid infusion of insulin and potassium [14].

Diabetic ketoacidosis is a much less frequent problem in adults but a potentially devastating one [13]. The patient with type I diabetes is much more prone to ketoacidosis and may develop this problem if glucose and insulin input are not regulated. The patient with very brittle diabetes may develop ketoacidosis very quickly and with little warning. Cerebral edema may intervene rapidly with fatal outcome. Precipitating factors include physiological stress due to infection, myocardial infarction, or pancreatitis, among others. These are all common problems in the elderly, and their occurrence would be cause for concern in the patient with type I diabetes.

COMORBID CONDITIONS IN THE PATIENT UNDERGOING STROKE REHABILITATION

Common comorbid conditions in the patient with stroke include pulmonary disease, gastrointestinal disease, renal disease, benign prostatic hypertrophy, and musculoskeletal disease.

As indicated earlier, the incidence of stroke increases dramatically with age and consequently the major comorbid conditions seen in the patient undergoing stroke rehabilitation become similar to a listing of the diseases that occur in the aging subject. The National Center for Health Statistics reported that the leading causes of disability in people over age 65 were heart disease, cancer, stroke, musculoskeletal disease, and diabetes, in descending order [11]. The leading causes of death, in descending order, for individuals over age 65 included heart disease, cancer, cerebral vascular disease, chronic obstructive pulmonary disease, pneumonia and influenza, diabetes, and atherosclerosis [11]. The prevalence of these conditions in an elderly population increases dramatically with each decade of age after 65 years and begins to approach more of a logarithmic than a linear progression. Each system in the body, however, demonstrates its own group of abnormalities associated with aging. It is worthwhile to review these, since this group of conditions represents many of the major problems with which the rehabilitation physician will have to cope.

Pulmonary Disease

The physiology of the aging lung by itself represents a problem limiting the effectiveness of rehabilitation. Pulmonary mechanics decline with age as manifested by a drop in forced expiratory volume at 1 sec (FEV1) from 4.5 L to 3.0 L between ages 20 and 80 [15,16]. There is a drop in arterial oxygenation with age as defined by the formula: $P_aO_2 = 100 - (0.34 \times age)$. This decline relates to changes in pulmonary mechanics and loss of gas exchange at the alveoli due to thicker alveolar membrane [15] and increased dead space due to declining pulmonary compliance.

In addition, the central control of respiration may be altered by aging and by disease [15]. The major changes are those of decreasing sensitivity to the three major stimuli for respiration: elevated CO_2, low O_2, and acidosis. This results in diminished pulmonary response to increased need for oxygen and may lead to poor respiratory response to demands of physical exercise.

Chronic obstructive pulmonary disease (COPD) can produce major problems for the patient undergoing rehabilitation. COPD is very common in the aging population. Estimates indicate that 7.5 million Americans have chronic bronchitis, 2 million have emphysema, while more than 6 million have asthma. Other surveys have suggested that 14% of men and 8% of women have chronic bronchitis, obstructive airway disease, or both [16]. These diseases are strongly related to smoking and to family history of COPD. Depending on location and occupation, other environmental factors may also play a role. In general, however, the three most important factors that have been identified are smoking, age, and family history of COPD [16].

The patient with severe COPD will have diminished maximum ventilatory capacity and diminished maximum oxygen consumption [16]. When these parameters are diminished, maximum tolerated physical activity is reduced and the patient is more prone to fatigue. As the process progresses, exhaustion takes place at lower levels of activity. Exhaustion occurs when there is conversion from aerobic to anaerobic metabolism for a prolonged period. If exhaustion occurs at a level of activity required for the rehabilitation program or for usual activities of daily living, this will produce significant additional disability and will seriously impair any attempt at rehabilitation therapy [16].

In addition to the condition itself, the medications used to treat COPD may interfere with the rehabilitation process. Commonly used medications include theophylline, topical beta-adrenergic receptor agonists, and expectorants. These agents can cause sedation, confusion, nausea, vomiting, or excessive fatigue and can slow progress with rehabilitation.

The patient with COPD is also more prone to pneumonia and influenza [16]. These complications are more likely to occur in patients who have limited physical mobility and, in turn, will further limit mobility. This leads to a situation in which there is a diminished capacity for physical activity and mental concentration, both of which delay the rehabilitation program.

Gastrointestinal Problems

The major problems seen with the gastrointestinal tract with aging relate to motility and endothelial lining [15]. Gastrointestinal motility tends to diminish with age. The endothelium of the gastrointestinal tract may become atrophic. Major causes of this atrophy include inflammatory responses or development of ulcers from acid–peptic disease or stress. Both of these conditions are aggravated by immobility and the stress of concurrent disease. Major disturbances in the gastrointestinal system can result in malnutrition, with inadequate carbohydrate and protein absorption and lead to declining tolerance to physical activity.

Following the movement of food down the gastrointestinal (GI) tract, the first problem is that of impaired swallowing. Swallowing is a complex motor process under direct control by the central nervous system. Local factors of esophageal and laryngeal control may interfere and produce dysphagia, a topic covered elsewhere in this book. The swallowing process triggers esophageal peristalsis. Poor esophageal motility may result in retention of food in the esophagus or megaesophagus and, in turn, interfere with the swallowing process. An incompetent gastroesophageal valve may result in gastroesophageal reflux. This reflux can cause significant and damaging acid–peptic disease at the gastroesophageal junction and lower esophagus [17]. Aspiration resulting in pneumonia can occur with gastroesophageal reflux.

Atrophic gastritis may occur in 25–33% of elderly patients [15]. The diminished output of gastric acid interferes with the digestion and late absorption of food in the small bowel. Parietal cell atrophy may lead to vitamin B12 deficiency and its subsequent complication of combined system disease. Poor gastric motility may occur from multiple causes including autonomic neuropathy or infiltration of gastric wall with tumor or amyloid. Delayed gastric emptying with early postprandial fullness can result in diminished caloric intake and poor nutrition.

Motility of the small intestine as well as its absorption capacity diminish with age [15]. Cholecystitis and pancreatitis increase in frequency with age. These may result in various acute syndromes, but the more chronic phase following multiple bouts may result in poor nutrition.

Motility of the large bowel may become a major problem. In the patient with significantly limited activity and increased time in bed, large bowel motility may be seriously impaired, leading to fecal impaction and obstipation [15,18]. These conditions may produce exacerbation of diverticulitis with development of focal colonic wall abscesses or perforations. Following acute diverticulitis, more indolent pelvic abscesses may also develop, resulting in longer-term debility. Studies have shown that in normal aging, large bowel motility is preserved. Inactivity, immobility, and lack of fiber contribute significantly to problems of large bowel motility [15]. These factors must be watched carefully in the patient receiving rehabilitation.

The diet of the patient on the rehabilitation service should be carefully monitored. Adequate caloric intake should be provided to match the increasing level of physical activity. The protein intake must be high enough to provide for tissue repair and increased activity. It is important to have adequate fiber content in the diet to help maintain gastrointestinal motility. Adequate vitamin intake must be ensured, since borderline vitamin deficiencies, especially of the water-soluble vitamins, are not uncommon. Periodic monitoring of hemoglobin, serum albumin, creatinine, and electrolyte levels may be needed to ensure adequate nutrition. In the case of patients with diabetes or other metabolic diseases, special diets may be needed. The participation of a dietician may be necessary for the provision of an optimal rehabilitation program.

Renal and Urogenital Systems

The renal system shows significant alterations with age [15]. Renal blood flow and glomerular filtration rate decline significantly with age. Creatinine clearance drops linearly at a rate of 8 ml/min/1.73 m body surface/decade. The creatinine clearance is usually 60–70 ml/min in the young, healthy person and may drop by 50% in the "healthy" geriatric patient of age 80. Further decline in renal function to a creatinine clearance below 15–20 ml/min will lead to symptomatic renal failure. The accompanying fatigue, malaise, alteration of nutrition, metabolic myopathy, and neuropathy will seriously impede the rehabilitation program.

Urinary incontinence may cause a great deal of difficulty in terms of disability as well as interfering with a rehabilitation program. Incontinence increases dramatically in the elderly over age 80. Incontinence has been noted in approximately 50% of institutionalized elderly patients and up to 20% of community-living elderly [19]. Incontinence will generally produce significant interference with the rehabilitation program because of the need to stop and change clothes or deal with catheters, penile clips, or adult diapers. Urinary incontinence is a major impediment to independent living or returning to the home environment in a semiindependent fashion [19,20]. Use of the adult diaper is helpful but problems of skin maceration and breakdown may occur. Chronic use of the diaper can be a significant expense.

Bacteriuria is common in the elderly [21]. It is often unclear if bacteriuria represents a significant infection or indicates a static and not acutely significant process. Bacteriuria should be evaluated carefully when first noted to determine if the infection is significant. If the infection is deemed insignificant, the patient with bacteriuria should be monitored periodically for subsequent development of symptomatic infection and renal impairment. Persistent bacteriuria may be associated with increase in mortality.

Benign Prostatic Hypertrophy

Benign prostatic hypertrophy increases in incidence with age and causes difficulty with voiding in the aging man. It is estimated that 10% of men will require prostatectomy to relieve urinary obstruction by age 80 [22]. The usual symptoms of BPH are diminished urinary stream and progressive strangury. This in turn leads to incomplete emptying of the bladder and may produce symptoms of urgency, frequency, and nocturia. With progression of the problem, this may lead to progressive dilation of the bladder and increasing postvoid residual urine volumes. Increased bladder residual can produce a milieu for bacteria, which eventually results in symptomatic bladder infection or pyelonephritis. In the patient with stroke, the problem is usually exacerbated by immobility. It is common for the older man who is having some difficulty with stranguria to have further increase in difficulty when immobilized for any reason. This may lead to complete or intermittent urinary obstruction with need for catheterization. The trauma from catheterization often exacerbates the problem. It is not uncommon that male patients with stroke will need to undergo a transurethral resection of the prostate during the course of the rehabilitation therapy because of difficulty with urination [23].

Musculoskeletal System

Osteoporosis and arthritis become increasingly common with age. Both produce significant problems for the patient receiving rehabilitation.

Osteoporosis is a problem of both men and women, but generally a more serious one in women. Both men and women begin to show a loss of cortical bone at about age 40, at a rate of 0.3–0.5% per year [24]. In postmenopausal women this rate of bone loss may accelerate to 2–3% per year for up to 10 years after menopause before returning to a slower rate. It has been estimated that 1.2 million fractures can be attributed to osteoporosis every year. The sites of fractures most commonly are the vertebrae, hip, distal forearm, pelvis, ribs, and other bones of the limbs. The incidence of hip fractures doubles each year after age 40. Another estimate suggests that by age 90 1:3 women and 1:6 men will have had a hip fracture [24]. Hip fractures are catastrophic and associated with a high death rate in the elderly [24,25]. In the population receiving rehabilitation it is necessary to be aware of this problem. A vigorous approach to stretching and manipulation in a patient with severe osteoporosis could result in fracture of a limb or vertebra and thus produce increased disability. Therapists must be careful with such programs in the "older" elderly (age > 80) or in chronically ill subjects.

The two major forms of arthritis, rheumatoid arthritis and osteoarthritis, are common problems but with somewhat variable manifestations. Rheumatoid arthritis is estimated to have a prevalence of 1–2% of the population [25]. The age at onset of the disease is between 25 and 55 years and it is usually a progressive problem that affects the smaller interarticular joints of the hands and feet, but may be associated with problems in the larger joints and spine. One of the major dangers in rheumatoid arthritis is pathological fracture of the odontoid, which, in turn may result in spinal cord injury at the cervicomedullary junction [25,26]. A history of falls or evidence of neck pain, limited range of neck motion, numb clumsy hands, or bilateral spasticity should alert the rehabilitation physician to a lesion of the cervicomedullary junction [26]. Cervical spine x-ray films with flexion and extension and odontoid views to evaluate neck stability should be done prior to initiating vigorous physical rehabilitation in these patients.

Osteoarthritis is a pleomorphic condition that is much more common than rheumatoid arthritis. Osteoarthritis tends to affect the large joints such as shoulders, hips, and knees. When affecting these joints, osteoarthritis can produce serious immobility for the patient and again interfere very significantly with the rehabilitation program.

The neuromuscular system shows significant changes in the elderly [27]. These include peripheral neuropathy, type II muscle atrophy, and decreased glycolytic metabolism (See Chap. 3). Autonomic neuropathy may also be significant, with development of orthostatic hypotension, poor cardiac response to exercise, and poor gastrointestinal motility. These factors, in turn, may significantly impair the rehabilitation process.

CONDITIONS OCCURRING DURING REHABILITATION THAT INTERFERE WITH THE REHABILITATION PROCESS

Table 3 provides a listing of the major problems that can develop while the patient is on the rehabilitation ward and may significantly interfere with the rehabilitation process. Most of these problems have been covered earlier in the chapter as pre-existing or coexisting conditions at the time of admission. In these situations, the management is essentially the same. Conditions that deserve additional comment are those of immobility, deep venous thrombosis, musculoskeletal problems, falls, and depression.

The problems of immobility and falling have similar background and associated factors [28,29]. Both are of diverse and often multifactorial cause, and both represent conditions that are not in themselves pathological. In these situations, the problem results from a distinctly unfavorable outcome related to the condition.

Immobility is associated with a host of problems and will exacerbate the pathological processes associated with all of the major organ systems. For the pulmonary system, there is increased tendency toward poor aeration of pulmonary segments and predisposition to pneumonia and hypoventilation. For the cardiac system, there may be loss of compensatory cardiac output mechanisms, and tendency for significant orthostatic hypotension when the patient becomes active again. For the gastrointestinal system, a number of problems may result in the upper part of the system; dysphagia and aspiration pneumonia are common problems. Gastric and bowel motility may be significantly diminished, leading to poor absorption of nutrients and poor nutrition. For the large bowel, poor motility may result with development of obstipation

Table 3 Conditions that may Occur While Patients Are on the
Rehabilitation Service

Immobility
Deep venous thrombosis
Pulmonary
  Pneumonia
  Pulmonary emboli
  Exacerbation of COPD
Cardiac
  Congestive heart failure
  Myocardial infarction
  Recurrence of hypertension
Gastrointestinal
  Dysphagia
  Poor esophageal motility
  Gastroparesis
  Gastric ulcer related to stress
  Poor colonic motility with constipation, obstipation, fecal impaction
Genitourinary
  Bacteriuria
  Pyelonephritis
  Bladder obstruction
Metabolic–Malnutrition
  Protein deficiency
  Avitaminosis, especially water-soluble vitamins (B complex and C)
Musculoskeletal
  Shoulder–hand syndrome
  Acromiohumeral subluxation
  Contractures
  Acceleration of osteoporosis
  Disuse atrophy
Skin: Decubitus ulcers
Falls
Depression

and fecal impaction followed by the other complications mentioned earlier.
With regard to musculoskeletal system, immobility can speed the development of osteoporosis and result in a type II muscle atrophy. Contractures may
develop in any immobile joint, making remobilization of the patient ever
more difficult. In addition, the contractures may be associated with significant pain and the development of complications such as the shoulder/hand
syndrome. Finally, the decubitus ulcer is much more likely to develop in the

patient with poor mobility due to prolonged periods of excessive pressure on areas of the skin overlying bony prominences.

The study by Dontas et al. [29] of a group of patients in a residential home highlights the problem of mobility. Modest decrease in mobility was defined as a patient requiring assistance to walk 20 stairs or 300 yards to an eating facility. This level of decreased mobility was associated with a doubling of the mortality rate. Increasing degrees of immobility are associated with even greater risks [28].

Risk factors associated with immobility in nursing home populations include dementia, poor vision, leg/hip fracture, and contractures [20]. Stroke and Parkinson's disease are also major factors. Selikson et al. comment that the problem of immobility is generally understated because most medical records do not reflect this as a part of the patient's condition [28].

While the goal of the rehabilitation process is to remobilize the patient, at times factors may appear that temporarily interrupt or negate remobilization. They may range from medical problems, such as deep venous thrombosis, to lack of motivation due to depression or dementia. The rehabilitation physician must be on guard for immobility and its consequences and be sure to remobilize patients as soon as possible.

Deep venous thrombosis (DVT) is a much feared complication that can lead to pulmonary embolization. Its incidence is low overall. Bromfield and Reding found this in 2.3% of 920 subjects [31] and McClatchie in 1.7% of 174 subjects [4]. The risk of DVT is greatest in patients who are nonambulatory with sensory loss in the limb [31]. Accurate measurement of calf circumference should be done daily in nonambulatory or minimally ambulatory patients. If asymmetry, erythema, or tender cords are noted, a Doppler study or venogram should be considered. Pulsating stockings should be used for patients with severe hemiplegia or paraplegia and virtually no limb movement. Subcutaneous heparin should be used in nonambulatory or minimally ambulatory subjects when not contraindicated by other conditions.

The decubitus ulcer or pressure sore can greatly complicate or prolong hospitalization. The prevalence of pressure sores has been reported to be 3–10% of hospitalized patients and up to 27% of populations in chronic care facilities [32,33]. Pressure sores are associated with multiple complications including osteomyelitis, pyarthroses, sepsis, anemia, and amyloidosis [32–35]. The patient with a pressure sore requires a longer period in the hospital, and the cost for the patient's care is much greater. Finally, the patient with a pressure sore will require up to 50% more nursing time.

Pressure sores develop over bony prominences where the skin is subjected to focal intense pressure between the contact point and the underlying bone. Constant pressure of 70 mmHg for 2 hr can produce tissue necrosis [36]. The higher the pressure, the less time needed to produce necrosis. A study of sitting patients showed pressures of up to 500 mmHg on the buttocks [36]. Foam padding only reduced this to 150 mmHg.

A second factor is that of shear force. Shear occurs when layers slide by each other and thus the blood supply may be disrupted. At the same time that shear forces are being applied to the skin, friction may damage the overlying skin, providing a double impetus for pressure sore production [36].

The major sites of involvement are the sacral and coccygeal regions and areas over the greater trochanter of the femur and the ischial tuberosity. The heels, lateral malleoli, elbows, scapulae, and occiput are also areas of importance [36].

The risk factors for pressure sores are listed in Table 4. The major risk factors are those involving immobility and poor nutrition [33,36].

The major approach to the pressure sore is prevention through skilled and dedicated nursing care. The physician and nurse must identify the high-risk patient and give close attention to areas of the skin subjected to pressure due to lying or sitting for prolonged periods of time. Bedbound patients should be rolled frequently to avoid development of decubitus ulcers on the hips, knees, ankles, shoulders, and scapulae. Bed covers should be soft and sponge mattress covers or even air mattresses should be employed. Attention must be given to the problem of shear forces, especially when the head of the bed is elevated and the patient has a tendency to slide towards the foot of the bed. The patient should be watched carefully for incontinence of stool or urine and kept clean and dry. The physician must be sure the patient has adequate caloric intake, avoids hypoalbuminemia, and does not have other metabolic problems such as hyperthyroidism, diabetes, anemia, or malnutri-

Table 4   Factors Associated with Pressure Sores

Altered level of consciousness
Bed- or chair bound
Impaired nutrition
Requiring total assistance with activities of daily living
Contracture
Fracture
Stroke
Fecal soiling
Urinary soiling
Diabetes
Hypoalbuminemia
Anemia, low hemoglobin
Increasing age

tion that may predispose to decubitus ulcers or interfere with healing of existing ulcers.

The final complication that should be mentioned is depression. This is a common problem in the patient undergoing rehabilitation and may occur at any time during the course of recovery. The physician should be aware of this complication and proceed with appropriate treatment. This topic is covered in detail elsewhere in the book. When treating depression, the physician should keep in mind the problems of using medications that cause sedation and diminished mobility. These complications must be balanced against the potential benefits of antidepressant medications.

In conclusion, this chapter presents a compendium of the multiple complications that may arise in the patient undergoing rehabilitation. It is, in many respects, a listing of the complications of geriatric medicine rather than specific problems relating to the patient undergoing rehabilitation. These complications, however, may produce significant interference with the rehabilitation process and diminish the patient's overall quality of life as well as speed of returning to maximum level of independence. These are common problems but they can interfere significantly with the overall outcome. For this reason, the rehabilitation physician must be aware of these problems in his daily interaction with the patient and the rehabilitation team. Caring for these problems on a daily basis may make the difference between success and failure in the goals of rehabilitation.

REFERENCES

1. B.H. Dobkin, *J. Neurol. Rehab.*, 1:3–7 (1987).
2. J.S. Feigenson, F.H. McDowell, P. Meese, M.L. McCarthy, and S.D. Greenberg, *Stroke*, 8:651–662 (1977).
3. M. Adler, D. Hamaty, C.C. Brown, and H. Potts, *J. Chron. Dis.*, 30:461–471 (1977).
4. G. McClatchie, *Med. J. Aust.*, 1:649–651 (1980).
5. W.M. Garraway, J.P. Whisnant, L.T. Kurland, and W.M. O'Fallon, *Stroke*, 10: 657–663 (1979).
6. P.A. Wolf and W.B. Kannel, *Semin. Neurol.*, 6:243–253 (1986).
7. W.B. Kannel, T.R. Dawber, P. Sorlie, and P.A. Wolf, *Stroke*, 7:327–331 (1976).
8. T. Harris, E.F. Cook, W.B. Kannel, and L. Goldman, *J. Am. Geriatr. Soc.*, 36: 1023–1028 (1988).
9. W.B. Applegate, *Textbook of Internal Medicine*, vol. 2 (W.N. Kelley, ed.), J.B. Lippincott, Philadelphia, pp. 2590–2593 (1989).
10. P.A. Wolf, R.D. Abbott, and W.B. Kannel, *Stroke*, 22:983–988 (1991).
11. L.G. Paulson, *Textbook of Internal Medicine*, vol. 2 (W. N. Kelley, ed.), J.B. Lippincott, Philadelphia, pp. 2569–2575 (1989).
12. R.J. Luchi, G.E. Taffet, and T.A. Teasdale, *J. Am. Geriatr. Soc.*, 39:810–825 (1991).

13. G.S. Eisenbarth, *Textbook of Internal Medicine*, vol. 2 (W.N. Kelley, ed.), J.B. Lippincott, Philadelphia, pp. 2222–2229 (1989).

14. C.R. Kahn, *Textbook of Internal Medicine*, vol. 2 (W.N. Kelley, ed.), J.B. Lippincott, Philadelphia, pp. 2216–2222 (1989).

15. J.W. Rowe, *Textbook of Internal Medicine*, vol. 2 (W.N. Kelley, ed.), J.B. Lippincott, Philadelphia, pp. 2584–2590 (1989).

16. T.L. Petty, *Textbook of Internal Medicine*, vol. 2 (W.N. Kelley, ed.), J.B. Lippincott, Philadelphia, pp. 1884–1889 (1989).

17. J.H. Walsh, *Textbook of Internal Medicine*, vol. 2 (W.N. Kelley, ed.), J.B. Lippincott, Philadelphia, pp. 500–513 (1989).

18. J.L. Barnett and W.J. Snape, Jr., *Textbook of Internal Medicine*, vol. 2 (W.N. Kelley, ed.), J.B. Lippincott, Philadelphia, pp. 513–519 (1989).

19. T.J. Wells and A.C. Diokno, *Semin. Neurol.*, 9:60–67 (1989).

20. Z. Khan, P. Starer, and V.K. Singh, *Semin. Neurol.*, 8:156–158 (1988).

21. B. Toye and A.R. Ronald, *Textbook of Internal Medicine*, vol. 2 (W.N. Kelley, ed.), J.B. Lippincott, Philadelphia, pp. 1757–1764 (1989).

22. C.B. Brendler, *Textbook of Internal Medicine*, vol. 2 (W.N. Kelley, ed.), J.B. Lippincott, Philadelphia, pp. 2599–2601 (1989).

23. D.A. Gelber, D.C. Good, L.J. Laven, and S.J. Verhulst, *Stroke*, 24:378–382 (1993).

24. K.W. Lyles, *Textbook of Internal Medicine*, vol. 2 (W.N. Kelley, ed), J.B. Lippincott, Philadelphia, pp. 2601–2607 (1989).

25. G.V. Ball and W.J. Koopman, *Textbook of Internal Medicine*, vol. 2 (W.N. Kelley, ed.), J.B. Lippincott, Philadelphia, pp. 974–981 (1989).

26. D.C. Good, J.R. Couch, and L.B. Wacaser, *Surg. Neurol.*, 22:285–291 (1984).

27. P.C.H. Baker, *Semin. Neurol.*, 9:50–59 (1989).

28. S. Selikson, K. Damus, and D. Hamerman, *J. Am. Geriatr. Soc.*, 36:707–712 (1988).

29. A.S. Dontas, A. Tzonou, P. Kasviki-Charvati, G.L. Georgiades, G. Christakis, and D. Trichopoulos, *J. Am. Geriatr. Soc.*, 39:641–649 (1991).

30. S.R. Lord, R.D. Clark, and I.W. Webster, *J. Am. Geriatr. Soc.*, 39:1194–1200 (1991).

31. E.B. Bromfield and M.J. Reding, *J. Neurol. Rehab.*, 2:51–57 (1988).

32. R.M. Allman, C.A. Laprade, L.B. Noel, J.M. Walker, C.A. Moorer, M.R. Dear, and C.R. Smith, *Ann. Intern. Med.*, 105:337–342 (1986).

33. D.R. Berlowitz and S.V.B. Wilking, *J. Am. Geriatr. Soc.*, 37:1043–1050 (1989).

34. R.J. Michocki and P.P. Lamy, *J. Am. Geriatr. Soc.*, 24:323–328 (1976).

35. B. Sugarman, S. Hawes, D.M. Musher, M. Klima, E.J. Young, and F. Pircher, *Arch. Intern. Med.*, 143:683–688 (1983).

36. J.B. Reuler and T.G. Cooney, *Ann. Intern. Med.*, 94:661–666 (1981).

V
SPECIFIC CONDITIONS

19
Stroke

Ronald Pak and Mary L. Dombovy

University of Rochester and
St. Mary's Hospital
Rochester, New York

EPIDEMIOLOGY

There are an estimated 400,000 new strokes per year and it remains a leading cause of death [1]. The incidence of stroke decreased in the 1960s and 1970s but there is evidence that the rate is no longer declining [2]. Mortality from stroke has also decreased [3]. Within the first 30 days poststroke, mortality is 17–25% for infarctions and 40–60% for hemorrhagic strokes [4,5]. Beyond this initial period of high mortality, survival is good, and by 18 months poststroke, survival is similar to that of the age- and sex-matched normal population [6,7]. Increased survival after stroke and the aging of the general population are contributing to an enlarging group of disabled stroke survivors.

When looking at functional loss after stroke, one needs to keep in mind the difference between neurological impairment (hemiplegia, aphasia) and disability (ability to ambulate, perform activities of daily living [ADLs], communicate). The two generally parallel each other but determinants of the latter are multifactorial. These may include medical comorbidities, psychosocial issues, and environmental factors, all of which can affect the way someone is able to adapt to his or her neurological impairment.

Studies of unselected stroke populations have demonstrated that within 1 week of stroke, 68–88% are dependent in some aspect of ADLs and mobility. At 6 months the percentage of survivors needing some assistance is

461

40–53%, and at 1 year 33% [6–8]. In general, four of five survivors will eventually become independent in ambulation (with or without assistive devices). Two of three will become independent in ADLs [9]. Beyond 1 year, functional status remains fairly constant for 5 years, after which more survivors experience functional deterioration along with increased rates of institutionalization [7]. This is likely related to cumulative medical and social factors associated with aging. Reports of institutionalization after stroke vary depending on when the assessment is done and what population is being studied, but have been reported at 15–29% [5,7,9,10].

Psychosocial adjustment poststroke is perhaps the most important determinant of quality of life for survivors of stroke. Although assessment methods vary, it is clear that a significant proportion of survivors experience decreased satisfaction with life. This proportion has been reported to be as high as 61–83% 4 years poststroke [11,12]. Not surprising is that decreased life satisfaction generally correlates with degree of functional deficit, however, even survivors with no disability report decreased satisfaction with their quality of life [11–13]. Other related factors included inability to return to work, decreased recreational/social activities, inaccessible transportation, and lack of community support. Decreased vocational status (employment, homemaking) at 6–12 months after stroke has been reported at 43–63% [6,9,13].

Depressive disorders are present in 30–50% of survivors and may persist for more than a year [6,14–16]. Symptoms of depression after stroke were previously thought to be an adjustment reaction to disability. However the high prevalence of long-term symptoms may represent an organic component related to the brain injury. There appears to be a higher incidence of depression in anterior left hemisphere and left basal ganglia strokes, and it does not necessarily correlate with degree of neurological impairment [14]. The widespread depletion of cerebral norepinephrine that occurs, particularly following anterior left hemisphere stroke, supports a neurochemical cause for poststroke depression [17]. There is evidence that depression is associated with decreased improvement in functional status [15,16,18]. This and the probable neurochemical cause underscore the need for pharmacological intervention. Despite this, few (< 8%) receive treatment [8,14,16], even though there is evidence that antidepressant therapy is beneficial [18,19].

PATTERNS OF NEUROLOGICAL RECOVERY

Recovery from hemiparesis tends to follow a sequential pattern described by Twitchell [20]. The initial stage is flaccidity. After this there is a return of reflexes and the development of spasticity. Return of voluntary movement follows, usually in a proximal to distal pattern. Initial voluntary movement occurs in a synergy pattern, with flexor synergies generally appearing first followed by extensor synergies. As a person is able to control and isolate movement better, there is usually an accompanying decrease in spasticity. These stages occur through a continuum and the degree to which each state is present may vary from person to person. Also the point at which recovery plateaus can differ. For instance, a few never progress beyond the flaccid stage. Many others develop severe spasticity and never get beyond synergistic movement. If voluntary movement is not present by 15 days or measurable grip strength by 1 month, the outlook for recovery of useful arm function is poor [20,21].

Motor recovery usually plateaus by 3 months [21–23]. The degree of recovery may vary depending on type of stroke. Intracerebral hemorrhages have a higher initial mortality; however, there is greater potential for later recovery [5]. The arm is usually more involved and has less complete recovery than the leg [22]. At 6 months after onset, 50–61% of survivors have some residual hemiparesis [6,24] and at 1 year the proportion is approximately 37% [6].

Aphasia has been reported in 24% of persons acutely after stroke [25,26]. Wade and colleagues [25] found that at 6 months only 12% had significant aphasia, but 44% of patients thought that their speech was still abnormal. Recovery from aphasia is generally fastest in the first 3 months; however, the total time course for recovery may be more prolonged with continued improvement possible beyond 1 year [27]. Different types of aphasia have different recovery patterns. Global aphasia has the worst prognosis for recovery, but more clinical improvement may be evident between 6 months and 1 year than in the first 6 months [28,29]. Comprehension is generally less affected and can improve more than expression [28].

Reports of sensory, perceptual, and cognitive deficits will vary depending on measures used. Neglect after right cerebral infarctions has been reported at 12–49% [30,31]. Gross neglect appears to resolve to a large extent in the majority of patients by 8–12 weeks [31,32]. More complex visuoperceptual deficits may recover incompletely, with deficits still present at 1 year [33]. Proprioception is a key factor in executing and relearning motor function. Smith [31] found proprioceptive deficits in 44% of testable patients after stroke. Eighty-seven percent of these who survived had recovered sense of proprioception by 8 weeks. Persistent cognitive and memory impairment has been reported in about 55–65% at 3 months and in 30–40% at 1 year [6].

Hemianopic visual field deficits have been reported at 17% acutely poststroke [34], but recovery has not been studied extensively. Gray and colleagues [35] evaluated stroke patients (infarcts and hemorrhages) with hemianopic field defects for 28 days. Forty-nine percent of those with complete field deficits detected by confrontation testing did not survive to 28 days. Among the survivors: 39% had persistent complete homonomous hemianosia, 27% had partial deficits, and 34% had recovered completely. Those who recovered completely did so by 2–10 days. They did not mention how the recovery patterns differed in hemorrhagic strokes vs. infarcts.

Swallowing problems may be as prevalent as 50% acutely after stroke [36,37]. Similar to other deficits, it appears that most recovery occurs in the first 3 months. Approximately 4% of 1 year survivors report persistent difficulty in swallowing [6].

NEUROPHYSIOLOGICAL MODELS OF RECOVERY

Neurophysiological mechanisms of recovery after stroke are not fully understood, but greater insight into this process is gradually emerging. Research in this area is of critical importance because through greater understanding there will be the opportunity for more directed, rational interventions aimed at minimizing effects of initial brain damage and promoting recovery. The following review touches on some of the theories regarding recovery after stroke that have support in animal or human subjects. More than one mechanism is operant during the recovery process. Recovery mechanisms can be broadly classified into resolution of acute affects of injury and dynamic functional and anatomical reorganization of brain.

Initial clinical improvement during the first weeks poststroke is attributed, in part, to resolution of edema and recovery of the surrounding ischemic penumbra. Interventions aimed at maximizing recovery of neural tissue at risk are discussed elsewhere in this text. Another effect of the acute injury is diaschisis or functional depression involving uninjured brain remote from the site of lesion [38]. Evidence in animal models indicates that this phenomenon correlates with alterations in the noradrenergic neurotransmitter system. Functional (metabolic) improvement in remote areas affected by diaschisis can take place over months, but it appears that the rate and degree of recovery can be affected by pharmacological agents [39]. The catecholaminergic drug amphetamine has been shown to promote recovery of remote functional depression and associated clinical deficits in animal models [40–42]. A preliminary study in human stroke victims reported improved motor recovery after treatment with amphetamines [43].

Other potential mechanisms of recovery involve dynamic functional and anatomical reorganization of intact brain to take over for the area of injured brain. Reports of functional return after hemispherectomy illustrate the ability of intact brain to adapt and take a greater role in function normally attributed to contralateral brain tissue [44]. A correlate of this using aphasia as a model is illustrated by Papanicolau's work [45], in which evoked potential monitoring showed greater right hemisphere activation in recovering adult aphasic compared to control patients.

Theories as to how intact brain might reorganize to "take over" function include unmasking or activation of previously inactive alternative pathways [46] and dendritic sprouting with synaptogenesis. Sprouting and synaptogenesis have been demonstrated in the mammalian central nervous system (CNS), even in the aged [47]. Its role in recovery, however, is unclear because electrophysiological integrity and functional correlation have not been adequately demonstrated. Sprouting may actually worsen outcome through maladaptive aberrant connections that may lead to seizures or learning problems [48,49].

The idea that experience can be the trigger for this adaptive brain reorganization is a key point from the standpoint of rehabilitation intervention. Evidence for experience- (i.e., "therapy") dependent brain plasticity has been demonstrated in a number of animal models [50–52]. Jenkins and Merzenich [53] have demonstrated through electrophysiological mapping studies in monkeys how topographical representations in the somatosensory cortex can reorganize based on repeated peripheral afferent input. When a small infarct is induced in an area that corresponds topographically to a portion of the monkey's hand, over a period of weeks to months, intact cortex surrounding the infarct takes over the sensory representation that had been in the infarcted area. The completeness of this reorganization is dependent on the degree of functional demand or use of the hand. It is postulated that a similar process could be occurring in other areas of neocortex to account for improvement in other deficit areas.

VALUE OF COMPREHENSIVE INPATIENT REHABILITATION

Ethical concerns and current practice make it unlikely that there will be a randomized controlled trial of comprehensive rehabilitation compared with no therapy whatsoever. A reasonable question to ask is: What are the benefits of comprehensive, interdisciplinary, focused rehabilitation programs in a designated rehabilitation unit compared with noncoordinated therapy efforts in a less structured setting? According to Feldman et al. [54], "The results suggest . . . that the great majority of hemiparetic stroke victims can be rehabilitated adequately on medical and neurologic wards (without formal rehabilitation services) if proper attention is given to ambulation and self care activities." In an earlier review of studies on stroke rehabilitation, Lind [55] concluded that spontaneous recovery accounted for most of the improvements in functional ability. However, he made two very important observations: although the functional improvements attributable to rehabilitation may be slight, they sometimes make the difference between institutionalization and return home; and carefully selected patients with "marginal functional impairment" may benefit from individualized and comprehensive rehabilitation.

Since these earlier reports, a number of additional studies have addressed the value of comprehensive rehabilitation, many of which are controlled prospective trials. In one study based on the population of Edinburgh, Scotland [56,57], patients with stroke were randomized a few days after onset to either a "stroke unit" or to a medical ward. Independence in ADL was assessed at discharge and found to be significantly greater in the patients on the stroke unit despite similar neurological deficits in the two groups. The length of hospitalization was shorter for patients in the stroke unit than for those on the medical wards. Patients in the stroke unit received physical therapy earlier and were more likely to receive occupational therapy and to receive it earlier. Other potentially important differences between the stroke unit and the medical ward included the presence of rehabilitation nursing, an interdisciplinary approach, and a functionally oriented atmosphere that may have encouraged patients and families to take a more active role, promoting consistent practice and carryover of skills.

Another similar, randomized community-based study from England [58] noted a higher proportion of patients from stroke units discharged home and a greater percentage independent in ADL at 1 year post-stroke (compared to patients receiving therapy on medical wards). In another prospective controlled population-based trial from Umea, Sweden, Strand et al. [59,60] compared the outcome for unselected patients with acute stroke in a stroke rehabilitation unit (n = 110) with patients receiving therapy on general medical wards (n = 183). Three months after onset only 15% of survivors admitted to the stroke unit compared with 39% from the medical wards were still in the hospital. A higher proportion of survivors from the stroke unit were independent in walking, personal hygiene, and dressing. In subgroups, with mild to moderate deficits or age <75, care in the stroke unit accelerated the process of rehabilitation. In groups with major deficits and age >75, stroke unit care enhanced the proportion of patients able to return home. Sievenius et al. [61], in another randomized trial (subjects drawn from a community stroke registrar in Kupio, Finland), found improved independence in ADL in a group of patients receiving intensive physical therapy (PT) in a designated rehabilitation unit compared to controls.

Dignan et al. [62], studying a large population of 774 patients in North Carolina, found no difference in Barthel scores at discharge, and 3, 6, 12 months after discharge in patients cared for in coordinated stroke program (an attempt to coordinate aspects of hospital and posthospital care) compared to patients in other hospitals without the program. Concluding from this study that coordinated care or interdisciplinary rehabilitation does not improve ADL may not be valid for the following reasons. This study was done in three separate hospitals where care might have been inherently different; there was a significantly higher number of initially comatose patients in the coordinated program (22.2% vs. 11.9%); outcome was measured at time since discharge and not at time since stroke onset. Patients admitted or discharged earlier from a rehabilitation unit are likely to have suffered a less severe stroke to begin with; little is known about the differences in duration and amount of therapy received by the two groups; and, as noted above, this study is not a trial of the effects of comprehensive rehabilitation but an attempt to improve and coordinate care.

Davies et al. [63] retrospectively matched for severity of stroke 30 patients admitted to the hospital with 31 patients managed at home from a community register in Oxfordshire of first strokes and found no difference in Barthel score at 5 months poststroke, despite the hospitalized group receiving more therapy. The hospitalized patients were not necessarily in a coordinated rehabilitation unit. The authors excluded all severely involved patients from analysis. In addition, the retrospective nature of the study limits the validity of the conclusions (e.g., the patients in the hospital may have been hospitalized because of medical complications that potentially could have interfered with recovery).

In a study from Canada [64], the benefits of team care appeared to be very limited. These researchers had a team of stroke specialists who consulted throughout the hospital. The patients were not situated in a defined unit, resulting in the loss of rehabilitation nursing and a rehabilitation focus and also probably leading to inconsistencies in care.

A recent study investigating the benefit of a comprehensive designated stroke unit providing both acute and rehabilitative care was undertaken at the University of Trondheim in Norway [65]. The University serves as the primary hospital for a population of approximately 200,000. Patients with onset of symptoms more than 1 week earlier, those living in a nursing home prior to stroke, those who were unconscious, and those who were not members of the community were excluded. Those with subarachnoid hemorrhage were also excluded. A total of 220 patients were randomized, 110 to the stroke unit and 110 to the general medical wards. There were no significant initial differences in demographics or function of the patients. At 6 weeks 56.7% of the patients in the stroke unit had returned home while only 32.7% of the patients in the medical unit were home (p = 0.0004). At 1 year poststroke 62.7% of patients in the stroke unit were home compared with 44.6 from the medical units (p = 0.002). Functional status as measured by the Barthel index was also significantly better in patients in the stroke unit at 6 weeks (p = 0.0014) and at 1 year (p = 0.001). This study also demonstrated an improvement in survival through use of a stroke unit. The differences in mortality were largely due to decreases in death from pneumonia, pulmonary embolus, and second or extension of stroke. Thus, the decrease in mortality may have resulted from earlier mobilization.

In light of the above studies on stroke rehabilitation, particularly the most recent study by Indredavik et al. [65], attention must be called to the practice of rehabilitation as it occurs in most settings in the United States. Most patients are initially admitted to a general medical or neurology ward where they remain for several days before being transferred to rehabilitation. In all of the above population-based, controlled studies, patients are randomized shortly after onset to either a stroke unit or to a medical unit. Although these investigators have had difficulty determining what aspects of treatment are important to recovery, any strategy to treat patients with stroke will face the problem of trying to isolate the specific therapies important to the improved outcome. In an integrated approach such as that of Indredavik et al. [65], acute treatment is standardized, systematic, and closely linked to early mobilization, intensive rehabilitation, and family education. They note that this systematically coordinated form of treatment would not be possible without a designated stroke unit.

OUTCOME PREDICTION AND ASSESSMENT FOR INPATIENT REHABILITATION

Patient assessment for a rehabilitation program is based on an estimate of the outcome that can be achieved. It is generally thought that patients with moderately severe impairment poststroke will likely benefit most from inpatient rehabilitation [66,67]. Ultimate outcome, however, is a complex issue that must be addressed on many levels: How much neurological recovery can occur? What functional level can be achieved? Will this person be able to return home? Return to work? Studies looking at factors predicting outcome after stroke have given some insight into contributing determinants, but there are no hard and fast rules that can be reliably applied to individual patients. This is because outcome determinants are multifactorial and go beyond intrinsic neurological recovery. How the neurological impairments interact with each other to contribute to functional deficits as well as premorbid intelligence and adaptability all may affect how a person responds to a rehabilitation program. Other underlying medical problems can also interfere with rehabilitation and recovery. Family support, socioeconomic status, and availability of outpatient services will be key factors in disposition. Each individual needs to be comprehensively assessed based on his or her own unique circumstances.

Clinical and neurological variables associated with functional outcome have been reviewed [68,69]. Methodological issues make it difficult to compare and interpret data across studies. However, factors reported as negative predictors of functional outcome include coma at onset, incontinence 2 weeks after stroke, poor cognitive function, no motor return within 1 month, previous stroke, spatial–perceptual deficits, significant cardiovascular disease, multiple neurological deficits, large lesions on computed tomogram (CT), and advanced age. Overall functional status at admission to rehabilitation, as measured by the Barthel Index, is one of the more reliable predictors of functional status at discharge [70,71]. Granger and colleagues [72] further identified a functional subset (bowel control, feeding, bladder control, grooming) that was not only predictive of discharge functional status but also predicted a 14-fold increase in the chance of living in the community at 6 month follow-up if a patient was independent in these functions. Other methods that may aid in predicting recovery include single photon emission commuted tomography (SPECT) [73,74] and electrophysiological testing with somatosensory and motor evoked potentials [75,76].

In addition to overall functional status, social support and economic status are key factors in determining disposition and become more important the greater the degree of patient disability. If a patient has a spouse, there is a greater chance of home discharge [7]. This correlation is stronger for stroke victims who are male rather than female, presumably because of the more traditional caretaker role of women [5,77].

Reports of return to work after stroke vary. In part, this appears to be related to the population studied and the definition of "work." As would be expected, better functional status correlates with return to work [78,79]. In a recent study, Black-Schaffer and Osberg [79] found that lower Barthel Index scores, longer rehabilitation stay, aphasia, and prior alcohol use were negative predictors of return to employment, homemaking, or studies.

In summary, in patients with a moderate degree of impairment poststroke inpatient rehabilitation can likely have the most impact and make the difference in facilitating discharge to the community. This has obvious advantages from both human and economic perspectives, when one considers the alternative of institutionalization. Outcome potential must be considered in the context of amount of neurological impairment, premorbid functional level, overall medical condition, psychosocial status, and economic considerations. Of critical importance is determining the patient's own goals for rehabilitation, because if a rehabilitation program can be tailored to meet those expectations, likelihood of "good outcome" based on increased life satisfaction is much greater.

REHABILITATION MANAGEMENT

Introduction

Rehabilitation is defined as the combined and coordinated use of medical, social, educational, and vocational services for retraining a person to the highest possible level of functional ability [80]. This comprehensive approach requires an interdisciplinary team generally consisting of a managing physician knowledgeable in stroke rehabilitation, rehabilitation nursing, physical therapy, occupational therapy, speech therapy, psychology, and social work services. Additional members can include recreation therapists, vocational counselors, nutritionists, and prosthetist/orthotists. There are two general components of rehabilitation management. The first includes preventive measures aimed at maintaining emotional, cognitive, and physical integrity and minimizing complications that will prevent or prolong functional return. These measures should begin immediately poststroke and continue as long as necessary. The second component is restorative treatment aimed at promoting functional recovery. This phase should begin as soon as the patient is medically and neurologically stable and has the cognitive and physical ability to participate actively in a rehabilitation program.

Rehabilitation Issues Immediately Poststroke

Preventive or maintenance rehabilitation measures are the primary issues immediately poststroke. Care should be taken to orient the patient to his or her surroundings and explain to both patient and family the nature and implications of their deficits. Physical, occupational, and, if indicated, speech therapists should become involved in the care as soon as the patient is stable. Range-of-motion exercises to all extremities should be performed at least twice a day through coordinated efforts of nursing and therapy staff. Attention to body positioning is critical to prevent pressure sores and contractures. Splinting of upper and lower extremities may also be needed to facilitate proper position and prevent hand–finger or ankle–foot contractures. Even if a patient does not experience significant neurological improvement, these problems can ultimately detract from patient comfort and care by causing pain, increasing spasticity, and interfering with positioning, transfers, dressing, and hygiene. For patients who are candidates for rehabilitation, the rehabilitation course becomes more prolonged since time, effort, and expense will be directed towards healing decubiti and correcting contractures.

Skin relief at vulnerable pressure points may be augmented through the use of water and eggcrate mattresses, as well as with elbow, knee, or heel pads. Additional mattresses may make bed mobility more difficult, but in the early stages skin protection is more important. The patient should initially be turned every 2 hr, with close attention to the affected side, which can be more prone to injury because of altered mental status, paresis, sensory deficit, and neglect. Ulnar and peroneal pressure neuropathies are also common on the involved side and should be prevented through padding and proper positioning.

The patient with a flaccid upper extremity is at risk for brachial plexus stretch injuries either through staff pulling on the affected arm or the patient trying to get up or move with the arm caught behind (e.g., in the bedrail). Patients with neglect are extremely prone to this problem. Prevention involves (a) staff education as to protection of the extremity by always making sure they do not pull on it or attempt to transfer the patient before positioning the patient's arm in front of them; (b) patient education and training (with much repetition for patients with neglect or sensory loss); (c) use of a sling during transfers.

Voiding status must be monitored. Initial concerns are to make sure that the bladder is emptying regularly without overdistention and that infection is avoided. Urinary incontinence poststroke is common and the cause is multifactorial. Impaired cognition, paresis, urinary tract infection, and loss of central control of detrusor function can all contribute to incontinence. Patients will often initially have an indwelling catheter that should be discontinued as soon as the patient is stable. Occasionally there may be urinary retention due to poor detrusor contractility, at which time a scheduled bladder catheterization program should be instituted until adequate spontaneous voiding occurs. The catheterization schedule and fluid intake should be designed to keep bladder volumes less than 500cc. The possibility of outlet obstruction must always be kept in mind. The neurogenic bladder pattern typically seen after suprapontine strokes is one in which the bladder fills and the detrusor autonomously contracts due to loss of central inhibition. Promoting increased awareness and subsequent voluntary control of voiding is done through a scheduled program of offering a bedpan or urinal every few hours. Postvoid residuals should initially be checked to ensure adequate emptying. Less than 100 ml is acceptable.

For men, other short-term solutions during training include propping the urinal for collection while in bed and using condom catheters. If the patient continues to have problems with frequency and urgency, and infection is not the cause, small amounts of oxybutynin (e.g., 5 mg twice daily) may be helpful. Conversely, patients with continued retention occasionally benefit from administration of urecholine. Tricyclic antidepressants and antihistamines may worsen urinary retention.

Bowel regularity and continence can be maintained through adequate fluid intake, diet, stool softeners, and suppositories when needed. The key is to start a bowel regimen before constipation and impaction become problems. Some severely constipated patients may require use of laxatives. If bowel incontinence is present, a scheduled bowel evacuation using a rectal suppository on a daily or every-other-day schedule can be effective in decreasing this.

Early assessment of swallowing and nutrition are also critical and will be discussed in a later section. The most common cause of death other than the stroke itself in the first 30 days poststroke is aspiration pneumonia and up to 40% of aspiration in stroke patients is silent and not detected at the bedside.

Cognition and Behavior

The presence of cognitive impairments after stroke will affect every facet of function, and is a key determinant in the patient's ultimate disability irrespective of the degree of physical impairment. Cognitive and neuropsychological dysfunction can include deficits in attention, alertness, orientation, memory and learning, reasoning, judgment, visual perception, affect, and mood. Language impairment, commonly associated with left hemispheric lesions, will be discussed separately. Neuropsychological evaluation including psychometric testing can be very helpful in identifying the presence and severity of specific cognitive deficits; identifying intact functions (i.e., areas of relative strength); and guiding development of appropriate restorative therapies and compensatory strategies.

Efficacy of rehabilitation for cognitive deficits after brain injury is somewhat controversial [81,82]. One area in cognitive rehabilitation that has shown some promise involves therapies directed at neglect and spatial perceptual deficits. These disorders are typically seen in right hemispheric injury and can profoundly interfere with all aspects of mobility and self-care from trying to orient clothing while dressing to driving a car. Techniques that can be effective in improving sensory awareness and visual perception include visual scanning, somatosensory awareness, sequencing, and spatial organization exercises [83,84].

There have been few studies of memory and learning dealing exclusively with patients with stroke. In general, attempts at restoring memory function after brain injury have not been successful [85,86]. Strategies for utilizing preserved learning ability to retain information include visual imagery, verbal elaboration, and spaced retrieval techniques, although there is some question as to whether these strategies can be used consistently in the brain-injured population [85–87]. Glisky and Schacter [88,89] have utilized a vanishing-cues technique to train patients with moderate to severe memory disorders specific complex computer skills that could be carried over to the workplace. Although this type of learning may not generalize well to the performance of other tasks, they argue that by addressing target domains that are practical and relevant for the patient, this will at least allow them to function better in everyday life. External aids can also be used to help with information storage and cuing. Such memory aids include alarm watches, calendars, posted schedules, and daily logs.

Changes in emotion and affect following stroke can include lability, anxiety, rage, and depression. Right hemispheric strokes are often associated with difficulty recognizing and expressing appropriate affect [90]. As mentioned before, depressive disorders after stroke appear to be quite prevalent and undertreated [14,16]. When depression is evident, treatment with pharmacological and psychotherapeutic intervention, should be initiated. There is evidence that nortriptyline and trazadone can be effective in poststroke depression [18,19].

Therapy Approaches for Motor Dysfunction

In addition to conventional therapy techniques such as range of motion, strengthening, and compensatory techniques to improve function, numerous neuromuscular retraining techniques have been described. These techniques are based on neurophysiological and developmental theories. Brunnstrom's approach [91] attempts to facilitate motor return using associated and primitive postural reactions to encourage movement through synergy patterns. Bobath's neurodevelopmental approach [92] focuses on normalization of muscle tone and inhibition of spasticity patterns using reflex inhibitory movement patterns and advanced postural reactions. The Rood technique [93] incorporates stimulation of cutaneous receptors to facilitate muscle contraction. Proprioceptive neuromuscular facilitation (PNF) [94] uses exercises in functional movement patterns and application of resistance to selected muscles in an effort to facilitate synergistic movement of associated weaker muscles.

These techniques are commonly incorporated into rehabilitation programs; however, their efficacy remains controversial. Numerous studies have reported no significant difference in outcomes between neurofacilitation techniques and more conventional therapies [95–98].

Another method used to promote neuromuscular recovery is electromyographic (EMG) biofeedback. Several studies have reported greater efficacy in upper extremity motor improvement with this technique than conventional therapies [99–101]. Basmajian and colleagues also compared neurodevelopmental techniques with an integrated program including behavioral therapy and EMG biofeedback [102]. They found that both techniques were associated with upper extremity functional improvement but that there was no significant difference in the two groups.

Functional electrical stimulation (FES) has also been used to promote muscle function, increase strength, and decrease shoulder subluxation. Merletti and colleagues [103] reported that after 1 month of FES to the peroneal nerve on the hemiplegic side for 20 min daily, there was a threefold difference in ankle dorsiflexion strength compared to controls who received just traditional PT. Positive results have also been reported through combining FES and biofeedback. Cozean and colleagues [104] found that serial use of both treatments resulted in greater improvement in gait than either treatment alone. Another technique reported to be beneficial is combining the two modalities using surface EMG over the involved muscles to trigger electrically augmented muscle contraction [105,106].

Mobility

Barriers to safe, independent mobility after stroke can include paresis, apraxia, incoordination, poor balance and postural control, cognitive and perceptual impairment, and sensory deficits. Other limiting factors such as deconditioning and medical comorbidities will also contribute.

Mobility retraining starts with learning how to move around in bed using the patient's unaffected side and progressing to balance and postural control activities while sitting. Transfer training is incorporated into the program to get the patient from the bed to other surfaces such as a wheelchair or commode. When the patient can stand with assistance, a stand pivot transfer is employed. Learning safe transfer technique is a critical step because of its importance in mobility independence, whether a patient will eventually walk or be wheelchair dependent. Training the family to assist with mobility, especially transfers, is a prerequisite for home passes and discharge.

Wheelchair mobility is achieved using a wheelchair low enough to the ground to allow the patient to use the uninvolved leg and arm to propel the chair. The paretic leg and arm are typically supported by a removable leg rest and arm board. Wheelchair mobility may take a significant amount of practice, especially if neglect or visual field deficits are present.

Progression towards ambulation starts with continued balance and postural control activities while standing. Because a person needs to bear some weight on the affected side during the gait cycle, weight shifting exercises are incorporated. When weight is shifted to the affected side, additional support can be given through weight bearing by the opposite upper extremity on a stable support such as parallel bars or other device such as a hemiwalker. During mobility training, an arm sling on the affected upper extremity can help with balance.

During these activities, feedback and repetition are critical. Motor learning is a process of execution and modification of an activity based on sensing and remembering the movements involved. This becomes more difficult in the person with impairments such as perceptual deficits, loss of proprioception, and impaired cognition and memory. Therefore, other techniques can be used to help improve feedback. One way this is done is through verbal repetition and cues from the therapist. This will have obvious limitations in the patient with language deficits. If a patient can utilize visual information, impaired proprioception may be offset by greater use of visual orientation and cues. A full-length mirror can be used for this purpose to show a patient immediately where his or her body is in space as he or she is performing an activity. Minimizing outside distractions is important to facilitate this feedback process and aid in concentration.

The key muscle group in the affected lower extremity for progression of ambulation is the hip extensors. Hip extension stabilizes the hip and advances the body during stance. It can also stabilize the knee by pulling it back into extension during stance phase despite weak quadriceps. Ankle dorsiflexors and everters are often slow to improve, therefore, an ankle–foot orthosis (AFO) is commonly used to support the foot in dorsiflexion. This facilitates foot clearance during swing phase and controls medial–lateral ankle instability. An AFO will also help control the knee during stance. If the knee tends to buckle during stance, increasing the amount of plantarflexion can bring the knee into earlier extension and prevent buckling. A maximum of 5–8 degrees is usually all that can be tolerated. If knee hyperextension is a problem, increasing the amount of AFO dorsiflexion can decrease knee hyperextension during stance, although greater quadriceps strength is required. To obtain the appropriate bracing, consultation between the physician, physical therapist, and an orthotist with expertise in hemiplegic bracing is highly recommended.

Spasticity often significantly affects ambulation training. Although a variety of patterns can be seen, it is common to see increased extensor tone at the knee and plantarflexion with inversion at the foot and ankle. This extensor synergy pattern may actually be helpful if it facilitates weight bearing on the affected side. However, an attempt at decreasing tone should be made if it is interfering with function or causing pain. This will be discussed further in a later section.

As ambulation improves, the patient progresses from the parallel bars to other devices as needed such as a hemiwalker, four-point cane, or straight cane. The goal is to achieve an energy-efficient reciprocal gait pattern. Eventually more complex ambulation training will be incorporated such as walking on uneven surfaces and in crowded areas. Negotiating stairs as well as transferring into and out of a car will also be very important for increasing independence and the return home. Reding and Potes [107] have shown that ambulating 150 feet with assistance is a reasonable goal for most patients with stroke, even in those with motor, sensory, and visual deficits although the time required to attain this goal may be longer.

Activities of Daily Living

Poststroke deficits in self-care and independent living skills can have an obvious impact on feelings of self-esteem. Rehabilitation interventions in this area can, therefore, significantly influence a person's concept of control and self-worth. These concerns are addressed initially by the occupational therapist starting with an ADL evaluation. Assessed are areas of basic self-care such as feeding, bathing, grooming, and dressing. Other areas that have an impact on independent living and quality of life are also addressed, such as leisure activities, homemaking, management of home finances, and child care skills, if appropriate. After assessment has been completed, individualized goals are formulated. These goals must take into account the wishes and expectations of the patient and family. In this way there is a greater chance of having the motivation to reach those targets.

The rehabilitation program generally includes upper extremity exercises for range of motion, strength, and coordination. Other methods to improve function often include neurofacilitation techniques, EMG biofeedback, and functional electric stimulation. Compensatory strategies are incorporated to help carry out tasks made difficult by neurological impairment. One-handed techniques can be used to address most areas of basic self-care. A wide array of adaptive equipment is available to help carry out tasks. These include items such as elastic shoelaces, weighted plates, dressing sticks, and reachers. Clothing modifications such as pantloops or Velcro closures may be added to aid in dressing. Home evaluations and subsequent modifications can significantly increase independence in the home. This may simply involve rearrangement of existing space. Other examples of home modifications to improve access could include widening doorways, adding a raised toilet seat, or adding shower grab bars.

Since cognitive and perceptual abilities are integral factors in independent living, occupational therapists will often be involved in testing and intervention. Therapies are geared toward practical applications such as meal planning, checkbook management and home finances, recreational activities, kitchen safety, and community living skills.

Nutrition and Swallowing

Many factors contribute to poor nutritional status after stroke. Decreased level of alertness, perceptual changes, hemiparesis, and dysphagia all interfere with adequate oral intake. Therefore, close monitoring of nutritional status must be a routine, integral part of care. Keeping track of calorie counts, weight, and results of laboratory tests will help guide nutritional support. The dietitian can be very helpful in addressing these issues. If oral intake is not thought to be safe or adequate, tube feedings via nasogastric or gastrostomy routes may be required initially.

Dysphagia after stroke may be as high as 50% [36,37]. Horner and Massey [36] found that 50% of those referred for a swallowing evaluation aspirated during videofluoroscopic evaluation. Of those who did aspirate, 54% aspirated silently. This underscores the high index of suspicion necessary for potential poststroke aspiration. Aspiration was more likely in the presence of combined cerebral–brainstem strokes and bilateral cranial nerve signs; however, it clearly also occurred in the setting of unilateral signs.

The most common problem after stroke is a delayed swallowing reflex [36,108]. Aspiration can then occur when material descends posteriorly, pools around the vallecula, and subsequently falls into the unprotected larynx. Other impairments such as neglect, poor attention, and oral muscle weakness can lead to pocketing of food and predispose to later aspiration. Since aspiration is often associated with pharyngeal phase abnormalities, it is difficult to diagnose on clinical examination alone. Dysphonia is often present in those who aspirate; however, absence of dysphonia does not rule it out. Dysphonia can occur as a weak, hoarse, or harsh sounding voice that may or may not sound wet. An impaired or absent gag reflex does not necessarily differentiate aspirators from those that do not aspirate [36,109]. Given the difficulty in diagnosing pharyngeal phase dysfunction, videofluoroscopic swallowing studies should be used when potential aspiration is a concern. This modified barium swallow procedure can determine if and why aspiration is occurring. It also helps to direct therapeutic intervention.

Swallowing therapies include exercise to improve oral strength and control. Laryngeal adduction exercises are aimed at protecting the airway. Thermal stimulation can be used to help trigger the swallowing reflex. If therapeutic feedings can be instituted without significant risk of aspiration, various compensatory strategies can be used to promote safe swallowing. These include proper positioning, controlling rate and bolus size during feeds, modification of food consistency, and repetitive swallowing with each bolus [110].

Communication

Poststroke communication deficits can be related to language or speech disorders. Impaired language can result from confusion or generalized intellectual impairment. This component may be especially prominent immediately after stroke. Aphasia may be present secondary to dominant hemisphere injury. Speech disorders are related to motor impairment and include dysarthria and verbal apraxia. As is often the case, the communication deficit may be due to a combination of the above. Management involves the coordinated efforts of the rehabilitation team including the speech and language therapist, neuropsychologist, and physician to identify the specific nature of the communication problem and institute appropriate therapy.

Treatment methods may be aimed at improving the specific impairment or using compensatory strategies to improve communication. Therapies to improve intelligibility and naturalness of dysarthric speech may include increasing respiratory control, phonation, velopharyngeal function, articulation, rate control, intonation, and phrasing [111]. Devices to augment or replace verbal communication such as communication boards or computers may be helpful in speech and language disorders, depending on the type of involvement and functional needs [112,113].

Studies generally support the efficacy of therapy for aphasia, although some have been criticized for methodological issues such as inadequate controls and lack of selection criteria [114–1116]. Therapy approaches include techniques to stimulate and facilitate language such as verbal repetition and sentence completion. Other methods attempt to utilize intact right brain function to enhance communication. Examples of this include melodic intonation therapy [117] and therapies that emphasize the use of visual symbols and gestures [118–120]. Using a more pragmatic framework, the promoting aphasics communicative effectiveness (PACE) technique promotes communication through putting therapy in a more natural communication setting. Principles of treatment include free use of any communication modality, such as gestures and facial expressions. Also, interaction between clinician and patient is more equal and conversational by alternating participation as sender and receiver [121].

Hemiplegic Shoulder

Shoulder pain and dysfunction on the involved side are very common after stroke. Because of the shoulder's complex anatomy and function, it is especially vulnerable to the poststroke effects of muscle weakness, sensory deficits, spasticity, and immobility. Van Ouweneller [122] found that 72% of stroke patients complained of shoulder pain at some time during the first year after stroke. The causes are not always clear and there is general agreement that further research in this area is needed [123,124].

Glenohumeral subluxation is often associated with shoulder pain; however, there is no conclusive evidence that it is causally related [123]. There is also controversy about whether current methods of reducing subluxation are effective in preventing pain [122,125]. Despite this, attempts are generally made to support the hemiplegic upper extremity because of potential adverse effects. Arm slings are often used when patients are ambulating; however, excessive use may promote unwanted flexion synergies and immobility [126]. When a patient is in a wheelchair, armboards allow more neutral rotation at the shoulder and elevation of the hand to prevent edema.

Reflex sympathetic dystrophy (RSD), or shoulder-hand syndrome, can occur in the hemiplegic upper extremity in 25% of stroke survivors [122,127].

Common clinical features include upper extremity swelling (particularly the hand and fingers), hyperpathia, vasomotor instability, and painful range of motion at the shoulder, wrist, and hand. Conservative management is often successful if the condition is diagnosed early. This includes nonsteroidal anti-inflammatory drugs (NSAIDs), aggressive range-of-motion exercise, and physical modalities. A short course of oral corticosteroids can be very effective [128]. Sympathetic blockade with stellate ganglion blocks, guanethidine bier blocks, or surgical sympathectomy may be necessary [123,129].

Prolonged immobility can lead to adhesive capsulitis or "frozen shoulder." Conditions that limit range of motion such as RSD and spasticity are often precursors to this problem. Proper positioning, range of motion exercises, and reducing muscle tone can prevent this complication.

Other conditions that can contribute to shoulder pain and dysfunction include degenerative joint disease, rotator cuff inflammation and rupture, subacromial bursitis, and biceps tendinitis [124,130]. Brachial plexus injury should be suspected in any patient with an unusual pattern of return of motor function in the upper extremity (e.g., no proximal movement in a patient with good return of function in the hand, or lack of finger flexion in a patient with good wrist and finger extension), absent or reduced reflexes, atrophy or patterns of sensory loss consistent with plexus injury [131].

Spasticity

In general, spasticity should be treated only if it is interfering with function or causing discomfort. In some cases, spasticity may be beneficial. For example, increased extensor tone in the hemiparetic leg may improve weight bearing ability during ambulation. Addressing spasticity begins with identifying contributing factors in the specific muscle groups involved. An increase in spasticity may be related to a nonneurological cause such as noxious stimulation from a poorly fitting orthosis or a skin ulcer. In the patient with stroke, problematic spasticity can often be isolated to unilateral regional areas such as elbow–wrist flexion or ankle plantar flexors. In this setting, initial therapy should be directed at the specific muscle groups and reflex loops involved, as opposed to systemic pharmacological therapy that may have detrimental side effects.

Treatment generally starts conservatively and progresses to more aggressive interventions depending on risk–benefit considerations. Range of motion and stretching exercises are an initial component of any spasticity treatment program. Not only does this prevent contractures but it can also have a prolonged effect on decreasing spasticity through decreasing reflex sensitivity [132]. Other ways of providing static stretch are through casting, splinting, and weight bearing. Additional methods of managing spasticity and joint deformity at specific sites include topical heat or cold and electrical stimulation [133,134]. Motor point and/or peripheral nerve blocks may be helpful in cases that do not respond to physical measures. The most commonly blocked nerves are the musculocutaneous (elbow flexion), median and ulnar (wrist and finger flexion), and posterior tibial (plantar flexion). The finger and wrist flexor muscles and the anterior tibialis muscle also may respond to intramuscular neurolysis. Diagnostic, temporary blocks with local anesthetic should be done before the semipermanent block with phenol is administered. The clinical benefit from the block often outlives the duration of action of the phenol and provides a window for aggressive, active therapy, and/or inhibitive serial casting. Botulinum toxin injection may prove to be an effective way to weaken specific spastic muscles [135].

Systemic pharmacotherapy has a limited role in treating patients with stroke with spastic hemiplegia. The main oral agents, baclofen, diazepam, and dantrolene, all have potential negative side effects that may be more prominent in brain-injured individuals. These include cognitive impairment, weakness, fatigue, and incoordination. If an oral agent is used, dantrolene is thought by some to be the preferred drug for cerebral spasticity [134,136]. It has relatively less cognitive effects and counteracts spasticity through peripheral action at the muscle. This occurs by blocking calcium release at the sarcoplasmic reticulum, thereby decreasing contractility. Because of potentially serious hepatotoxic effects, liver function must be monitored carefully [137].

Psychosocial Issues

Psychosocial variables are crucial factors in overall outcome after stroke. Unless there is psychological adjustment, full functional potential cannot be realized. As mentioned previously, poststroke depression is a significant problem and can be negatively associated with functional capacity and maintenance of gains [16,138,139]. Psychosocial adjustment of the family/caretaker is another main area that affects outcome. The family has to deal not only with the patient's emotional adjustment but also their own. The altered family dynamics creates new roles and responsibilities and resultant stresses often contribute to deteriorating relationships and depression in the caregivers [140].

Since the whole family system is affected by stroke, psychosocial concerns need to be addressed with those who will be a part of the recovery and adjustment process. Psychosocial assessments of the patient and family should be done to identify potential areas of dysfunction [141,142]. Identified depression should be treated with psychotherapy and/or pharmacotherapy [18,19]. Open communication with the patient and family throughout the rehabilitation process is critical. There should be opportunities for education and counseling. Education is beneficial not only for learning about stroke consequences and patient care skills but also for learning about coping and problem solving skills [143]. Thorough, coordinated discharge planning with appropriate services and follow-up can ease the transition to home. Encouraging contact with social supports outside the family can also be helpful. These can include groups such as church organizations or stroke support groups.

Sexual Function

Sexuality continues to be an important aspect of life as people grow older [144,145]. Despite this, the issue of sexual function after stroke is often neglected. A significant number of patients with stroke experience sexual dysfunction. Problems that have been reported include erectile and ejaculatory dysfunction in men, decreased vaginal lubrication and difficulty achieving orgasm in women, as well as decreased sexual satisfaction, decline in libido, and less frequent sexual activity in both [146–150].

The causes of sexual dysfunction after stroke have not been extensively studied, but psychological factors are thought to be significant contributors. Depression, anxiety, and loss of self-esteem are related to lessened sexual desire, insecurities about own desirability, and uncertainty about ability to participate sexually. Stroke patients report fears of increasing blood pressure and having a recurrent stroke if they have sex [138]. The emotional adjustment of the stroke patient's partner may also be interfering with resumption of sexual activity [151].

Functional deficits in the areas of motor function, sensation, perception, communication, cognition, and continence can also contribute to decrease sexual activity. Medications may play a role in sexual dysfunction. Many cardiovascular and psychoactive medications are known to have a detrimental effect on libido, erectile function, and ability to achieve orgasm [152,153].

Addressing sexual function after stroke can occur on several levels. First, it needs to be routinely discussed in a way that lets the patient and partner know that a return to sexual activity can be a component of poststroke function. Once sexual concerns and problems are identified, interventions aimed at underlying factors can range from counseling about self-image or sexual activity modification to adjusting medications. Depending on the expertise and comfort level of the rehabilitation team members in dealing with sexuality issues, referrals may be appropriate to certified sex therapists, psychologists, or other clinicians knowledgeable in this area. It certainly may be that the patient and partner are not ready to address the area of sexual function, especially during the inpatient phase. In this case there needs to be the opportunity to explore this issue further as an outpatient if necessary.

From a physiological perspective, it is unclear whether specific limitations should be put on certain types of sexual activity. In healthy and post-myocardial infarction subjects, there are elevations in heart rate and blood pressure during sexual intercourse that are variable and transient [154,155], but since reports of recurrent stroke during sex are lacking, the general message about resumption of sexual activity should be reassuring. In theory, patients with hemorrhagic strokes should perhaps be more cautious. More research in this area is needed.

Outpatient Care

The purpose of outpatient rehabilitation services is to help integrate the stroke patient back into the community and to continue addressing issues contributing to disability and handicap. Depending on the stroke patient's needs and available resources, outpatient management may range from routine physician follow-up to assess progress and maintenance of gains, to involvement in a comprehensive interdisciplinary rehabilitation program. Physician follow-up visits are an opportunity to reassess a number of functional and medical issues. Mobility and self-care status should be explored, psychosocial issues addressed, equipment checked, and medications reviewed. Continuing therapies and the home program should be reviewed with respect to content, progress, and goals. A functionally oriented physical examination should be documented. If a patient with stroke is not doing well functionally, it may take an in depth exploration to determine underlying physical or psychological factors that are contributing.

Outpatient therapies may be administered at home or at an outpatient facility. Determinants of therapy options and duration include availability of facilities and services, transportation, economic resources, and the person's individual needs. Since functioning in the home is more environment-specific, in-home therapies may be more effective in certain cases, although adequate, consistent, and appropriate in-home therapy is often difficult to arrange. Outpatient facilities can range from offering single therapies like PT to offering a full rehabilitation team in a comprehensive program. Other programs in the community can also be very helpful. These may include day care programs or exercise and recreation groups. A key aspect of the outpatient program is to continue to shift the emphasis toward having the patient and family take over responsibility for therapies and maintenance of functional status.

The potential for driving an automobile often becomes an issue in the outpatient setting. Being able to get around in a car is of obvious importance for one's sense of independence. Many patients with stroke can return to this activity. Hemiplegia can generally be compensated for. Some vehicle modifications may be necessary, such as steering wheel spinner knobs, automatic transmission, power steering, and extenders on turn signals and gear shifts. Cognitive, sensory, and perceptual deficits are more significant barriers. Those who have had a right cerebrovascular accident (CVA) generally have more problems trying to drive than those who have had a left CVA [156,157]. The greater difficulty is related to neglect, spatial perceptual deficits, and attentional problems. Impairments in memory, reasoning, and judgment after stroke also have obvious implications for driving. Whether someone can return to driving or not is best assessed through a driver rehabilitation program. Evaluations may include neuropsychological testing and driving assessments in simulators and on the road. Driver retraining and vehicle modifications can then be instituted if appropriate.

Vocational Aspects

Some patients can and do continue with vocational activities after returning home regardless of age [158,159]. Whether the occupation is employment, homemaking, or going to school, participation can significantly enhance feelings of self-worth and reduce the extent of handicap caused by disability. Vocational issues need to be considered early in the context of the type and severity of deficits present, as well as what type of work the person was doing and would want to return to. This can help in directing therapy and counseling the patient as to what is realistic. The state vocational rehabilitation agency can be of assistance in counseling, job preparation, and placement.

MEDICAL ISSUES
Thromboembolic Disease

Prophylaxis and monitoring for thromboembolic disease are imperative after stroke. Without prophylaxis, deep venous thrombosis (DVT) can occur in up to 73% of patients after stroke [160]. Approximately 25% of patients with untreated DVT will go on to develop pulmonary embolism [161]. Viitanen and colleagues [162] examined autopsy-verified causes of death after stroke and found that pulmonary embolism was the most common cause of death 2–4 weeks after stroke. A high index of suspicion must be maintained because clinical examination is notoriously insensitive to DVT [161,163]. Also the patient may not be able to report subjective symptoms because of cognitive, sensory, or hemiattentional deficits. Subtle changes in leg circumference, temperature, color, or superficial veins may be tip-offs that further examination is indicated with venography or ultrasound. DVT usually occurs on the hemiparetic side, but may also be present in the uninvolved leg [161].

In the absence of contraindications, low-dosage subcutaneous heparin started within 48 hr of stroke can be effective in decreasing the incidence of

DVT and pulmonary embolism (PE) [160,164]. In the patient with potential for bleeding complications, pneumatic compression stockings are an alternative [165,166].

Use of aspirin has had equivocal results in preventing DVT [167,168]. Anticoagulation for 3–6 months is indicated for treatment of DVT and PE [169]. Hull and colleagues [170] have demonstrated the efficacy of an anticoagulation regimen starting with 5 days of intravenous heparin and beginning oral anticoagulation with warfarin on day 1.

Seizures

The risk of seizures at the onset of stroke is about 4–5% for infarcts and 15–20% for intracerebral or subarachnoid hemorrhages [171]. It is difficult to predict which patients that have early seizures will go on to have late seizures [172]. Considering all stroke types, the risk of developing recurrent seizures (epilepsy) is about 5–10% [171]. This risk appears to be substantially higher for those who develop late-onset seizures (> 80%) or who have lobar hematomas (60%) [173,174]. In general, anticonvulsants are not used simply for seizure prophylaxis in the absence of a history of seizures.

For those who require continued anticonvulsant therapy, the main consideration from a rehabilitation perspective, is the potential for side effects relating to motor and cognitive function. All anticonvulsant medication can have adverse effects on these areas, depending on blood levels. In comparing various anticonvulsant agents, there are numerous reports that carbamazepine is associated with less cognitive and motor disturbance than phenytoin or phenobarbital [175–177]. If someone is taking anticonvulsants, this needs to be considered when there appears to be deterioration or failure to progress in rehabilitation. Dosing schedules and serum levels should be checked as possible contributors.

Cardiac Disease

Stroke and ischemic heart disease often coexist as manifestations of systemic atherosclerosis [178,179]. In those who survive stroke, the leading late cause of death is heart disease [180]. Manifestations of cardiac disease such as congestive heart failure (CHF), angina, or arrhythmias can complicate rehabilitation and limit functional gains [9,181]. Monitoring for signs and symptoms of heart disease can be more difficult in the elderly stroke patient because communication deficits or silent ischemia may be present. These factors underscore the importance of addressing cardiac considerations in overall planning, implementation, and monitoring of the rehabilitation program.

Activities such as hemiplegic ambulation require more total energy; however, the rate of energy of expenditure is about the same as that of normal ambulation. This is accomplished through a much slower pace [182]. In general, the low level of exertion involved allows most patients to participate in stroke rehabilitation and begin a conditioning program. Efforts to optimize the medical regimen should be undertaken and proper precautions observed as the patient's response to initial therapies is monitored [183]. Further noninvasive diagnostic tests, electrocardiographic monitoring, or cardiology consultation may be indicated to help guide rehabilitation therapies if there is a high degree of concern regarding the patient's ability to tolerate exercises.

Stroke Prevention

Persons who have had a stroke are clearly at risk for a recurrence. Data from the Framingham cohort showed a 42% 5-year cumulative recurrence rate of atherothrombotic brain infarction in men, and a 24% recurrence rate in women [184]. Therefore, efforts at trying to prevent recurrent stroke is a crucial part of poststroke care. The rehabilitation phase is an excellent time to address this. The prolonged contact with the patient and family during this time affords the opportunity to educate them further about risk factors and management strategies. Dietary habits, smoking cessation, and sedentary lifestyle can be addressed. Physiological parameters such as blood pressure, serum glucose, and lipid levels can easily be monitored. When appropriate, medications can be started or adjusted with an opportunity to monitor response.

REFERENCES

1. M. Goldstein, *Stroke*, *21*:373–374 (1990).
2. J. Broderick, S. Phillips, J. Whisnant, W. O'Fallon, and M. Bergstrahl, *Stroke*, *20*:577–582 (1989).
3. W.M. Garraway, J.P. Whisnant, and I. Drury, *Stroke*, *14*:699–703 (1983).
4. W.M. Garraway, J.P. Whisnant, and I. Drury, *Mayo Clin. Proc.*, *58*:520–523 (1983).
5. M. Kelly-Hayes, A. Wolf, W. Kannel, P. Sytkowski, R. D'Agostino, and G. Gresham, *Arch. Phys. Med. Rehab.*, *69*:415 (1988).
6. M. Kotila, O. Waltimo, M. Niemi, R. Laaksonen, and M. Lempinen, *Stroke*, *15*:1039 (1984).
7. M.L. Dombovy, J.R. Basford, J.P. Whisnant, and E. Bergsthralh, *Stroke*, *18*: 830–836 (1987).
8. D. Wade, R. Langton-Hewer, *J. Neurol. Neurosurg. Psychiatry*, *50*:177–182 (1987).
9. G.E. Gresham, T. Phillips, P. Wolf, P. McNamara, W. Kannel, and T. Dawber, *Arch. Phys. Med. Rehab.*, *60*:487 (1979).

10. J. Lehman, B. Delateur, R. Fowler, Jr., C. Warren, R. Amhold, G. Schertzer, R. Hurka, J. Whitmore, A. Masock, and K. Chambers, *Arch. Phys. Med. Rehab.*, 56:375–382 (1975).

11. M. Niemi, R. Laaksonen, M. Kotila, and O. Waltimo, *Stroke*, 19:1101–1107 (1988).

12. M. Viitanen, K. Fugl-Meyer, B. Bernspang, and A. Fugl-Meyer, *Scand. J. Rehab. Med.*, 20:17–24 (1988).

13. C. Granger, B. Hamilton, and G. Gresham, *Arch. Phys. Med. Rehab.*, 69:506–509 (1988).

14. R. Robinson and T. Price, *Stroke*, 13:635–641 (1982).

15. R. Robinson, P. Bolduc, and T. Price, *Stroke*, 18:837–843 (1987).

16. D. Sinyor, P. Amato, D. Kaloupek, R. Becker, M. Goldenberg, and H. Coopersmith, *Stroke*, 17:1102–1107 (1986).

17. R. Robinson, L. Starr, and T. Price, *Br. J. Psychiatry*, 144:256–262 (1984).

18. M. Reding, L. Orto, S. Winter, I. Fortuna, P. DiPonte, and F. McDowell, *Arch. Neurol.*, 43:763 (1985).

19. J. Lipsey and R. Robinson, *Lancet*, 2:297 (1984).

20. T. Twitchell, *Brain*, 74:443–480 (1951).

21. D. Wade, R. Langton-Hewer, V. Wood, C. Skilbeck, and H. Ismail, *J. Neurol. Neurosurg. Psychiatry*, 46:521–524 (1983).

22. D. Smith, A. Akhtar, and M. Garraway, *Age Aging*, 14:46–48 (1985).

23. T. Olsen, *Stroke*, 21:247–252 (1990).

24. R. Bonita and R. Beaglehole, *Stroke*, 19:1497–1500 (1988).

25. D. Wade, R. Langton-Hewer, R. David, and P. Enderby, *J. Neurol. Neurosurg. Psychiatry*, 49:11–16 (1986).

26. J.C. Brust, S. Shafer, R. Richter, and B. Bruun, *Stroke*, 7:167–174 (1976).

27. C. Skilbeck, D. Wade, R. Langton-Hewer, and V. Wood, *J. Neurol. Neurosurg. Psychiatry*, 46:5–8 (1983).

28. G. Demeurisse, O. Demol, M. Derouck, R. DeBeuckelaer, M. Coekaerts, and A. Capon, *Stroke*, 11:455–458 (1980).

29. M. Sarno and E. Levita, *Stroke*, 10:663–670 (1979).

30. K. Fullerton, D. McSherry and R. Stout, *Lancet*, 1:430–432 (1986).

31. D. Smith, A. Akhtar, and W. Garraway, *Age Aging*, 12:63–69 (1983).

32. A. Sunderland, D. Wade, and R. Langton-Hewer, *Int. Disabil. Studies*, 9:55–59 (1987).

33. S. Egelko, D. Simon, E. Riley, W. Gordon, M. Ruckdeschel-Hibbard, and L. Diller, *Arch. Phys. Med. Rehabil.*, 70:297–302 (1989).

34. W. Isaeff, P. Waller, and G. Duncan, *Ann. Ophthalmol.*, 6(10):1059–1069 (1974).

35. C. Gray, J. French, D. Bates, N. Cartlidge, G. Venables, and O. James, *Age Aging*, 18:419–421 (1989).

36. J. Horner, E. Massey, J. Riski, D. Lathrop, and K. Chase, *Neurology*, 38:1359–1362 (1988).

37. C. Gordon, R. Hewer, and D. Wade, *Br. Med. J.*, 295:411–414 (1987).

38. D. Feeney and J. Baron, *Stroke*, 17:817–830 (1983).

39. D. Feeney and R. Sutton, *CRC Crit. Rev. Neurobiol.*, 3:135–197 (1987).
40. D. Feeney, A. Gonzalex, and W. Law, *Science*, 217:855–857 (1982).
41. D. Feeney and D. Hovda, *Brain Res.*, 342:352–256 (1985).
42. M. Boyeson and D. Feeney, *Pharmacol. Biochem. Behav.*, 35:497–501 (1990).
43. E. Crisostomo, P. Duncan, M. Propst, D. Dawson, and J. Davis, *Ann. Neurol.*, 23:94–97 (1988).
44. P. Glees, *Recovery of Function: Theoretical Considerations for Brain Injury Rehabilitation* (P. Bach-y-Rita, ed.), University Park Press, Baltimore (1980).
45. A. Papanicalaou, B. Moore, H. Levin, and H. Eisenberg, *Arch. Neurol.*, 47: 521–524 (1987).
46. P.D. Wall, *Recovery of Function: Theoretical Considerations for Brain Injury Rehabilitation* (P. Bach Y Rita, ed.), University Park Press, Baltimore (1980).
47. S. Buell and P. Coleman, *Brain Res.*, 214:23–41 (1981).
48. L. Harrell, T. Barlow, and J. Davis *Exp. Neurol.*, 82:379–390 (1983).
49. D. Tauck and J. Nadler, *J. Neurosci.*, 5:1016 (1985).
50. K. Chow and D. Stewart, *Exp. Neurol.*, 34:409–433 (1987).
51. M. Rozenwieg, D. Krech, E. Bennett, and M. Diamond, *J. Comp. Physiol. Psychol.*, 55:429–437 (1962).
52. D. Krech, M. Rosenzweig, and E. Bennett, *J. Comp. Physiol. Psychol.*, 55:801–807 (1962).
53. W. Jenkins and M. Merzenich, *Prog. Brain Res.*, 71: 249–266 (1987).
54. D.J. Feldman, P. R. Lee, J. Unterecker, et al., *J. Chron. Disabil.*, 15:297–310 (1962).
55. K. Lind, *J. Chron. Disabil.*, 35:133–149 (1982).
56. W.M. Garraway, A.J. Akhtar, R.J. Prescott, et al., *Br. Med. J.*, 280:1040–1043 (1980).
57. W.M. Garraway, A.J. Akhtar, D.L. Smith, et al., *J. Epidemiol. Commun. Health*, 35:39–44 (1981).
58. R.S. Stevens, N.R. Ambler, and M.D. Warren, *Age Aging*, 13:65–75 (1984).
59. T. Strand, K. Asplund, S. Eriksson, et al., *Stroke*, 16:29–34 (1985).
60. T. Strand, K. Asplund, S. Eriksson, et al., *Stroke*, 17:377–381 (1986).
61. J. Silvenius, K. Pyorala, O. Heinonen, et al., *Stroke*, 16:928–931 (1985).
62. M. Dignan, G. Howard, J. Toole, et al., *Stroke*, 17:382–386.
63. P. Davies, J. Bamford, and C. Warlow, *Int. Disabil. Studies*, 11:40–44 (1989).
64. S. Wood-Dauphinee, S. Shapiro, E.R. Bass, et al., *Stroke*, 15:864–872 (1984).
65. B. Indredavik, F. Bakke, R. Solberg, et al., *Stroke*, 22:1026–1031 (1991).
66. H. Ring, J. Schwartz, B. Elazar, N. Berghaus, Y. Luz, P. Solzi, and T. Najenson, *Scand. J. Rehab.*, (Suppl.)12: 143 (1985).
67. M. Garraway, *Stroke*, 16: 178 (1985).
68. M. Dombovy, A. Burton, M. Sandok, and J. Basford, *Stroke*, 17:363 (1986).
69. L. Jongbloed, S. Stacey, and C. Brighton, *Stroke*, 17:765 (1986).
70. C. Granger, L. Lewis, N. Peters, C. Sherwood, and J. Barrett, *Arch. Phys. Med. Rehabil.*, 60:14 (1979).
71. J. Hertanu, J. Demopoulos, W. Yang, W. Calhoun, and H. Feinstein, *Arch. Phys. Med. Rehabil.*, 65:505 (1984).

72. C. Granger, B. Hamilton, G. Gresham, and A. Kramer, *Arch. Phys. Med. Rehabil.*, *70*:100 (1989).
73. D. Bushnell, S. Gupta, A. Mlcoch, and W. Barnes, *Arch. Neurol.*, *46*:665 (1989).
74. G. Defer, J. Moretti, P. Cesar, A. Sergent, C. Raynaud, and J. Degos, *Arch. Neurol.*, *44*:715–718 (1987).
75. R. MacDonnell, G. Donnan, and P. Bladin, *Ann. Neurol.*, *25*:68 (1989).
76. B. Zeman and C. Yiannikas, *J. Neurol. Neurosurg. Psychiatry*, *52*:242–247 (1989).
77. G. Dejong and L. Branch, *Stroke*, *13*:648 (1982).
78. G. Howard, J. Till, J. Toole, C. Matthews, and L. Truscott, *JAMA*, *253*:2 (1985).
79. R. Black-Schaffer and S. Osberg, *Arch. Phys. Med. Rehabil.*, *71*:285–290 (1990).
80. World Health Organization: WHO, *WHO Tech. Rep. Ser.*, *419*:1–23 (1969).
81. S. Berrol, *Arch. Neurol.*, *47*:219–220 (1990).
82. B.T. Volpe and F.H. McDowell, *Arch. Neurol.*, *47*:220–222 (1990).
83. J. Weinberg, L. Diller, W. Gordon, L. Gerstman, A. Lieberman, P. Lakin, G. Hodges, and O. Ezrachi, *Arch. Phys. Med. Rehabil.*, *60*:491–496 (1979).
84. W.A. Gordon, M. Ruckdeschel, S. Egelko, L. Diller, M. Shaver, A. Lieberman, and K. Ragnarsson, *Arch. Phys. Med. Rehabil.*, *66*:353–359 (1985).
85. D.L. Schacter, *Clinical Neuropsychology of Intervention* (B.P. Uzzel and Y. Gross, eds.), Martinus Nijhoff, Boston, pp. 257–282 (1986).
86. B. Wilson, *Rehabilitation of Memory*. Guilford Press, New York (1987).
87. D.L. Schacter, *J. Clin. Exp. Neuropsychol.*, *7*:79–96 (1985).
88. E. Glisky and D. Schacter, *Neuropsychologia*, *26*:173–178 (1988).
89. E. Glisky and D. Schacter, *Neuropsychologia*, *27*:107–120 (1989).
90. L.M. Binder, *Stroke*, *15*:175–177 (1984).
91. S. Brunnstrom, *Movement Therapy in Hemiplegia*. Harper and Row, New York (1970).
92. B. Bobath, *Adult Hemiplegia. Evaluation and Treatment*, ed. 2. Heinmann, London (1978).
93. S.L. Stockmeyer, *Am. J. Phys. Med.*, *6*:900–955 (1967).
94. D.R. Voss, *Proprioceptive Neuromuscular Facilitation*, ed. 3. Harper and Row, Philadelphia (1985).
95. P.H. Stern, F. McDowell, J. Miller, and M. Robinson, *Arch. Phys. Med. Rehabil.*, *51*:526–531 (1970).
96. R. Dickstein, S. Hocherman, Pillar, and R. Shaham, *Phys. Ther.*, *8*:1233–1238 (1986).
97. J.P. Lord and K. Hall, *Arch. Phys. Med. Rehabil.*, *64*:364–367 (1986).
98. M.K. Logigian, M. Samuels, and J. Falconer, *Arch. Phys. Med. Rehabil.*, *64*:364–367 (1983).
99. J.V. Basmajian, C. Gowland, M. Brandstater, L. Swanson, and J. Trotter, *Arch. Phys. Med. Rehabil.*, *63*:613–616 (1982).
100. L.P. Ince, H. Zaretsky, M. Lee, and P. Kerman-Lerner, *Arch. Phys. Med. Rehabil.*, *68*:645 (1987).

101. J. Ingles, M. Donald, and T. Monga, *Arch. Phys. Med. Rehabil.*, 67:755–759 (1984).

102. J. Basmajian, C. Gowland, M. Finlayson, A. Hall, L. Swanson, P. Stratford, J. Trotter, and M. Brandstater, *Arch. Phys. Med. Rehabil.*, 68:267–272 (1987).

103. R. Merletti, F. Zelaschi, D. Latella, M. Galli, S. Angeli, and M. Sessa, *Scand. J. Rehab. Med.*, 10:147–154 (1987).

104. C. Cozean, W. Pease, and S. Hubbell, *Arch. Phys. Med. Rehabil*, 69:401–405 (1988).

105. B. R. Bowman, L. Baker, and R. Waters, *Arch. Phys. Med. Rehabil.*, 60:497–502 (1979).

106. van Overeem and G. Hansen, *Scand. J. Rehab. Med.*, 11:189–193 (1979).

107. M. Reding and E. Potes, *Stroke*, 19:1354 (1988).

108. S. L. Veis and J. Logemann, *Arch. Phys. Med. Rehabil.*, 66:372–375 (1984).

109. P. Linden and A. Siebens, *Arch. Phys. Med. Rehabil.*, 64:281–284 (1983).

110. J. A. Logeman, *Evaluation and Treatment of Swallowing Disorders.* College Hill Press, San Diego (1983).

111. K. M. Yorkston, D. R. Beukelman, and K. Bell, *Assessment of Intelligibility of Dysarthric Speech.* College Hill Press, San Diego (1987).

112. K. M. Colby, D. Christinaz, R. Parkinson, S. Graham, and C. Karpf, *Brain and Language*, 14:272 (1981).

113. D. F. Johns, *Clinical Management of Neurogenic Communicative Disorders.* Little, Brown and Company, Boston/Toronto (1985).

114. A. Basso, E. Capitani, and L. Vignolo, *Arch. Neurol.*, 36:190–196 (1974).

115. C. Shewan and A. Kertesz, *Brain Language*, 23:272–299 (1984).

116. R. T. Wertz, D. Weiss, J. Aten, R. Brookshire, F. Garcia-Bunuel, R. Brannegan, H. Greenbaum, R. Marshall, D. Vogel, J. Carter, N. Barnes, and R. Goodman, *Arch. Neurol.*, 43:653–658 (1986).

117. M. L. Albert, R. Sparks, and N. Helm, *Arch. Neurol.*, 29:130–131 (1973).

118. H. Gardner, E. Zurif, T. Berry, and E. Baker, *Visual Communication in Aphasia* (1976).

119. N. Helm-Eastbrook, P. M. Fitzpatrick, and B. Barresi, *J. Speech Hearing Disord.*, 47:385–389 (1982).

120. H. Johanssen-Horback, B. Cegla, U. Mager, and B. Schempp, *Brain Lang.*, 24: 74–82 (1985).

121. G. A. Davis and M. J. Wilcox, *Adult Aphasia Rehabilitation: Applied Pragmatics.* College Hill Press, San Diego (1985).

122. C. Van Ouweneller, P. M. LaPlace, and A. Chantraine, *Arch. Phys. Med. Rehabil.*, 67:23–26 (1986).

123. C. Roy, *Clin. Rehab.*, 2:35–44 (1988).

124. J. Griffin, *Phys. Ther.*, 66:1885–1893 (1986).

125. M. Hurd, K. Farrell, and G. Waylonis, *Arch. Phys. Med. Rehabil.*, 55:519–523 (1974).

126. B. Bobath, *Adult Hemiplegia: Evaluation and Treatment.* Heinmann, London (1978).

127. P.S. Tepperman, N.D. Greyson, L. Hilbert, J. Jiminez, and J.I. Williams, *Arch. Phys. Med. Rehabil.*, 65:442–447 (1984).

128. S.W. Davis, C.R. Petrullo, I.D. Eichberg, and D.S. Chu, *Arch. Phys. Med. Rehabil.*, 58:353–356 (1977).

129. S. Bonelli, G. Conoscente, P.G. Movilia, L. Restelli, B. Francucci, and E. Grossi, *Pain*, 16:297–307 (1983).

130. T. Najenson, E. Yacubovich, and S. Pikielini, *Scand. J. Rehabil. Med.*, 3:131–137 (1971).

131. J. Meredith, G. Taft, and P. Kaplan, *Am. J. Occup. Ther.*, 35:656 (1981).

132. I. Odeem, *Scand. J. Rehabil. Med.*, 13:93–99 (1981).

133. M.B. Glenn and J. Whyte, *The Practical Management of Spasticity in Children and Adults*. Lea & Febiger, Philadelphia/London (1990).

134. R.T. Katz, *J. Neurorehab.*, 5(Suppl. 1):S5–S12 (1991).

135. B. Snow, J. Tsui, M. Bhatt, M. Varelas, S. Hashimoto, and D. Calne, *Ann. Neurol.*, 28:512 (1990).

136. W.B. Ketel and M.E. Kolb, *Curr. Med. Res. Opin.*, 9:161–169 (1984).

137. C.H. Chan, *Neurology*, 40:1427–1432 (1990).

138. R. Robinson, P. Bolduc, and T. Price, *Am. J. Psychiatry*, 143:1238–1244 (1986).

139. R. Evans, D. Bishop, A. Matlock, S. Stranahan, G. Smith, and E. Halar, *Arch. Phys. Med. Rehabil.*, 68:513–517 (1987).

140. G.J. Kinsella and F. Duffy, *Scand. J. Rehabil. Med.*, 11:129–132 (1979).

141. R.L. Evans, D. Bishop, A. Matlock, S. Stranahan, E. Halar, and W. Noonan, *Arch. Phys. Med. Rehabil.*, 68:508–512 (1987).

142. C. Tompkins, R. Schulz, and M. Rau, *J. Consult. Clin. Psychol.*, 546:502–508 (1988).

143. R. Evan, A. Matlock, D. Bishop, S. Stranahan, and C. Pederson, *Stroke*, 19:1243–1249 (1988).

144. G. Newman and C.R. Nichols, *JAMA*, 173:33–35 (1960).

145. E. Pfeiffer, A. Verwoerdt, and H.S. Wang, *Arch. Gen. Psychiatry*, 19:753–758 (1968).

146. K. Sjogren and A.R. Fugl-Meyer, *J. Psychosom. Res.*, 26:409–417 (1982).

147. A.R. Fugl-Meyer and L. Jaasko, *Scand. J. Rehab. Med.*, 7:158–166 (1980).

148. T.N. Monga, J.S. Lawson, and J. Inglis, *Arch. Phys. Med. Rehabil.*, 67:19–22 (1986).

149. G.P. Bray, R.S. DeFrank, and T.L. Wolfe, *Arch. Phys. Med. Rehabil.*, 62:286–288 (1981).

150. H.B. Coslett and K.M. Heilmann, *Arch. Neurol.*, 43:1036–1039 (1986).

151. B. Emick-Herring, *Rehabil. Nursing*, 10(2):28–30 (1985).

152. C. Papadopoulos, *Arch. Intern Med.*, 140:1341–1345 (1980).

153. G.S. Tardif, *Arch. Phys. Med. Rehabil.*, 70:763–766 (1989).

154. J.L. Larson, M.W. McNaughton, J.W. Kennedy, and L.W. Mansfield, *Heart Lung*, 9:1025–1030 (1980).

155. J.G. Bohlen, J.P. Held, O. Sanderson, and R.P. Patterson, *Arch. Intern. Med.*, 144:1745–1748 (1984).

156. F.L. Quigley and J.A. DeLisa, *Am. J. Occup. Ther.*, 37:473–478 (1983).

157. J. Bardach, *Arch. Phys. Med. Rehabil.*, 52:328–332 (1971).
158. A.K. Coughlin and M. Humphry, *Rheumatol. Rehab.*, 21:115–122 (1982).
159. G. Howard, J.S. Till, J.F. Toole, C. Matthews, and B.L. Truscott, *JAMA*, 253: 226–232 (1985).
160. S.T. McCarthy and J. Turner, *Age Aging*, 15:84–88 (1986).
161. C. Warlow, D. Ogsten, and A.S. Douglas, *Br. Med. J.*, 1:1178–1183 (1976).
162. M. Viitanen, B. Winblad, and K. Asplund, *Acta Med. Scand.*, 222:401–408 (1987).
163. B.K. Prasad, A.K. Banerjee, and H. Howard, *Age Aging*, 11:42–44 (1982).
164. S.T. McCarthy, J.J. Turner, D. Robertson, and C.J. Hawkey, *Lancet*, 2:800–801 (1977).
165. A.G.G. Turpie, A. Gallus, W.S. Beattie, and J. Hirsh, *Neurology*, 27:435–438 (1977).
166. J.J. Skillman, R.E. Collin, N.P. Cole, B. Goldstein, R. Shapiro, N. Zervas, M. Bettmann, and E. Salzman, *Surgery*, 83:354–358 (1978).
167. W.H. Harris, E.W. Salzman, C.A. Athanscoulis, A.C. Waltman, and R.W. DeSanctis, *N. Engl. J. Med.*, 297:1246–1249 (1977).
168. G.K. Morris and J.R.A. Mitchell, *Br. Med. J.*, 1:535–537 (1977).
169. T.M. Hyers, R.D. Hull, and J.G. Weg, *Chest*, 95(Feb. Suppl.):37S–51S (1989).
170. R.D. Hull, G.E. Raskob, D. Rosenbloom, A.A. Panju, P. Brill-Edward, J.S. Ginsberg, J. Hirsch, G.J. Martin, and D. Green, *N. Engl. J. Med.*, 322:1260–1264 (1990).
171. C. Armon, R.A. Radtke, and E.W. Massey, *Clin. Neuropharmacol.*, 14:17–27 (1991).
172. C.J. Kilpatrick, S.M. Davis, B.M. Tress, S.C. Rossiter, J.L. Hopper, and M.L. Vandendriesen, *Arch. Neurol.*, 47:157–160 (1990).
173. C.Y. Sung and N.S. Chu, *J. Neurol. Neurosurg. Psychiatry*, 52:1273–1276 (1989).
174. S. Louis and F. McDowell, *Arch. Neurol.*, 17:414–418 (1967).
175. D.B. Smith, R.H. Mattson, J.A. Cramer, J.F. Collins, R.A. Novelly, and A. Craft, *Epilepsia*, 28(Suppl. 3):S50–S58 (1987).
176. M.R. Trimble, *Epilepsia*, 28(Suppl. 3):S37–S45 (1987).
177. D.G. Andrews, L. Tomlinson, R.D.C. Elwes, and E.H. Reynolds, *Acta Neurol. Scand. Suppl.*, 99:23–30 (1984).
178. R. Rokey, L.A. Rolak, Y. Harati, N. Kutka, and M.S. Verani, *Ann. Neurol.*, 16: 50–53 (1984).
179. N.R. Hertzer, J.R. Young, E.G. Beven, R.A. Graor, P.J. O'Hara, W.F. Ruschhaupt, V.G. deWolfe, and L.C. Maljovec, *Arch. Intern. Med.*, 145:849–852 (1985).
180. N. Matsumoto, J.P. Whisnant, L.T. Kurland, and H. Okazaki, *Stroke*, 4:20–29 (1973).
181. E.J. Roth, K. Mueller, and D. Green, *Stroke*, 19: 42–47 (1988).
182. D. Hash, *Orthop. Clin. North Am.*, 9:372–374 (1978).
183. C.N. Leach and J.A. Leach, *Phys. Med. Rehabil.*, 3(Aug):611–618 (1989).
184. R. Sacco, P. Wolf, W. Kannel, and P. McNamara, *Stroke*, 13:290–295 (1982).

20
Traumatic Brain Injury

Douglas I. Katz and Michael P. Alexander

Braintree Hospital
Braintree, and
Boston University School of Medicine
Boston, Massachusetts

INTRODUCTION

Traumatic brain injury (TBI) is among the most common of neurological disorders. The incidence rate of 200:100,000 exceeds even that of stroke (130:100,000) [1]. If one recognizes that the age distribution is skewed toward the younger end of the population and that TBI often produces long-lasting problems, it is certainly one of the most important chronically disabling neurological disorders. A significant minority of cases (7–25%) [2] fall into the "severe" TBI category and will receive hospitalized rehabilitation and perhaps months to years of rehabilitation services. The majority of patients with TBI fit into the "mild" category (130:100,000) [2] and will generally not require in-hospital rehabilitation. Nevertheless, this group of patients often presents important issues for neurological diagnosis and rehabilitation management to promote timely restoration to a functional, productive level.

This chapter is organized according to a framework suggested by the neuropathology of TBI. TBI produces a variety of pathological consequences, some focal and some diffuse, that have independent clinical effects (Table 1). Understanding the neuropathology of TBI clarifies the clinical phenomena of TBI, including the course of recovery and prognosis. Deviations from the expected pattern of recovery will identify secondary complications that might be reversible.

A complete neurological diagnosis in the rehabilitation setting should

Table 1 Cerebral Pathological Classifications of TBI

Focal
  Focal cortical contusion (FCC)
  Deep hemorrhages
  Focal hypoxic–ischemic injury (FHII)
Diffuse
  Diffuse axonal injury (DAI)
  Diffuse hypoxic–ischemic injury (DHII)
Indirect pathological conditions and secondary phenomena
  Extracerebral hematomas
  Herniation syndromes
  Hydrocephalus
  Chronic subdural hematomas
  Hygromas

include the following elements (Table 2): a characterization of the types of brain damage and their severity; identification of any neurological, medical, or psychological complicating factors; staging recovery in the context of the natural history of the disorder; characterization of impairments and capacities in a manner useful to planning appropriate interactions and treatments; and estimation of short- and long-term functional capability and outcome.

Integration of these five neurological elements of TBI diagnosis will guide rehabilitation management. The clinical profiles of specific TBI pathologies evolve in recognizable patterns over coarsely predictable periods of time. Some will improve spontaneously, and some will not improve beyond certain limits whatever the rehabilitation interventions. Specific neuropathological injuries, severity of those injuries, and time postinjury all constrain expectations for treatment and recovery. For instance, amnesia 3 weeks following a severe diffuse TBI presents a completely different set of

Table 2 Elements of Neurological Diagnosis to be Considered in Planning Rehabilitation

Types of brain damage and severity
Neurological, medical, and psychological complicating factors
Stage of recovery
Specific impairments and functional capacities
Short- and long-term prognosis

Table 3 Principles of Rehabilitation Management

Goals and interventions should:
Be consistent with the diagnosis and natural history of the neuropathological profile.
Have real-life functional relevance to a patient's needs and stage of recovery.
Conform to available resources and environmental demands.
Recognize that not all problems require treatment.

rehabilitation problems than amnesia 3 months postinjury in a patient with a left posterior cerebral artery infarct associated with an epidural hematoma. These memory disorders will evolve with a substantially different time course and outcome.

Several principles should guide rehabilitation management (Table 3). Interventions should be consistent with specific neurological diagnosis and the expected natural history of the particular neuropathological profile. Goals should have a real-life functional basis and should be relevant to a patient's needs at a given stage of recovery. Goals should be consistent with available resources and environmental demands, anticipating the setting in which the patient will be living. Not all problems require treatment; some have no functional relevance, some will get better on their own, some are over-shadowed by other problems, and some may never be remediable.

The most consistent and pervasive problems following TBI are in the realm of cognition and behavior and these problems will be emphasized throughout this chapter. Various other neurological problems occur such as disorders of motor control, tone, balance, gait, eye motility, swallowing, and incontinence. These problems are more variable and less predictable; they occur with increased frequency and severity in more severe injuries. Motor problems will be mentioned along with more ubiquitous neurobehavioral and neuropsychological dysfunction but a more complete discussion of motor function, spasticity, gait, and bladder function may be found elsewhere in this text.

We will use the term TBI synonymously with closed head injury. Although penetrating brain injuries, such as gun shot wounds, present issues similar to other focal brain injuries, there are some particular features that will not be discussed in this chapter.

This chapter is organized into three parts: the pathophysiology of TBI; the clinical effects of TBI, including course of recovery and rehabilitation strategies; and outcome. Each of these parts will consider the focal and diffuse effects separately.

PATHOPHYSIOLOGY OF TBI

Focal Pathology

There are several types of focal pathology. Focal cortical contusion (FCC) is the most common and familiar. Deep hemorrhages, usually in the basal ganglia area, and focal hypoxic–ischemic lesions (HII-focal) or strokes are other focal pathologies associated with trauma.

Focal Cortical Contusion

FCC can occur directly underlying a point of impact, sometimes associated with skull fracture, or more commonly as a result of inertial movement of the brain relative to the skull in acceleration injuries. FCC at the area of contact are often termed coup contusions. If bony fragments tear the arachnoid and pia, brain lacerations may occur. Most of what are referred to as contracoup contusions actually result from acceleration injuries and occur primarily at the anterior and inferior surfaces of the frontal and temporal lobes [3,4]. The relative movement and distortion of these areas of brain against ridged portions of the anterior and middle fossae make them particularly susceptible to FCC. Holbourn's [5] classic experiment using gelatin models in the shape of the brain demonstrated that angular acceleration produces the greatest strains in these same areas.

Table 4   Neuropathological Diagnosis

FCC	FHII	DAI	DHII
		Principal means of diagnosis	
Neuroimaging	Neuroimaging	History (acceleration mechanism, immediate loss of consciousness) Neuroimaging (swelling, petechial hemorrhage, subarachnoid hemorrhage, or normal scan)	History (cardiopulmonary compromise or severely increased ICP)
		Determinants of severity	
Location Size Bilaterality	Location Size	Depth and duration of coma PTA Rostral brainstem signs	Depth and duration of coma PTA Signs attributable to hypoxic lesions (e.g., persistent amnesia, proximal limb weakness, transcortical aphasia, movement disorders)

The typical appearance of FCC is of localized hemorrhage, swelling, and tissue disruption. In late stages they appear as shrunken brown scars [4]. The depth and size of the hemorrhagic component vary from superficial, at the crest of gyri, to the entire thickness of cortex, to involvement of subcortical areas. Lesions may be single or multiple and are often bilateral.

Diagnosis of FCC depends almost entirely on static neuroimaging: computed tomography (CT) or magnetic resonance imaging (MRI) (Table 4; see Figs. 1, 2). MRI has some advantage in demonstrating superficial lesions that may be obscured by bony artifact. The critical diagnostic features are location, size (particularly depth of lesion), and bilaterality, especially if in homologous areas. Lesion size may change substantially over time as hemorrhage and swelling resolve. Later scans (more than 2 months after injury) are best for long-term clinical pathological correlation.

Deep Hemorrhages

These are distinct from FCC in that they are defined collections of blood and do not arise at the cortical surface [6]. They may be difficult to differentiate

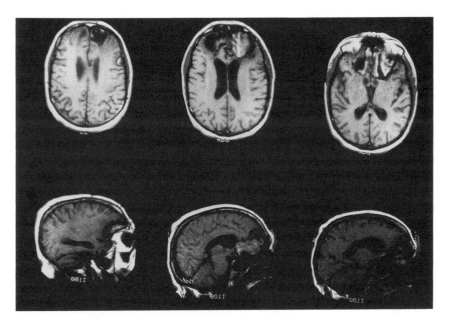

Figure 1 Focal cortical contusion (FCC): MRI 5 months after injury demonstrates bilateral orbital frontal FCC (axial and sagittal views). A 47-year-old man fell 4 feet; patient had severe persistent disinhibition and poor social judgement.

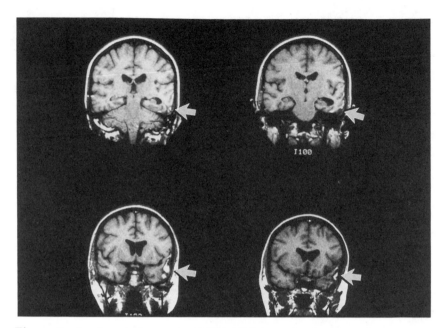

Figure 2   Focal cortical contusion (FCC): MRI 4 months after injury demonstrates left temporal FCC (arrows). A 33-year-old woman fell down ravine while skiing; patient had anomic aphasia.

from FCC on neuroimaging [6], but they are much less common than FCC, occurring in no more than 3% of cases [7–10]. Deep hemorrhages frequently occur in the basal ganglia area, likely resulting from rupture of deep penetrating vessels such as the lenticulostriate or anterior chorioidal arteries [9,10]. They usually occur with diffuse, acceleration-induced injuries and are distinctly larger than the punctuate hemorrhages in white matter, corpus callosum, and dorsolateral midbrain that often occur with diffuse axonal injury (DAI) (Fig. 3) (see below).

Focal Hypoxic–Ischemic Injury

These are areas of infarction that occur as a result of compromise in a particular arterial territory or localized vascular bed. The most common FHII lesion is infarct in the territory of the posterior–cerebral artery following transtentorial herniation (Fig. 4). Anterior cerebral artery strokes may occur with transfalcine herniations and upper brainstem strokes may result from compromise of basilar artery perforators during herniation [11].

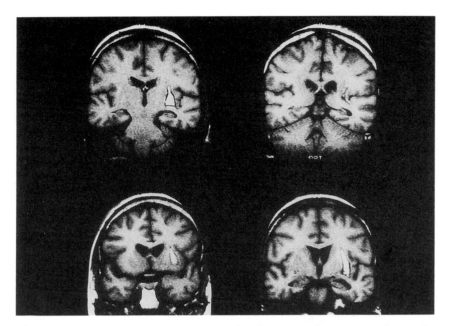

Figure 3   Deep hemorrhage: MRI 3 months after injury demonstrates deep right basal ganglia area hemorrhage. A 24-year-old man was involved in a motor vehicle accident; patient had recovering hemiparesis, left spatial neglect, and delusional thinking.

Diffuse Pathology

Diffuse Axonal Injury

DAI occurs in conjunction with acceleration injuries. DAI is much more common in motor vehicle accidents than falls [12–14]. Acceleration causes deformations of the brain as its motion lags relative to the skull. Deformation or strain causes brain damage as the viscous and elastic limits of neural and vascular tissues are exceeded. Of the three types of strains, compressive (pushing together), tensile (pulling apart), and shear (deformation parallel to adjacent layers), tensile and shear strain are potent causes of axonal damage. The magnitude and velocity of displacement (strain and strain rate) are the critical mechanical factors determining the amount of DAI and related pathology [15–17].

Most of our understanding of DAI is derived from animal models of TBI and human autopsy studies. Gennarelli's studies [18,19] on primates using a device that produced nonimpact acceleration injuries caused the same pathology (DAI) observed in humans [12,20,21]. A fluid percussion model creating a

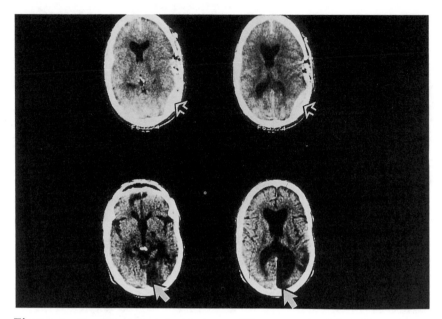

Figure 4 Focal hypoxic ischemic injury following epidural hematoma (EDH). Immediately after injury, CT scan (top) shows left EDH with mass effect (open arrows); 2 months after injury (bottom) it shows left PCA infarct (solid arrows). A 33-year-old man was assaulted with a bat; patient was left with right hemianopia and alexia.

transient pulse of intracranial pressure has also simulated axonal pathology [22–25].

DAI is defined by its characteristic microscopic appearance (Fig. 5). Axonal swellings and retracted broken ends of axons called "retraction balls" appear early (days); later (weeks), microglia surround and "clear" areas of damaged axons and, still later (months), Wallerian-type axonal degeneration predominates. Axonal rupture probably occurs as a delayed (hours to days) process, not as an immediate mechanical interruption. The mechanical stress causes a disruption of axonal cytoskeleton and transport, leading to a "backup" of intra-axonal components; local axonal swellings result and these progress to complete separation [25–27]. This delay raises the prospect of a therapeutic window during which the process may be halted or reversed.

The distribution of DAI is widespread in the cerebrum, brainstem, and cerebellum but appears to distribute along a centripetal gradient from surface to deeper areas. With injuries of greater severity the concentration of DAI increases in deeper regions of the cerebrum and brainstem [18,19,28].

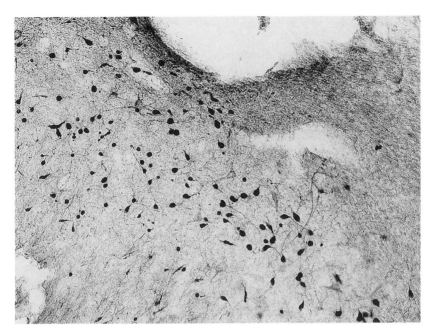

Figure 5   Diffuse axonal injury shows reactive swellings (retraction balls) in damaged axons in hippocampus from a patient who survived for 88 hr (stained with antibodies targeted to neurofilament subunit, ×125; courtesy of John T. Povlishock, Ph.D., Medical College of Virginia; reproduced with permission).

DAI also appears to concentrate in the frontal parasagittal areas, and an anterior to posterior gradient may also occur.

The complete pathophysiological picture of diffuse injury includes vascular injury as well as axonal disruption. The vascular injury has a range of appearances. These include small hemorrhages, local and diffuse brain swelling, and even breakdown of the blood–brain barrier [29]. The small hemorrhages occur in the cerebral white matter, in the corpus callosum, usually just off the midline, and in the rostral brainstem, usually in the dorsolateral quadrants [12,18,30]. The number of hemorrhages does not correlate with severity [31] but callosal and brainstem hemorrhages tend to occur in the more severe injuries [18,30]. Small subarachnoid and intraventricular hemorrhages are also common.

Brain swelling is an important delayed secondary problem often associated with diffuse injuries. It can result from increased intravascular volume due to loss of vasoregulation and from cerebral edema, with increased interstitial or intracellular fluid [32]. It is an important cause of morbidity and mortality and can lead to secondary hypoxic–ischemic injury due to swelling and mass effect.

Whether initiated by axonal or vascular injury there are numerous neurochemical derangements leading to delayed neuronal death. The neuro-chemical changes include surges of excitatory neurotransmitters, such as acetylcholine, glutamate, and aspartate. A cascade of intracellular processes occurs that disrupts function and may go on to destroy neurons [33,34]. Even if not directly cytotoxic, these phenomena lead to heightened sensitivity to other secondary insults such as hypoxia [35]. Various strategies to halt these processes to prevent neuronal death are under investigation [36–38].

Since DAI is directly defined by its microscopic axonal pathology, clinical diagnosis is indirect and sometimes problematic (Table 4). There are as yet no reliable clinical biological markers of severity. Neuroimaging is useful in demonstrating concomitant phenomena such as small white matter, intraventricular, and subarachnoid hemorrhages and edema, but these are not reliable gauges of severity. These features constitute the typical CT pattern of DAI [39,40], but a negative scan does not exclude DAI. MRI has some advantage in the demonstration of small hemorrhages long after injury (Fig. 6). There is an association of severity with depth of lesion observed on MRI, consistent with the distribution gradient noted previously [14,31]. Atrophy and ex-vacuo ventricular enlargement on late scans also correlate with severity [41].

Diagnosis of DAI rests mainly with its clinical features (Table 4): a mechanism of injury compatible with significant acceleration; a history of unconsciousness immediately from time of injury [12], features on neuro-imaging compatible with the diagnosis. Severity is also determined by clinical criteria: depth and duration of coma; signs of rostral brainstem injury; duration of posttraumatic amnesia (PTA). In primate studies, duration of coma correlated with level of recovery, and both correlated with the magnitude of DAI at post-mortem [18,28]. In human studies the Glasgow Coma Score (Table 5), dura-tion of coma, and PTA all have well-known correlations with outcome [42–45].

In summary, DAI results from acceleration injuries and has a recog-nized clinical profile. The severity of clinical consequences and rate of recovery directly relate to the amount of pathology and are qualitatively similar across the spectrum of severity. Axonal disruption is observed even in mild injuries [23,25,46] and the number of physiologically impaired and destroyed axons increases proportionally with increasingly severe levels of clinical impairment [19].

Diffuse Hypoxic Ischemic Injury

Evidence of hypoxic damage is common in more severe injuries and was present in more than 90% of autopsy cases [47], with severe hypoxic pathol-ogy noted in 27% of these cases [4,47]. Patients with severely increased

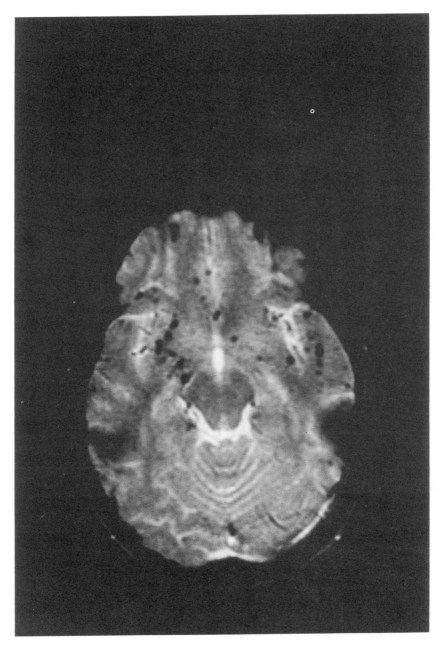

Figure 6 Magnetic resonance imaging 1 month after injury shows multiple deep hemorrhages in a 17-year-old girl with DAI following a motor vehicle accident. Dark, low-signal spots are areas of iron deposition from hemorrhages (gradient echo technique [178]).

Table 5 Glasgow Coma Scale

	Score
Eye opening	
Spontaneous	4
To speech	3
To pain	2
None	1
Best motor response	
Obeys commands	6
Localized to pain stimuli	5
Withdraws from pain stimuli	4
Decorticate flexion	3
Decerebrate extension	2
None	1
Verbal response	
Oriented	5
Confused conversation	4
Inappropriate words	3
Incomprehensible sounds	2
None	1

Scores can range from 3 to 15.
Source: From ref. [89].

intracranial pressures (ICP) (sustained ICP, over 20 mmHg) are at added risk of DHII, since high intracranial pressure impedes cerebral perfusion. The severity and location of DHII are highly variable but certain distributions are characteristic: hippocampus, basal ganglia, diffuse cortical necrosis, infarctions in arterial border zone ("watershed") areas, cerebellum. Diagnosis may be difficult because, again, there are no specific biological markers other than frank infarction on neuroimaging (Table 4). The diagnosis is suspected in cases with documented systemic hypotension and sustained increased ICP; clinical signs compatible with particular distributions of DHII noted above also suggest the diagnosis (see next section).

Clinical–Pathological Diagnosis

A meaningful diagnosis in the rehabilitation setting must incorporate all of the diagnostic possibilities. Several pieces of information are necessary to formulate the clinical–pathological profile and estimate severity:

1. Cause of injury
2. History of immediate coma versus lucid interval

3. Depth of coma after stabilization: Glasgow Coma Score
4. Duration of coma: usually time to first signs of cerebral responsiveness, such as following commands
5. Duration of PTA
6. Neuroimaging
7. Early signs of herniation, such as 3rd nerve palsy
8. Other brainstem signs
9. History of secondary complication such as severe increased ICP or systemic hypotension

With this information the rehabilitation clinician can make a reasonable estimate of the contributions of focal pathologies, diffuse pathologies, and secondary complications to the clinical picture (Table 4).

A neuropathologically based diagnosis might appear as follows: "severe diffuse axonal injury (coma: 6 days, PTA: 7 weeks), large right frontal contusion (involves orbital frontal cortex and deep prefrontal white matter), and possible diffuse hypoxic–ischemic injury (pulseless, resuscitated in ambulance)"; or "acute left subdural hematoma, small left anterior temporal contusion, herniation syndrome (acute fixed, dilated left pupil), and resulting left posterior cerebral artery infarct (focal HII)." This diagnostic effort sets a clear neurologically based context to understand the presenting clinical problems, predict the evolving course of recovery, recognize late complications, such as hydrocephalus or chronic subdural collections, and project long-term outcome.

Indirect and Secondary Pathologies

Acute Extracerebral Hemorrhages

These are hemorrhages that arise outside the brain among its membranous linings. Epidural hematomas occur outside the dura and usually result from rupture of meningeal arteries with skull fractures (Fig. 4). Subdural hematomas occur between the dura and arachnoid membranes when the veins bridging the subdural space are ruptured. These hemorrhages, especially subdural, have a high associated mortality, over 50% in some studies [6]. They affect the brain by localized mass effect, local or diffuse increased intracranial pressure, and by herniation syndromes. Morbidity from subdural and epidural hematomas varies and depends entirely on their secondary effects on the brain. If these lesions are surgically evacuated before irreversible secondary damage occurs, long-term clinical consequences will be negligible.

Herniation Syndromes

Herniation is a shift in a portion of the brain out of its usual cranial compartment to another as a result of mass lesions or asymmetrical swelling.

The major types are temporal lobe (uncal) herniation, transtentorial (central) herniation, and transfalcine (cingulate) herniations [11]. The clinical consequences of herniation are due to vascular or neural compressions producing infarction in the territory of major arteries (posterior cerebral or anterior cerebral) (Fig. 4), small hemorrhages or infarctions in the brainstem and diencephalon, and direct localized damage to a variety of basal neural tissues (e.g., medial temporal lobes, midbrain, hypothalamus, 3rd cranial nerve). Although the acute clinical effects of herniation syndromes are well described [11], prediction of some of the longer-term consequences is less completely understood.

Hydrocephalus

Ventricular enlargement associated with atrophy is common in severe diffuse injuries [48], but is a secondary effect not requiring treatment. A much smaller percentage, about 4% in one series [49] of patients develops communicating or noncommunicating hydrocephalus resulting from an interruption of cerebrospinal fluid (CSF) flow or absorption. There is often a history of subarachnoid hemorrhage or intraventricular hemorrhage. Treatment involves temporary ventricular drainage or a ventriculoperitoneal shunt. Identification of cases that might benefit from a shunt is a problem. The neuroimaging pattern of large ventricles (out of proportion to cerebral atrophy), with distended anterior horns and periventricular lucency from transudatation of CSF is quite supportive of this diagnosis. Other techniques such as radionucleotide cisternography or lumbar punctures to remove large volumes of CSF (20–30 ml) are not well proven [50,51]. There may be more promise in newer methods: CSF flow characteristics using MRI [52] and CSF dynamic perfusion studies [53]. A further issue is the choice of shunt valve pressure; a low pressure shunt valve may be necessary to benefit some patients, although risk of subdural hematoma is higher [54].

Chronic Subdural Hematoma and Hygromas

Chronic subdural hematomas are those that present more than 20 days after injury and likely result from slowly accumulating or recurrent hemorrhages in the subdural space [6]. They are much more common in the elderly, probably because of associated brain atrophy. They have a hypodense or mixed density appearance on CT. Treatment is usually surgical removal. Hygromas are subdural CSF collections, but they may have a similar CT appearance to chronic hematomas. They probably result from leaks through arachnoid tears or effusion from injured capillaries. Treatment is usually conservative since they most often resolve spontaneously; a small percentage that remain symptomatic or increase in size require surgical removal or subdural shunting [6].

Posttraumatic Seizures

The overall lifetime risk of seizures after TBI is around 2–5% [55,56]. This risk is dramatically increased in certain subgroups: patients with severe TBI, regardless of pathology (13% risk) [56]; with a depressed skull fracture (17% risk) [55]; or with a documented focal injury such as FCC (35% risk)[55]. Early seizures (first seizure within a week of injury) have a different substrate than late seizures (first seizure more than a week postinjury), but the occurrence of an early seizure is another factor that increases the risk of a late seizure (25%) [55].

Focal motor seizures are common in early epilepsy. Although focal signs also occur in about 40% of late seizures, the majority of late seizures generalize, with loss of consciousness [55]. Complex–partial seizures are a common late type. As with any cause of seizures, diagnosis rests mainly on clinical grounds: history or direct observation of seizures. Electroencephalography (EEG) and other electrophysiological studies merely support clinical suspicion; an abnormal EEG does not diagnose epilepsy, unless electrical seizures are recorded, and a negative EEG does not rule out epilepsy.

Treatment is similar to any cause of seizures, but there is added concern over the possible cognitive side effects of anticonvulsants compounding the cognitive effects of the brain injury. Although the relative detriment of various anticonvulsants remains inconclusive, phenobarbital appears to be the worst offender, even in a study that demonstrated relatively little difference among anticonvulsants [57]. Carbamazepine and valproic acid may have the fewest cognitive effects [58,59]. Dikmen and co-workers [60] found worse neuropsychological performance in patients with severe TBI treated prophylactically with phenytoin than in nontreated controls. Whether long-term recovery is affected by any of these anticonvulsants is unknown.

Prophylactic anticonvulsant treatment is also controversial. Temkin and colleagues [61] demonstrated that phenytoin had a benefit in preventing seizures only in the first week postinjury; beyond the first week there was no difference between treated and nontreated controls regardless of injury severity and pathology type. Others [62] have also failed to show a benefit of prophylactic use of phenytoin. Other anticonvulsants have not been well studied in this regard.

Risk decreases with time postinjury; in one series over one-quarter of patients had their first seizure within 3 months postinjury and nearly three-quarters had had their first seizure within the first year [55].

Medication Effects

Side effects from, or enhanced sensitivity to, centrally acting medications are common causes of slowed or regressed recovery. The common offenders in patients with TBI are toxic levels of anticonvulsant medications, cumulative effects of sedative medications, or use of medications, such as phenobarbital or methyldopa, with potent central nervous system (CNS) depressant effects.

Medical Illnesses

Although there is scant evidence for this assertion, most clinicians (including us) believe that many medical illnesses, even apparently trivial ones, may complicate recovery and enhance impairments at any stage of recovery. In hospitalized patients, urinary tract infections, thrombophlebitis, and pneumonia are the most common.

CLINICAL CONSEQUENCES AND REHABILITATION STRATEGIES

The sequelae of TBI may be described using many dimensions, such as time postinjury, severity, or categories of dysfunction (cognition, behavior, perceptual–motor function). Our approach is to utilize each, but subsumed in the pathophysiological categories just outlined.

Focal Lesions

FCC

As with focal lesions of any cause, the profile of impairments from focal traumatic brain injury corresponds to the area of brain involved (see below). Several general principles govern the effects of focal traumatic lesions.

First, owing to their usual location in the anterior and inferior portions of the frontal and temporal lobes, the common long-term effects of FCC involve higher-order behavioral, emotional, and cognitive functions (Table 6). These portions of brain contain paralimbic and multimodal or heteromodal association areas [63], both highly connected to limbic structures and sensory and motor association areas. Functions represented in more posterior portions of the cerebrum such as language, praxis, visual perception, and motor control are not usually directly affected by FCC.

Second, the size of the lesion, particularly the depth of subcortical involvement, is an important determinant of long-term effects. FCC with greater subcortical involvement interrupt more short and long cortical–cortical connections with more widespread deafferentiation and de-efferentiation of cortical and subcortical areas. Superficial cortical lesions may ultimately have minimal or negligible consequences. Furthermore, small differences in location, particularly in deeper structures, can make an enormous clinical difference by disrupting critical structures and pathways. For instance, whether or not a FCC in the deep left frontal white matter involves the anterior

Table 6   Focal Lesions: Typical Locations and Consequences

Lesions	Location	Consequences
Focal cortical contusion	Frontal polar and orbital frontal	Alterations in affect and behavior (apathy or disinhibition), higher-level intellectual abilities (processing, executive functions, self-awareness)
	Anterior–inferior temporal	Alterations in affect and behavior, auditory association deficits (e.g., aphasia) visual association deficits (e.g., agnosia)
Deep hemorrhages	Basal ganglia area	Hemiparesis, discoordination, hypertonia, movement disorders, aphasia (left), neglect, visuospatial problems (right)
Focal hypoxic–ischemic injury	Posterior cerebral artery infarct	Hemianopia, amnesia, aphasia (alexia and anomia; left), hemispatial neglect, topographical disorientation, prosopagnosia (right)

periventricular region might determine the presence of muteness or non-fluent speech during early recovery [64].

Third, the early appearance of FCC on neuroimaging may be quite different than its later appearance owing to the degree of resolution of hemorrhage, edema, and other early effects. The corresponding clinical consequences should parallel this resolution.

Fourth, FCCs are often multiple and sometimes bilateral. Multiple FCC have, not surprisingly, a worse prognosis than single lesions [39]. Multiple unilateral lesions have a worse outcome than multiple bilateral lesions, apparently because of a greater propensity for temporal lobe herniation. Bilateral lesions in homologous areas, however, carry a grim prognosis. One could consider the well-documented differences in recovery of memory after unilateral or bilateral medial temporal injuries or the differences between residual visuoperceptual function in unilateral (hemifield neglect) versus bilateral (Balint's syndrome) parietal lesions [65–67].

Fifth, combinations of pathologies are common, and the localizable clinical effects of FCC are often intermixed with problems attributable to other pathologies, such as DAI. The specific clinical effects of FCC may be masked. For instance, it is usually impossible to evaluate "focal," modality-specific deficits while patients are in a confusional state, when attentional difficulties still predominate. Even in the absence of DAI, the early course of focal lesions may be primarily a confusional state of uncertain pathophysiological mechanism.

Frontal FCC   The prefrontal areas (exclusive of primary motor and motor association areas) have important ties to both sensory association areas and the limbic system. In an overall sense, the prefrontal areas assimilate highly integrated multimodal sensory information with information about a person's internal state (e.g., emotions, drives) and use this information to initiate, govern, and modify appropriate goal-directed behavior [63]. Therefore, traumatic prefrontal focal lesions lead to alterations in three interdependent domains: affect, higher-level intellectual abilities, and complex behavior (Table 6). The emotional and intellectual deficits reflect the inability of the damaged frontal regions to regulate and monitor other, generally preserved, functional brain networks such as those for language, perception, visual–spatial functions, and somatosensory functions [68]. Rather than causing modality specific deficits, frontal lesions interrupt the integrated working of these functional networks in novel situations.

There is no universally accepted model of frontal regulatory processes, but the theories of Stuss are representative of most models [69–71]. He identified four large categories of frontal regulation that may be impaired. Drive is the capacity to activate and channel attention to information. Processing is the supramodal organization and temporal ordering of information. Executive functions are modality-independent representations of complex actions that allow anticipation, selection, or inhibition of behavior. Self-analysis and awareness are highly abstract mental representations of behavior and past, and future, information. The dysfunctional clinical manifestations of frontal lesions include poor initiation of behavior; impaired organization, sequencing, and planning of behavior; deficient inhibition of irrelevant behaviors; and failure to anticipate the consequences of behavior. Emotional and personality alteration tend toward either apathy (affective blunting, withdrawal, and poor initiative) or disinhibition (irritability, impulsiveness, and overactivity). In either case, mood is shallow and rapid changes in mood and deportment may occur with apparently trivial triggers. Emotional responses may extend long past the associated event.

Confabulation is a particularly troublesome behavior that may emerge after frontal injury. Variable and inconsistent confabulative responses are quite common during confusional states associated with a variety of focal and diffuse pathologies (see below); confabulating after confusion has cleared has a high association with focal frontal (especially right frontal) pathology [72–74]. These confabulations can take on extraordinary or grandiose proportions [72]. They are often based in some part on true personal history or on misinterpretation of an actual situation. These "frontal" confabulations are often fixed and unshakable, resistant to logical arguments or even physical proof; that is, they take on the behavioral structure of delusions. Fixed confabulative beliefs may persist long after resolution of the period of active confabulation. Attempts at "treatment" of confabulation through confrontation or reality orientation are generally futile, although patients sometimes learn to suppress confabulative responses [75]. Neuroleptic medication sometimes lessens confabulation of a more paranoid or psychotic flavor.

Focal frontal lobe lesions are not the exclusive cause of "frontal" clinical signs in TBI. Diffuse pathology can be associated with identical signs in the absence of focal pathology (see below), likely owing to "disconnection" or deafferentiation of prefrontal projections. Frontal signs may parallel both the extent of focal pathology and the severity of diffuse pathology [76].

Temporal FCC Traumatic temporal lobe lesions also involve connections between tertiary sensory association areas and limbic structures (Table 6). The typically anterior–inferior location of temporal FCC causes damage to paralimbic temporal neocortex that is highly connected to prefrontal areas. These regions may well function as a unit involved in emotional regulation of behavior [63]. Although the amygdalae and hippocampi are not usually directly affected by temporal FCC, the amygdalofugal pathways may be damaged, further disrupting emotional regulations.

Medial temporal and more posterior inferior temporal regions may occasionally be directly damaged or compressed by local mass effect and herniation. If hippocampal projections are sufficiently disrupted, prominent memory problems result. Bilateral anterior medial temporal lesions damaging the amygdala and sensory–limbic connections lead to severe defects in the attribution of significance to environmental stimuli [63]. At the extreme is the Kluver-Bucy syndrome, first described after bilateral temporal lobectomy in rhesus monkeys [77]. Fragments of this syndrome have been described in humans after traumatic anterior temporal injury and include placidity, compulsive exploratory behavior, bulemia, and altered sexual behavior [78].

Lesions that extend more posteriorly in the temporal lobe can affect auditory, visual, or bimodal association areas. When posterior association areas of the left hemisphere are involved, language impairments occur. Anomic aphasia is the most frequent problem, but, depending upon depth and extent, transcortical sensory aphasia or Wernicke's aphasia may occur. Bilateral lesions extending posteriorly to the inferior temporal occipital junction produce visual recognition problems (the various visual agnosias). Delusional thinking may be seen with temporal focal lesions as well, but the mechanism is not based on confabulation. Paranoid delusions are most typically associated with left temporal lesions [73,74]. These may be quite persistent and resistant to any therapeutic intervention, but neuroleptic medication, such as haloperidol, may lessen their expression [75].

Focal HII

The most common manifestation of focal HII is infarction in the posterior cerebral artery territory producing clinical signs attributable to posterior medial occipital and temporal injury (Table 6). Visual field defects are common. If damage is left-sided, various combinations of amnesia, anomic aphasia, alexia, transcortical sensory aphasia, and possibly visual agnosia can occur [67]. If damage is right-sided, hemispatial neglect, nonverbal amnesia, topographical disorientation, or prosopagnosia may occur. Bilateral lesions obviously compound the findings.

Recovery from Focal Lesions

Recovery patterns from focal traumatic lesions have not been well described. Their clinical natural history should be defined by the same factors noted before: location, size, bilaterality, and concomitant pathological factors. Recovery from traumatic lesions should not differ substantially from acute focal lesions of other causes, particularly other vascular causes. There is an acute phase, when problems may appear more widespread and less localizable, reflecting in large part the extent of localized reactive pathophysiological processes and diffuse pathologies. Patients may be frankly confused. There is a subacute phase when localizing effects may be more distinct; and a chronic or residual phase with relatively stable deficits, which are direct consequences of a fixed lesion. The time to reach a stable chronic phase is variable, depending on numerous factors specific to the injury and patient, but is probably sooner than after diffuse pathology. The point of stability may be reached in months. Of course, even after reaching a pathophysiological endpoint, new learning, proceduralization of compensatory skills, and overall plasticity of brain functions will allow functional change beyond that point [79].

Measuring Focal Impairments

Focal impairments are best measured by instruments aimed at the operational deficits produced by the lesion. For instance, specific language batteries such as the Western Aphasia Battery [80] or Boston Diagnostic Aphasia Evaluation [81] will be useful to track aphasia from left hemisphere lesions. Most of the focal lesions associated with TBI, however, produce problems not well characterized by traditional neuropsychological batteries. Evaluations such as the Wechsler Adult Intelligence Scale [82] will fail to capture functions typically altered by frontal and temporal lesions. Tests more sensitive to frontal lobe function (e.g., Wisconsin Card Sorting Test [83] or the Stroop test [84]) can be more useful, but these tests can also be affected by nonfrontal lesions. Informal evaluation should include tests of abstract reasoning, such as proverb and idiom interpretations, tests of sustained performance, word list generation, and tests of sequencing and ordering, such as accounts of familiar multistep tasks (e.g., tire changing).

Few instruments are available to capture characteristic emotional and behavioral disorders. Innovative measures of planning deficits in real-life settings after frontal lesions have been recently developed but are not broadly applied [85]. Observations of patients' performance during mental status testing or during formal neuropsychological testing are as good as any available measure. Assessment of distractibility, impulsivity, susceptibility to interference, ability to shift set, plan, anticipate, self-monitor, initiate, and sustain performance will provide a profile of the relevant functions, if not an objective score. At later points family observations and detailed accounts of daily activities will give important clues to these functions.

Treatment Strategies: Focal Lesions

Several principles govern rehabilitation of focal lesions. First, earlier intervention may be warranted since recovery from focal pathology may evolve and plateau more quickly, and behavior patterns may become established earlier than diffuse pathology. For instance, "frontal" behavioral disorders may improve over a long period of time following diffuse injury, whereas identical problems following large frontal FCC may have a limited late recovery. Second, specific interventions may be useful for specific focal deficits. For instance, language therapies may benefit patients with aphasia. Third, some persistent, fixed impairments following focal lesions will not improve despite any sort of intervention. Substitution of function using preserved abilities may aid in functional adaptation in some cases. For example, all the memory remediation strategies available will not alleviate dense amnesia resulting from bilateral hippocampal lesions; however, exploiting preserved capacities such as procedural learning may aid in teaching new skills and adaptations [86].

Diffuse Pathology

Pattern of Recovery

As we emphasized above, it is the quantity of DAI that determines its severity and in turn determines its clinical consequences. The clinical course is qualitatively similar across the range of severities from most mild to severe, and a recognizable pattern of recovery defines the clinical course whatever its duration (Table 7, Fig. 7). Loss of consciousness (in all but the mildest cases) occurs immediately, without lucid interval [12,13]. Emergence from unconsciousness is followed by a proportionally longer period of confusion and amnesia; when confusion and amnesia clear, a yet longer period of residual impairment and restoration of function occurs. The duration of each of these

Table 7   Diffuse Axonal Injury: Clinical Consequences

Relative to quantity of damaged axons
Immediate coma (no lucid interval)
Confusional state (PTA)
Residual attention, higher-level cognitive, behavioral impairments
Other
  Dorsolateral midbrain: cerebellar motor deficits
  Rostral brainstem: ocular motility disturbances
  Parasagittal: muteness, hypokinesia

periods is unequivocally related to severity of DAI. Briefer durations and rapid transitions characterize mild diffuse TBI: unconsciousness, if at all, lasting seconds to minutes, confusion and PTA extending minutes to hours, and residual dysfunction usually up to days or several months. The process evolves more slowly in severe DAI: days to weeks of unconsciousness, weeks

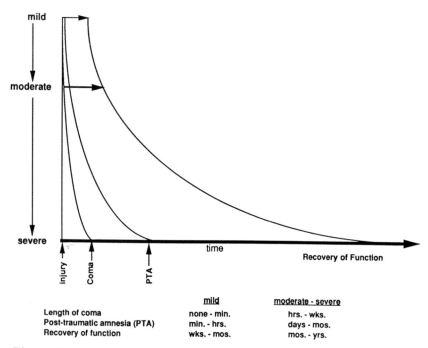

Figure 7   Course of recovery from DAI at different severities (from ref. [45]; reproduced with permission).

to months of confusion (PTA), months to years of residual dysfunction. In the most severe injuries the clinical evolution may be incomplete and patients may remain at an intermediate level (e.g., persistent vegetative state).

A number of schemes have been developed to define the natural history of diffuse TBI. The Rancho Los Amigos scale [87] is commonly used (Table 8). There are eight levels; the first three describe unconsciousness and emerging responsiveness, the next three describe confusion, and the last two represent the residual recovery period.

Another scheme previously described by one of the authors [88] will be used to illustrate the recovery process in more detail (Table 9). This model more closely follows traditional neurological concepts along with levels of general social functioning. The description of these stages is more applicable to patients with moderate or severe diffuse injuries; again, patients with mild diffuse injuries pass through analogous stages, but more rapidly. (The particular clinical consequences and management problems of mild injury are discussed separately below.)

Coma

DEFINITION   This stage is defined by absent cerebral responsiveness or verbalization with eyes remaining closed, even with stimulation. Reflex or automatic motor responses may occur based on brainstem or spinal cord functions. Limb movements may be completely absent at the lowest levels, or may be decerebrate or decorticate postures, or reflex withdrawal at progressively higher stages. The Glasgow Coma Scale [89] is a valuable measure of this progression (Table 5).

TREATMENT STRATEGIES   Patients rarely begin active rehabilitation at this stage. Strategies applicable to the next stage are probably

Table 8   Rancho Los Amigos
Levels of Cognitive Functioning

Level	Clinical Findings
I.	No response
II.	Generalized responses
III.	Localized responses
IV.	Confused: agitated
V.	Confused: inappropriate
VI.	Confused: appropriate
VII.	Automatic: appropriate
VIII.	Purposeful and appropriate

Source: From ref. [87].

Table 9 Stages of Recovery from DAI

Coma: unresponsive, eyes closed

Unresponsive vigilance–vegetative state: no cognitive responsiveness gross wakefulness, sleep–wake cycles

Mute/low-level responsiveness: purposeful wakefulness, responds to some commands

Confusional state: recovered speech, amnesic (PTA), severe attentional deficits, agitated, hypoaroused, or labile behavior

Evolving independence: resolution of PTA, cognitive improvement, achieving independence in daily self-care, improving social interaction; developing independence
at home

Intellectual/social competence: recovering cognitive abilities, goal-directed behaviors, social skills, personality; devleoping independence in community; returning to
academic or vocational pursuits

appropriate at this stage as well. The main focus is on ensuring basic life
support and managing acute medical and neurological problems (such as
intracranial pressure) that may be life-threatening or cause further damage.

Unresponsive Vigilance/Vegetative State

DEFINITION   Transition to this stage usually occurs within 4 weeks
[11] and is marked by restoration of eye opening and gross wakefulness;
sleep–wake cycles may resume. There is still no cognitive activity, and some
continue to term patients in this state "comatose." This first signs of cerebral
activity heralding transition to the next stage may be visual fixation and
tracking.

TREATMENT STRATEGIES   The main issue of management is to
recognize when cerebral responsiveness has begun. Appropriate conditions
will maximize chances of responsiveness. Patients must be wakeful and
allowed some "warm-up" time. They must be given enough time to respond,
with adequate interstimulus intervals. Rapid fatiguing of responses is common. Purposeful responses need to be differentiated from automatic, generalized, or reflex responses. Those most familiar to patients (i.e., family) and
those who spend most time with patients will inevitably be the first to
recognize purposeful behavior. Factors that may inhibit responsiveness
should be alleviated when possible. Late secondary neurological problems
(e.g., hydrocephalus), medical problems, or medications such as narcotic pain
medications, benzodiazepines, and barbiturates may all suppress responses.

Stimulation at some level is probably beneficial. The value of elaborate,
intensive, personalized sensory stimulation programs remains dubious. They
do provide systematic means of recognizing, tracking, and establishing the
time and stimulus dimensions of responsiveness.

Ensuring the best possible general medical health, preventing complications such as contractures and skin breakdown, and alleviating iatrogenic problems are the main treatment strategies to promote recovery to further stages. Some patients will not progress beyond low-level response states and less intensive therapy in appropriate longer-term institutions may be necessary.

Mute/Low-Level Responsiveness

DEFINITION Patients begin to demonstrate cognitive responsiveness, usually marked by ability to follow commands, prior to spontaneous speech output [90]. Some may remain mute for some time, perhaps related to the frontal parasagittal preponderance of DAI [18] interrupting supplementary motor area projections necessary for speech initiation [64]. A smaller proportion of patients verbalize before reliably following commands [90]; focal left hemisphere lesions may contribute to delays in language-based responsiveness.

TREATMENT STRATEGIES Establishing some level of yes/no responsiveness and other communication through an appropriate response modality is a major goal during this stage. Oral feeding may often begin at this time; assessment of swallowing to avoid complications is necessary.

Confusional State

DEFINITION Although verbal communication is established, it is degraded, along with other cognitive operations, by severe attentional disturbances that define this stage. Patients have difficulty focusing and sustaining attention for appreciable periods of time and are extremely distractable. Any modality-specific cognitive evaluation will be contaminated by attentional deficits, so detailed cognitive batteries are not useful during this stage.

Dense anterograde PTA continues; virtually no encoding of episodic events or new learning occurs. Patients are disoriented and have little or no insight into their problems. The end of this stage is marked by resumption of continuous day-to-day memory and by restoration of orientation, first to place, then to time in most [91]. The Galveston Orientation and Amnesia Test (GOAT) is a useful tool to track this process [92].

Behavior disorders are ubiquitous during this period. Patients may be hyperaroused or hypoaroused or erratically either one. Hyperaroused agitation can be the most disturbing and difficult to manage problem at this time. Hypoaroused patients are apathetic, amotivational, and hypokinetic. Patients may evolve from one state to another or may vary over the course of the day, based on environmental and internal factors.

TREATMENT STRATEGIES Appropriate levels of stimulation are most important at this stage. Hyperaroused patients may require quieter, less stimulating environments, and shorter treatment sessions. Staff and family may need to back off and decrease demands if patients become overaroused and agitated. Hypoaroused patients may benefit from greater levels of stimulation and added encouragement to promote better initiation and participation. Stimulant medications or dopamine agonists such as bromocriptine may benefit some such patients [93]. Familiar persons and objects may help with both types of confused patients. Interactions and communication should respect that attentional disturbances predominate; lengthy and complex directions, simultaneous conversations, and distracting environments should be avoided.

Fatigue may add to confusion. Regulation of sleep/wake cycles and appropriate pacing of activities and rest periods during the day may reduce confusional problems. Patients may need to be kept awake later in the day, and sleeping medications may be necessary to promote adequate sleep. If used, an adequate dosage of medications should be given at bedtime to ensure therapeutic effect and to avoid morning hangovers from later repeat doses.

Much of the work of inpatient rehabilitation is simply to allow patients to pass through the confusional state as smoothly and safely as possible. Setting up the patient's environment appropriately, and providing abundant structure, support, and reassurance, will go a long way in ensuring an easier transition through this stage.

Evolving Independence

DEFINITION   Resolution of PTA and marked improvement in attention allow a much greater awareness and more meaningful and appropriate interaction with caretakers. Patients become continent, take on more responsibility for self-care, and have greater appreciation of physical limitations and safety. Despite profound improvement in attention and memory, higher-level attention and cognitive problems still abound. Although largely aware of their situation, patients still do not recognize the extent of their cognitive problems. Instrumental deficits related to focal damage, such as aphasia, become more apparent and better evaluated. Severe agitation and lability usually resolve, but behavior problems and personality alterations, often in the form of disinhibition, are usually present.

As levels of independence in activities of daily living (ADL) and mobility improve, patients become ready for discharge from inpatient rehabilitation settings. Limitations in ADLs and mobility become less dependent on mental impairments and more on residual physical problems (e.g., weakness, tone problems, balance and gait disorders, orthopedic injuries).

TREATMENT STRATEGIES   The main goals are promoting as much independence in self-care as possible, enhancing awareness of functional limitations and safety, and encouraging greater levels of personal responsibility. Restoring appropriate social skills through group and family activities is also important.

Facilitating transition to home, as smoothly as possible, is one of the major management goals during this stage. An appropriate discharge plan ensuring a safe environment, supervision, assistance with any necessary equipment, and available outpatient programs to continue rehabilitation goals should be formulated. Family involvement is especially important at this time; family sessions with staff, community visits, and day passes will aid in this transition.

Some level of structure and consistency to patients' days is still important at this stage. Patients should be encouraged, however, to be more engaged in their rehabilitation treatment. They should follow their own schedules. They should contribute to their own treatment goals. Sedative and sleep medications may no longer be necessary.

Some patients will have very limited evolution through this stage. They may have a persistently high level of dependency. Discharge to a longer-term treatment facility may be appropriate and support continued, while there is any, albeit slow, improvement. For some slowly recovering patients, home discharge with extensive support and outpatient programs may be preferred.

Intellectual/Social Competence

DEFINITION   This stage takes up the proportionally longer period of time during which patients attempt to regain some level of social independence and, if possible, return to personal, academic, and vocational roles. The evolution of this process can take years and many patients with more severe injuries stall at this stage. Persistent disturbances in higher-level attention, memory, and higher order cognitive functions, such as planning, are the usual impediments. Personality changes (disinhibited or apathetic) and degraded complex social interactions are other important limitations. If depression occurs, it usually presents sometime during this stage.

Recovery at this stage may also be limited by residual physical and motor control problems. Fatigue and decreased stamina are complaints in the majority of patients and will exaggerate all residual problems. Other stressors, exogenous or endogenous, will also tend to amplify deficits (e.g., alcohol, medical illness, psychological stress).

TREATMENT STRATEGIES   The main goal is enhancing personal independence in the home and community. When possible, supervision should be gradually withdrawn, first at home, and then outside the home.

Patients usually continue in outpatient rehabilitation programs and some may benefit from reentry or transitional living programs. Despite this programming, patients usually have problems coping with large amounts of unstructured time. Pursuit of hobbies, interests, and home responsibilities should be encouraged; structured scheduling may be helpful.

There may be significant stress on family and other relationships. Impaired social skills and behavior problems are a particular burden and group therapies, individual and group psychological counseling, and specialized behavior programs in refractory cases are useful interventions. Excess fatigue after both mental and physical activity and at the end of the day is a typical persistent complaint. Ensuring adequate sleep, avoiding boredom, pacing activities, maintaining a physical conditioning program, screening for alcohol use, removing unnecessary sedating medications, and treating depression (if present) are important steps to managing fatigue.

When recovery is adequate, return to work or school may be contemplated. Neuropsychological and vocational assessments, physical capacity evaluations, school and special needs assessments will help to specify residual problems and aid in appropriate planning. Volunteer work or "work trials" may help to re-establish work skills. Return to work or school should be graded, with daily performance closely monitored. Job modifications or school modifications may be necessary. Job coaches or supported work programs may be useful; lower-level occupations may be necessary. In school such compensations as resource rooms, tutors, reduced class load, assistance of note takers, and relaxation of time constraints on examinations are important measures to prevent early failures. Hasty, premature return to work or school can have potentially disastrous consequences and produce difficult secondary psychological problems.

When recovery is more limited, return to work or meaningful academic activity may not be possible. Treatment should focus on time management, recreational activities, and abilities to participate socially and in the community at some level.

Return to driving is a frequent decision at this stage. In some, physical or mental limitations preventing safe driving will be obvious. In others, capacity to drive will be fairly apparent and initial observation and supervision by a trusted, experienced driver will be all that is necessary. In the rest, a more formal evaluation of driving skill should be undertaken, including tests of perception and reaction time and an on-the-road evaluation.

Specific Impairments of Diffuse Injury (Moderate to Severe)

Now that we have considered the overall pattern of recovery after diffuse injury in the previous section, the following section contains a more complete discussion of cognitive, behavioral, and physical problems that occur in the residual period (evolving independence and intellectual/social competence) after resolution of confusion and PTA. Problems associated with moderate to severe diffuse injury will be considered separately from mild diffuse injury, since they may require distinct diagnostic and management strategies.

Cognitive Problems After Diffuse Injury Beyond issues of arousal, the principal cognitive deficits of diffuse TBI involve attention, memory, and higher-level processes, such as organization and planning. Problems in these areas occur in different forms at various stages of recovery and are the most likely components of any residual cognitive disorder. Other areas involving well-established information stores and patterns of behavior, such as semantic knowledge and praxis, are relatively less affected.

ATTENTION   Once the profound disruption of the more basic elements of attention resolves, and confusion and PTA clear, more complex attentional processes still remain affected. Subjective complaints and observations include poor concentration, distractibility, slowness, and difficulty focusing on more than one task at a time. Objective measures of the performance of patients with TBI on tasks probing one or more subcomponents of attention have demonstrated some typical problems. More severely injured patients have generally slower reaction times, and slowing is sensitive to the complexity of the task. Reaction times are particularly slowed in tasks requiring some response decision or choice [94]. The rate of information processing is slowed, and the Paced Auditory Serial Addition Test (PASAT), which requires addition of numbers presented at progressively faster rates [95], is an excellent measure for this problem. The aspect of attention most sensitive to TBI is probably divided attention [96]. Patients have difficulty handling two or more tasks or subtasks at a time, as demanded by many everyday activities (e.g., driving and carrying on a conversation at the same time). Susceptibility to distractibility and interference in the middle of a mental operation is another well demonstrated attention disorder in patients with TBI [97].

MEMORY   Memory impairment is a salient feature of early and late recovery from diffuse TBI and is among the most common persistent subjective complaint [98]. Acquisition and retrieval of new information are profoundly disturbed in early stages until confusion and PTA resolve. Memory deficits are still evident after this point, and the degree of persistent impairment is related to severity of diffuse injury [99]. In some patients the memory disturbance remains prominent and disproportionately greater than other cognitive problems [100]. Focal left temporal lobe pathological involvement or hypoxia associated with diffuse pathological changes is most likely to account for a large portion of this subgroup [100,101].

The neuropsychological structure of the memory problem after DAI has been well characterized. In the early stages it cannot be meaningfully differentiated from attentional deficits. Immediate or working memory recovers more quickly than delayed recall [99] and is probably at a normal level in most cases by the time PTA clears. Learning remains inefficient for several reasons long after PTA has cleared. Learning is more susceptible to distractions or interference from other stimuli [96]. Patients with TBI have more difficulty with "automatic" learning, that is, learning that normally occurs without active strategies or effort [102]. When active learning is attempted, patients with TBI tend not to use effective strategies, such as semantic clustering on word list learning [99].

Various memory compartments may be differentially affected. There is a relative preservation of semantic memory or knowledge stores even when episodic memory (information linked to recollection of events) is severely degraded. Procedural memory (recall of motor skills and cognitive operations) is also relatively preserved [103]. Patients with TBI are able to acquire specific motor and other skills even when little or no declarative learning (acquiring new information) is occurring [103,104]. This observation has important implications for teaching new skills to patients in rehabilitation during PTA.

HIGHER COGNITIVE ABILITIES   Evaluations of general cognition and intelligence have demonstrated long-term impairments, particularly in more severe diffuse injuries [105]. These tests, such as the Wechsler Adult Intelligence Scale–Revised (WAIS-R) [82], evaluate a broad range of capacities, some of which may be more or less affected by TBI. Mandelberg's [106] observation of earlier recovery of verbal scores than performance scores on the WAIS is likely a reflection of the sensitivity of the performance tasks to attention and speed of processing. At the same time the WAIS-R may not adequately tap some of the more salient features of long-term cognitive dysfunction, such as those related to frontal "executive" functions. Problems in planning, reasoning, and decision-making frequently persist after general intellectual abilities approach normal. Tests of executive abilities, such as the Wisconsin Card Sorting Test [83], can better capture some of the longer-term cognitive deficits [107,108]. Newer strategies of problem solving may also capture residual deficits [85].

As is the case with focal pathology, some cognitive functions are better preserved after diffuse TBI. Although complex verbal skills are frequently affected, specific language disorders are relatively uncommon in diffuse injury [109]. Most who show signs of aphasia early in recovery (usually naming difficulties) show resolution [110]. Specific perceptual and visuo-spatial functions also recover relatively well [107].

OTHER FACTORS   A number of related factors need to be considered in evaluation of the cognitive effects of TBI. More important than particular scores on neuropsychological tests is how a person is functioning compared to their preinjury status. Premorbid intellectual capacity, including areas of talent and learning disability, must be determined. Behavior and affective disorders may affect cognition. A patient who is unmotivated and apathetic may not initiate or sustain mental activities despite preservation of those capacities. Depression may interfere with attention, and poor motivation is a frequent cause of "deterioration" of cognition. Fatigue is the most common cause of deteriorated performance. Patients often complain that problems emerge or worsen after periods of strenuous activity and toward the end of the day. Overall variability and inconsistency of performance are other recognized features of cognitive impairments, whether due to fatigue or some other cause [97]. Exogenous factors of various sorts may also have an impact on mental performance. Centrally acting substances, such as alcohol or some medications, other concomitant brain disorders or medical illnesses, and psychological stressors may all adversely affect cognition.

TREATMENT STRATEGIES   Rehabilitation management of cognitive impairments can largely be classified under the rubric of cognitive rehabilitation. This refers to a generally unstandardized set of procedures aimed at reducing cognitive deficiencies or promoting compensatory strategies. Approaches may be more or less systematic and may incorporate more or less real-world functional tasks. Some specific procedures aimed at specific impairments have demonstrated benefits [111]. Some programs incorporating cognitive rehabilitation strategies have reported improved status of patients completing these programs [112]. Programs that work on entirely functionally based activities, without any specific cognitive rehabilitation strategies have, however, reported similar success [113]. A comparison of structured neuropsychological treatment with nonstructured supportive, stimulating treatment demonstrated improvement in both groups [114]. The overwhelming majority of cognitive remediation techniques remain unsubstantiated, with unclear indications and benefits and uncertain generalization to real-life situations. A complete discussion of this topic is beyond the scope of this chapter.

Behavioral Problems After Diffuse Injury   Behavioral abnormalities and personality changes rarely occur independently of cognitive impairments. Behavioral and cognitive disturbances are related to a common neuropsychological substrate. The same mechanisms leading to disinhibited, impulsive behavior might underlie the inability to organize, anticipate, and plan when performing complex cognitive operations. Furthermore, the degree of cognitive deficit is related to the amount of emotional disturbance [115].

The behavioral and personality alterations after DAI are often described in psychiatric diagnostic terms. This psychiatric taxonomy, while descriptive by analogy to traditional psychiatric disorders, sometimes betrays lack of appreciation of the underlying neurological determinants. Diagnoses such as "schizophrenia-like psychosis" and "organic personality syndrome" do not capture the full nature of these disturbances.

PERSONALITY CHANGE   In general, personality changes associated with diffuse injury distribute along the same lines as that described for focal frontal brain lesions. This is understandable in the context of disrupted frontal projections by DAI, as previously described. Personality changes tend toward either passive, unmotivated, and apathetic or active, disinhibited, and aggressive [116]. Assessment of the stage of recovery during which a behavioral disturbance is occurring is critical for understanding and managing the problem. Aggressive behavior, for instance, is quite common in a confusional state but is often transient and quickly resolves as confusion clears. Personality changes observed at later stages may be more enduring. The occurrence of personality disturbance is not clearly related to severity of injury, but more lasting problems occur in the most severe injuries [117]. With diffuse pathology the pattern of recovery of personality and behavioral alterations probably parallels that for cognitive functions, evolving in a time course proportional to severity. Persistent behavioral problems or particular disturbances, such as paranoia (see below), depend also on the presence of fixed lesions, typically frontal or temporal contusions.

Aside from the injury factors (pathology, severity, stage of recovery), two other sets of interacting factors are needed to explain fully and appropriately manage the behavioral problem. First, all behaviors must be understood in the context of pretrauma personality style, second, environmental factors provide both antecedent and consequent determinants of behavior.

At all stages of recovery, posttrauma behavior disorders will be shaped by previously established patterns of emotional and motivational responses [118]. Indeed, some of the typically observed pretrauma patterns are themselves risk factors for injury, further loading the potential for characterological disturbances in patients with TBI. Personality changes often present as exaggerations of previous patterns of behavior [74]. Families often observe that a patient's personality is the same but that he or she seems "even more short-tempered" or "sillier than ever" after injury.

Sometimes families will blame all behavior problems on the injury even when these problems were clearly present premorbidly. The clinician is obliged to sort out the relationship between premorbid personality, preexisting disorders, and injury effects to determine prognosis and appropriate management goals. Age and developmental level need also be considered. Psychological development, previous social learning, neurological maturation, and gender- and hormone-specific interactions are all powerful, age-related, determinants of behavior. Some behaviors may be more or less appropriate in certain age-determined contexts and not be entirely viewed as a consequence of injury.

Environmental effects on behavior must be examined at all levels of recovery. Excessive levels of stimulation or particular events may set off aggressive behavior during a confusional state. Overwhelming environmental demands, which tax reduced intellectual capacities, may lead to irritability, belligerence, withdrawal, or depression at later stages of recovery. Manipulation of environmental factors is the most important strategy in managing behavior problems.

Aside from personality changes, a number of other behavioral problems should be mentioned. Confabulation, delusional thinking, and paranoia have already been discussed in the context of focal lesions. These problems may occur with diffuse injuries as well, but usually emerge during or just following resolution of confusion and PTA [119]. Persistent problems are more likely related to focal pathology or very severe levels of diffuse pathology. Premorbid tendency to suspiciousness and paranoid thinking is probably another factor in development of this symptom in some patients with TBI.

DEPRESSION AND MANIA   Depression, ranging from dysphoric mood to major depression, is common after head injury and may be more common after milder injuries [74]. A combination of premorbid personality traits, cerebral injury, and reactive environmental factors must account for the cause. Focal brain lesions, particularly left frontal, and specific patterns of monoamine alterations have been associated with depression after head injury and other neurological disorders [120]. Depression most often occurs as other functions are improving, and insight and concern become established [119] (e.g., intellectual and social competence stage). Although criteria from the *Diagnostic and Statistical Manual of Mental Disorders*, 3rd edition (revised) (DSM-III-R) are useful in establishing the diagnosis, presentations may be atypical because of brain injury-induced personality changes, impaired awareness of mood states, altered prosody, and emotional expression. A premature plateau or regression in recovery or cognitive performance may suggest the diagnosis.

Mania and hypomania are less common than depression and have a higher association with right-sided limbic structures and with premorbid or family histories of mania [121]. Mania tends to occur earlier in recovery (e.g., emerging independence stage) than depression [119]. It appears closely linked to disinhibited unregulated behavior that is also highly associated with frontal injury, especially on the right. Verbosity, pressured speech, grandiosity, irritability, euphoria, and sleep disruption are typical of these patients.

AGGRESSION   Aggressive behavior and agitation are common and are the behavioral disorders that receive the most attention from staff. Aggressive disorders should be interpreted and managed in the context of stage of recovery. Periods of verbal and physical aggression are almost ubiquitous during confusional states with hyperarousal. As with other behavioral alterations, aggressiveness usually largely resolves when confusion clears. The temporary nature of this form of agitation along with its association with profound attention and memory disturbances suggests a treatment strategy. The general strategies employed at this stage (support and reassurance, use of familiar objects and caretakers, and environmental manipulation to decrease levels of stimulation) are often effective. Adjusting schedules to prevent excessive fatigue and overstimulation is usually necessary. Regulating sleep by preventing excess daytime napping and, if necessary, use of adequate dosages of sedative medication at bedtime, will sometimes reduce agitation. Complex and long-term behavioral management strategies such as token economies or operant conditioning are not appropriate in managing confusional aggression. When behavioral strategies are not adequate, judicious use of medication should be guided by the usually temporary nature of this form of aggression, and the primary goal should be the patient's and caretakers' safety. When aggression is expected to be a short-term problem, we sometimes use neuroleptic medications or benzodiazepines at times of agitation or to prevent agitation that consistently occurs at particular times. One must recognize potential problems of increased restlessness (akathesia) or parkinsonian effects caused by the former and paradoxic agitation caused by the latter. The effect of those medications on recovery remains controversial.

When confusional aggression is expected to last longer (e.g., very severe DAI with coma durations exceeding 2 weeks), regular dosages of medications may be useful. Although beta-blockers, tricyclic antidepressants, anticonvulsants, lithium, and neuroleptics are among the medication classes used, there is limited evidence to support meaningful choices. A full discussion of the pharmacological treatment of aggression is beyond the scope of this chapter [122].

Aggression that occurs in the stages following confusional state demands a different approach. Irritability and short temper are common persistent problems and often do not require specific management. More serious forms of aggression can occur, and these are frequently associated with focal limbic lesions. Premorbid histories of aggression are sometimes identified; other possible triggers such as alcohol or other substances must be identified. Behavioral management techniques should be employed [123]. First, antecedent conditions need to be identified, and the frequency and duration of aggressive behaviors assessed. Direct or indirect reinforcements of aggression should be removed and appropriate behaviors should be positively reinforced; attention itself may be a potent reinforcer. Group treatment to train and reinforce appropriate social skills may help reduce the tendencies toward aggression. Systematic behavioral techniques such as "time-out" and "token economies" have been used successfully. Specialized behaviorally oriented programs that employ these techniques to deal with intransigent and severe aggressive disorders are available in some regions. Pharmacotherapy using the medication classes described above is often required for persistent problems.

SOCIAL RELATIONSHIPS AND FAMILY Disintegration of social skills and breakdown of social relationships are common consequences of maladaptive behaviors and of cognitive impairments. Social awareness and social judgment are as dependent on cognitive operations as any other complex perceptual or problem solving task. Deteriorated social functioning is characterized by loss of friendships, decline in leisure activities, and increased loneliness [124]. Social isolation is one of the main complaints of patients with severe TBI late in recovery. The degree of social disintegration is related to severity of diffuse injury and significantly worse in those with PTA lasting longer than 7 days [124].

Behavioral dysfunction and personality change are the major contributors to long-term family stress after head injury [124]. This stress leads to a high incidence of psychological disorders such as depression and severe anxiety in family members [125,126]. Even the relationships between family members (excluding the head-injured patient) may deteriorate [125–127]. Of course, just as patients with TBI may have a higher incidence of premorbid psychosocial problems, families of patients have a higher rate of preinjury dysfunction. The degree of subjective family burden and the prevalence of severe anxiety were related to severity of injury particularly with durations of PTA greater than 2 weeks [128,129]. The severity of personality and behavior alteration is an even better predictor of family dysfunction than severity of injury [127]. Family malfunctioning is usually delayed, occurring beyond 6 months post injury [127]. The degree of perceived burden may intensify with time, even years after the injury [128].

Physical Problems After Diffuse Injury   Physical disorders following moderate to severe diffuse brain injury are less consistent and predictable than the characteristic cognitive and behavioral problems. A host of physical problems occur and are more prevalent and severe in patients with more severe injuries. The most common problems are discussed below.

MOTOR IMPAIRMENTS   DAI is generally associated with a mix of motor deficits attributable to diffuse, bilateral disruption of multiple motor systems. The usual patterns of distribution of DAI (e.g., predilection for parasagittal frontal areas and dorsolateral quadrant of the midbrain) and the varying density and mixtures of preserved versus destroyed axons in affected areas of the brain differentiate the characteristic motor dysfunctions of DAI from more focal motor system lesions. There is not a clear correspondence between the severity of cognitive or behavioral deficits and motor impairments, but more severe injuries (i.e., more DAI) are associated with more severe and lasting motor impairment. The more severe injuries not only produce more concentrated amounts of axonal loss, but there is also more likely involvement of converging motor pathways deeper in the neuraxis, including the brainstem.

Several patterns of motor dysfunction may be observed. Deficits are usually bilateral but asymmetrical. Some form of balance or gait problem is common, even in less severe injuries. Dysfunction in one or more sensory or motor systems may contribute: proprioceptive, vestibular, visual, postural motor control [130]. Poorly coordinated limb movements, impaired fine motor control, dysmetria, and other patterns usually attributed to cerebellar system dysfunction are frequently observed. Limb weakness and spasticity may occur in a hemiparetic or quadriparetic distribution. Various movement disorders occur but less commonly. Tremors, dystonia, myoclonus, choreoathetosis, ballismus, tics, and parkinsonism have all been documented after trauma [131,132]. Again, bilateral mixtures of motor problems are common; dense focal deficits are more exceptional. Along with compromised control of limb and trunk muscles, bulbar muscles are also commonly affected (paresis, ataxia, akinesia, or tremor) causing articulation and swallowing problems. Diffuse pathology may also compromise bowel and bladder motor control with loss of voluntary control of striatal sphincter muscle and disinhibition of bowel and bladder reflex control. It justifies re-emphasis: there is no single, typical pattern of motor impairment after DAI. Dense, single-system focal deficits are less common than mixed, bilateral, multisystem deficits.

Motor behavior may also be disrupted by deficits at superordinate levels, such as praxis, initiation, or motivation. For instance, lack of awareness and concern related to cognitive and behavioral disturbances (e.g., during confusional state) often override bowel and bladder motor problems. High-level ambulatory goals and interventions may be useless, even when no motor problems preclude walking, if a patient is too unmotivated and apathetic to get out of a chair.

Other confounding problems include peripheral nerve injuries, orthopedic injuries, contractures, and other joint limitations (e.g., heterotopic ossification). Appropriate intervention requires accurate diagnosis after all of these factors have been considered.

Once an appropriate diagnosis is formulated, some specific interventions may be targeted at certain motor problems. (A more complete discussion of some of these interventions may be found elsewhere in this text.) As in any aspect of rehabilitation planning, motor interventions should aim at realistic goals with some functional value consistent with the larger picture of deficits, the natural history of the disorder, and environmental constraints.

SPASTICITY   Spasticity should be managed with a multifaceted approach that may include serial casting, inhibitive casting, splinting, pharmacological treatments, neurolytic blocks, and, in more extreme cases, rhizotomy and tendon releases. New treatments presently under investigation that have some promise include injections of C. botulinum toxin to decrease neuromuscular transmission in selected spastic or dystonic muscles [133,134] and installation of intrathecal baclofen by indwelling pump [135]. Medications, including baclofen, diazepam, and dantrolene sodium, are of limited success in treating spasticity of cerebral origin [136] and sedation may be particularly detrimental to patients with TBI (see Chapter 12).

VESTIBULAR AND POSTURAL CONTROL PROBLEMS These problems can now be assessed by a number of sophisticated techniques in addition to the clinical examination. Dynamic electromyography [137] and dynamic posturography [130] are two such methods. The latter analyzes the organization of the sensory components (visual, proprioceptive, and vestibular) of balance. In addition to traditional balance and gait techniques, strategies aimed at habituating the vestibular response or enhancing adaptation of the vestibular system (e.g., training greater reliance on one or another sensory components) may be beneficial.

SWALLOWING AND ARTICULATION DISORDERS These may occur separately, and their incidences are proportional to severity of injury [138]. Dysarthria often persists in later stages of recovery, whereas dysphagia resolves in the majority of patients after resolution of confusion [138]. Swallowing disorders present a particular problem because of the risk of aspiration. A comprehensive swallowing evaluation includes a bedside assessment of oral motor and sensory functions; observation of swallowing and protective mechanisms (e.g., cough); laryngeal examination; and, most importantly, barium swallow videofluorographic examination [139]. Evaluation of the gag reflex alone is not adequate to predict functional swallowing or risk of aspiration. Treatment strategies include various head and neck posturing techniques, volitional alterations of swallowing, and thermal stimulation to trigger the pharyngeal reflex [139]. The best strategy is usually to allow time for recovery and to supply nutrition through gastric tube feedings to prevent aspiration. Feeding trials may begin when reassessment demonstrates minimal risk of aspiration. Diet modifications are sometimes necessary.

Specific Impairments of Diffuse Injury: Mild Head Injury

Mild TBI is often treated in textbooks as though it is an entirely different disorder from severe TBI with no important features in common. As outlined above, however, experimental models of TBI are unambiguous that TBI is a single disorder that may generate distinct pathological profiles [18]. DAI is the pathology produced by inertial forces, and it is the central problem of all patients with acceleration–deceleration trauma, from the mildest "ding" to the most severe injury. Animal studies [18] have demonstrated the quantitive relationship between pathological changes and behavioral/neurological deficits at even the mildest end of the experimental injury spectrum. Even secondary effects of excitatory neurotransmitter release are qualitatively similar [25,33,140]. At the very mildest level there may be no actual disruption of axons, only transient functional impairment. At more severe (still mild, however) levels there may be scattered axonal damage and loss, following the same time course and cerebral topography as described above for severe cases. With more and more severe physical disruption, the behavioral/ neurological effects become progressively more severe.

At the clinical level, the stages of evolution of DAI described for severe cases are also probably seen after mild TBI, but the initial stages may all be condensed into a few minutes: length of coma (LOC) of seconds or minutes, mute responsiveness for seconds, and PTA for minutes or hours. The subsequent evolution occurs over weeks and months [141,142] rather than months and years for severe cases (see Fig. 7). The long-term achievement of good recovery is quicker and more complete the less severe the injury.

The American Congress of Rehabilitation Medicine has adopted a cutoff between minor and moderate TBI at LOC for 1 hr and PTA of 1 day [143]. It is our opinion that this captures an excessive range of severity. The modal concussion case is unconscious less than 1 min and amnesic less than 30–60 min. Others [144] have suggested that initial GCS definitions of mild (GCS 13–15), moderate (10–12), severe (7–9), and very severe (3–6) TBI have prognostic significance. However, this is only effective if a specific time postinjury is utilized and if patients with focal lesions are excluded. In summary, since there is no experimental, pathological, or clinical measure capable of splitting the population into fundamentally different processes, we recommend viewing DAI as a continuum with appropriate guidelines for expected outcome based on all available measures of severity: GCS, LOC, PTA, and CT/MRI. This view is as appropriate for mild as it is for severe DAI.

Now, having lumped in principle, we will split in practice. Patients at the milder end of DAI experience a much different illness than patients at the severe end. Because the former are often alert, oriented, and apparently intact by the time they are first evaluated, they frequently are managed as though their problem is trivial. Symptoms related to nonneurological injury may take precedence acutely and obscure the signs of DAI. Because PTA and retrograde amnesia may be brief, the patients may have much more recall of the circumstances of injury, with all the attendant psychological distress that may entail. For these reasons, minor TBI is best viewed as an interaction of three separate types of injury: neurological, peripheral, and psychological (Table 10).

Table 10   Categories of Mild Head Injury

Neurological: problems with arousal/attention, memory, behavior
Peripheral: headache, cervical pain, vestibular dysfunction
Psychological: depression, anxiety, posttraumatic stress disorder

All three types of injury may contribute to the postconcussive syndrome.

The Neurological Injury   This was reviewed above in the definition and description of mild TBI. After PTA clears, the primary clinical manifestations are deficits in arousal/attention, in memory and in behavior. These are present in all cases, at least transiently.

Regarding arousal/attention, patients may complain of excessive time sleeping or restless, shallow sleep. They may complain of distractibility and poor concentration. The appropriate clinical assessment is directed at attention. In the office, simple tasks such as digit span, serial subtractions, or novel manipulations of otherwise simple activities, such as reciting the months in reverse order, may suffice.

Regarding memory, patients complain of memory loss. They often paradoxically can recall in detail the experience or event that they claim to have forgotten earlier. They may complain that they cannot remember what they have read, especially if there has been noise or disturbance around them, but they can describe the disturbance exactly. Thus, their episodic memory is quite erratic and seems, overall, to reflect diminished efficiency of learning with susceptibility to interference, perhaps in part due to attentional defects. They are not amnesic in the usual sense. Clinical assessment can focus on new learning but must be more challenging than the neurologist's usual shorthand of remembering 3 words for 3 min. Efficiency of learning a 10-word list over 5 trials and then recalling the 10 words in 5 min will be more informative.

Behavioral disturbances in the first days after minor TBI are protean. Irritability, poor tolerance of noise or commotion, and withdrawal are all common. Patients may also experience fragments of posttraumatic stress, such as avoidance behavior (refusing to drive), reliving the injury (even in nightmares), and significant anxiety. Clinical assessment demands a careful history.

The time course of neurological recovery after mild injury remains imprecise. There is evidence that very mild injuries may recover in days [145]. More severe, though still "mild," injuries may take months; studies of patients seen in emergency rooms indicate recovery of attention and memory may extend up to 1 [141], 3 [142], or 6 months [96]. In addition to the clinical assessments described above, neuropsychological measures can document this progress. The proper assessment tools are those that measure complex aspects of memory and attention [96,97,142,146], not those that measure language, intelligence, problem solving, or other abilities. The behavioral problems are more complex. Their natural history can become hopelessly entangled in other aspects of injury such as chronic pain, depression, unemployment, and so on. Tests of so-called executive functions (see above) may illuminate the cognitive deficiencies that parallel behavioral change, but the interpretation of these tests is fraught with hazards in these patients.

Perhaps because the time course of recovery is imprecise, it is often both under- and overestimated. Patients in the emergency room or at their doctor's office in the days after injury are often just told to rest for "a few days," but, except for the mildest "dings," "a few days" is not long enough; weeks to months are required. There exists no model to guide physicians in working with patients, employers, schools, and other institutions in the construction of a gradual schedule for return. At the other end, patients with mild injury who are symptomatic months to years later are often assumed to have incomplete neurological recovery because they are symptomatic. This is a failure in clinical logic.

Peripheral Injury   Patients with mild CHI often have severe scalp, facial, cervical, or vestibular injury. Thus, they may have pain, headache, neckache, or dizziness. The severity of any of these symptoms has no mandatory correlation with the neural injury. When several of these symptoms co-occur after mild CHI, the resulting clinical problems is called the postconcussive syndrome (PCS). In most patients (and clinical reports) the neural symptoms (attention, memory, and behavior) are also considered part of the PCS.

The most common complaints are headache, insomnia, memory problems, fatigue, and irritability [144]. Patients with mild CHI also frequently endorse items suggesting depression [147]. The natural history of this syndrome has been difficult to establish, in part, no doubt, because it is so polytypic. In the vast majority of symptomatic patients, the syndrome resolves over several weeks but, in some, symptoms may be more prolonged [148]. The components of the syndrome may vary. In some cases, it may be migraine that prolongs recovery. In others it may be positional vertigo and in others, anxiety, or back pain; indeed, any combination of these problems may contribute. At 1 year after injury the incidence of PCS (about 10–15%) is probably not greatly different from the percentage of normal controls who would endorse similar complaints [149].

The mechanism for persistent postconcussive symptoms (PPCS) is unclear. Underestimation of injury severity and psychological factors have been suggested. Underestimation of severity may be due to failure to diagnose a focal contusion that need not be associated with prolonged LOC or PTA (see above). Age greater than 60 (perhaps even greater than 40) may also be a substantial reason for prolonged and incomplete recovery from apparently mild CHI.

Severe migraine headaches or balance disorder may also emerge out of PCS and produce lasting symptoms. Headache is reported by large numbers of patients with PPCS. Two mechanisms of headache are common. First, many patients with mild CHI suffer whiplash or other injuries to the neck. The free movement of the cervical spine may absorb much of the inertial force in deceleration. Soft tissue damage is generated that may produce muscle spasm and disruption of normal muscular and ligamentous architectures of the neck. It is exceedingly difficult to rest the cervical muscles because of their antigravity role. Injuries are susceptible to inadvertent aggravation during sleep. In addition to the orthopedic injury and pain, the chronic cervical pain is a potent trigger of migraine. The second cause of headache after mild CHI is, of course, migraine. Many patients first experience migraine after mild CHI. Classic migraine is uncommon. Chronic daily headache without associated focal neurological or ophthalmological symptoms is more common. In our study of patients with PPCS compared to patients with severe TBI, chronic daily headache was significantly more frequent in the mild cases [150]. Headache is usually considered a symptom of PCS, but it is likely to be a cause of PPCS.

Psychological Injury As noted above, patients with PPCS complain of fatigue and irritability. They also frequently endorse symptoms of depression and anxiety [147]. Investigation of factors that might predict PPCS have been identified: "older age, female gender, low socioeconomic class, ineffective coping style, poor social support network, low social competence, low self esteem, and negative labelling of stressful or ambiguous events" [151]. Because of significant early neurological deficits or peripheral problems, many patients with mild CHI are out of work and unable to participate in their usual recreations. They may face legal or financial problems. They may be at home in an unaccustomed role or attempting to return to work when they are incapacitated. They have had their "few days rest." To their families and even their doctors they appear well. In all probability, no one has performed an examination of attention or learning efficiency. They are taking analgesics, possibly ones with opiates that further blunt attention.

They believe that they have rested their aching necks because they have not gone to work, but they spend the day straightening up the house or helping out by doing errands. They appear well to family, friends, teachers, and co-workers. If they have returned to work (out of necessity or at the doctor's urging), they realize how marginal their performance might be and how much energy even simple activities require, but no one else does. In the evening, they may be exhausted, only to have families expect them to be helpful because, after all, they had their "few days rest." That psychological factors emerge in these patients should not be surprising. That psychological factors emerge more commonly in the postacute phase of mild CHI than severe has two explanations. First, patients with mild cases remember much more of the injury circumstances. Second, during the interval of resolution of symptoms, patients with severe cases are hospitalized, in rehabilitation, and followed in established and very supportive programs; patients with mild cases are at home getting "a few days rest." By the time that symptoms and signs of the neural injury are resolving, the patient may be out of work, angry, depressed, and in daily pain. It seems, in our experience, that these patients often feel least recovered about the time that they have recovered.

Depression is the most common psychiatric diagnosis. Anxiety and even posttraumatic stress disorder are sometimes seen [147]. Patients will meet DSM-III-R criteria for major depressive episode or dysthymic disorder, although "organic" exclusions, must be ignored. As with headaches, the symptoms of depression or anxiety are often considered symptoms of PCS. In patients with PPCS, depression or anxiety may be the cause. Depression alone may have marked detrimental effect on cognitive functions [152].

There are occasional patients who appear to be malingering. Three patterns of malingering have been described. There are patients with some "crippling" peripheral problem: migraine and neck pain, typically, who are nevertheless able to dance, garden, and cavort when not being observed by physicians. The second pattern is a picture of crippling neural problems: profound memory loss and severe inattention, a virtual dementia. This pseudodementia may even worsen with time. The third pattern is "classical" nonphysiological neurological signs: nonphysiological weakness, tunnel vision, pseudoseizure, and others. Any of these patterns of frank malingering are, in our experiences, uncommon.

The critical clinical message is that PPCS does not mean neural damage. The same symptoms are common in patients with chronic migraine [152], with depression [153], with anxiety [154], and with normal stresses in life [149].

Treatment Strategies   Management of mild CHI is a mixture of symptomatic treatment, psychological treatment, education, and social work. Patients must be given a reasonable time-frame for recovery, from days for the mildest "dings" to weeks for an uncomplicated brief LOC to months for a LOC of minutes. All of these time frames must be increased for patients of increasing age. They must also be given sensible advice about restriction of activities and demands. This advice may differ for patients with different life requirements. For example, a concussed neurosurgeon may be aware of problems and of fatigue for a very long time [155] and may respond to that demanding life much differently than someone in a less demanding role. During the period of recovery, impaired attention may leave a patient at increased risk for a second injury. Driving, use of equipment, dangerous recreations, and other activities should be reviewed. Employers, schools, and families should allow sufficient time before expecting recovery. It is probably the physician's role to clarify this need.

Patients need some education about premorbid habits that may prolong symptoms: inadequate rest, overloaded schedules, excessive caffeine intake, use of alcohol, as examples. Any disruption of schedules may precipitate a crisis (unrelated directly to the injury) that had previously been controlled: financial problems, absence of family support, and other events. These crises cannot be helped by prescribing amitriptyline. The inevitable sleep disorders should be reviewed. Careful sleep hygiene, analgesics, or temporary use of hypnotics may control the problem.

Aggressive treatment of acute cervical soft tissue injury with rest, cervical pillows, and intensive physical therapy should be instituted. Management of headache is fundamentally similar to management of any migraine patient. It is not known yet if the new generation of serotonin receptor-specific agents will have any special usefulness in post-traumatic headache, but there is no reason to doubt that they will be equally useful in cases with CHI. Recovery of vestibular symptoms may be improved with habituation exercises. There is no need to treat depression directly in PCS. Anxiety and insomnia may, however, benefit from temporary symptomatic treatment. Management of these traditional medical domains obviously requires accurate differential diagnosis of the severity of neural injury and the exact nature of peripheral injuries. It also requires an understanding of the complex psychosocial difficulties that simple "medical" treatment will not resolve.

OUTCOME

Predicting outcome after TBI is a seemingly daunting task. The heterogeneity of TBI and the multiplicity of interacting factors that affect recovery impede straightforward prognostication and study. A number of predictor variables and outcome criteria are typically used in clinical investigations. Other critical factors in understanding outcome are the study population and the timing of predictor and outcome measures. Study samples drawn from a hospitalized neurosurgical population, for instance, may provide enormously different information than one drawn from a postacute rehabilitation facility [156]. Regarding timing, a GCS at the scene of an accident may have completely different implications than GCS postresuscitation, hours later; Glasgow Outcome Scale (GOS) scores at 6 months may underestimate longer-term outcome levels in patients with more severe injuries.

Outcome Measures

There are generally three types of outcome criteria: mortality or survival, measures of neuropsychological functions, and measures of functional outcome, either global or in specific areas of social functioning and disability. We will not consider mortality.

Neuropsychological Outcome

Neuropsychological evaluation has been discussed earlier in this chapter. Most outcome studies use batteries of tests across various neuropsychological domains. In general, tests of attention, memory, and various levels of information processing yield the most information, since these show the greatest impairments over the longer term [107]. Outcome based on neuropsychological measures may vary drastically based on the particular measures and injury severity. Dikmen and colleagues [44] reported improvements in all neuropsychological measures in the first year but improvements in only some measures and only in the more severely injured patients in the second year postinjury. Mandelberg [106] observed that WAIS verbal IQ scores plateaued 5 months post injury whereas performance scores did not plateau until 13 months post injury. We have reviewed the specific results of more focused assessments in this chapter. Well-constructed neuropsychological testing best captures the residual neurological deficits, but the neuropsychological measures are, themselves, only, at best, indirectly related to functional outcome.

Functional Outcome

Global Measures   The GOS is the most widely used global social adaptation measure [157]. Its five levels gauge level of dependency and return to previous activities (Table 11). Death and vegetative state are the lowest levels. Severe disability implies dependence on another person for some or all of a 24 hr period; moderate disability indicates some reduced capacity but ability to function independently, for instance, at a level commensurate with riding public transportation; good recovery implies return to near premorbid capacity but some impairments may remain. Outcome categories are broad; the GOS sacrifices specificity for good reliability.

Other commonly used global outcome/disability measures in TBI include the Disability Rating Scale [158] and the Functional Independence Measure (FIM) [159]. The latter is in increasing use in rehabilitation facilities and was developed to create a uniform data collection system for medical rehabilitation.

Vocational Outcome   Return to work is a frequently used social outcome measure. Gradations include proportion of full-time work and occupational level compared to premorbid functioning.

A number of factors, preinjury, injury, and postinjury, are important in predicting vocational outcome [160,161]. Of preinjury factors, age and pre-

Table 11   Glasgow Outcome Scale

Classification	Clinical Findings
Good recovery	Return to premorbid capacities but may have minor residuae
Moderate disability	Largely independent at home and in community, but disabled
Severe disability	Dependent on others for all or some of a 24 hr period
Vegetative state	Unresponsive with gross wakefulness
Death	

Source: From ref. [157].

vious occupational level seem most important. Probability of return to work diminishes considerably after age 40 probably because of both worse recovery and social factors [160,162]. Those with higher-level occupations premorbidly had a better chance of returning to work in one study [160].

Severity of injury as measured by criteria such as duration of coma or PTA predicts return to work, however, certain psychosocial consequences are even more predictive [160]. Cognitive functioning, in particular verbal memory [107,160] and speed of information processing [160], are also very important predictive variables. Behavioral and emotional problems, identified in one study as deficits in "personal hygiene," "taking responsibility," "control of anger," and mood disorders, are also important predictors of successful employment [160].

Predictor Variables

Outcome measures are only meaningful when applied to a specific population sample or when related to certain predictor variables. The number of potential variables is huge, and some contribute more weight than others. Furthermore, interactions are unpredictable but surely important. Again, sample population and time postinjury make a difference; injury factors, for instance, become less and less important with increasing time after injury.

Acute Indices

In an acute neurosurgical population, several early injury and demographic variables have been consistently important. GCS score (Table 5) or GCS motor score alone, pupillary abnormalities, and age are always among the best predictors [163–166]. These three variables may account for up to 83% of the variance in predicting mortality [163].

Severely increased intracranial pressure (ICP) and hypotension are other important early predictors. Marmarou and colleagues [166] found that severely elevated intracranial pressure (ICP) (>20 mm) and hypotension (<80 mm) taken with the 3 variables above, predicted 53% of the variance of global outcome using the GOS. In contrast, Levin and co-workers [107,167], looking at a group selected from the same patient population and screened for "testability," found no significant effect of elevated ICP on neuropsychological measures and GOS 1 year postinjury. This may indicate that the elevated ICP is not an absolute marker of severe secondary brain damage. Increased ICP may have very deleterious effects (mortality or severe reductions of mental capacity) or few effects.

Age

Among factors not directly related to injury, age is the most important predictor of outcome. Older patients with TBI have higher mortality and morbidity following head injury, and this is not a simple matter of a greater frequency of premorbid or postmorbid nonneurological systemic disorders in older patients [168]. Injuries in older patients are more likely to be caused by falls and pedestrian accidents rather than passenger motor vehicle accidents [168–170]. The elderly are more prone to SDH and hemorrhage associated with FCC, and hemorrhages tend to be larger [168,169,171]. Recovery tends to be slower in older patients, with notably slower resolution of PTA and confusion [43,169]. Overall outcome is worse in older survivors [162,168,169, 172]. Whether the effect on recovery is continuous or more marked at certain ages is not known. Greater risk of mortality, prolongation of confusion, and worsening of outcome has been noted by the 5th decade by several investigators [55,163,168,169]. In a series of 661 patients from the Traumatic Coma Data Bank with severe injuries (GCS 8 or less), only 4% of patients over 45 made a good recovery by 6 months postinjury whereas 29% of those 45 or less achieved a good recovery [168]. In a series of 244 patients from a rehabilitation population, no patients over 40, comatose more than 1 hr, achieved a good recovery at 1 year although almost 50% of those under 20 made a good recovery [169]. The effect of age on recovery has clear implications for rehabilitation. Treatment planning should account for longer periods of confusion and higher levels of dependency expected in an older population.

Neuropathological Variables

The clinicopathological model provided throughout this chapter can serve as a framework to conceptualize prognosis and outcome. Few studies frame outcome directly according to neuropathological variables, but important information in this regard can be derived from existing studies.

Focal Pathology   As previously discussed, location, size of lesion, and secondary problems from mass effect are the main issues determining outcome from focal pathology (see Figs. 1–4). The specific effects of focal pathology on outcome are difficult to study in large groups of patients with TBI because important fine clinical distinctions based on anatomical location are lost in large group studies and these effects are often embedded in clinical phenomena associated with diffuse pathology. A few relatively specific effects of location of focal lesions have been demonstrated, such as verbal versus nonverbal problems and the side of lesion [173] or differentially worse memory impairments in patients with focal temporal lobe lesions [42]. Existing studies of focal lesions generally consider only their contribution as mass lesions, and extracerebral and intracerebral lesions may be lumped together.

Any attempt to capture the specific effects of focal lesions on outcome are most likely to be successful if it keeps clear the lesions' characteristics (location, depth, etc.) and the natural history of associated clinical syndromes.

Recovery from TBI focal lesions will resemble focal lesions of other acute causes, and information from stroke populations may serve as a model. There are several general observations. Recovery from focal lesions tends to evolve more rapidly and reach an earlier plateau than severe diffuse pathology. Bilateral focal lesions in homologous areas produce more profound lasting effects than unilateral lesions. Small differences in location and particularly depth of lesion can make an enormous difference in syndrome characteristics and prognosis.

Diffuse Pathology   Depth and duration of coma and duration of PTA, markers of the early course of diffuse pathology, serve as important predictors of outcome. Most outcome studies do not differentiate other causes of coma such as brainstem compression from focal mass lesions; however, diffuse pathology is the cause of immediate coma in the vast majority of cases. A recent report of patients from the Traumatic Coma Data Bank did identify patients with diffuse injury based on neuroimaging criteria. Extrapolating from their data, they found 40% dead or vegetative, 31% severely disabled, and 29% with moderate disability or good recovery at the time of discharge [174]. Signs of cerebral swelling or shift (without focal lesion) on CT scan worsened the prognosis.

GCS scores in the first few hours or days are clearly related to outcome. Outcome is much worse with GCS scores below 6. Of patients from the Traumatic Coma Data Bank with GCS scores less than 6, 16% had good recoveries or moderate disability at last follow-up and of those with GCS scores of 6–8, 63% achieved a good recovery or moderate disability [174]. Similar findings were noted from the International Coma Data Bank Study; only 11% of those patients with a best score of 5 achieved a good recovery or moderate disability and 97% with a best score of 4 died or remained vegetative [175].

Coma duration also strongly relates to outcome. Carlsson and co-workers [172], using verbal responsiveness as the endpoint of coma, found an almost linear relationship between coma duration and recovery time. Prognosis was closely related to duration of coma in patients with CT patterns consistent with DAI without focal lesions [39]. In our experience with 119 consecutive patients with DAI admitted to a rehabilitation facility (thus, only survivors), outcomes were proportionally worse at 1 year with increasingly longer coma (measured by first ability to follow commands) [45]. Of those comatose 1 day to 1 week, 58% had a good recovery and 37% were moderately disabled; no patient comatose over 2 weeks achieved a good recovery and 62% of those comatose more than a month were severely disabled (Fig. 8).

Duration of PTA probably has an even stronger relationship with outcome. Of patients collected from an acute neurosurgical population by the International Coma Data Bank, there were 83% with good recovery and none

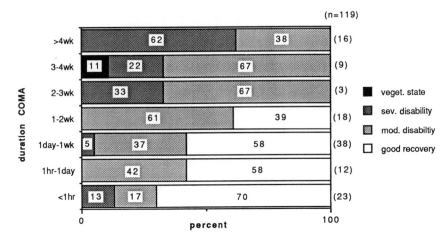

Figure 8 Glasgow outcome scores 1 year after injury at various coma durations in patients with DAI (numbers on bars are percentages; total number of patients in groups are in parentheses) (from ref. [45]; reproduced with permission).

with severe disability among those with PTA less than 2 weeks; in those with PTA exceeding 1 month, 27% had a good recovery and 30% were left with severe disability [175,176]. In a series of 114 patients with DAI admitted to a rehabilitation facility, PTA of less than 2 weeks was compatible with 80% good recovery and 13% moderate disability and PTA between 4 and 8 weeks with 46% good recovery and 54% moderate disability. None with PTA exceeding 12 weeks achieved a good recovery [45] (Fig. 9).

Mild Diffuse Injury   For mild TBI, overall outcome is generally good, but within the narrow range of clinical measures (LOC, PTA, etc.) there is no correlation with outcome. The weakness of this correlation is probably due to two factors. First, the measurement of small differences in LOC or even PTA is probably not reliable. Even if it could be clearly established that PTA lasted 31 min or 17 min, both would likely be called less than an hour. Would it matter if such differences could be measured? Second, the important factors in functional outcome at 3–6 months after injury are only partially (and, with the progress of time, probably vanishingly) the neural ones. They are, instead, the peripheral and psychological ones. The overall sense of the literature is that fewer than 20% of patients have anything less than good outcome at 1 year. In those cases, there will be a few with underestimated injury and a large number with headaches, depression, and anxiety.

Combination of Pathology   Combinations of different types of pathological damage are the rule rather than the exception. Outcome is more difficult to

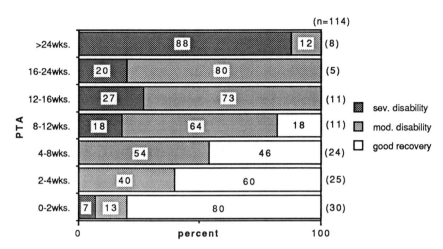

Figure 9   Glasgow outcome scores at 1 year after injury at various PTA durations in patients with DAI (numbers on bars are percentages; total number of patients in groups are in parentheses) (from ref. [45]; reproduced with permission).

predict. Early, global outcome will usually be related to the severity of diffuse injury, and specific problems secondary to focal lesions will be observed among signs attributable to the evolving course of diffuse pathology. Consider a specific example: patients with traumatic basal ganglia area hemorrhages (TBGH). Overall outcome is related to the severity of DAI not simply the TBGH, but the individual disturbances in motor or language functions depend on the specific anatomical distribution of the TBGH [9].

As already discussed, the addition of diffuse HII significantly worsens prognosis. Looking at patterns of recovery of verbal learning, Ruff and colleagues [101] noted that a subgroup with a flat recovery curve had disproportionately more patients with hypoxia. If the same markers of acute severity are used for diffuse HII and DAI, apparently equivalent measures have a much more ominous prognosis in patients with diffuse HII. When one examines recovery from purely diffuse HII, for instance, patients comatose over 1 week have virtually no chance of recovery better than severe disability [177], whereas the majority of patients with DAI comatose 1–4 weeks reach a moderate disability or good recovery [45].

Determining Prognosis in the Clinical Setting

There does not exist as yet any formula that allows reliable prediction of the outcome of any individual case, but there are group correlations that allow actuarial predictions. It is this level of probability that the neurorehabilitation clinician should bring to the assessment of the patient with TBI. Physicians should be comfortable with this type of knowledge and its conversion from groups (in which it is accurate) to individuals (for whom it may not be accurate). To say that a patient with stage IV adenocarcinoma of the lung has a 50% chance of surviving 6 months is clinically and personally helpful, even if the individual only happens to live 1 month or is still doing well 12 months later. It is unlikely that all of the heterogeneity of premorbid qualities and capacities, of neurological injury variables, of postinjury management, and of personal and social resources will ever be harnessed in a regression formula that predicts individuals' outcomes.

To establish the actuarial expectations for any patient requires that clinicians manipulate some fearsome mental algebra. Has there been DAI? If so, how severe? Has there been FCC or focal HII? If so, where and how severe? Can the effects be detected through the DAI? Was there diffuse HII? If so, was it severe enough to now dominate the whole clinical picture? What secondary or indirect brain injuries might have occurred—hydrocephalus, seizures, or others? What are the premorbid factors that will be important: age, work history, social history, prior injury? What are the comorbid factors that influence recovery: depression, chronic pain, family distress? In this review we have tried to outline the clinical steps taken in solving these problems even if no specific algebraic formula yet exists and may never exist. We have also attempted to demonstrate how the answers to these same questions produce the theory behind the rehabilitation and medical management of TBI.

REFERENCES

1. J.F. Kurtzke and L.T. Kurland, *Clinical Neurology* (A.B. Baker and R.J. Joynt, eds.), Harper & Row, Philadelphia, pp. 1–143 (1987).
2. J.F. Kraus, *Head Injury*, 2nd edition (P.R. Cooper, ed.), Williams & Wilkins, Baltimore, pp. 1–19 (1987).
3. C.B. Courville, *Pathology of the Central Nervous System*, Pacific, Mountain View, CA (1937).
4. D.I. Graham, J.H. Adams, and T.A. Gennarelli, *Head Injury* (P.R. Cooper, ed.), Williams & Wilkins, Baltimore, pp. 72–78 (1978).
5. A.H.S. Holbourn, *Br. Med. Bull.*, 3:147–149 (1945).
6. P.R. Cooper, *Head Injury*, 2nd edition (P.R. Cooper, ed.), Williams & Wilkins, Baltimore, pp. 238–284 (1987).
7. C. Rivano, M. Barzone, F. Carta, and G. Michelozzi, *J. Neurosurg. Sci.*, 24:77–84 (1980).
8. K.G. Jamieson and J.D.N. Yelland, *J. Neurosurg.*, 37:528–532 (1972).
9. D.I. Katz, M.P. Alexander, G.M. Seliger, and D.N. Bellas, *Neurology*, 39:897–904 (1989).

10. P. MacPherson, E. Teasdale, S. Dhaker, G. Allerdyce, and S. Galbraith, *J. Neurol. Neurosurg. Psychiatry*, 49:29–34 (1986).

11. F. Plum and J.B. Posner, *The Diagnosis of Stupor and Coma*, F.A. Davis, Philadelphia (1980).

12. J.H. Adams, D.I. Graham, L.S. Murray, and G. Scott, *Ann. Neurol.*, 12:557–563 (1982).

13. J.H. Adams, D.I. Graham, T.A. Gennarelli, and W.L. Maxwell, *J. Neurol. Neurosurg. Psychiatry*, 54:481–483 (1991).

14. L. Levi, J.N. Guilburd, A. Lemberger, J.F. Soustie, and M. Feinsod, *Neurosurgery*, 27:429–432 (1990).

15. D.C. Viano, General Motors Research Laboratories, GMR4989R (1985).

16. D.C. Viano, Society of Automotive Engineers, Warrendale, Pennsylvania (1988).

17. D.C. Viano, General Motors Research Laboraties Publication, Warren, Michigan, GMR 6885 (1989).

18. T.A. Gennarelli, L.E. Thibault, J.H. Adams, D.I. Graham, C.J. Thompson, and R.P. Marcincin, *Ann. Neurol.*, 12:564–574 (1982).

19. T.A. Gennarelli, *J. Head Trauma Rehab.*, 1:23–29 (1986).

20. S.J. Strich, *J. Neurol. Neurosurg. Psychiatry*, 19:163–185 (1956).

21. S.J. Strich, *J. Clin. Pathol.*, 23 (Suppl 4):154–165 (1970).

22. L. Rinder, *Acta Physiol. Scand.*, 76:352–361 (1969).

23. J.T. Povlishock, D.P. Becker, J.D. Miller, L.W. Jenkins, and W.D. Dietrich, *Acta Neuropathol*, 47:1–12 (1979).

24. J.T. Povlishock, D.P. Becker, C.C.Y. Cheng, and G.W. Vanghan, *J. Neuropathol. Exp. Neurol.*, 42:225–242 (1983).

25. J.T. Povlishock and T.H. Coburn, *Mild Head Injury* (H.S. Levin, H.M. Eisenberg, and A.L. Benton, eds.), Oxford University Press, New York, pp. 37–53 (1989).

26. J. Povlishock and D. Becker, *Lab. Invest.*, 52:540–552 (1985).

27. J. Povlishock, *Acta Neuropathol*, 70:53–79 (1986).

28. A.K. Ommaya and T.A. Gennarelli, *Brain*, 97:633–654 (1974).

29. J. Povlishock, *Central Nervous System Status Report* (D. Becker and J. Povlishock, eds.), Byrd Press, Richmond, pp. 443–452 (1985).

30. P.C. Blumbergs, N.R. Jones, and J.B. North, *J. Neurol. Neurosurg. Psychiatry*, 52:838–841 (1989).

31. J.E. Wilberger, W.E. Rothfus, J. Tabas, A.L. Goldberg, and Z.L. Deeb, *Neurosurgery*, 27:208–213 (1990).

32. R.A. Clasen and R.D. Penn, *Head Injury* (P.R. Cooper, ed.), Williams & Wilkins, Baltimore, pp. 285–312 (1987).

33. R.L. Hayes, H.H. Stonnington, B.G. Lyeth, C.F. Dixon, and T. Yamamoto, *J. Cent. Nerv. Syst. Trauma*, 3:163–173 (1986).

34. R.L. Hayes, L.W. Jenkins, and B.G. Lyeth, *J. Head Trauma Rehab.*, 7:16–28 (1992).

35. L.W. Jenkins, W. Lewett, K. Moszynski, B.G. Lyeth, R.L. Hayes, D.S. DeWitt, S.E. Robinson, A. Allen, J. Opoka, A. Marmarou, and H.F. Young, *Soc. Neurosci. Abstr.*, 13:153 (1987).

36. L.W. Jenkins, B.G. Lyeth, W. Lewell, K. Moszynski, D.S. DeWitt, S.E. Robinson, A. Allen, J. Opoka, A. Marmarou, and H.F. Young, *J. Neurotrauma*, 5:275–287 (1988).

37. E.D. Hall, P.A. Yonkers, J.M. McCall, and J.M. Brauchler, *J. Neurosurg.*, 68: 456–461 (1988).

38. S.E. Karpiak, Y.S. Li, and S.P. Mahadik, *Brain Inj.*, 1:161–170 (1987).

39. R.D. Lobato, F. Cordobes, J.J. Rivas, M. De la Fuente, A. Montero, A. Barcena, C. Perez, A. Cabrera, and E. Lamasa, *J. Neurosurg.*, 59:762–744 (1983).

40. L.F. Marshall, S.B. Marshall, M.R. Klauber, et al., *Neurosurgery*, 75 (Suppl):14–17 (1991).

41. H.S. Levin, C.A. Meyers, R.G. Grossman, M. Sarwar, *Arch. Neurol.*, 38:623–629 (1981).

42. H.S. Levin, A.L. Benton, and R.G. Grossman, *Neurobehavioral Consequences of Closed Head Injury*, Oxford University Press, New York (1982).

43. W.R. Russell and A. Smith, *Arch. Neurol.*, 5:4–17 (1961).

44. S.S. Dikmen, J. Machamer, N. Temkin, and A. McLean, *J. Clin. Exp. Neuropsychol.*, 12:507–517 (1990).

45. D.I. Katz, *J. Head Trauma Rehab.*, 7:1–15 (1992).

46. D.R. Oppenheimer, *J. Neurol. Neurosurg. Psychiatry*, 31:299–306 (1968).

47. D.I. Graham, J.H. Adams, and D. Doyle, *J. Neurosci.*, 39:213–234 (1979).

48. H.S. Levin, C.A. Meyers, R.G. Grossman, and M. Sarwar, *Arch. Neurol.*, 38: 623–629 (1981).

49. P.R. Kishore, M.H. Lipper, J.D. Miller, A.K. Girevendulis, D.P. Becker, and F.S. Vines, *Neuroradiology*, 16:261–265 (1978).

50. C.M. Fischer, *Lancet*, 7:37 (1978).

51. C. Wikkelso, H. Andersson, C. Bloomstrand, et al., *Acta Neurol. Scand.*, 73: 566–573 (1986).

52. W.G. Bradley, A.R. Whittenmore, K.E. Kortman, et al., *Radiology*, 178:459–466 (1991).

53. B. Beyerl and P.M. Black, *Neurosurgery*, 15:257–261 (1984).

54. G.M. Seliger, D.I. Katz, M. Seliger, and M. DiTullio, *Brain Inj.*, 6:71–73 (1992).

55. B. Jennett and G. Teasdale, *Management of Head Injuries*, F.A. Davis, Philadelphia (1981).

56. J.F. Annegers, J.D. Grabow, R.V. Groover, E.R. Laws, L.R. Elveback, and L.T. Kurland, *Neurology*, 30:683–689 (1980).

57. K.J. Meador, D.W. Loring, K. Huh, B.B. Gallagher, and D.W. King, *Neurology*, 40:391–394 (1990).

58. R. Gallassi, A. Morreale, S. Lorusso, G. Procaccianti, E. Lugaresi, and A. Baruzzi, *Arch. Neurol.*, 45:892–894 (1988).

59. J.S. Duncan, S.D. Shorvon, and M.R. Trimble, *Epilepsia*, 31:584–591 (1990).

60. S.S. Dikmen, N.R. Temkin, B. Miller, J. Machamer, and H.R. Winn, *JAMA*, 265:1271–1277 (1991).

61. N.R. Temkin, S.S. Dikmen, A.J. Wilensky, J. Keihm, S. Chabal, and H.R. Winn, *N. Engl. J. Med.*, 323:497–502 (1990).

62. B. Young, R.P. Rapp, J.A. Norton, D. Haack, P.A. Tibbs, and J.R. Bean, *J. Neurosurg.*, *58*:236–241 (1983).
63. M.M. Mesulum, *Principles of Behavioral Neurology* (M.M. Mesulum, ed.), F.A. Davis, Philadelphia, pp. 1–70 (1985).
64. M.P. Alexander, D.F. Benson, and D.T. Stuss, *Brain Lang.*, 37:656–691 (1989).
65. N. Butters, *Human Neuropsychology* (K.M. Heilman and E. Valenstein, eds.), Oxford University Press, New York, pp. 439–474 (1979).
66. D.Y. von Cramon, N. Hebel, and V. Schuri, *Brain*, *111*:1061–1077 (1988).
67. E. DeRenzi, A. Zambolin, and G. Crisi, *Brain*, *110*:1099–1116 (1987).
68. J.M. Fuster, The Prefrontal Cortex: Anatomy, Physiology and Neuropsychology of the Frontal Lobes, Raven Press, New York (1989).
69. D.T. Stuss and D.F. Benson, *The Frontal Lobes*, Raven Press, New York (1986).
70. D.T. Stuss, *Neurobehavioral Recovery from Head Injury* (H.S. Levin, J. Grafman, and H.M. Eisenberg, eds.), Oxford University Press, New York, pp. 166–177 (1987).
71. D.T. Stuss, *Awareness of Deficit After Brain Injury* (G.P. Prigatano and D.L. Schacter, eds.), Oxford University Press, New York, pp. 63–83 (1991).
72. D.T. Stuss, M.P. Alexander, A. Lieberman, and H. Levine, *Neurology*, *28*: 1166–1172 (1978).
73. J. Cummings, *Br. J. Psychiatry*, *146*:184–197 (1985).
74. W.A. Lishman, *Organic Psychiatry: The Psychological Consequences of Cerebral Disorder*, Blackwell Scientific Publications, Oxford (1978).
75. G.P. Prigatano, K.P. O'Brien, and P.S. Klonoff, *J. Head Trauma Rehab.*, 3:23–32 (1988).
76. A. Wirsen, Chronic Effects of Traumatic Frontal Lesions: Clinical, Neuropsychological and Neurophysiological Aspects, University of Lund, Lund, Sweden (1991).
77. H. Kluver and P.C. Bucy, *Arch. Neurol. Psychiatry*, *42*:979–1000 (1939).
78. R. Lilly, J.L. Cummings, F. Benson, and M. Frankel, *Neurology*, 33:1141–1145 (1983).
79. S. Finger and D. Stein. *Brain Damage and Recovery: Research and Clinical Perspectives*, Academic Press, New York (1982).
80. A. Kertesz, *Aphasia and Associated Disorders*, Grune & Stratton, New York (1979).
81. H. Goodglass and E. Kaplan, *The Assessment of Aphasia and Related Disorders*, Lea & Febiger, Philadelphia (1972).
82. D. Wechsler, *Wechsler Adult Intelligence Scale*, Psychological Corporation, New York (1955).
83. E.A. Berg, *J. Gen. Psychol.*, *39*:15–22 (1948).
84. J.R. Stroop, *J. Exp. Psychol.*, *18*:643–662 (1935).
85. T. Shallice and P.W. Burges, *Brain*, *114*:727–741 (1991).
86. E.L. Glisky, D.L. Schacter, and E. Tulving, *Neuropsychologia*, *24*:313–328 (1986).
87. C. Hagen, D. Malkmus, and P. Durham, *Levels of Cognitive Functioning*, Ranchos Los Amigos Hospital, Downey, CA (1972).

88. M.P. Alexander, *Psychiatric Aspects of Neurologic Disease* (D.F. Benson and D. Blumer, eds.), McGraw-Hill, New York, pp. 251–278 (1982).

89. B. Jennett and G. Teasdale, *Lancet*, 1:878–881 (1977).

90. A. Bricolo, S. Turazzi, and G. Feriotti, *J. Neurosurg.*, 52:625–634 (1980).

91. W.M. High, H.S. Levin, and H.E. Gary, *J. Clin. Exp. Neuropsychol.*, 12:703–714 (1990).

92. S.L. Levin, V.M. O'Donnell, and R.G. Grossman, *J. Nerv. Ment. Dis.*, 167: 675–684 (1979).

93. C.T. Gualtieri and R. W. Evans, *Brain Inj.*, 2:273–290 (1988).

94. A.H. Van Zomeren and B.G. Deelman, *J. Neurol. Neurosurg. Psychiatry*, 41: 452–457 (1978).

95. D. Gronwall and P. Wrightson, *J. Neurol. Neurosurg. Psychiatry*, 44:889–895 (1981).

96. D.T. Stuss, P. Ely, H. Hugenholtz, M.T. Richard, S. LaRochelle, C.A. Poirier, and I. Bell, *Neurosurgery*, 17:41–47 (1985).

97. D.T. Stuss, L.L. Stethem, H. Hugenholtz, T.W. Picton, J. Pivik, and M.T. Richard, *J. Neurol. Neurosurg. Psychiatry*, 52:742–748 (1989).

98. M. Oddy, T. Coughlan, A. Tyerman, and D. Jenkins, *J. Neurol. Neurosurg. Psychiatry*, 48:564–568 (1985).

99. H.S. Levin, *J. Clin. Exp. Neuropsychol.*, 12:129–153 (1989).

100. H.S. Levin, F.C. Goldstein, W.M. High, and H.M. Eisenberg, *J. Neurol. Neurosurg. Psychiatry*, 51:1294–1301 (1988).

101. R.M. Ruff, D. Young, T. Gautille, L.F. Marshall, et al., *J. Neurosurg.*, 75 (suppl):50–58 (1991).

102. H.S. Levin, F.C. Goldstein, W.M. High, and D. Williams, *Brain Cognitions*, 7: 283–297 (1988).

103. J. Ewart, H.S. Levin, M.G. Watson, and Z. Kalisky, *Arch. Neurol.*, 46:911–916 (1989).

104. B.A. Wilson, A.D. Baddeley, and J.M. Cockburn, *Cortex*, 25:115–119 (1989).

105. H.S. Levin, R.G. Grossman, J.E. Rose, and G. Teasdale, *J. Neurosurg.*, 50: 412–422 (1979).

106. I.A. Mandelberg, *J. Neurol. Neurosurg. Psychiatry*, 39:1001–1007 (1976).

107. H.S. Levin, H.E. Gary, and H.M. Eisenberg, *J. Neurosurg.*, 73:699–709 (1990).

108. D.T. Stuss and L. Buckle, *J. Head Trauma Rehab.*, 7:40–49 (1992).

109. M.T. Sarno, *J. Nerv. Ment. Dis.*, 168:685–692 (1980).

110. H.S. Levin, R.G. Grossman, and P.J. Kelly, *J. Neurol. Neurosurg. Psychiatry*, 39:1062–1070 (1976).

111. M.M. Sohlberg and C.A. Mateer, *J. Clin. Exp. Neuropsychol.*, 9:117–130 (1987).

112. G.P. Prigatano, D.J. Fordyce, H.J. Zeiner, J.R. Roueche, M. Pepping, and B.C. Wood, *J. Neurol. Neurosurg. Psychiatry*, 47:505–513 (1984).

113. V.M. Mills, T. Nesbeda, D.I. Katz, and M.P. Alexander, *Brain Inj.*, 6:219–228 (1992).

114. R.M. Ruff, C.A. Baser, J.W. Johnston, L.F. Marshall, et al., *J. Head Trauma Rehab.*, 4:20–36 (1989).

115. R.A. Bornstein, H.B. Miller, and J.T. Van Schoor, *J. Neurosurg.*, 70:509–513 (1989).
116. P. Eames, *J. Head Trauma Rehab.*, 3:1–6 (1988).
117. H.S. Levin and R.G. Grossman, *Arch. Neurol.*, 35:720–727 (1978).
118. G.P. Prigatano, *Neurobehavioral Recovery from Head Injury* (H.S. Levin, J. Grafman, and H.M. Eisenberg, eds.), Oxford University Press, New York, pp. 215–231 (1987).
119. M. Bond, *Closed Head Injury: Psychological, Social and Family Consequences* (N. Brooks, ed.), Oxford University Press, Oxford, pp. 148–178 (1984).
120. R.G. Robinson and Szetela, *Ann. Neurol.*, 9:447–453 (1980).
121. R.G. Robinson, J.D. Boston, S.E. Starkstein, and T.R. Price, *Am. J. Psychiatry*, 145:172–178 (1988).
122. C.T. Gualtieri, *Brain Inj.*, 2:101–129 (1988).
123. P. Eames and R. Wood, *J. Neurol. Neurosurg. Psychiatry*, 48:613–619 (1984).
124. M. Oddy, M. Humphrey, and D. Uttley, *Neurol. Neurosurg. Psychiatry*, 41: 611–616 (1978).
125. M. Oddy, M. Humphrey, and D. Uttley, *Br. J. Psychiatry*, 133:507–513 (1978).
126. M.G. Livingston, D.N. Brooks, and M.R. Bond, *J. Neurol. Neurosurg. Psychiatry*, 48:870–875 (1985).
127. M.G. Livingston, D.N. Brooks, and M.R. Bond, *J. Neurol. Neurosurg. Psychiatry*, 48:876–881 (1985).
128. D.N. Brooks, L. Campsie, C. Symington, A. Beattie, and W. McKinlay, *Head Trauma Rehab.*, 2:1–13 (1987).
129. W.W. McKinlay, D.N. Brooks, M.R. Bond, D.P. Martinage, and M.M. Marshall, *J. Neurol. Neurosurg. Psychiatry*, 44:527–533 (1981).
130. A. Shumway-Cook and R. Olmscheid, *Head Trauma Rehab.*, 5:51–62 (1990).
131. W.C. Koller, G.F. Wong, and A. Lang, *Mov. Disord.*, 4:20–36 (1989).
132. D.I. Katz, *J. Head Trauma Rehab.*, 5:86–90 (1990).
133. J. Jankovic and M.F. Brin, *N. Engl. J. Med.*, 324:1186–1194 (1991).
134. B.J. Snow, J.K.C. Tsui, M.H. Bhatt, et al., *Ann. Neurol.*, 28:512–515 (1990).
135. R.D. Penn, S.M. Savoy, D. Corcus, M. Latashi, G. Gottlieb, B. Parke, and J.S. Kroin, *N. Engl. J. Med.*, 320:1517–1521 (1989).
136. R.R. Young and B.J. Delwaide, *N. Engl. J. Med.*, 304:28 (1981).
137. R.L. Waters, J. Frazier, D. Garland, C. Jordan, and J. Perry, *J. Bone Joint Surg.*, 64A:284–288 (1982).
138. K.M. Yorkston, M.J. Honsinger, P.M. Mitsuda, and V. Hammen, *J. Head Trauma Rehab.*, 4:1–16 (1989).
139. J.A. Logemann, *Head Trauma Rehab.*, 4:24–33 (1989).
140. R.L. Hayes, B.G. Lyeth, and L.W. Jenkins, *Mild Head Injury* (H.S. Levin, H.M. Eisenberg, and A.L. Benton, eds.), Oxford University Press, New York, pp. 37–53 (1989).
141. D. Gronwall and P. Wrightson, *Lancet*, 2:605–609 (1974).
142. H.S. Levin, S. Mattis, R.M. Ruff, H.M. Eisenberg, et al., *J. Neurosurg.*, 66: 234–243 (1987).
143. American Congress of Rehabilitation Medicine, Mild Traumatic Brain Injury

and Committee, *Definition of Mild Traumatic Brain Injury*, Head Injury Interdisciplinary Special Interest Group Publications (1991).

144.　R.W. Rimel, B. Giordani, J.T. Barth, T.J. Boll, and J.A. Jane, *Neurosurgery, 9*: 221–228 (1981).

145.　J.T. Barth, W.M. Alves, T.V. Ryan, S.N. Macciocchi, R.W. Rimel, J.A. Jane, and W.E. Nelson, *Mild Head Injury* (H.S. Levin, H.M. Eisenberg, and A.L. Benton, eds.), Oxford University Press, New York, pp. 257–275 (1989).

146.　M. Gentilini, P. Nichelli, and R. Schoenhuber, *Mild Head Injury* (H.S. Levin, H.M. Eisenberg, and A.L. Benton, eds.), Oxford University Press, New York, pp. 163–175 (1989).

147.　R. Schoenhuber and M. Gentilini, *J. Neurol. Neurosurg. Psychiatry, 51*:722–724 (1988).

148.　W.H. Rutherford, J.D. Merrett, and J.R. McDonald, *Injury, 10*:225–230 (1978).

149.　S. Dikmen, A. McLean, N. Temkin, and A. Wyler, *J. Neurol. Neurosurg. Psychiatry, 49*:1227–1232 (1986).

150.　M.P. Alexander, *J. Head Trauma Rehab., 7*:60–69 (1992).

151.　S.S. Dikmen, N. Temkin, and G. Armsden, *Mild Head Injury* (H.S. Levin, H.M. Eisenberg, and A.L. Benton, eds.), Oxford University Press, New York, pp. 229–241 (1989).

152.　F.D. Sheftell, *Neurology, 42* (suppl. 2):32–36 (1992).

153.　H. Weingartner, R.M. Cohen, D.L. Murphy, et al., *Arch. Gen. Psychiatry, 38*: 42–47 (1981).

154.　L.M. Binder, *J. Clin. Exp. Neuropsychol., 8*:323–346 (1986).

155.　L.F. Marshall and R.M. Ruff, *Mild Head Injury* (H.S. Levin, H.M. Eisenberg, and A.L. Benton, eds.), Oxford University Press, New York, pp. 276–280 (1989).

156.　S.S. Dikmen and N. Temkin, *Neurobehavioral Recovery from Head Injury* (H.S. Levin, J. Grafman, and H.M. Eisenberg, eds.), Oxford University Press, New York, pp. 191–205 (1987).

157.　B. Jennett and M. Bond, *Lancet, 1*:480–487 (1975).

158.　M. Rappaport, K.M. Hall, K. Hopkin, I. Bellaza, and D.N. Cope, *Arch. Phys. Med. Rehab., 63*:118–123 (1982).

159.　B.B. Hamilton, C.V. Granger, F.S. Sherwin, M. Zielezny, and J.S. Tashman, *Rehabilitation Outcomes: Analysis and Measurement* (M.S. Fuhrer, ed.), Paul H. Brooks Publishing, Baltimore, pp. 137–147 (1987).

160.　N. Brooks, W. McKinlay, C. Symington, A. Beattie, and L. Campsie, *Brain Inj., 1*:5–19 (1987).

161.　M. Oddy, *Closed Head Injury: Psychological, Social and Family Consequences* (N. Brooks, ed.), Oxford University Press, Oxford, pp. 108–122 (1984).

162.　O. Heiskanen and P. Sipponen, *Acta Neurol. Scand., 46*:343–348 (1970).

163.　R.K. Narayan, R.P. Greenberg, J.D. Miller, G.G. Engs, S.C. Choi, P.R.S. Kishore, and J.B. Selhorst, *J. Neurosurg., 54*:751–762 (1981).

164.　D.M. Stablein, J.D. Miller, S.C. Choi, and D.P. Becker, *Neurosurgery, 6*:243–248 (1980).

165.　R. Braakman, G.J. Gelpke, J.D.F. Habbema, A.I.P. Maas, and J.M. Minderhoud, *Neurosurgery, 6*:362–370 (1980).

166. A. Marmarou, R.L. Anderson, J.D. Ward, et al., *J. Neurosurg.*, 75 (suppl):59–66 (1991).
167. H.S. Levin, H.M. Eisenberg, H.E. Gary, et al., *Neurosurgery*, 28:196–200 (1991).
168. D.G. Vollmer, J.C. Torner, J.A. Jane, et al., *Neurosurgery*, 75 (suppl):37–49 (1991).
169. D.I. Katz, G.J. Kehs, and M.P. Alexander, *Neurology*, 40 (suppl):276 (1990).
170. A.L. Amacher and D.E. Bybee, *Neurosurgery*, 20:954–957 (1979).
171. B. Pentland, P.A. Jones, C.W. Roy, and J.D. Miller, *Age Aging*, 15:193–202 (1986).
172. C.A. Carlsson, C. von Essen, and J. Lofgren, *J. Neurosurg.*, 29:242–251 (1968).
173. B.P. Uzzell, R.A. Zimmerman, C.A. Dolinskas, and W.D. Obrist, *Cortex*, 15:391–401 (1979).
174. L.F. Marshall, T. Gautille, M.R. Klauber, et al., *Neurosurgery*, 75 (suppl):28–36 (1991).
175. B. Jennett, G. Teasdale, R. Braakman, J. Minderhand, J. Heiden, and T. Kurze, *Neurosurgery*, 4:283–289 (1979).
176. B. Jennett, G. Teasdale, R. Braakman, et al., *Lancet*, 1:1031–1034 (1976).
177. D.E. Levy, J.J. Caronna, B.H. Singer, R.H. Lapinski, H. Frydman, and F. Plum, *JAMA*, 253:1420–1426 (1985).
178. S.W. Atlas, A.S. Mark, R.I. Grossman, and J.M. Gomori, *Radiology*, 168:803–807 (1988).

21

Multiple Sclerosis

Randall T. Schapiro

Fairview Multiple Sclerosis Center and University of Minnesota
Minneapolis, Minnesota

Laurie Laven

National Rehabilitation Hospital
Washington, D.C.

INTRODUCTION

The physician who manages and directs the care of people with multiple sclerosis (MS) must comprehend that MS is a disease of diversity involving more than myelin and the immune system. It is, in fact, a disease of people. The rehabilitation of these people begins at the time of diagnosis. At the time of diagnosis patients are most vulnerable, frightened, and impulsive. Calm and education should prevail. When the clinician mentions the feared abbreviation, "MS," the patient may be unable to process further information, unable to think of anything except "when does the wheelchair come?"

One approach is initially to discuss what MS is in simple terms and provide educational materials, and then to set up a second educational session a week later. Topics to be covered during the second educational session include types of MS, management strategies, and epidemiology. It should be stressed that most patients with MS lead relatively normal lives, with over two-thirds ambulatory and one-third employed 25 years after diagnosis [1]. A physician who believes there is "nothing to be done" for a patient with MS should refer the patient to an MS specialist.

Patients should also be referred to a national MS organization for educational materials. A regular source of scientific information and a sensitive physician will help a patient deal with adversity and avoid becoming desperate to "try anything" [2]. Patients with MS are repeatedly victimized by glowing media reports of preliminary studies of treatments that ultimately prove useless. They are easy prey for advertised miracle cures such as chelation, nutritional supplements, and removal of dental fillings.

As in any neurorehabilitation program, a multidisciplinary team approach is critical in reducing MS-related handicaps such as physical, psychosocial, vocational, and recreational barriers. Some of the roles of team members will be referred to in this chapter, but the full roles of physical, occupational, recreational, and speech therapists; social workers; rehabilitation nurses, and neuropsychologists are beyond the scope of this chapter.

GENERAL HEALTH ISSUES

Introduction

All patients should understand the importance of a generally healthy life style for people with chronic disease. There is no scientific evidence that proper diet and exercise change the course of MS, but clearly a person who is trim and fit and develops a new motor deficit stands a greater chance of achieving independent mobility and activities of daily living (ADLs) than an obese patient with chronic obstructive pulmonary disease (COPD). The argument that smoking and eating are "the only pleasures left" must be rejected.

Exercise

Although muscle fatigue has been shown to increase with inactivity in patients with upper motor neuron dysfunction [3], studies of exercise in MS are rare. Aquatic exercise has been shown to reduce fatigue and increase strength, work, and power as measured by a dynamometer [4]. A safe protocol for cardiovascular testing and exercise prescription has been developed by the Jimmy Heuga Center [5], and patients exercising according to this protocol show modest improvement in work load achieved [6]. The patients exercise at 60–70% of maximum ability, avoiding increased body temperature and hyperventilation, for at least 20–30 min three times per week. A study of the effect of a long-term aerobic exercise program on fatigue and functional status is in progress.

Stress Management

There is no evidence that stress causes exacerbations of MS [7]. Nonetheless, stress management is critical in coping with any chronic disease and minimizing disabilities in the face of fluctuating impairment. The difficulty in diagnosing MS, the unpredictable nature of the disease, and the significant fatigue in patients who "look healthy" are additional stresses to patients.

Educational pamphlets on stress management are available from the National MS Society. Patients should be referred for counseling as needed.

Smoking

Avoidance of tobacco is even more critical in patients with MS than in the healthy population. Respiratory muscle weakness is well documented in MS [8]. In addition, nicotine causes a transient worsening of motor function in patients with MS.

Life Expectancy

Studies of suicide in MS patients have inconsistent results, finding no increase in suicide [10] or a frequency 2–14 times that of the general population [11,12]. Excluding suicide, case fatality ratios for patients with an expanded disability status score (EDSS) greater than 7.5 (essentially restricted to wheelchair, cannot self-propel chair for full day, and need assistance to transfer) is almost 4 times the control population, while that for patients with EDSS less than 7.0 (essentially wheelchair-restricted, wheel self, and transfer alone) is about 1.5 [13]. Overall life expectancy for patients with MS is 6–7 years less than that of the insured population in Canada [13].

Diet

Despite therapeutic claims for low-fat, high-fat, gluten-free and other diets, and megavitamin therapy, there is no scientific evidence that any diet alters the outcome or symptoms of MS. The generally accepted healthy diet has added significance for the person impaired by MS. Proper diet helps to prevent further weakness due to anemia and protein depletion, and promotes wound healing and regular bowel movements. Obesity is common in patients with MS, particularly those confined to a wheelchair. It is extremely difficult for patients with severe paraparesis to burn large amounts of fat and calories. The emphasis should be on preventing obesity by early dietary counseling and exercise prescription.

SYMPTOM MANAGEMENT

Introduction

Symptom management is a major treatment approach in MS. Primary symptoms, caused by actual demyelination, include spasticity, weakness, sensory disturbance, neurogenic bladder/bowel, cognitive changes, and others. Secondary problems include contractures and urinary tract infections. Depression may be primary or secondary; the basis of one of the most disabling symptoms, fatigue, is unknown. The rehabilitative approach to MS is not limited to symptomatic treatment, but also attempts to minimize the resultant disabilities and handicaps. The physician's role is to maximize medical management and to identify symptoms that warrant referral to other rehabilitation professionals. A frequent error among physicians is to delay referral to therapists because the patient is not "bad enough yet."

Spasticity

Spasticity is very common in MS. Its presence is not a reason for treatment. Most physicians treat spasticity when it impairs function or causes pain. There is inadequate recognition, however, of the role of spasticity in fatigue of the ambulatory patient, leading to undertreatment.

The energy cost of walking is twice normal in patients with MS, with motor involvement of the legs an important factor in fatigue. Multivariate regression analysis demonstrates that this increased energy cost is related to spasticity, not to ataxia and weakness [14]. In some patients, however, spasticity is beneficial by allowing stabilization of the knees for transfers and walking. Overtreatment, therefore, can cause functional decline.

Mild to moderate spasticity may be managed with stretching exercises and inhibitive positioning, which are best taught by a physical therapist. Stretching exercises should be performed daily by the patient although, in some cases, family members or caretakers must be instructed. Since spasticity increases after prolonged rest, many patients find daily stretches followed by exercise critical in decreasing spasms and stiffness. Other physical measures include the use of cold packs and electrical stimulation [15].

If more aggressive treatment is necessary, baclofen is the drug of choice (5–80 mg daily). It is most useful in spasticity of spinal origin and is less likely than dantrolene to cause weakness and fatigue. A common clinical error is to give up on this medication too early. It may take up to 1 month to become effective and the dosage should be increased as needed and tolerated to 80 mg daily. Diazepam or clonazepam may be used with baclofen, but these are rarely effective when used alone. Tizanidine, an antispasticity drug with central effects, is currently in clinical trials. Clonidine transdermal system has also been effective in relieving spasticity of spinal cord origin [15]. Painful nocturnal spasms may also respond to treatment with carbamazepine.

For a local decrease in spasticity, phenol motor point blocks have been used. A new technique is electromyographically (EMG) guided application of C. botulinum toxin [16]. For severe spinal spasticity that is not responsive to oral medications, continuous infusion of intrathecal baclofen is extremely effective [17,18].

Weakness

An overly aggressive strengthening program may be counterproductive by increasing fatigue. However, a moderate strengthening program is effective in preventing deconditioning and disuse atrophy and in decreasing spasticity. Guidelines for the appropriate intensity of exercise may be assessed by the cardiovascular test protocol previously described.

A cooling vest that lowers core body temperature 1°C (Mark VII Microclimate System) has been reported to improve walking and quality of life in a single small study [19]. Treatment with the aminopyridines, a group of potassium channel blockers that allow more efficient conduction in demyelinated nerves, has been reported to result in clinical improvement in persons with MS. The improvement is greatest in pyramidal function, and occurs primarily in patients with progressive disease and heat-sensitive symptoms [20].

Fatigue

Fatigue in MS is poorly understood, frequently disabling, and often undertreated. Up to 80% of patients with MS complain of fatigue that prevents sustained activity, worsens with heat, interferes with daily function, and correlates poorly with depression [21]. Reports of elevated interleukin 2 levels in fatigued patients with MS are conflicting [22,23].

As noted above, deconditioning and the high energy cost of spastic gait contribute to fatigue, which improves with exercise and management of spasticity. Another type of fatigue associated with MS is best described as lassitude and is not directly associated with physical activity. Medications may be of benefit for this type of fatigue. Amantadine, 100 mg twice daily, can improve general energy level, concentration, problem solving, and sense of well-being [24]. Pemoline, 18.75–75 mg daily, may be effective, but must frequently be discontinued due to adverse effects [25]. There are anecdotal reports of the efficacy of fluoxetine, 20–40 mg daily.

Tremor and Ataxia

Tremor and truncal ataxia are also very disabling and poorly treated MS symptoms. While medications may be of slight benefit for tremor (clonazepam, diazepam, propranolol, isoniazid), physical means of management may be more effective. These include weighting the wrists or utensils to decrease the amplitude of the intention oscillations and supporting the elbows (i.e., resting on a table) to use the hands.

A walker or crutches may provide bilateral support and balance for an ataxic patient, but often the patient will fall with the assistive device. Ataxic patients with good strength and endurance may improve gait with a weighted walker. There is no effective medication for truncal ataxia.

Visual Symptoms

Of Kurtzke's functional system scales, visual dysfunction correlated most strongly with quality of life in one study of patients with MS [26]. Poor visual acuity may be partially corrected with glasses. An eye patch is useful for diplopia and should be alternated between eyes daily. Large print books and following written text with a finger or a straight edge by patients with adequate strength and coordination are beneficial. Fatigue of the eyes is reduced with frequent rests.

Neurogenic Bowel and Bladder

Early evaluation and treatment of bladder symptoms was identified as a key factor in avoiding hospitalization of patients with MS [27]. A frequent clinical error is the prescription of an anticholinergic agent for a patient complaining of frequency and urgency, without checking renal function, urinalysis and culture, or postvoid residual (PVR). Most authorities recommend fluid regulation and timed voiding if PVR is less than 100 ml and a cystometrogram (CMG) to guide therapy in patients who cannot adequately empty the bladder (see Chapter 18). Kornhuber and Schutz, however, argue that CMGs are unnecessary, since detrusor–sphincter dyssynergia and detrusor hyperactivity are secondary to, not the cause of, urinary retention that is overcome with catheterization [28]. They have been successful in weaning patients from catheters with a program of frequent intermittent catheterizations followed by trials of voiding using suprapubic taps and Credé maneuvers. Catheterization is then decreased on the basis of ultrasound-measured PVRs. No CMGs are obtained. All bladder retraining to free persons with MS from catheters requires the patient to be highly motivated, willing to adhere to a rigid voiding and fluid schedule, and willing to accept intermittent catheterization during the training period [29]. Care must be taken in asking a spouse or child to perform the catheterizations since it may lead to an alteration in family relationships.

Patients with frequent urinary tract infections require a full evaluation of kidney and bladder function and diagnostic studies to rule out stones or other sources of urinary tract infections. Caution must be exercised in prescribing prophylactic antibiotics that may lead to infection with resistant organisms. Foods that help to acidify the urine, which may reduce bacterial growth, include cranberry juice, prunes, and prune juice. Vitamin C, 2000–4000 mg daily, also acidifies the urine. Adequate fluid intake (1800–2000 ml) reduces infection by preventing concentration of urine.

An indwelling catheter is necessary if there is skin breakdown in an incontinent patient, inability to adhere to a program of intermittent catheterization, or in certain travel situations.

Diarrhea is rare in MS. Constipation is managed with a 45 g fiber diet, adequate fluids (2000 ml), bulk formers, and stool softeners as needed. Patients should attempt to void every 2–3 days, preferably at a standard time 30–60 min after a large meal. Laxatives, enemas, and suppositories are the last line of therapy.

Sexual Dysfunction

Patients are too often embarrassed to complain spontaneously of sexual dysfunction. Others believe that the symptom cannot be treated and so do not mention it. Physicians must ask if sexual problems exist and explain treatment options. Physicians uncomfortable in discussing or treating sexual dysfunction should offer referrals to specialists.

The most common symptom of primary sexual dysfunction in female patients with MS is impaired sensation, which may be increased by use of a vibrator or oral stimulation. Poor vaginal lubrication can be treated with water-soluble vaginal lubricants. Fluids should be decreased for 2–3 hr before intercourse and the bladder emptied immediately before sexual activity.

In male patients with MS, failure to achieve and sustain an erection may be primary or secondary. Chronic erectile problems may be managed with prostheses, injections, or external vacuum pump devices. All patients benefit from symptomatic treatment of depression, fatigue, adductor spasticity, and pain. Education on sexuality may allow for alternative gratifying means of expressing affection.

Pain

Trigeminal neuralgia and other lancinating, burning neuropathic pains occur occasionally in MS and often respond to treatment with carbamazepine, amitriptyline, capsaicin, and other drugs used for neuropathic pains. It is a common clinical error, however, to assume all pain in a person with MS is due to MS without adequate investigation or treatment for other problems such as tendinitis or degenerative joint disease.

Depression and Cognitive Decline

Depression in MS may be primary, due to MS plaques, or secondary, in reaction to diagnosis or functional decline. The symptom should never be left untreated because "the patient has reason to be depressed." Depression may lead to greater disability than that due to neurological impairment and can be successfully treated with medication and counseling.

Cognitive decline is of functional significance in about 20% of people with MS, but may be reversible if due to depression. Memory aids such as memory logs and regularly scheduled activities are adaptive techniques. Family training is essential but frequently not addressed. Some families benefit from attending other dementia or brain injury support groups.

Speech and Swallowing Dysfunction

Functionally significant dysarthria occurs in fewer than 10% of people with MS [30] and aphasia in fewer than 1% [31]. These patients are best referred to speech pathologists. Breath support for speech production can be increased by diaphragmatic exercise and treatment of any coexisting pulmonary disease.

Published reports of videofluoroscopy and dysphagia in MS are rare. The largest study to date included 50 patients and demonstrated that clinical scales of disease severity such as the Expanded Disability Status Scale were highly correlated with radiological abnormalities, but symptoms were not [32]. Voice quality did not correlate with aspiration demonstrated on videofluoroscopy. Treatment of aspiration and frequency of pneumonia were not reported. Since patients with severe MS frequently require tube feedings to maintain nutrition and frequently develop pneumonia, this is clearly an area in which further studies are needed.

Sensory Deficits and Skin Care

No treatment exists to improve impaired sensation. Patients with sensory ataxia may compensate by visual and auditory cues (watching the feet and hearing the foot hit the floor). Adaptive equipment improves ADLs in those with sensory deficits of the hands. Precautions to minimize injury and pressure sores are similar to those for spinal cord injured patients (see Chapter 22).

SUMMARY

For physicians experienced in rehabilitation, the benefits of a multidisciplinary approach to treating people with MS are well accepted. Most patients with MS, however, are primarily treated by neurologists or family physicians with little experience in MS and even less in team treatment. Referrals to physical and occupational therapists are frequently delayed because patients "are not bad enough yet," and symptomatic depression and fatigue are dismissed as inevitable consequences of the disease. Early education and evaluation of a person newly diagnosed with MS by a full rehabilitation team is essential to maximize that person's function and independence.

REFERENCES

1. A.K. Percy, F.T. Nobregu, H. Okazaki, E. Glattie, and L.T. Kurland, *Arch. Neurol.*, 25:105–111 (1971).
2. R.P. Erickson, M.R. Lie, and M.A. Wineinger, *Mayo Clin. Proc.*, 64:818–828 (1989).
3. A.J.R. Lenman, F.M. Tully, et al., *Muscle Nerve*, 12:938–942 (1989).
4. G.M. Gehlsen, S.A. Grigsby, and D.M. Winant, *Phys. Ther.*, 64:653–657 (1984).
5. D.K. Kosich, B. Molk, J. Feeney, and J.H. Petajan, *J. Neurol. Rehab.*, 1:167–170 (1987).
6. R.T. Schapiro, J.H. Petajan, D. Kosich, B. Molk, and J. Ferry, *J. Neurol. Rehab.*, 2:43–49 (1988).
7. P.F. Nisipeanu and A.D. Karczyn, *Neurology*, 42 (Suppl. 3):384 (1992).
8. R. Olgiati, J. Jacquet, and E. DiPrompero, *Am. Rev. Respir. Dis.*, 143:1005–1010 (1986).
9. M. Emre and C. deDecker, *Arch. Neurol.*, 49:1243–1247 (1992).
10. D. McAlpine, C.E. Lumsden, and E.D. Acheson, *Multiple Sclerosis. A Reappraisal*, 2nd ed., Williams & Wilkins, Baltimore, pp. 179–184 (1972).
11. E. Kahana, U. Liebowitz, and M. Alter, *Neurology*, 21:1179–1185 (1971).
12. N.S. Stenager, E. Stenager, N. Koch-Henriksen, H. Broxnnum-Hansen, K. Hyllested, K. Jensen, and H. Bille-Brahe, *J. Neurol. Neurosurg. Psychiatry*, 55:542–545 (1992).
13. A.D. Sadovnick, G.C. Ebers, R.W. Wilson, and D.W. Paty, *Neurology*, 42:991–994 (1992).
14. R. Olgiati, J. Bergunder, and M. Mumenthaul, *Arch. Phys. Med. Rehabil.*, 69:846–849 (1988).
15. J.H. Petajan, *J. Neurol. Rehab.*, 4:219–224 (1990).
16. B.J. Snow, J.K. Tsui, M.H. Bhatt, M. Varelas, M.A. Hashimoto, and D.B. Calve, *Ann. Neurol.*, 28:512–515 (1990).
17. R.D. Penn, S.M. Savoy, D. Corcos, M. Latash, G. Gottlieb, B. Parke, and J.S. Kroin, *N. Engl. J. Med.*, 320:1517–1521 (1989).
18. P.G. Loubur, R.K. Narayan, K.J. Sandin, W.H. Donovan, and K.D. Russell, *Paraplegia*, 29:48–64 (1991).
19. A. Woldanski, K. Syndulka, R.W. Baumhefner, and W.W. Tourtellotte, *Neurology* (abstr.) In press (1993).
20. H.A.M. Dieman, C.H. Polman, T.M.M.M. VanDongen, A.C. VanLoenen, J.J.P. Nanta, M.J.B. Taphoorn, H.K. VanWalbeek, and J.C. Koetsier, *Ann. Neurol.*, 32:123–130 (1992).
21. L.B. Krupp, L.A. Alvarez, N.G. LaRocca, and L.C. Scheinberg, *Arch. Neurol.*, 45:435–437 (1988).
22. R.A. Rudick and B.P. Barna, *Arch. Neurol.*, 47:254 (1990).
23. K. Mohr, P.K. Coyle, L.B. Krupp, and C. Doscher, *Neurology*, 42 (Suppl. 3):384 (1992).
24. R.A. Cohen and M. Fisher, *Arch. Neurol.*, 46:676–680 (1989).

25. B.G. Weinshenker, M. Penman, B. Bass, G.C. Ebers, and G.P.A. Rice, *Neurology*, *42*:1468–1471 (1992).
26. R.A. Rudick, D. Miller, J.D. Clough, L.A. Gragg, and R.G. Farmer, *Arch. Neurol.*, *49*:1237–1242 (1992).
27. D.N. Bourdette, A.V. Prochazka, D.J. Mitchell, P. Licari, and J. Burks, *Arch. Phys. Med. Rehabil.*, *74*:26–31 (1993).
28. H.H. Kornhuber and A. Schultz, *Eur. Neurol.*, *30*:260–267 (1990).
29. J.L. Opitz, *Mayo Clin. Proc.*, *51*:367–372 (1976).
30. G.H. Kraft, J.E. Freal, and J.K. Coryell, *Arch. Phys. Med. Rehabil.*, *67*:164–168 (1968).
31. A. Achison, I. Ziv, R. Djaldetti, H. Goldberg, A. Kuritzky, and E. Melamed, *Neurology*, *42*:2195–2196 (1992).
32. W. Herrera, B. Zeligman, J. Gurber, M. Jones, R. Panther, R. Wriston, M. Cain, T. Prescott, N. Cobble, and J. Burks, *J. Neurol. Rehab.*, *4*:1–8 (1990).

22

Spinal Cord Injury

Mindy L. Aisen

Cornell University Medical College
The Winifred Masterson Burke Rehabilitation Hospital, Inc.
White Plains, New York

Spinal cord injury (SCI) acutely, and often permanently, produces profound disability that has an impact on an individual's ability to move, feel, control bowel and bladder function, and engage in sexual and reproductive activities. Despite the devastating physical, social, and emotional consequences of SCI, appropriate rehabilitation and medical management can often enable its victims to function comfortably, independently, and productively at home as well as in the workplace.

SPINAL CORD TRAUMA

SCI occurs when there is sudden compression, hyperextension, or extensive flexion of the spinal column. Such forces disrupt bony integrity by producing fracture and/or dislocation. The spinal cord, which is normally supported and stabilized by the spinal column, may then experience transient or lasting tension, torsion, and compression, leading to crush, hemorrhage, and infarction. It is rare for the cord to be transected during this sort of trauma; transection is more often the result of a direct penetration wound such as a knife or bullet would produce.

The spinal column is most vulnerable at the points of greatest mobility, particularly when such regions reside adjacent to less mobile structures [1]. These areas are the atlantoaxial joint, the low cervical region, and the thoracolumbar junction.

Epidemiology

The incidence of SCI in the United States is approximately 50 per million population per year; the estimated prevalence is 250,000–500,000 [2]. More males are affected, with the male to female ratio varying from 2.4:1 to 4.3:1 [3,4]. Teenagers and young adults are at greatest risk. Eighty percent of patients who sustain SCI are under the age of 40 and the median age of onset is 25 years [2,5]. Quadriplegia is most often caused by motor vehicle accidents, followed in frequency by sporting injuries, falls, and penetrating wounds [2,6,7]. Paraplegia is most commonly associated with penetrating wounds, motor vehicle accidents, and falls [7]. Most injuries occur after midnight.

Clinical Syndromes

The incidence of quadriplegia and paraplegia is approximately equivalent, as is the incidence of complete and incomplete injuries [5,7]. A complete lesion describes the syndrome in which there is absolute loss of functional motor activity or sensory perception below the level of injury. In an incomplete lesion, some motor and/or sensory function is preserved below that level. The level of injury refers to the anatomically lowest functional motor or sensory segment, and lesions are often defined by separate description of motor and sensory level and severity.

Many patients with incomplete lesions will experience some degree of neurological recovery, and improvement may occur up to 5 years after injury [8]. Approximately 95% of patients with complete lesions will have permanent impairment [6].

The incomplete spinal cord syndromes include the central cord, anterior spinal cord, and Brown-Sequard syndromes [9]. The central cord syndrome is most often seen in patients over the age of 50 who have sustained hyperextension injuries. Cervical spondylosis is a significant risk factor [10–12]. In this syndrome, upper extremities are more severely affected than lower extremities; patients who are ultimately ambulatory may suffer permanent upper limb disability. Deficits are referable to damage of the central gray matter and medial portions of the corticospinal and spinothalamic tracts, and include weakness, spasticity, and often severe dysesthesia.

In the anterior spinal cord syndrome, posterior column function is preserved while corticospinal and spinothalamic tracts suffer transverse damage. When induced by trauma, this syndrome is associated with cervical flexion injuries, particularly in the setting of cervical canal narrowing and atherosclerotic involvement of the anterior spinal artery.

The Brown-Sequard syndrome is produced by cord hemisection, resulting in ipsilateral corticospinal and posterior column and contralateral spinothalamic dysfunction. Causes include penetrating wounds and, less often, rotational closed injuries.

REHABILITATION: MANAGING THE SYMPTOMS AND COMPLICATIONS OF SCI

It is useful to classify symptoms as primary, secondary, and tertiary. Primary symptoms are directly attributable to the nervous system lesion, and include weakness, spasticity, neurogenic bowel and bladder symptoms, autonomic dysfunction, neuropathic pain, impotence, and infertility. The secondary findings are the medical and surgical complications that develop as a result of the chronic neurological deficits. These include urinary tract infections and stones, respiratory infections, decubitus ulcers, deep vein thromboses, and tendon contractures. Tertiary complications are the emotional, social, and financial difficulties that the individual with SCI must face for a lifetime.

Weakness

Functional abilities are dictated by the level of injury and regions of preserved motor power. The goals of physical and occupational therapy are to maintain range of motion in all limbs, increase muscle strength and endurance in groups with preserved innervation, train the patient to compensate for motor loss by substituting motions of preserved muscle, and assess orthotic and equipment needs. Table 1 summarizes spinal segmental levels, preserved motor function at those levels, and potential functional abilities. An appropriate program of physical and occupational therapy should enable most patients with SCI to perform the activities outlined. Most patients learn to use their upper extremities to perform the work of locomotion, often substituting shoulders for hips as the weight-bearing joint. Strengthening is achieved by employing traditional weight lifting and resistive exercise programs.

Functional electrical stimulation (FES), a technique that produces contraction in paralyzed muscle by applying electrical current to peripheral nerves, is used increasingly to exercise paralyzed limbs or limb segments. FES exercise increases the bulk and strength of deconditioned muscle, and may enable paretic muscle groups to perform at a functional level. FES can also be incorporated into a conditioning program. Although the technique is still considered experimental, there is evidence that patients with SCI improve endurance and oxygen consumption when FES-induced lower extremity exercise is added to an upper body exercise program [13,14]. Another use of FES involves producing functional movement in paralyzed muscle, including grasp and ambulation. Surface as well as implanted electrodes have

Table 1 Spinal Segmental Levels, Preserved Motor Function, and Potential Functional Abilities in SCI

Spinal Level	Key Innervated Muscles/ Motor Function	Functional Abilities	Useful Equipment
C4	Diaphragm Trapezii (neck motion, shoulder elevation)	Cough Steer motorized wheelchair Type/turn pages Activated electronic appliances: telephone, computer, television	Abdominal binder Chin control Mouth stick Puff and sip switch or environmental control unit (ECU)
C5	Deltoid Biceps (shoulder motion, elbow flexion)	Feeding Grooming Typing Page turning Manage manual wheelchair Pressure relief/assist with transfers Drive	Mobile arm support Hand cuff for adapted utensils Wheel projections Wheelchair gloves Sliding board Hand controls Manual switch for ECU
C6	Extensor carpi radialis Rotator cuff (shoulder control, wrist extension, tenodesis grasp)	Limited grasp Self-catheterization Wheelchair propulsion Sliding broad transfers	Universal cuff Adapted utensils Wheelchair gloves Sliding board
C7	Triceps Flexor carpi radialis Extensor pollicis longus (extend elbow, flex wrist, mass grasp)	Transfer with depression lift technique Insert rectal suppositories Inspect skin Stand with bracing and assistance at parallel bars	Raised seat Tub bench Inserter Mirror Long leg braces
C8	Hand extrinsics (some active finger flexion and extension)	Transfer from wheelchair to all surfaces	Standard wheel rims Grab bars
T1	Full functional hand use	Function from wheelchair as a paraplegic	
T2–12	Abdominal Intercostal Paraspinals	As the level drops, there is increasing respiratory function and truncal control and balance. Those with lower thoracic lesions can stand and take steps.	Wheelchair Long leg braces Walker
L1–2	Rectus abdominus Iliopsoas (hip hikers, hip flexors, hip adductors)	Ambulate short distances with braces	Walker Crutches Long leg braces

Table 1 Continued

Spinal Level	Key Innervated Muscles/ Motor Function	Functional Abilities	Useful Equipment
3–4	Quadriceps (knee extension)	Functional ambulation with bracing	Cane(s) Short leg braces
5, 1–2	Tibialis anterior Soleus Partial hamstring (ankle control, knee flexion)	Functional ambulation without bracing	Canes
3–5	Lower extremities fully functional	Continued bowel and bladder disability	

been successfully used for these purposes in a limited number of patients [15]. Commercially available FES ambulation systems have recently been marketed in the United States, although their efficacy in the general population with SCI has not yet been documented. Muscle fatigue, electrode failure, and skin irritation at the electrode site have been limiting factors. Muscle fatigue may be compensated for by combining FES with appropriate bracing. As technology advances, partial FES/orthotic systems will probably become an increasingly popular alternative, although patients with substantial proprioceptive deficits will always be limited in their ability to ambulate effectively.

Adaptive equipment can enhance independence in performing activities of daily living, for example, by interfacing with electronic equipment that can control the environment (environmental control unit [ECU]), or aiding in dressing, grooming, and eating. Braces and splints can substitute for weak muscle groups, enhancing function as well as protecting vulnerable joints from injury. Prescribing leg orthoses requires careful consideration of the patient's and clinician's goals, level of injury, and function below the level of injury. Bracing the lower limb can be used to protect joints, allow therapeutic standing and walking, or permit functional ambulation. The patient with an injury above T11 will require bilateral Scott-Craig orthoses, shown in Figure 1, to stand, coupled with a lordotic posture to maintain stability. For a reciprocal gait, excessive lateral trunk flexion and pelvic rotation or elaborate mechanical cable system, such as the reciprocating gait orthosis, to advance the limb is required. Functional ambulation generally cannot be achieved. With lower injuries, knee–ankle–foot (L2,3) or ankle–foot (L4,5) orthoses may be used, shown in Figures 2 and 3. Less than one-half of patients requiring knee or hip support consistently use their braces after discharge from rehabilitation centers. Ambulation with orthotics expends at least four times the energy required for normal gait. In addition,

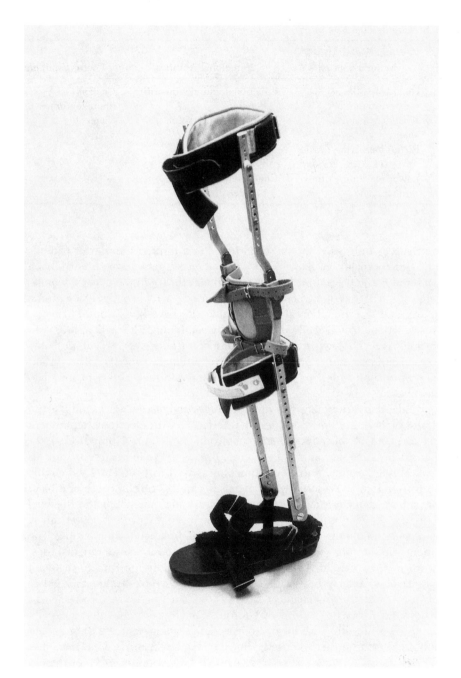

Figure 1   Scott-Craig orthosis.

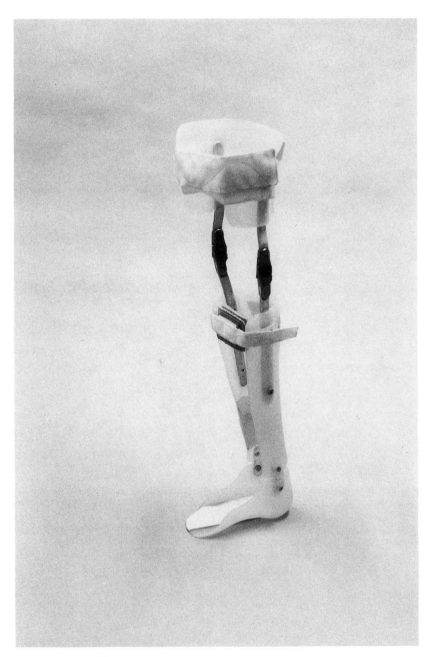

Figure 2 Knee–ankle–foot orthosis.

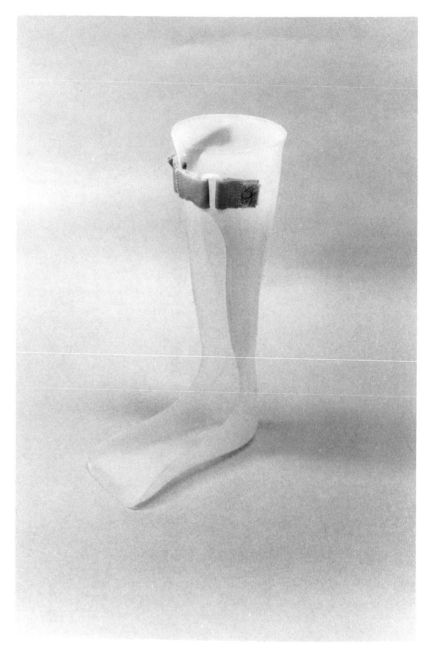

Figure 3   Ankle–foot orthosis.

lower limb braces are expensive, bulky, time-consuming to apply properly, and can lead to skin breakdown. However, most patients have strong, albeit unrealistic, desires and opinions about the potential benefits of bracing, which are often difficult to resist. In addition, theoretical, although unproven, benefits include preserved range of motion, improved cardiovascular tone, decreased risk of skin breakdown, and prevention of osteoporosis. Lower extremity bracing is most often successful in the young motivated patient with an incomplete lesion, preserved proprioceptive function, and limited spasticity. It is often advisable to emphasize transfer training, upper body conditioning, and wheelchair skills in the early phases of rehabilitation, reserving orthotic evaluation for the outpatient stage.

Spasticity

Spasticity is a disorder of motor function seen in patients with SCI when supraspinal control of spinal cord activity is impaired. To varying degrees, accentuated segmental reflexes, velocity-dependent increases in resistance to passive muscle stretch, dyssynergic patterns of muscle contraction, and involuntary flexor or extensor spasms are seen [16,17].

The presence of spasticity does not necessitate its treatment, since a moderate degree of hypertonicity may enhance standing or improve transfer independence. In addition, occasional flexor or extensor spasms can improve circulation and decrease venous pooling. Intervention is indicated when spasticity impairs function, restricts voluntary movement, or induces pain. Severe unchecked hypertonia can lead to tendon contracture or joint deformity.

Spasticity is amenable to treatment by physical as well as pharmacological therapy. Often eliminating nociceptive stimuli such as tight clothing, distended bowel or bladder, urinary tract infection or stone, or skin irritation will alleviate spasticity. Physical therapy, particularly sustained stretching, decreases hypertonicity and prevents contractures. Limb cooling with ice packs decreases tone by slowing nerve conduction velocity and increasing excitation–contraction coupling time and is a useful adjunct to physical therapy in cases of severe spasticity [18]. Functional electrical stimulation has been advocated as a treatment of spasticity, and is occasionally a useful supplementary therapy. The mechanism of its effect may be through activation of inhibitory synapses, or presynaptic neurotransmitter depletion [19].

Spasticity results largely from hyperactivity of alpha- and gamma-mediated reflex arcs. Drugs that decrease excitability of spinal reflexes, depress muscle contractility, or block transmission at the neuromuscular junction can alleviate spasticity. Glycine and gamma-aminobutyric acid (GABA) are the major inhibitory neurotransmitters in the spinal cord [17]. Glycine is released by inhibitory interneurons and Renshaw cells; GABA's most important function is presynaptic inhibition of primary afferent fibers. GABA agonists represent the most widely used class of drugs in the treatment of spasticity.

Baclofen is the first-line pharmacological therapy in patients who have disabling spasticity. It activates GABA-B receptors in primary sensory afferents, producing presynaptic inhibition of the sensory arc of spinal stretch reflexes. It may, in addition, augment Renshaw cell activity and depress fusimotor activity [17]. It effectively decreases spasms and muscle tone. Its side effects include sedation, nausea, constipation, urinary incontinence, and peripheral edema. High dosage oral baclofen treatment, with dosages as high as 240 mg/day, has recently been documented to treat severe spasticity safely and effectively. However, this must be done with caution in patients with impaired renal function, since baclofen clearance may be impaired [20]. Intrathecal baclofen continuously infused by pump is gaining acceptance as a treatment for refractory patients [21].

Second-line drugs include benzodiazepines and dantrolene sodium. Benzodiazepines bind to classic GABA receptors on the terminals of primary sensory afferents, enhancing the receptor's affinity for GABA and enhancing presynaptic inhibition [17]. Although these agents are effective in reducing spasticity, the known sedating, habituating, and addicting potential of benzodiazepines limits their clinical utility. Dantrolene sodium inhibits muscle contractility by reducing the release of calcium ions from the sarcoplasmic reticulum [17]. Its clinical usefulness is limited by side effects such as increased motor weakness and hepatotoxicity, but when used judiciously it is often a useful clinical adjunct.

Chemical denervation by motor point block is a method that can selectively reduce spasticity, for example, when excessive adductor tone interferes with bladder catheterization. Phenol is injected intramuscularly at motor points as defined by EMG. The effect is immediate but temporary, generally reversing over months. C. botulinum toxin has recently been advocated to produce specific local spasticity control similarly [22,23]. Although its clinical effect is primarily due to neuromuscular junction blockade, there is experimental evidence that the toxin is transported in a retrograde manner to the spinal cord via axon, where it may block Renshaw cell inhibition. This is a technique that warrants further evaluation in persons with SCI.

Autonomic Dysfunction: Neurogenic Shock and Autonomic Dysreflexia

Patients with complete motor lesions experience acutely a state of flaccid paralysis associated with absent deep tendon reflexes. This condition is known as spinal shock. It resolves 1–4 months after injury, at which point upper motor neuron signs develop [6]. Neurogenic shock refers to a condition also present during the acute and subacute periods of cervical and high thoracic SCI, and is due to disrupted communication between the sympathetic nervous system and higher centers.

In the neurologically intact person, blood pressure is maintained when an upright posture is assumed through a reflex loop consisting of afferent baroreceptor input to the central nervous system (CNS) through the ninth and tenth cranial nerves, and sympathetic efferent responses. In persons who have sustained SCI, blood pressure regulation is dependent upon vagal responses, increased activity in the renin–angiotensin system, and increased vasopressin release [24,25]. Early after injury, patients with SCI experience low resting systolic pressures and heart rates. Orthostatic hypotension is often coupled with hypertension and rapid diuresis upon assuming a supine posture, due to aldosterone-induced expanded intravascular volume. Hyperactive vagal responses are common, and are accentuated by hypoxia. Patients may experience hyperactive responses to vasoactive drugs, and surgical procedures requiring general anesthesia should be avoided during this time. Although neurogenic shock usually resolves spontaneously, some quadriplegic patients will experience chronic orthostatic hypotension and poikilothermia. In most cases adequate symptomatic control is achieved through gradual mobilization, firm support hosiery, and avoidance of extreme fluctuations in ambient temperature.

The autonomic dysreflexia syndrome is due to uninhibited spinal sympathetic reflexes leading to excessive sympathetic activity. SCI breaks the connection between the inhibitory baroreceptor response and the sympathetic nervous system, while vagal parasympathetic pathways continue to function. When sympathetic reflexes are triggered by nociceptive afferent spinal cord inputs (e.g., bladder distention, decubiti, bowel impaction, peptic ulcer), profound blood pressure surges coupled with bradycardia result. Other symptoms include gooseflesh, throbbing headache, and sweats; complications include seizures and hypertensive hemorrhage. Treatment must be provided rapidly, and consists of removing the triggering stimulus and elevating the head to lower blood pressure. Nitropaste or sublingual nifedipine may be useful in the acute phase, and recurrent dysreflexia may respond to chronic alpha-blocking therapy.

Neurogenic Bladder

Bladder dysfunction is very common in persons with SCI and is due to interruption of innervation to the detrusor (cholinergic) and internal sphincter (alpha-adrenergic) muscles. Patients report symptoms of urinary retention, frequency, urgency, and incontinence.

The bladder may fail to empty completely when there is inadequate detrusor pressure, typically seen during spinal shock and in cauda equina lesions. Inadequate voiding also occurs in the setting of sphincter hyperactivity or mechanical outlet obstruction. Failure to store urine occurs when there is hypertonicity of the detrusor muscle and/or sphincter insufficiency, generally seen in upper motor neuron lesions, frequently during the chronic phase of SCI. Detrusor sphincter dyssynergia is also an upper motor neuron syndrome. It produces urinary retention coupled with incontinence and potential turbulent flow and reflux.

Defining the nature of bladder dysfunction occasionally requires formal urodynamic testing. Frequently, however, postvoid residual volume measurement provides adequate information. A postvoid residual greater than 100 ml or 20% of the total bladder volume indicates a need for an intermittent catheterization regimen, which will decrease the risk of infection, urolithiasis, and hydronephrosis. Intermittent catheterization will also allow patients with retention to use anticholinergic agents to control urinary frequency and incontinence [26].

The drugs useful in the management of the neurogenic bladder are agents such as propantheline bromide (Probanthine), which relax the detrusor muscle by antagonizing the effects of acetylcholine at muscarinic receptors, and cholinergic agents such as bethanechol (Urecholine), which improve detrusor contraction [26,27].

Tricyclic antidepressants such as imipramine hydrochloride (Tofranil) promote bladder storage, probably through both anticholinergic detrusor action and adrenergic effects on the internal urinary sphincter [28]. Alpha-adrenergic blocking agents such as phenoxybenzamine (Dibenzyline) and terazosin hydrochloride (Hytrin) decrease outflow resistance by relaxing the internal sphincter. Baclofen, by relaxing the pelvic floor, may also help to limit outflow resistance.

As spinal shock resolves, some degree of spontaneous bladder emptying occurs. At that stage the female patient with SCI usually opts for urinary continence through a regimen of intermittent catheterization and anticholinergic agents. Men, particularly quadriplegics who are unable to self-catheterize, usually prefer a condom catheter in combination with cholinergic and alpha-blocking agents to enhance voiding. Sphincterotomy surgery may be required for the male with chronic urinary retention despite pharmacological intervention.

The most common complication of the neurogenic bladder and the most common infection seen in patients with SCI is urinary tract infection (UTI). The entry route for bacteria is the urethra, which is normally colonized by organisms such as *E. coli*, enterococci, *Proteus* species, *Klebsiella*, and *Pseudomonas* [29]. Indwelling or intermittent catheterization or simply sphincter hyperactivity can allow retrograde bacterial migration. Coincident urinary retention further promotes infection, since stagnant urine serves as a culture medium, and the chronically distended bladder loses its epithelial antibacterial defenses [30]. Detrusor hyperactivity or the manual Credé maneuver may lead to upper urinary tract involvement (pyelonephritis, sepsis) through retrograde urinary flow.

In patients with SCI the acute UTI may go unrecognized because it is asymptomatic. However, it can manifest itself by aggravating seemingly unrelated neurogenic symptoms such as dysreflexia, dysesthesias, weakness, or spasticity, rather than producing traditional local symptoms. Frequent surveillance urinalyses are more useful than cultures, since they help to differentiate cystitis from colonization; antibiotic therapy should be reserved for the setting in which pyuria is seen. When antibiotics are indicated, a 7–10 day course is generally necessary to eradicate infection in the setting of associated urodynamic abnormalities.

Persistent UTIs may reflect recurrence, reinfection, or chronic infection. Recurrent UTI with the same bacterial strain is often due to insufficient antibiotic dosage. Reinfection with a different organism is common and may be related to catheterization technique. In chronic cystitis the infection involves deeper layers of the bladder wall, and increases the risk of squamous cell carcinoma of the bladder [29]. Chronic infection may indicate underlying structural pathological conditions (tumor, calculi, diverticuli). Cystoscopy and intravenous pyelography are useful diagnostic procedures.

Prophylaxis against UTI may be provided by maintaining a urine pH less than 6.0. Urinary acidifying agents such as vitamin C (1 g four times per day) in combination with urinary antiseptics such as methenamine mandelate (1 g four times per day) or hexamine hippurate (1 g twice a day) should be prescribed for the patient with neurogenic bladder. Cranberry juice consumption should also be encouraged, since it is the only fruit juice that consistently reduces urine pH. Recurrent UTI in the absence of underlying structural pathological conditions may require chronic low-dosage antimicrobial therapy, such as nitrofurantoin 50 mg twice a day [31].

Urinary calculi commonly develop in persons with SCI. Factors that contribute to stone formation include urine alkalinity, related to infection with urea-splitting bacteria, hypercalcemia, and urinary stasis. Stone prevention therefore includes minimizing infections, treatment with urinary acidifiers, mobilization, high-fluid intake, and intermittent catheterization. Calculi may be asymptomatic or may produce hematuria, infection, recurrent dysreflexia, or pain.

Neurogenic Bowel

Constipation and incontinence are exceedingly common symptoms. Scrupulous attention to bowel function must be provided in order to avoid complications such as impaction and obstruction. A program consisting of daily stool softeners, laxatives, high-fiber diet, and adequate fluid intake coupled with alternate-evening disimpaction followed by a suppository will suffice as a bowel routine. The goal is to provide adequate stool evacuation every other day to prevent episodes of incontinence. Quadriplegics will frequently readily respond to a bowel regimen. Paraplegics, particularly those with cauda equina injuries, have a far more difficult time. Bowel routines often must be individually tailored to achieve satisfactory results.

Sexuality and Fertility

Male

The organs of male sexual and reproductive function are supplied by spinal segments T10 through S4. Parasympathetic erectile and genital afferent fibers travel through pelvic nerves that emanate from S2–S4 segments, the site of the erectile reflex center. The sympathetic motor supply to structures involved in psychogenic erection run in T10–L2 roots. Somatic supply controlling ejaculation travels from S2 to S4 through the pudendal nerves [32]. In patients with lesions above T10, reflex and spontaneous erections are common. Reflex ejaculation may also begin approximately 6 months after injury, particularly if a powerful stimulus, such as a vibrator, is applied [33,34]. Erection and ejaculation are substantially less common in patients with lumbar lesions, perhaps because parasympathetic fibers are connected to a small segment of isolated cord or because damage may have extended to sacral cord. It is not surprising that an incomplete functional lesion portends a better prognosis than does a complete lesion.

Prior to the advent of pharmacological and electroejaculation techniques, more than 90% of patients with upper motor neuron or incomplete lower motor neuron lesions and approximately 25% of patients with complete cauda equina lesions had erections. Coitus was reportedly attempted in 80% and was successful in 50%. Ejaculation occurred in 5–70% of men with SCI, but the incidence of fertility was only 1–10% [32]. Sterility in spinal cord injured men has been ascribed to ejaculatory dysfunction, genital ductal blockage secondary to recurrent genitourinary infections and nondrainage of the reproductive tract, and impaired spermatogenesis due to local testicular temperature elevations [35].

Adequate sexual and reproductive function are very important issues to the population affected by SCI. It is estimated that 29% are married at the time of injury and in 78% the marriage endures. Another 12% marry during the 5 years after injury [5]. Patients should be routinely questioned about sexual dysfunction, since they often feel inhibited about broaching the subject. A careful history may identify contributing factors such as psychological or pharmacological (e.g., anticholinergic or antidepressant medications) mechanisms. Referral to a urologist with appropriate expertise is indicated when neurological dysfunction is responsible for impotence. Men with SCI benefit from such a referral when they wish to improve quality and duration of erections for sexual intercourse, obtain semen for insemination, or improve semen quality.

Treatment of erectile dysfunction by injection of vasoactive drugs directly into the penis has now gained worldwide acceptance [36,37]. Papaverine, phentolamine, and prostaglandin E1, alone or in combination, increase tumescence or produce an erection when injected into the corpus cavernosum, and produce satisfactory results in a majority of patients. Side effects include local hematomas, penile fibrous changes, and priapism. This treatment should not be used more than twice per week. It should only be offered if 24 hr emergency care is available to deal quickly with complications and if the patient agrees to undergo monthly examination.

Assisted reproductive technology such as the use of vibrators or electro-ejaculation to obtain semen for artificial insemination now enables an increasing number of men with SCI to father children. High-frequency vibratory stimulation produces an ejaculation rate of 57%, but semen quality is generally inadequate [5,34]. Complications include autonomic dysreflexia, and pretreatment with nifedipine is advised [5].

Electrical rectal stimulation is a technique borrowed from veterinary medicine: to induce ejaculation, postganglionic sympathetic nerves are electrically stimulated with electrodes attached to a rectal probe. Depending on the degree of preserved sensation, general anesthesia may or may not be necessary. Repeated ejaculation generally leads to improved sperm counts. Patients typically ejaculate anterograde and retrograde. Although anterograde semen is more viable, retrograde can also be used. Although the number of patients is small, pregnancy rates of up to 50% have been reported [5,38]. As in the case of vibratory stimulation, autonomic dysreflexia may complicate the procedure.

Female

Women of childbearing age may experience a disruption of the menstrual and ovulatory cycle in the acute stage following SCI, as produced by many other major systemic stressors. This generally resolves during the first year; if it fails to, referral to a gynecologist for endocrine evaluation is advisable. Long-term female reproductive capacity is not impaired by SCI [39].

Sexual function is frequently impaired following SCI, and is related to the neural structures that have been damaged. The parasympathetic pelvic nerves (S2–S4) control tumescence of the clitoris and vaginal secretion.

Sympathetic splanchnic nerves (T10–L2) innervate the smooth muscle of the fallopian tubes and uterus. Contraction of the pelvic floor is controlled by somatic pudendal nerves emanating from S2–S4. Sexual dysfunction generally consists of impaired lubrication, often amenable to treatment with lubricating jelly, and intercourse-induced urinary tract infections, which may be controlled by advising patients to void or use bladder catheterization immediately after intercourse.

Because fertility is not impaired, counseling concerning the need for birth control measures, if the patient wishes to avoid pregnancy, may be indicated. Pregnancy and delivery may be problematic for the patient with SCI because of impaired bowel and bladder function, diminished abdominal wall strength, and the risk of autonomic dysreflexia. A team approach between an neurologist, anesthesiologist, and an experienced "high-risk" obstetrics team is advantageous to the patient.

Pain

Following spinal cord injury, patients commonly experience pain, which may be musculoskeletal or neuropathic in origin. Musculoskeletal problems typically occur in shoulders and wrist due to compensatory weight bearing assumed by the upper body, and in the lumbar region in paraplegics who assume lordotic postures while standing. Bursitis and tendinitis are common, and are generally amenable to treatment with nonsteroidal anti-inflammatory agents, heat, massage, and other modalities such as phonopheresis. Steroid injection is rarely required. Patients are susceptible to shoulder–hand syndrome, and it is crucial to provide proper positioning and shoulder alignment, frequent range-of-motion exercise, and hand massage as needed to minimize edema.

Neuropathic pain ranges from paresthesias to disabling dysesthesias and may be chronic or paroxysmal. It results from root entrapment (which may be helped by appropriate surgical intervention) or from cord injury. Combined counterirritant therapy, tricyclic and other antidepressant agents, carbamezepine, phenytoin, and transcutaneous nerve stimulation are at times effective in controlling pain. New onset of pain or sudden escalation in pain severity may signal the presence of a new structural lesion (e.g., posttraumatic syringomyelia) or other systemic pathological change (e.g., urinary tract disease, bowel impaction). Pain management continues to present a difficult and challenging aspect of the care of persons with SCI.

SECONDARY SYMPTOMS

Secondary symptoms are complications that develop as a result of chronic neurological disability. In addition to diseases of the urinary tract, these include decubitus ulcer, deep vein thrombosis, and respiratory complications.

Decubitus Ulcer

Decubitus ulcer is a common clinical problem. Impaired sensation and mobility, incontinence, and spasticity increase susceptibility by producing sustained pressure, friction, and moisture. Training patients in pressure relieving and appropriate transfer techniques, prescription of appropriate cushions and seating systems, and adequate bowel and bladder care are key preventative measures. Patients should be taught to inspect their skin regularly and should be instructed in the use of handheld mirrors. Pressure is the most significant causative element in the formation of decubitus ulcers. It has been shown that a constant skin pressure of 70 mmHg applied for more than 2 hr results in irreversible tissue damage. However, if pressure is alternated at 5 min intervals, damaged does not occur [40]. Pressure under the buttocks adjacent to the ischial tuberosities when seated in a wheelchair may exceed 500 mmHg [41]. Persistent external pressure on the skin leads to ischemia and exudation of fluid from capillaries. Shearing forces aggravate ischemic changes by angulating blood vessels in the dermis, and friction and moisture contribute to superficial skin loss.

Treatment of pressure sores consists of removal of superficial devitalized tissue and complete avoidance of weight-bearing, friction, and moisture on the lesion. Stage I and II lesions will respond to aggressive local care. Stage III and IV sores often require surgical intervention, such as excision of necrotic tissue and bony prominences followed by closure with myocutaneous flaps.

Deep Vein Thrombosis and Pulmonary Embolism

Deep vein thrombosis (DVT) and pulmonary embolism (PE) are frequent complications of SCI. The incidence of thromboembolism has been reported to be as high as 70–100%, although in our institution DVT occurs in approximately 20% and PE in about 5% [42]. DVT tends to occur within the first 6 months after injury, related to the immobility and venous stasis that are particularly prevalent during the spinal shock phase, as well as possible posttraumatic hypercoagulability. Prophylaxis with low-dosage subcutaneous heparin and antiembolism stockings are conventional therapy during the acute and subacute stages. However, thrombotic or hemorrhagic complications develop in approximately 35% of patients treated with low-dosage heparin prophylaxis. Low-molecular-weight heparin is reportedly a superior treatment, but remains experimental at this time [42].

DVT and PE are common and potentially life-threatening. The caregiver must, therefore, not only vigilantly monitor lower limb diameter, but should also consider these diagnoses when increased spasticity, unexplained fever, cough, or breathlessness occur.

Other Pulmonary Complications

Respiratory dysfunction results from diaphragmatic paralysis (lesion above C4) and impaired intercostal muscle performance (lesion above T12) [43]. Gastric distention may interfere further with diaphragmatic movement. As a result, patients develop respiratory fatigue, atelectasis, pneumonias, and acute bronchial obstruction by mucus plugs. Tracheal suctioning may induce profound bradycardia during the neurogenic shock phase, particularly if there is attendant hypoxemia.

Chest x-rays, measurement of arterial blood gases, and vital capacities are useful parameters to monitor. Vital capacity may be increased by applying an abdominal binder that will push abdominal contents higher on inspiration and allow greater diaphragmatic excursion on expiration. Daily use of incentive spirometry should be encouraged to prevent atelectasis. A program of chest wall percussion and vibration will help to mobilize secretions. The clavicular portion of the pectoralis major muscle plays a major role during coughing in the quadriplegic patient, and cough effectiveness may be improved by a combination of muscle training and abdominal binding [44].

Despite the use of preventive measures, quadriplegic patients remain at increased risk for developing respiratory infections. Systemic infections (most notably UTI) may seed the lungs, producing localized pulmonary infections, and bacterial pneumonia is associated with acute viral upper respiratory infections. Vaccination against influenza is recommended for patients who are at increased risk of pneumonia. Diagnosis of pneumonia depends on recognition of characteristic clinical and laboratory signs, and treatment consists of appropriate antibiotic and aggressive respiratory therapy.

Disorders of Bone Metabolism: Hypercalcemia and Heterotopic Ossification

Osseous demineralization with hypercalcemia due to prolonged immobilization is described not only in spinal cord injury, but following femur fracture, Guillian-Barré syndrome, and poliomyelitis [45–48]. Hypercalcemia is a metabolic complication of SCI that occurs most often during the acute and subacute stages. Risk factors include male sex, age less than 21 years, complete and high cervical injuries, dehydration, prolonged immobilization, renal dysfunction, and increased milk intake [45]. Patients may be asymptomatic or may experience lethargy, weakness, nausea, mood changes, and anorexia. Appetite changes prevent adequate oral intake, thereby aggravating dehydration and hypercalcemia. As the serum calcium level rises, vomiting, bowel impaction, polyuria and polydipsia, confusion, and cardiac arrhythmias may develop. Therapy consists of mobilization and vigorous hydration. If necessary, saline infusion and furosemide may be used. In severe cases, treatment with calcitonin and steroids have been advocated. The condition is always self-limiting, rarely occurring beyond 12 months after injury. Passive standing (with a tilt table) may decrease serum calcium during the early stages following acute SCI; its effects are controversial in the chronic stages [49].

Heterotopic Ossification

Ectopic bone histologically indistinguishable from normal bone develops in para-articular regions below the level of injury in 20–30% of patients with SCI [50]. Hips are the most commonly affected joints. Although functional immobility appears to be a causative factor, the stimulus for osteogenesis is unknown. Its onset is usually within 1–4 months of injury.

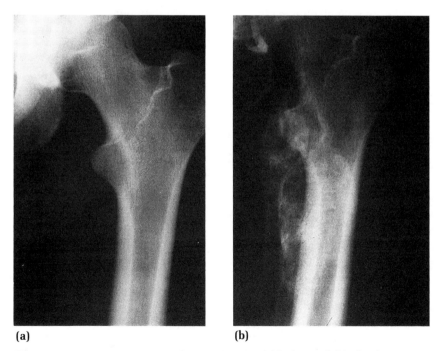

(a)   **(b)**

Figure 4   The left hip of a quadriplegic patient (a) before and (b) after heterotopic ossification.

Heterotopic ossification may be clinically asymptomatic or may cause local erythema, warmth, and pain, which symptoms mimic cellulitis and thrombophlebitis. Laboratory tests that may be useful in its diagnosis are measurements of serum alkaline phosphatase (which is elevated in some patients during active ossification), triphasic bone scan (which may demonstrate a vascular blush before radiographically apparent calcification has occurred), and plain x-ray. Figure 4 shows the x-ray changes typical of heterotopic ossification in the left hip of a 17-year-old quadriplegic boy.

Treatment options are reviewed elsewhere in this volume. Conventional therapy includes disodium etidronate prophylaxis, early and consistent range-of-motion exercises, and surgical removal of mature ectopic bone if substantial loss of range of motion has resulted.

TERTIARY COMPLICATIONS

The person living with the chronic sequelae of SCI experiences financial, social, and emotional changes. Problems include vocational difficulties, shifts in family status, social isolation, and diminished self-esteem. Difficulty obtaining and maintaining employment may result from inability to perform specific physical aspects of job requirements, but is more often related to discrimination, architectural barriers, and transportation difficulties. The demands and expense of providing care for a dependent and disabled individual often results in the breakdown of domestic relationships.

Employment

SCI most often occurs at an age critical to job training and earning potential. The majority of those successful in obtaining and maintaining employment are engaged in managerial or professional activities, since the physical demands are substantially less than skilled labor positions require. Therefore, it is helpful to advise patients to seek education and job skills that will enable them to secure positions in less physically demanding fields. They should be referred to appropriate agencies for vocational rehabilitation. The physician should periodically reassess the patient's functional status and prescribe medical interventions that may augment work capacity. A multidisciplinary approach involving not only social workers and therapist, but also attorneys is often required, in order to help obtain disability benefits, remove architectural barriers, overcome discrimination in the work place, and allow patients to be cognizant of their rights according to law.

The Americans with Disabilities Act (ADA) of 1990, Public Law 101-336, was enacted July 26, 1990. Title I of the ADA will go into effect in July, 1992. It specifies that employers cannot discriminate against a qualified individual with a disability in regard to hiring, training, compensation, or discharge. The ADA provides remedies available under Title VII of the Civil Rights Act of 1964, including back pay and court orders to stop discrimination. Employers with 25 or more employees must comply, effective July 26, 1992; those with 15–24 employees must comply, effective July 26, 1994.

The Act stipulates that requiring pre-employment physical examinations or inquiry concerning presence of disability is prohibited. However, inquiries pertaining to the ability of an applicant to perform job-related functions are permitted and once employment is offered, voluntary medication examinations are allowed. Employers may reject applicants or fire employees who pose a threat to the health or safety of co-workers.

Employers will be required by law to provide "reasonable accommodation" to individuals with disabilities. This includes steps such as:

1. Making existing facilities (offices, lounges, bathrooms, cafeterias) used by employees readily usable by people with disabilities
2. Restructuring job (part-time or modified work schedules; changes in training materials)
3. Acquiring new equipment or assistive devices, or modifying presently owned equipment, to better enable disabled individuals to perform necessary duties
4. Adjusting qualifying examinations and hiring and promotion policies

Employers are not required to provide accommodations that impose an "undue hardship" on business operations. It is important that the physician maintain a referral network encompassing appropriate ancillary services. Independence and continued employment must be encouraged.

At Home

A comfortable and safe home environment is a fundamental necessity. Structural modifications such as bathroom grab bars, widened doorways, ramps, and stair lifts all improve accessibility. Early after injury, the occupational therapist should evaluate the home situation to provide the patient and family with structural recommendations as well as lists of appropriate vendors, contractors, and funding sources.

SCI has many effects on family life and interpersonal relationships. Financial and physical issues interfere with leisure activities, children's education, and vacations, adversely affecting all family members. Patients experience depression, loss of self-esteem, and difficulty coping with increased dependence. The physician can help by maintaining a referral network to available community services such as support groups and visiting nurse associations. Emotional disturbances may require clinical intervention.

Realizing this, the primary care physician should monitor depressive signs and symptoms, and maintain an atmosphere that encourages dialogue about emotional problems.

Independent living centers are often an invaluable resource for the SCI outpatient community. They are nonresidential, consumer-controlled, not-for-profit organizations that employ persons with disabilities whenever possible. Funding is derived from federal, state, and private sources. Services vary among states, but may include individual advocacy, systems advocacy, peer counseling, accessibility advice, recreational activities, vocational training, and housing assistance.

SCI is a complex condition that has an impact on all aspects of the patient's life. A multidisciplinary and interdisciplinary approach is important. Although specific neurological function may not change as a result, longevity will be increased and quality of life will be enhanced.

REFERENCES

1. T.N. Byrne and S.G. Waxman, *Spinal Cord Compression*, F.A. Davis, Philadelphia (1990).
2. J.F. Krauss, *Central Nervous System Trauma Status Report 1985* (D.P. Becker and J.R. Povlishock, eds.), NIH, Washington, DC, pp. 313–322 (1985).
3. M.B. Bracken, D.H. Freeman, and K. Hellenbrandt, *Am. J. Epidemiol.*, *133*: 615–622 (1981).
4. P.R. Fine, K.V. Kuhlemeier, M.J. Devivo, and S.L. Stower, *Paraplegia*, *17*:237–250 (1970).
5. C. Bennett, R. Robinson, and D.A. Ohl, *Contemp. Urol. Nov*:25–28 (1990).
6. B.A. Green and I.A. Magana, *Handbook of the Spinal Cord* (R.A. Davidoff, ed.), Marcel Dekker, New York (1987).
7. G.M. Yarkony, E.J. Roth, A.W. Heinemann, Y. Wu, R. Katz, and L. Lovell, *Arch. Neurol.*, *44*:93–96 (1987).
8. J.M. Piepmeier and N.R. Jenkins, *J. Neurosurg.*, *69*:399–402 (1988).
9. L. Guttmann, *Spinal Cord Injuries: Comprehensive Management and Research*, Blackwell Scientific, Oxford (1976).
10. R.C. Schneider, G. Cherry, and H. Pantek, *J. Neurosurg.*, *11*:564 (1954).
11. R.C. Schneider, J.M. Thompson, and J. Bebin, *J. Neurol. Neurosurg. Psychiatry*, *21*:216 (1956).
12. D. Foo, *Paraplegia*, *24*:301 (1986).
13. R.M. Glaser, J.R. Strayer, and K.P. May, *Proceedings of the Seventh Annual Conference of the IEEE Engineering in Medicine and Biology Society*, Chicago, IL, pp. 308–313 (1985).
14. S.F. Pollock, K. Axen, and N. Spielholz, *Arch. Phys. Med. Rehabil.*, *70*:214–219 (1989).
15. P.H. Peckham, *Paraplegia*, *25*:279–288 (1987).
16. E. Knutsson and A. Martensson, *Scand. J. Rehabil. Med.*, *12*:93–106 (1980).

17. R.A. Davidoff, *Neurology*, *17*:107–116 (1985).
18. E. Knuttson, *Scand. J. Rehabil. Med.*, *2*:159–163 (1970).
19. T. Petersen and B. Kelmar, *J. Neurol. Rehab.*, *2*:103–108 (1988).
20. M.L. Aisen, M.A. Dietz, J.K. Cedarbaum, and H. Kutt, (1991).
21. R.D. Penn, S.M. Savoy, and D. Corcos, *N. Engl. J. Med.*, *320*:1517–1521 (1989).
22. B.J. Snow, J.K.C. Tsui, M.H. Bhatt, M. Varelas, S.A. Hashimoto, and D.B. Calne, *Ann. Neurol.*, *28*:512–515 (1990).
23. J. Jankovic and M.F. Brin, *N. Engl. J. Med.*, *324*:1186–1194 (1991).
24. A.F. Sved, F.H. McDowell, and W.W. Blessing, *Neurology*, *35*:78–82 (1985).
25. C.J. Mathias, N.J. Christensen, J.L. Corbett, H.C. Frankel, T.J. Goodwin, and W.S. Peart, *Clin. Sci. Mol. Med.*, *49*:291–299 (1975).
26. J. Lapides, A.C. Diokno, S.J. Silber, and B.S. Lowe, *Trans. Am. Assoc. Genito-urin. Surg.*, *63*:92–96 (1971).
27. J. Lapides, *Urol. Clin. North Am.*, *1*:81–97 (1974).
28. A.J. Wien, *Surgery of Female Incontinence* (S.L. Stanton and E.A. Taragho, eds.), Springer Verlag, Heidelberg, pp. 185–199 (1980).
29. T. Hald and W.E. Bradley, *The Urinary Bladder: Neurology and Dynamics*, William & Wilkins, Baltimore (1982).
30. R.M.L. Mehrotra, *J. Pathol. Bacteriol.*, *65*:78–89 (1953).
31. W.E. Stamm, *Ann. Intern. Med.*, *92*:770–775 (1980).
32. E. Bors and A.E. Comarr, *Urol. Surv.*, *10*:191–222 (1960).
33. G.S. Brindley, *Male Infertility* (T.B. Hargreave, ed.), Springer Verlag, Berlin, pp. 261–279 (1983).
34. G.S. Brindley, *Paraplegia*, *19*:299–302 (1981).
35. S. Ver Voort, *Urology*, *29*:157–165 (1987).
36. Intracavernous injections for impotence, *Med. Lett.*, *29*:95–96 (1987).
37. A. Zorgniotti, *Med. Aspects Hum. Sexuality* Jan:28–30 (1991).
38. C.J. Bennet, J.W. Ayers, and J.F. Randolph. *Fertil. Steril.*, *48*:1070–1072 (1987).
39. H.S. Talbot, *J. Urol.*, *73*:91 (1985).
40. S.M. Dinsdale, *Arch. Phys. Med. Rehabil.*, *55*:147 (1974).
41. J.D. Shea, *Clin. Orthop.*, *11*:89–100 (1975).
42. D. Green, M.Y. Lee, A.C. Lim, J.S. Chimiel, M. Vettes, T. Pant, C. Chen, L. Fenton, G.M. Yarkony, and P.R. Meyer, *Ann. Intern. Med.*, *113*:571–574 (1990).
43. E.J. Campbell, E. Agostoni, and J. Newson Davis, *Mechanics and Neural Control*, 2nd ed., W.B. Saunders, Philadelphia (1970).
44. M. Estenne and A. De Troyer, *Ann. Intern. Med.*, *112*:22–28 (1990).
45. F. Maynard, *Arch. Phys. Med. Rehabil.*, *67*:41–44 (1986).
46. L. Hyman, G. Boner, J. Thomas, and W. Segar, *Am. J. Dis. Child.*, *124*:723–727 (1972).
47. W. Clouston and H. Lloyd, *Clin. Orthop. Rel. Res.*, *216*:247–252 (1987).
48. F. Plum and M. Dunning, *Arch. Intern. Med.*, *101*:528–536 (1958).
49. R. Kaplan, W. Roden, E. Gilbert, L. Richards, and J. Goldschmidt, *Paraplegia*, *19*:289–293 (1981).
50. J.M. Connor, *Soft Tissue Ossification*, Springer Verlag, Great Britain (1983).

23

Rehabilitation of Parkinsonism, Other Movement Disorders, and Ataxia

Bala V. Manyam

Southern Illinois University School of Medicine
Springfield, Illinois

Disorders of movement affect both axial and appendicular structures. Movement disorders are usually caused by disturbances of the extrapyramidal system, cerebellum, and other parts of the central nervous system (Table 1). Movement disorders may be defined as "diseases or syndromes secondary to either structural or biochemical alteration in the basal ganglia, certain thalamic nuclei, substantia nigra, certain brain stem nuclei, or cerebellum that produces nonepileptic involuntary movements without loss of consciousness." The causative factors may be genetic, toxic, immunological, degenerative, vascular, traumatic, and metabolic (Figure 1). With the exception of ballismus and palatal myoclonus, all involuntary movements disappear in sleep and are exacerbated by anxiety. To assess the true degree of disability, several observations of the patient may be necessary. Removal of ill-fitting dentures and chewing gum before assessing oral-facial movements is important.

Various descriptive terms are used to designate the involuntary movements that occur (Table 2). These may be broadly classified into akinetic (hypokinetic) or hyperkinetic disorders. Parkinsonism is the best example of a hypokinetic movement disorder. Diseases such as Huntington's disease, Tourette's syndrome, dystonia, essential tremor, Wilson's disease, and others in which hyperkinesia is present are grouped under hyperkinetic movement disorders.

In parkinsonism, more than one form of movement disorder, including

Table 1 Anatomical Structures Directly or Indirectly Associated with Movement Disorders

Cerebral cortex: Diffuse, poorly delineated, mainly from frontal lobe
Caudate nucleus ⎤ Striatum ⎤
Putamen ⎦ (neostriatum)
⎥ Corpus striatum
Globus pallidus ⸺ Pallidum ⎦
(paleostriatum)
Substantia nigra
Red nucleus
Subthalamic nucleus
Thalamus: ventrolateral and anterior nuclei
Cerebellum
Reticular formation

tremor, dyskinesia, dystonia, myoclonus, and akinesia, occurs; hence, this is an ideal example of a movement disorder. It is also the most common. For these reasons, major discussion will be focused on parkinsonism. Other movement disorders in which rehabilitative measures have application will be highlighted.

PARKINSONISM

Parkinsonism is a clinical syndrome characterized by bradykinesia, tremor, loss of postural reflex mechanisms, and gait disturbance. It has several causes (Table 3) but the majority of cases are idiopathic. Pharmacotherapy, especially with dopaminergic drugs, improves the majority of symptoms of parkinsonism. Rehabilitative measures play a significant role, since symptoms are either not fully amenable to drug therapy or supplementation with rehabilitative measures improves the quality of life for the patient. In Parkinson's Plus, pharmacotherapy is often not effective, thus rehabilitation becomes the major means of therapy.

Bradykinesia affects all activities of the patient: every movement is considerably slowed down, contributing to severe disability. This is manifested in decreased expression of facial movements (hypomania): the patient does not readily respond to emotional changes. Blinking becomes less frequent, often resulting in a staring expression (reptilian stare). Rigidity affects the entire body but is manifest mostly in the limbs, thus interfering with all activities. Truncal rigidity and loss of postural reflexes result in decreased balance when standing and walking. Stooped posture may be an attempt to compensate for this loss of stability by lowering the center of gravity. The

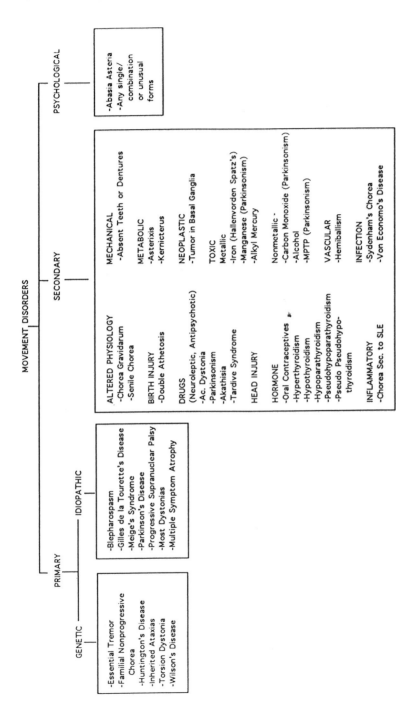

Figure 1 Classification of movement disorders based on cause.

Table 2   Definition of Abnormal Movements

Term	Definition
Akathisia	Unable to sit still. An inner restlessness relieved by moving about.
Ataxia	Ataxia or asynergia is a disturbance, quite independent of any motor weakness, due to breakdown of normal coordinated execution of voluntary movement. The direction and extent of voluntary movement are altered and the sustained voluntary or reflex muscle contractions are impaired.
Akinesia	Lack of spontaneous movements despite the potential ability to make the movement. Bradykinesia refers to decreased ability.
Athetosis	Slow writhing, bizarre movements in an irregular sequence, primarily involving the distal portion of the extremities; however, occasionally appendicular structures such as neck, face, and tongue could be involved. It should be considered a form of choreic movement since it usually occurs in combination with chorea.
Ballism	Very large amplitude, poorly patterned, purposeless wildly flinging movement involving the proximal axial musculature of appendicular structures. Most frequently it is unilateral and is referred to as hemiballismus.
Cogwheel rigidity	Intermittent yielding of the muscles to stretching, and/or passive motion or against muscular tension. The resistance is interrupted at regular intervals in a jerky fashion, and the muscles seem to give way in a series of steps, as if the manipulator were moving a limb attached to a heavy cogwheel or pulling it over a ratchet. Typically seen in parkinsonism.
Dystonia	Twisting, movements that tend to be sustained at the peak of the movement, frequently repeated, and often progresses to prolonged abnormal posture involving both axial and appendicular musculature.
Myoclonus	Quick movement due to muscular contractions (positive myoclonus) or inhibitions (negative myoclonus). Asterixis is the most common form of negative myoclonus. Myoclonus can be triggered by sudden stimuli such as sound, light, visual threat, or movement. Myoclonus can be present during sleep, as in palatal myoclonus.
Rigidity	Resistance to active or passive movement, in all directions.
Spasticity	A state of sustained increase in tension of a muscle when it is passively lengthened. The tension is caused by an exaggeration of the muscle stretch reflex and occurs in association with lesions involving the so-called pyramidal system and has been ascribed to the loss of, or release from, the normal inhibiting action of the pyramidal cortex on the anterior horn cells.
Tardive dyskinesia	Encompasses a series of abnormal involuntary movements, usually of the lower face, jaw, and tongue.

Table 2 Continued

Term	Definition
Tics	Clonic, rarely chronic, sterotyped, coordinated movements occurring repeatedly in attacks often with rhythmic intervals. They can be motor tics or phonic tics (involved with sounds).
Titulsation	To and fro movement of trunk and head.
Tremor	Rhythmic, involuntary oscillations around the plane. Can be regular or irregular in rhythm and amplitude. Tremor may be present at first or with action. The term "intention tremor" means that the tremor worsens as the limb approaches the target, as seen in cerebellar diseases.

patient loses the ability to initiate walking, cannot suddenly change direction or speed, and is unable to stop suddenly. All of this leads to a disturbed righting reflex, resulting in falls.

The characteristic tremor in parkinsonism is a resting tremor. Anxiety can increase tremor and often results in action tremor. Cogwheel rigidity is not specific for parkinsonism. Minor symptoms also contribute to the overall well being of the patient. The functional performance of patients with parkinsonism may show remarkable fluctuation throughout the day or from one day to another. Sometimes, the changes may last for several days to weeks, requiring that medication be altered. Factors such as anxiety and depression may also affect the patient's performance.

Levodopa alone or in combination with dopadecarboxylase inhibitor (carbidopa, benserazide), has a remarkable effect on most symptoms of parkinsonism, but tremor may not be fully controlled. Gait disturbance is not fully responsive to levodopa treatment or, for that matter, to any drug. Tremor responds to many antitremor drugs including centrally acting beta-blockers (propranolol) and anticholinergics. Diphenhydramine has both a sedative and an anticholinergic effect and is often beneficial to patients whose tremor increases due to anxiety. It can also be a good hypnotic for a parkinsonian patient. Some patients may require tranquilizers in addition to antiparkinsonian drugs to control symptoms such as tremor that are exaggerated by emotional stress.

The clinical course of Parkinson's disease may be classified into five stages (Figure 2) according to the severity of symptoms and the degree of disability [1].

In Stage I, unilateral disease usually manifests as tremor. Tremor is usually seen in one of the upper extremities and early changes in the patient's handwriting (micrographia) of the involved hand may be seen. There may or

Table 3 Differential Diagnosis of Parkinsonism

Parkinsonism	
Idiopathic	Synonyms: Parkinson's disease
	Paralysis agitans
	Shaking palsy
Postencephalitic	Encephalitis lethargica (Economo's disease)
	Other viral encephalitides
Drug-induced	Reserpine
	Neuroleptics (including metaclopramide)
Toxin-induced	MPTP
	Manganese
	Carbon monoxide
	Carbon disulfide
	Cyanide
Metabolic	Hypothyroidism
	Hypoparathyroidism with basal ganglia calcification
Degenerative	Striatonigral degeneration
	Fahr's disease
Hereditary disorders	Wilson's disease
	Striatonigral degeneration

Parkinson plus
Progress supranuclear palsy
Shy-Drager syndrome
Olivopontocerebellar atrophy
Parkinson's–amyotrophic lateral sclerosis–dementia complex of Guam

Parkinsonian features may be associated with	
Degenerative	Alzheimer's disease
	Corticobasal ganglionic degeneration
	Primary pallidal atrophy
	Huntington's disease (hypokinetic rigid form)
	Hallervorden-Spatz disease
	Neurocanthocytosis
	Dystonia/parkinsonism
	Normal-pressure hydrocephalus
Vascular	Multi-infarct
	Binswanger's disease
	Arteriovenous malformation
Structural	Basal ganglia: tumor, abscess
Infection	Creutzfeldt-Jakob disease
Trauma	"Punch-drunk syndrome"
	Subdural hematoma

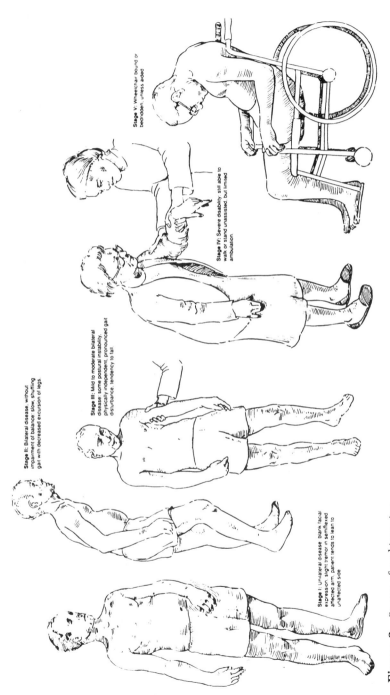

Figure 2 Stages of parkinsonism.

may not be minimal changes in posture, locomotion, facial expression, and speech. A mild degree of rigidity on the involved side and mild bradykinesia may be present. No major functional impairment is present at this stage. The patient may continue to participate in activities of daily living and remain gainfully employed. In an occasional patient, the involvement may remain unilateral, which is referred to as hemiparkinsonism. Although the patient's symptoms involve only one side, impairment of balance and gait sometimes occurs. This is referred to as stage I.5.

Bilateral involvement without impairment of balance is the next level of progression (stage II). The rate at which patients enter stage II may vary and often they are unaware of it. Sometimes the patient will state that the disease has started involving both sides of the body. In stage II, there are definite signs of rigidity, impaired gait, hypomania, and even change in the speech pattern. Patients are able to perform activities of daily living at an adequate level and continue to remain gainfully employed, even though performance of all their activities may be slower. This stage may last for a long time. Walking begins to be affected, and especially the ability to turn may be impaired. Patients do not have any difficulty maintaining their righting reflex.

The first signs of impaired righting reflex occur in stage III in addition to bilateral progression of the disease. As a result, patients may suffer moderate generalized disability. In some, tremor may be minimal with rigidity more prominent. There is definite postural abnormality and gait is definitely impaired. Despite dopaminergic therapy, patients may have significant difficulty with their righting reflex. They may be capable of independent living but mild to moderate disability will be present as they are functionally restricted. They may be able to maintain some gainful employment, depending on the nature of the occupation.

In stage IV, significant disability with progression of the disease occurs to an extent that the patient can stand and walk for short distances unaided, but is markedly incapacitated. The patient is no longer able to live alone without supervision and requires assistance in completing the ordinary activities of daily living. Turning over in bed and rising from a sitting position become difficult and the patient may have frequent falls. The gait is slow and both propulsion and retropulsion may be severe. The patient is largely confined indoors. Activities such as buttoning, putting on clothes, and others are cumbersome and can no longer be performed without help. The patient's eating habits may have to be changed; food has to be in smaller pieces and modified utensils may be needed.

Stage V entails complete invalidism. The disease is now severely advanced. The patient is confined to a wheelchair or bed and is totally disabled. It may be possible for her or him to stand and take a few steps without assistance. Speech is severely impaired and is soft.

Dopaminergic treatment will modify the clinical pattern of progression and the natural history of the disease, yet in stages III–V there may be added motor fluctuations complicating the patient's clinical condition. While the "wearing off" phenomenon (in which the duration of therapeutic benefit of a given dosage of levodopa is progressively reduced) may be controlled by increasing the frequency of doses, the "on–off" phenomenon (in which abrupt, unpredictable shifts in the motor response to a given dosage of levodopa occur) is difficult to control. Superimposed on this, dyskinesia and dystonia occur that can also be incapacitating. "Freezing," especially when the patient has to go through a narrow passage, adds to the disability. For example, when the patient needs to get into or out of an elevator, unless someone holds the door, by the time the patient is able to initiate the movement the automatic door closes. Advancing dementia and depression will interfere with rehabilitative measures and need to be addressed. While depression is amenable to pharmacotherapy, no significant treatment is available for dementia. Other complications such as hallucinations may be treated to some extent with appropriate pharmacotherapy.

Drooling requires special mention, since this is not due to excess production of saliva but to impaired swallowing mechanisms. As a result, saliva, instead of draining backwards, drools forwards. No drug is known to control drooling effectively. As a result, use of a cotton bib may be helpful. A hand towel may be used to cover the pillow at night. Radiographic studies of swallowing in patients with parkinsonism have demonstrated neuromuscular incoordination of the pharyngeal musculature. Normally, during swallowing the cricopharyngeal muscle (inferior constrictor of the pharynx) must first relax and then contract as the bolus of food enters the hypopharynx. This action of the hypopharyngeal musculature forces the bolus of food into the upper esophagus. In patients with parkinsonism, relaxation of the inferior constrictor muscle of the pharynx is delayed, causing difficulty in swallowing. As dysphagia progresses, the patient can no longer maintain adequate caloric intake and starts losing weight. Eventually, aspiration may occur in the very advanced stages of the disease. If the patient survives aspiration pneumonia, he or she may require a percutaneous gastric feeding tube. Gastrointestinal hypomotility occurs due to autonomic nervous system involvement in parkinsonism resulting in constipation. Constipation is exacerbated by reduced fluid and food intake and anticholinergic medication. After adequate fluid and fiber intake has been provided, constipation in parkinsonism is best treated by mild stimulant drugs such as senna concentrates.

Orthostatic hypotension in the form of lightheadedness can rarely be symptomatic and interfere with the patient's functions. Dopaminergic drugs could exacerbate orthostatic hypotension and, as a result, the patient's posture and walking could be further impaired. It is best treated with adequate salt intake and salt-retaining drugs such as fludrocortisone. Pressure stockings such as Jobst or Sigvoris, are difficult to use due to the patient's disability. As a result, patients often do not wear them.

Lack of motivation due to depression and fatigue is a major concern in the rehabilitation process of the parkinsonian patient. The patient is not motivated to go for a walk, which is often the best form of exercise. Fatigue is a common complaint in parkinsonism, especially in the later stages of the disease. The reason for this is unclear. Like bradykinesia, fatigue may be another consequence of impaired central dopaminergic neurotransmission. It may result in part from less efficient activation of skeletal muscle (leading to greater metabolic "cost"). A recent study from a standardized exercise task suggests that less efficient utilization of skeletal muscles during exertion may be one factor contributing to the fatigue perceived by parkinsonian patients [2]. Although no effective treatment is known for fatigue, amantadine is often helpful. No studies have been done on the role of amantadine in the fatigue of parkinsonism, but studies done in patients with multiple sclerosis have shown definite benefit [3,4].

Rehabilitation of the parkinsonian patient requires a multidisciplinary team approach coordinated by a physician well versed in all aspects of parkinsonism and with knowledge of available rehabilitative resources. Physical therapy, occupational therapy, speech therapy, dietetics, social services, psychological counselors, and the support group all play an important role, in addition to administration of adequate and appropriate pharmacotherapy, in the total well-being of the patient. Instruction of the caregiver and other interested persons in rehabilitative measures is extremely important in order to maximize the benefit to the patient. A rehabilitation program for patients with parkinsonism, especially in stages III and IV, is best undertaken in an inpatient setting. The patient's antiparkinsonian medications should first be stabilized, either before or at the beginning of their stay on the rehabilitation ward. Patients are evaluated by the entire team of professionals mentioned above. Based on the individual evaluations, appropriate therapy is initiated. Group meetings between the various therapists and the physician are held to assess progress. The physician and the family will have the opportunity to observe the patient's performance during various therapy sessions. Often family members, especially the caregiver, are trained. Before the patient is discharged, a family conference is held, the patient's home is visited by the occupational therapist to suggest changes to be made, and all assistive devices are provided to the patient. In our experience, most patients require about 2 weeks in the rehabilitation unit. At the end of the stay, their functional disability shows marked improvement over what dopaminergic drugs could alone accomplish. Similar findings are reported by others [11].

Physical Therapy

Long before the availability of levodopa, physical therapy was used in the treatment of parkinsonism [5,6]. The goals of physical therapy in parkinsonism include increased movement and range of motion, maintaining or improving chest expansion, improving equilibrium and balance and maintaining functional abilities and independence as long as possible. Additional goals are to prevent contractures and normalize the patient's disturbed movement patterns. Physical therapy is used in conjunction with pharmacotherapy, even though conclusive evidence regarding the effectiveness of physical therapy has never been established by controlled studies. Subjective reports of benefits exist, which generally attribute decreases in bradykinesia to physical therapy exercises [7–11]. Studying the benefit of physical therapy in the treatment of Parkinson's disease has been hampered by the lack of adequate objective measures. For example, in one study there was no measurable effect from a 12 week program of physical therapy [12]. In this study, simultaneous electromyographic (EMG) recordings were made at different angular velocities and peak torque area and EMG area were calculated for concentric and eccentric contractions of the ankle flexors. It is debatable whether these measures were appropriate because measuring only strengths (peak torque production) during muscle contraction (confirmed by EMG) probably does not accurately reflect the physiological changes that must occur for a parkinsonian patient to improve performance. In parkinsonism, the automatic execution of learned complex movements is disturbed. The selection of an appropriate simple movement to initiate voluntary locomotion is delayed and is sometimes even impossible. Furthermore, the amplitude of the simple movement is too small and the coordinated simultaneous or sequential execution of the multiple simple movements needed to compose a complex movement is disturbed. As a result, it takes a long time to switch from one movement to the next. This results in bradykinesia, akinesia, and start hesitation. Superimposed on this is rigidity, which is a form of isometric muscle activity. It is unclear which of these parameters changes as a result of physical therapy and what is the best way to measure these changes. This leads to contradictory results. One small trial did not confirm the efficacy of physical therapy [13] while another [14] suggested that participation in regular physical exercise was associated with a lowered (but not significantly lowered) risk of developing parkinsonism, thereby implying a slight protective effect of physical exercise. Nonetheless, physical therapy continues to be an integral part of the treatment plan for patients with parkinsonism [10,15–19].

It is important to emphasize that physical therapy should be undertaken only after optimal pharmacotherapy has been established in order to achieve the maximum benefit from the medication. Physical therapy needs to be undertaken at a time when the maximum therapeutic benefit is present. All exercise programs should be individualized to the needs of the patient. In stages I and II, when the patient is functioning adequately, the conventional wisdom is to encourage the activities and exercises normally undertaken by any healthy individual. However, for ambulatory parkinsonian patients, it is better to correct and prevent the musculoskeletal complications with an exercise program based on the patient's individual needs identified by a physical therapy assessment [20,21]. Since parkinsonism is a progressive disease, as motor problems increase, exercises may have to be supervised in an outpatient setting or group setting. In patients with advanced disease, inpatient rehabilitative programs may become necessary.

There is some evidence that outpatient exercise programs are helpful. Palmer et al. [10] quantitatively measured the strength, coordination, and speed of movement, as well as long latency and stretch reflexes following a 12 week exercise program. They found improvement in gait, strength, and coordination of fine motor tasks. However, there was no change in movement that required speed, suggesting that bradykinesia was unaffected by their exercise program. In a home-based exercise project, a weekly home exercise regimen for ambulatory patients with parkinsonism was taught by nursing students and results were compared to control patients with the same disease who did not participate in the program. The results indicated that those patients who participated in the exercise program had better mobility, feeding ability, and self-care skills than patients who did not participate. There was also improvement in recent memory, diminished nausea, improved sucking ability, and less urinary retention and incontinence in the group who exercised [22]. Some of the latter components may be related to patients' improved motivation.

Individualized and structured outpatient physical therapy, along with an educational program to improve flexibility, posture, and gait, provided significant benefits to patients with stage II and III parkinsonism [23]. For these ambulatory patients, an independently performed home-based exercise program that addressed the areas of joint range of motion, posture, locomotion and lung capacity achieved similar results to a three-times weekly one-on-one outpatient physical therapy program [24]. Harris et al. [25] reported 56% of patients with stages I and II exercised compared to 32% of patients in stages III–V. The incidence of depression was less in those who exercised. Economic status of the patient also appeared to influence whether the patient exercised or not. Those with perceived economic hardship tended not to exercise. Once the patient is in stage III or later, some of the exercises recommended in published manuals [26,27] may be practiced, but some require the help of a trained caregiver, or the involvement of a trained physical therapist to individualize patients' particular needs. The focus should be on active and passive movements for control of rigidity, gait training, and use of assistive devices such as a walker and cane. Later training may include use of a wheelchair, transfer from wheelchair to bed, and so on. No specific physical therapy is aimed at tremor, since tremor is mainly resting and pharmacotherapy is most effective in controlling it. Wrist weights may result in some reduction in tremor amplitude. Most current physical therapy programs begin with rhythmic symmetrical movements of increasing amplitude. The rhythm and auditory cues facilitate continuous movement. Exercise programs should be individualized to meet the needs of the patient, with emphasis placed on speed, mobility, and continued motion of the face, neck, trunk, and limbs. Neck and trunk rotation exercises using wide arcs of motion with the patient seated in an armless swivel rocker are also useful. Many of the exercises may be performed with the patient seated or lying down, while some require standing and walking positions. For example, since many functional motions (such as rolling to get out of bed) require neck and trunk rotation, seated exercises using wide arcs of motion are helpful to improve range of motion and balance, while the rhythmic repetitive motion can help with initiating movement. In patients with severe gait disturbance, walking balance may be practiced with a rolling walker (Figure 3), in parallel bars or marching in place. Exercise instruction often involves spouses to enhance socialization and to motivate patients. Family supervision can also improve and correct exercise performance at home.

Breathing exercises stressing both the inspiratory and expiratory phases may be undertaken to improve lung capacity. This promotes relaxation and improves voice projection. Facial exercises performed while the patient is seated in front of a mirror can be part of the program.

Dishwashing (pots and pans too!) is an excellent form of physical therapy for the hands and can be done two to three times a day. What variety this activity offers when compared to repeatedly pressing a tennis ball or clay (how boring). If done standing at the sink, dishwashing also becomes a balancing activity.

Assistive devices such as canes (straight or quad canes) and standard or rolling walkers can be helpful to stabilize patients or prevent an excessive forward lean. While the use of a cane is a sign of being a "gentleman" in certain cultures, North American patients resist the use of a cane since it is considered a sign of aging. Use of these devices needs to be properly evaluated and taught so that they improve gait, not exacerbate it. For example, when patients attempt to use a quad cane, they may not know how to coordinate the cane with their walking or the introduction may increase incoordination by unbalancing the weight distribution between the two sides of the body. Canes and walkers can "get in the way," increasing the likelihood of falling. A standard walker may increase "start hesitation" while

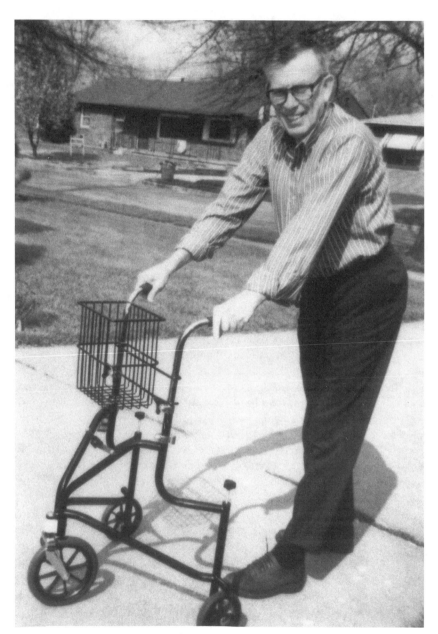

Figure 3 A patient with ataxia using a three-wheeled walker ("Rajowalt").

wheeled walkers sometimes encourage excessive speed, accentuating the illusion of the patient "catching up to her center of gravity."

On the other hand, assistive devices may help with partial instability and a wheeled walker may improve the fluidity of movement. In some patients, the height of the walker may be shortened to shift the center of gravity forward, counteracting the patients' tendency to lean back while walking. However, overcorrecting this problem may result in balancing the patient forward, increasing forward speed or causing forward falls. Therapists take all these factors into account when they evaluate the need for assistive gait devices.

Proper clothing and footwear are important. Leather-soled shoes move much more easily than rubber-soled ones. Sweat suits with elastic waist pants or Velcro closures facilitate dressing and undressing.

Compliance may become a problem after the initial month or two of the rehabilitation program. After awhile there is gradual decline in motivation. The daily discipline an exercise program requires does not seem worth it when the patient cannot see the regression prevented. Even if positive changes occur, and they usually do, they occur so gradually that the patient may not notice them and then sees no benefit from the exercise efforts. Therefore, periodic visits to physical therapists, at least once every 6 months, are helpful to assess changes and remotivate the patient. Therapists will also adjust or correct exercise performance and assess additional needs of the patient, including the need for assistive devices. In general, once physical therapy is initiated, it should be a continuing process and not a one-time event. This is because the patient's needs will change as the disease progresses. As with antiparkinsonian drugs, frequent monitoring of rehabilitative measures is necessary.

Gait Disturbance

Walking is a learned skill, and the one most valued by all individuals. Therefore, gait disorders, or the inability to walk properly, constitute a major challenge to rehabilitation professionals. Although impairments frequently affect both the swing and stance phases of gait, the most disabling impairments occur during the stance phase [28]. Regardless of the cause of the walking impairment, it is frequently associated with the inability of the affected lower extremities to accept, bear, and transfer the weight of the body forward. Postural stability is an essential component for stable walking. The pathophysiology of postural instability is not well understood, complicating the development of an effective treatment. Movements of the trunk and arms in a standing human subject are preceded by preparatory muscular activity in postural trunk and leg muscles [29,30]. This preparatory activity seems to be an integral part of a particular motor program: it provides destabilization of the center of gravity due to limb or trunk movements. The question remains whether this preparatory motor activity is centrally programmed as a unit and processed in parallel pathways, or whether it reflects a hierarchy of an organized motor pattern [31]. The center of gravity in normalized posture lies 3–8 cm anterior to the ankles. Sensory input provides information about deviations in the center of gravity from its normal position over the feet. The body responds to the deviations with a series of coordinated automatic motor responses aimed at correcting the deviation in the center of gravity that include anticipatory reactions: events that occur in anticipation of an alteration in the center of gravity; compensatory righting reflexes: events that occur at the time of unacceptable deviation from the normal center of gravity; rescue reactions: a final attempt to restore equilibrium if falling is imminent; protective reactions: events to reduce the impact of the fall [32].

Postural control is the ability to maintain equilibrium in a gravitational field by keeping or returning the center of body mass over its base of support. Execution of postural control requires a smooth coordination between three basic functional components of the postural control system. These are the biomechanical components that execute the motor act of balance: bones, muscles, ligaments, and others; the sensory organization components that carry internal and external sensory information to the central nervous system: the visual, vestibular, and proprioceptive systems; and the motor coordination components, which are the least understood of the three and refer to the wide repertoire of autonomic postural reactions orchestrated by the central nervous system dealing with expected and unexpected destabilizing situations [33]. In parkinsonism, there is a primary abnormality of postural control mechanisms. Hypokinesis causes decreased range of motion which may impair the body's motor response to deviations from the normal center of gravity. Simian posture shifts the center of gravity. Thus, falling is a serious problem in parkinsonism since it can lead to severe injury. In one study, 38% of patients reported falls; of these 13% fell more than once a week. Fractured bones occurred in 13%; hospitalization in 18%, and permanent confinement to wheelchair in 3%. Incidents of falling are related to the age of the patient, severity of the disease, postural instability, bradykinesia and rigidity, but not to tremor. Frequency of falls and postural stability is not influenced by dopaminergic therapy [34]. Risk factors for fall may be grouped as extrinsic or intrinsic. Extrinsic factors are environmentally related, and include poor lighting, stairs that do not have a side rail, throw rugs, and furniture being closely arranged. Intrinsic risk factors include the disease itself, drug-induced dyskinesia, cognitive impairment, and defective vision, including difficulty with accommodation due to anticholinergic drugs. Navigating through narrow spaces, for example, a hallway or getting in and out of an elevator, can precipitate "freezing" (akinesia paradoxica), which may result in a fall. Patients tend to hurry in order to maintain the speed necessary to "catch up self with balance," while getting in and out of an elevator, and other movements. Unfortunately, this increases the risk of a fall.

It is difficult to teach balance to patients but training by a rehabilitation team is desirable. A home visit may be very helpful to minimize or eliminate environmental risks of falling. Patients can be trained to assume the best posture for optimal upright balance and to practice dynamic balance exercises, including leaning from side to side and doing rotary hip exercises. Exercise helps patients learn to adjust their balance for a greater sense of security. Pointers on such simple things as getting out of a chair or bed by getting closer to the edge, and using the bedside table as a support to rise, are often as important in preventing falls as gait improvement. Patients with orthostatic hypotension should be taught to sit at the edge of the bed or chair for a short period of time before getting up to minimize or eliminate the orthostatic component causing lightheadedness.

Gait improvement is an important part of the rehabilitation training program. The emphasis is placed on promoting arm swing, lengthening stride, turning, starting and stopping. A long board, 10–15 cm wide, can be placed on the floor so the patient can practice walking with a wider base of support, placing one foot on each side of the board. Teaching a family member to hold a gait belt tied to the patient's waist provides additional security in helping the patient walk. Canes and walkers, discussed earlier, frequently provide increased stability as do railings in the hallway. Yet some patients may require assistance by holding onto another person when they walk. In one study practicing oriental T'ai Chi exercises resulted in significant improvements in balance [33]. It may be helpful to teach patients to improve their stability through Asian self-defense arts like karate and Judo, or exercises like T'ai Chi that emphasize a wide-based stance in combination with slight flexion at the knee and hip.

Exercise that promotes general fitness should be encouraged in patients with mild parkinsonism. Walking is the widest single choice for most patients. This is not only a good form of exercise but is also relaxing. In colder climates, walking may be undertaken in the morning in a shopping mall, big department store, or even in the airport, since these places are heated and adequate security is present. Swimming could be one of the best forms of exercise since it lessens wear and tear on the joints, but is less accessible to most people than walking. However, because of bradykinesia, swimming should be undertaken in shallow water in the presence of a lifeguard. Ballroom dancing is an excellent way to improve one's ability to shift weight, a necessary component of balance. Dancing can also help with coordination of the extremities and with trunk rotation.

The general consensus is that physical therapy is helpful in reducing the incidence of falling [8,10,17,34–37]. Prevention is obviously the best means of avoiding the many problems associated with falls. When a fall itself cannot be prevented, attempts can be made to minimize injury. In fact, karate, judo, T'ai Chi, and similar techniques teach "safe" falling. There are other more expensive and specialized mechanical devices available, such as an overhead trolley that is able to roll along a ceiling-molded track (Figure 4). For a patient with severe cerebral ataxia, the father, who was a paratrooper, developed such a system using a parachute harness that helped the patient to walk in the basement at home. However, a device such as this requires installation and mobility is limited. A more advanced device uses a trolley attached to a special vest-like garment that a person wears. If the person falls, the system catches and lowers the patient gently to the floor. Another system uses "active air bags" with carbon dioxide cartridges similar to those found in life jackets, which are inserted into special garments. When sensors detect the onset of a fall, the cartridges eject gas into the air bag around the hips and knees, thus minimizing the injury [38]. Other devices include a pneumatic system mounted over a conductive walkway placed between parallel bars [39]. This device, of course, had significant limitations because it requires parallel bars.

Occupational Therapy

The purpose of occupational therapy is to teach patients to use their "intrinsic motivation" to influence their social and physical environment through purposeful activity. Occupational therapists provide teaching and practice in learning new or compensatory techniques for doing familiar things, as well as analyzing the process involved so that a skill may be retaught, step-by-step. Assistive devices to ease or make possible the accomplishment of specific tasks are sometimes provided together with instruction on how to use the device. The need for occupational therapy services may be identified by anyone who recognizes such functional problems as difficulty in self-care, poor balance, trouble in dressing or bathing, poor judgment, and declining safety practices. An occupational therapist would evaluate the patient's limitations, evaluate strengths and deficits and plan a program that best suits the patient's pursuit of a life of the highest possible quality, keeping in mind individual parameters of lifestyle, culture, leisure values, and education and social experiences [40]. Early intervention will assist in overcoming problems as they arise due to changes in the patient's condition, and may reduce the likelihood of accidents. A liaison between physician, physical and occupational therapists will be important in planning some of the activities for the patient.

A visit to the patient's home by an occupational therapist is often

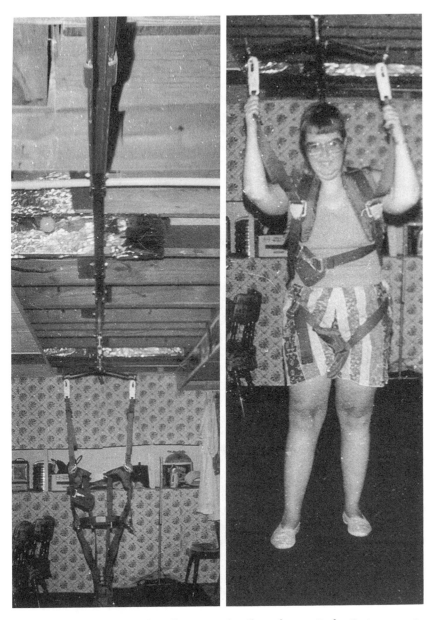

Figure 4   Left: Overhead trolley-assisted walking device. Right: Patient wearing parachute harness.

beneficial to the patient and the family. The therapist evaluates environmental factors, such as home set-up, floor plan, presence of stairs, pattern of the bathroom, and others, and can recommend physical changes that should be made to accommodate the patient and encourage maximum independence. Access from the street to the patient's home should be suitable. If there are steps, it may be necessary to install a hand rail or, if a wheelchair has to be used, a ramp may have to be built. It is desirable for the patient to have the kitchen, living room, bedroom, and bathroom at street level. The house should be well lit, including the bedroom and bathroom. Since one of the major risks in parkinsonism is a fall, some furniture to hold on to or a handrail should be provided at all appropriate areas for patients to get around the house. A number of additional devices can be helpful to both the patient and caretaker. In the bathroom these include grab bars at the tub, toilet and shower; bath seat or a bench for tub or shower; power toothbrush (battery or electric) or a handle for the toothbrush; sports ring hung from the ceiling and chained at transfer points to toilet or tub. A raised toilet seat is helpful. In some cases, caregivers find that a Hoyer lift has saved their backs in getting the patients from bed to commode or wheelchair. The bathroom should be large enough in which to move around. In the kitchen, adaptive suggestions may include grab bars beside stove and work areas, a lap board (such as a large wooden cutting board) to carry items from the stove to the sink while seated in a wheelchair, food processor, plastic placemats to keep plates from sliding off the table, silverware with large handles, spill-proof cups and straws for drinking, attachments for handles on tableware, and a plate guard. Adaptations for the bedroom include a light that can be turned on and off from the bed, and a night light. Top bed sheets that are oversized will stay tucked in better. Satin sheets are desirable, since they make moving in bed much smoother. Pajamas and night gowns can be made of either satin or silk for added benefit. A firm mattress makes it easy to get in and out of bed. A waterbed should be avoided. A bicycle water bottle that will not spill can be kept on the bedside table if medications are to be taken. Some patients may require a bedside commode. A hospital bed is desirable, depending on the stage of the disease. A twin bed that the patient can get in and out from either side is more desirable than a king- or queen-sized bed. Many spouses find it difficult to sleep in the same bedroom because patients generally tend to get up several times at night. A telephone should contain large numbers and one with a speaker may be easier to use. Sometimes, an amplifier can be added to the telephone. Some patients find the use of a suction machine invaluable if a serious swallowing problem exists. A caregiver must be thoroughly trained to use such a device by a qualified therapist after a doctor's prescription has been obtained. The living room could contain a firm chair with a high back to support the head. Some patients may find a lift chair, especially a "Lazy Boy" type more desirable since the patient is likely to spend several hours in a chair. The television should have a larger screen with a remote control; the remote should have a larger button panel and be simple in design. For communication, especially since handwriting is affected, a typewriter or, even better, a computer such as a portable "lap-top," would be highly desirable. With such a device, the patient could be independent and deal with correspondence. When walking becomes difficult in stage IV, and the patient must use a wheelchair for community outings, a wheelchair with arms, a seat belt, and a chest belt is desirable. A bicycle water bottle and a bracket can be attached to the wheelchair. A wheelchair caddie can be added to the top of an automobile to carry the wheelchair or a van can be equipped with a wheelchair lift.

Loose clothes or sweat suits, with elastic waist bands or Velcro closures, are desirable. Comfortable pants for persons sitting in wheelchairs are available. Western shirts with snaps are a consideration. Otherwise, buttons on shirts can be replaced with snaps. If a tie must be worn, a clip-on is desirable. A button aid to help with buttons may be needed in some cases. Boots with zippers or elastic shoe laces might be used. A long-handled shoe horn is recommended. Sometimes a dressing stick is helpful. The American Parkinson's Disease Association has published a book listing many of the above items with appropriate illustrations [41]. Very occasionally, a urinal may need to be carried with the patient when going outdoors. All of the above may not be applicable for every patient; choices are based on each patients' needs.

Employment

Most patients can continue their current occupation after they are diagnosed as having parkinsonism. Some readjustment in the nature of the occupation may have to be made, especially in occupations that involve heights, handwriting, or fine coordinated handwork. While in the majority of patients the disease starts in the fifth to seventh decade of life, in some the disease may start earlier. Hence, the ability to remain employed becomes an important issue. Sidney Dorros, author of *Parkinson's: A Patient's View*, acquired the disease at age 38, remained employed for a long period of time, and continued to participate actively in Parkinson's disease support groups. It is desirable to let the employer know about the disease, as well as family and friends, since sooner or later the symptoms of the disease are visible and they will find out. If they are not knowledgeable about the symptoms of parkinsonism, they may become suspicious that something is wrong. Some patients have been misunderstood to be alcoholic or "on drugs." Despite the fact that the most consistent thing about parkinsonism is its inconsistencies, it is not unusual for a patient to remain gainfully employed for several years. Each patient should be assessed individually. Many individuals have continued to retain their employment for a long period of time. When the patient can no longer function adequately, he or she should be able to receive medical disability or take early retirement.

Driving

Driving may be considered a combination of a continuous tracking task and a multiple choice reaction time task, requiring actions involving sequential movements of limbs and joints. Judgment, planning, perception, and attention are also critical for safe driving. Many of these abilities may be impaired in patients with parkinsonism [42]. Yet in order to maintain independence, driving is necessary in many American communities and elsewhere in the world. Study of a small sample of patients with parkinsonism in Britain revealed that most individuals had given up driving a car but only a third of the group had notified the driving and vehicle licensing department of their disorder. Most patients likewise had not informed their insurance companies of their diagnosis. A small number of patients admitted that parkinsonism had been a contributory factor in an accident involving another vehicle. Giving up driving exacerbated the premature social aging often encountered by patients with parkinsonism [43]. Dulsimsky et al. [42], in an interview based study of patients with parkinsonism, found that with increased disability a smaller percentage of patients drove, with fewer miles traveled but proportionally more accidents occurring. Although the disability scores did not correlate well with driving ability, there were significantly more accidents among subjects with more severe parkinsonism. In another study, a computerized driving simulator was used to examine the effect of parkinsonism on driving abilities. Patients were compared to age- and gender-matched healthy controls. Both the simulated driving reaction time and the accuracy of steering were significantly impaired in the group with parkinsonism compared to the controls. Parkinsonian patients missed the highest number of red traffic lights [43]. These simulated test results should be interpreted with caution, since patients who volunteer for such studies could be those with more confidence than others who have a greater degree of impairment. Several additional factors need to be considered, including where the patients may be driving (rural or urban area), degree of bradykinesia, and presence of any dementia. Termor itself may not be a major factor in determining driving ability. Presence of "on–off" phenomenon could have a major impact on driving abilities because of the inability to predict when the "off" effect may happen. Questions regarding ability to drive are among those most frequently asked by patients. In the absence of any definite guidelines to determine whether the patient should drive or not, physicians and families often tend to lean towards safety considerations, and recommend that the patient not drive. Patients, however, are likely to insist on maintaining driving privileges.

Speech Disorders

In an early prevalence study, 73% of all parkinsonian patients were observed to have some form of speech disturbance [44]. Subsequent studies have shown an incidence of about 45–49% [45,46]. As the disease progresses toward its later stage, the prevalence of speech disturbance increases to almost 100%. Speech disturbances in patients with parkinsonism include deviations of phonation producing monotony of pitch, monotony of loudness, and a breathy or mildly harsh voice; disturbances of rate or cadence, resulting in slow or extremely fast rate of speech, periodic rhythm changes with inappropriate silences, or repetition of sounds and syllables giving the impression of stuttering speech; articulatory disorder with distortion of the sounds of speech; and alterations in loudness, and decay of voice. All of this combined has been referred to as "hypokinetic dysarthria." In addition, many patients may present with palilalia: an involuntary, compulsive repetition of sentences or phrases [47].

The initial defect in patients with parkinsonism is a failure to control respiration for the purpose of speech. Following this, there is a forward progression of articulatory symptoms involving the larynx, pharynx, tongue, and finally, the lips. These is evidence that integration of speech production is organized asymmetrically at the thalamic level. Experimental or therapeutic lesions in the region of the inferior medial portion of the ventrolateral thalamus may influence initiation, respiratory control, prosody, and process of speech. The thalamus may also be involved in the integration of higher language functioning [48]. More than 100 muscles are normally involved in articulation, producing phonemes at a rate of 14/sec. Thus, several hundred individual muscle events of contraction, relaxation, and maintenance of tone occur every second [49]. In parkinsonism, the most common defect in articulation is an unnatural regulatory and equality of articulatory movement produced by stiffness of facial, oral, buccal, and pharyngeal muscles [50] resulting in a hypokinetic dysarthria [51].

Levodopa has some beneficial effect on speech. Clonazepam in low dosages is reported to be effective in parkinsonian dysarthria [52]. Yet the benefit of drugs may be minimal rather than substantial, and speech therapy plays a definite role. One should make sure that the patient has no associated hearing impairment before beginning speech therapy. A main goal of treatment is to assist the patient to achieve maximum effectiveness of communication within the limits of their speech production mechanisms. It has been suggested that patients should adopt an erect posture, take a deep breath before initiating speech, speak only a few words with each breath, and speak facing the listener. Patients should also practice reading aloud. Music therapy for parkinsonian patients is strongly encouraged, since this may help voice volume by increasing vocal projection ability. Music may also help patients to synchronize movement when they develop akinesia paradoxica ("freezing"), since they can easily "walk to music." Music acts as a stimulus connecting thought process to action. Another interesting treatment involves the use of a pocket-sized delayed auditory feedback (DAF) device, which has been helpful in decreasing the frequent blocking and hesitation that sometimes makes speech totally unintelligible. In one study, short delay in feedback of 50 msec showed a dramatic improvement, resulting in a slowing of the speech so that the syllables became clearly separated [53]. However, these changes occurred only through continuous use of DAF; periodic use of the device did not result in any noticeable carryover of the reduction of speech rate. In other studies, daily speech therapy (prosodic exercises) resulted in significant improvement of speech [54]. Certain exercises may be practiced for speech improvement; these are well presented in a booklet published by the American Parkinson's Disease Association [55]. In patients with serious hypophonia, the underlying cause is often bowing of the vocal folds. The bowing is effectively treated by injecting collagen into the vocal folds, which increases amplitude and duration of phonation.

In an occasional patient these efforts do not work. In these situations, communication charts (alphabetical chart, printed word communication chart, picture communication chart) may be tried. A typewriter, or a computer with printer or screen, preferably a portable one ("lap top"), is sometimes helpful. More sophisticated devices, including augmentative communication systems, may be appropriate for selected patients.

Dysphagia

Dysphagia and a variety of swallowing abnormalities are well-recognized complications of parkinsonism. The subjective discomfort, difficulty in handling oral medications, nutritional problems, and, most importantly, the high incidence of fatal bronchopulmonary pneumonia attest to the clinical importance of this problem [1]. Drooling, which occurs early in the disease, is an example of an impaired swallowing mechanism. This improves to some extent with dopaminergic treatment. A few studies have addressed the effects of levodopa therapy, but the results are controversial [56–58]. As the disease advances, patients develop increased difficulty with swallowing. It is suggested that the patient make a conscious effort to swallow often, including before attempting to speak. When eating, tucking the chin closer to the chest during swallowing reduces the risk of aspiration. In those patients with poor control of neck muscles, reclining at 60 degrees with head support has been found to result in improved oral intake with reduced risk of aspiration as demonstrated by videofluoroscopy. This is considered to be due to greater body and neck support, reduced anxiety, and possibly reduced fatigue of muscles of mastication (Victoria S. Mlacknik, MS, CCC-SLP, personal communication). Eating small bites of food, chewing well, and swallowing before taking another bite of food is recommended. Smooth solids and thick liquids are easier to swallow. It is desirable for the caregiver to learn the Heimlich maneuver, in the event that the patient has a choking episode.

Nursing Care

Once the patient reaches stage IV and V, nursing care gains importance. The intensity of nursing care may vary from a caregiver assisting with basic care to nursing home professionals administering care around the clock. Nursing care includes help with feeding, making sure adequate liquid is consumed, help in the shower, help with personal hygiene and getting dressed, providing adequate mobility, and, for a bedridden patient, turning the patient periodically to prevent pneumonia, deep vein thrombosis, and pressure ulcers. A patient is generally encouraged to self-feed and any needed modification of silverware and utensils may be provided by an occupational therapist. Patients will generally be slower to eat than others. While the rest of the diners are ready for dessert, the patient may still be eating the soup or salad. For that reason, going out for dinner gradually becomes less desirable. Better control of symptoms is facilitated by taking dopaminergic medication about 30 min before mealtime.

General personal hygiene such as showering will certainly need attention. Constipation is a common problem. Use of a mild stimulant laxative is recommended, but the diet should contain adequate fluids and fiber. Fecal incontinence is uncommon, but if it occurs the cause may be the patient's immobility. Urinary incontinence is not uncommon. Side effects from use of dopamine agonists (bromocriptine, pergolide) should not be overlooked. If symptoms persist after use of the dopamine agonist is stopped, local causes should be excluded. Severe bradykinesia should be considered if no other causes are found. The use of a bedside urinal, especially at night, should be encouraged.

Patients often do not sleep continuously at night because they nap several times during the day. This often becomes a main concern of the family. The major reason this occurs is that it is extremely difficult, even for a normal person, to sit still and do nothing; for example, during a long-distance airplane flight more than 50% of the "normal" passengers doze off after a period of time. This interferes with the rest of the family members' ability to get adequate sleep, especially the spouse, who is often the main caregiver. Sometimes the patient may not be able to sleep with the spouse in the same bedroom. Occasionally, tremor can keep the patient from falling asleep. If this happens, use of diphenhydramine is recommended, since it acts as a sedative and controls the tremor enough to aid sleep. Depression can cause insomnia and should be evaluated. In patients with associated dementia, nightmares, hallucinations, and what is referred to as "sundown" syndrome may develop. All may require proper management with pharmacological agents.

In most communities, home health care is available to supervise patients at home. When this is no longer possible, placement in a skilled care nursing home facility may become necessary. A great majority of patients with parkinsonism have a spouse for support. Occasionally, a patient without family support may need a nursing home facility at a premature stage, because living independently becomes impossible. Some patients can be managed at a senior citizen retirement facility where the patient lives in a studio apartment or a room with maid service, in-house dining facilities, transportation, and other support services.

Studies done after levodopa became available suggested that levodopa, through its action on the hypothalamic–pituitary–gonadal axis, resulted in increased sexual desire in male patients that was unrelated to improvement in locomotor function [59]. However, further observation suggests that problems with sexual function are a more common complaint from patients with parkinsonism [60,61]. No large studies have been done to estimate prevalence rate. Many things may affect sexual function in a parkinsonian patient, including autonomic nervous system involvement, depression, motor disabilities, and feeling unattractive or having a negative self-image. The patient's partner may interpret the unemotional expression on their loved one's face as a lack of sexual interest. In one small study [60] of patients who had had parkinsonism for an average of 10 years or longer, patients and partners were evaluated for sexual satisfaction, frequency, avoidance, lack of sensuality, premature ejaculation, impotence, vaginismus, and anorgasmia. Although some cases could be attributed to the disease, psychological and social factors affecting both the patients and their partners were more commonly involved, and no single factor could be identified. In a small number of patients, hypersexuality is reported [62].

Diet and Nutrition

A well-balanced diet is encouraged for the proper well-being of all individuals, including patients with parkinsonism. However, the average American's diet contains about 100 g protein, which is far in excess of the needs of a patient with parkinsonism, the major concern being that excess protein consumption may interfere with absorption of levodopa. Deterioration in levodopa effectiveness may be due to the erratic delivery of levodopa to the dopamine-depleted brain in advanced parkinsonism, while in the early stages of the disease there is still some capacity by the brain to store dopamine [63]. The factor responsible for this is considered to be the large neutral amino acids (LNAAs), which include phenylalanine, tyrosine, leucine, isoleucine, valine, tryptophan, and methionine. There appears to be no difference in percentage of total LNAAs derived from various sources of protein, whether animal or plant. No data are available on the minimum daily amount of dietary protein needed to interfere with absorption. One study [64] showed that a daily protein intake of 50 g/day for men and 40 g/day for women resulted in statistically significant improved performance. Berry et al. [65] found that plasma LNAAs were stable for 2 hr following a balanced meal, but the 2 hr mean plasma levodopa level was higher from a high-carbohydrate diet than either a balanced diet or a high-protein diet. The motor performance tests used were not standardized to evaluated parkinsonian performance and hence no definite conclusions can be drawn from this study.

When dietary protein is restricted, it should be replaced by carbohydrates without making much change in fat consumption. Because patients are more active during the day and their protein absorption may interfere with levodopa absorption, the major protein in the diet is taken at the evening meal. Breakfast and lunch are high in carbohydrates and very low in protein [66]. This is called a "protein redistribution diet." The diet should, of course, contain adequate fiber in the form of fresh fruits and vegetables. A well-planned diet should provide all the necessary vitamins and minerals. However, it is important to avoid ingesting excessive amounts of vitamin B6 (pyridoxine), since it may interfere with levodopa metabolism. A low-dosage vitamin B6 multiple vitamin preparation is available if needed, but it is expensive. As the disease advances, the patient's regular food may be replaced by semisolids and soft foods. Because of the complex nature of the nutritional needs of the patient with parkinsonism, it is best to consult a clinical dietitian to plan an adequate diet to maintain optimal nutritional status.

Social Services

Parkinsonism is an expensive disease. The cost of the medications alone is significant. One study revealed that the median cost for caring for an uncomplicated patient with parkinsonism was $2,820.00 per year [25]. Add to this the cost for medical care, nursing, rehabilitation, and other needs, and expenses can quickly surpass the patient's financial resources. Furthermore, finding a suitable skilled care facility convenient for family visits is also important, as is the need for assistive devices. A social service worker is an invaluable source for information about financial aid, local skilled care facilities, and the many other health care services available to patients with Parkinson's disease and their families. Social workers often begin working with patients at the onset of the disease and continue throughout the duration of the illness.

Support Groups

There are several Parkinson's disease support groups organized at local, state, and national levels. These organizations help patients and their families with problems arising from parkinsonism, and disseminate information relating to the illness. They also collect funds for Parkinson's disease research. Information is distributed in the form of newsletters, and lectures on various topics of interest are presented at meetings by various experts in the field. The support group serves as a platform for socialization and provides valuable contact for patients and their families. The groups publish small booklets on the disease itself, on physical therapy, occupational therapy, and other topics of interest. These organizations play a vital role in the social rehabilitation of the patient.

HUNTINGTON'S DISEASE

Huntington's disease, which is inherited in an autosomal dominant fashion, results in dementia and chorea. In the great majority of patients, symptoms first appear in adult life. However, in a small percentage of patients, hypokinesia and rigidity appear in place of chorea. This is referred to as the Westphal variant, and is especially seen in patients who are younger at the onset of disease. Patients with the hypokinetic rigid form look like parkinsonian patients and many of the items discussed above apply to them. In classic Huntington's disease, in addition to chorea, significant gait abnormalities are common. Dysarthria, dysphagia, cachexia, and progressive dementia occur. Functional disability in Huntington's disease usually results from a combination of movement disorders, intellectual decline and psychopathological changes. Of these, intellectual impairment seems to be the major problem, reducing functioning capability in the early stages of the disease [67]. Rehabilitative efforts should focus on occupational therapy, speech therapy, swallowing, nursing, and social services. Support groups for patients with Huntington's disease are available in many communities. Chorea itself does not improve with physical therapy. Chorea is actually an exercise, consuming excessive calories, and if coupled with inadequate calorie intake, may result in significant weight loss. Gait training is important, since gait disturbances in Huntington's disease do not respond to pharmacotherapy. Many of the issues related to rehabilitation in parkinsonism discussed earlier also apply to Huntington's disease. Similar principles apply to the management of hemichorea and other types of chorea.

DYSTONIA

Dystonia is characterized by involuntary spasms or muscle contractions that induce abnormal movements and sustained posture. Dystonic spasms may affect one part of the body, such as the eyes, neck, or a limb (focal dystonia); a larger region, such as the neck and arms (segmental dystonia); many parts of the body (multifocal dystonia); the arm and leg on the same side (hemidystonia); or the whole body (generalized dystonia). Dystonic syndromes can be primary (idiopathic) or secondary (symptomatic). Most focal dystonias respond to injections of *botulinum* toxin. Hemidystonia and multifocal and generalized dystonias respond only slightly to pharmacotherapy (high dosages of trihexyphenidyl), so rehabilitation efforts, especially occupational therapy, are important. Physical therapy for the dystonias is of limited value because of the sustained muscle contraction usually accompanying these conditions. However, persons with generalized dystonia may benefit from gait and other mobility training, including instruction in wheelchair use for patients with advanced disease.

ESSENTIAL TREMOR

Essential tremor is an autosomal dominant inherited disorder that can cause considerable disability due to a sustained tremor that interferes with patient's function. The majority of tremors respond to pharmacological treatment and rehabilitative measures are usually limited to occupational therapy. Wrist weights can dampen the amplitude of tremor but are of limited value.

OTHER MOVEMENT DISORDERS

In patients with tics, ballismus, and myoclonus, rehabilitation benefits are limited, but an occasional patient may benefit from occupational therapy. In those with tardive dyskinesia, in which the symptoms are usually drug induced, rehabilitative efforts may be limited by the presence of an underlying psychotic disturbance. Nevertheless, some patients may benefit, so each case should be assessed individually.

ATAXIAS

The term "ataxia," from the Greek, means "without order." Today, the word is used to mean incoordination. Ataxia is independent of any motor weakness. It alters the direction and extent of voluntary movements and impairs the sustained voluntary or reflex muscle contractions necessary for maintaining posture and equilibrium. Ataxia generally refers to disorders involving the cerebellum and its connections. However, a patient may be ataxic from lesions of the peripheral nerve, dorsal root, spinal cord, brainstem, vestibular system, frontal lobe, or partial lobe. The group of diseases that cause ataxia also feature other symptoms of cerebellar dysfunction including dysmetria, intention tremor, hypotonia, dysarthria, dysphagia, and fatigue. There are often associated skeletal deformities such as kyphosis or foot deformities. Both inherited and acquired conditions cause ataxia, the latter including infectious, toxic, metabolic, and other causes.

Pharmacotherapy for ataxias is not satisfactory [68]. Rehabilitative measures are most important in the management of patients with ataxia. Early rehabilitation goals include maintaining safe ambulation and independence in activities of daily living. As ataxia progresses, use of assistive devices, such as a walker, may be necessary to maintain balance. Use of lower extremity orthotic devices may occasionally be beneficial in stabilizing the ankle and in increasing proprioceptive input. When ataxia progresses to involvement of the trunk and upper extremities, patients typically become wheelchair-bound. At this point, proper wheelchair seating is paramount to optimize self care and prevent such complications as pressure sores and compressive nerve palsies. A molded seat with posterior lumbar support, low thoracic lateral supports, and slight posterior inclination of the seating system is recommended [69]. To aid upper extremity functioning, stabilization of the proximal joints and distal weighting may be used. The occupational therapist may devise a built-up handle for pencil, toothbrush, spoon, fork, and other tools to make the patient as independent as possible. Home modifications, such as wheelchair access, toilet riser, shower bars, and modified wash basin may be used as necessary. Speech therapy may be beneficial in facilitating improvement in articulation and swallowing function. If severe dysarthria develops, use of a communications board may be necessary. A typewriter or a personal computer has been found to be helpful for some patients. As the disease progresses further, joint contractures may develop as mobility becomes increasingly limited. At this point, it is most important to maintain adequate range of motion in all joints through an aggressive stretching program. Family members can often be integrated into the rehabilitation process to continue these programs at home.

Many hereditary forms of ataxia begin during adolescence and result in progressive deterioration, so patients and their families require considerable psychological support.

SUMMARY

The neurorehabilitative management of patients with parkinsonism, movement disorders, and ataxias require a multidisciplinary approach. Through careful evaluation and follow-up, our patients' lives can be made much more comfortable. In the meantime, researchers will continue to try to unlock the mysteries surrounding these diseases' causes and pharmacological treatment.

ACKNOWLEDGMENT

The author acknowledges the critical review and valuable suggestions on the sections on parkinsonism, physical therapy, and gait disturbance by Denise E. Herrmann, and editorial assistance by Stacey J. Warren and Linda S. Stevenson.

REFERENCES

1. M. Hoehn and P.A. Yahr, *Neurology*, 17:427–442 (1967).
2. A. Bharucha, I. Chitrit, S. Patil, C. Takis, B. Pichurko, and P. LeWitt, *Neurology*, 42 (Suppl. 3):309 (1992).
3. T.J. Murray, *Can. J. Neurol. Sci.*, 12:251– 259 (1985).
4. G.A. Rosenberg and O. Appenzeller, *Arch. Neurol.*, 45:1104–1106 (1988).
5. L.J. Hurwitz, *Lancet*, 2:953–955 (1964).
6. J. Brumlik, *Am. J. Phys. Med.*, 46:536–543 (1967).
7. W. Murray, *Phys. Ther. Rev.*, 36:587–594 (1956).
8. F.B. Gibberd, G.R. Page, K.M. Spencer, and J.B. Williams, *Research Progress in Parkinson's Disease* (F.C. Rose and R. Capildeo, eds.), Pitman Medical, Tunbridge Wells, pp. 401–403 (1981).
9. K.R. Gustavsson and L.W. Nilsson, *Sjukgymnasten*:19–21 (1983).
10. S.S. Palmer, J.A. Mortimer, D.D. Webster, R. Bistevins, and G.L. Dickinson, *Arch. Phys. Med. Rehabil.*, 67:741–745 (1986).
11. J.M. Cedarbaum, L. Toy, M. Silvestri, A. Green-Parsons, A. Harts, and F.H. McDowell, Tenth International Parkinson's Disease Symposium 145 (1991).
12. S.E. Pedersen, B. Öberg, A. Isulander, and M. Vretman, *Scand. J. Rehab. Med.*, 22:207–211 (1990).
13. E.B. Gibberd, N.G.R. Page, K.M. Spencer, E. Kinnear, and J.B. Hawksworth, *Br. Med. J.*, 282:1196 (1981).
14. A.J. Sasco, R.S. Paffenbarger, Jr., I. Gendre, and A.L. Wing, *Arch. Neurol.*, 49: 360–365 (1992).
15. M. Greer, *Geriatrics*, 31:89–96 (1976).
16. S.J. Perlik, W.C. Koller, W.J. Weiner, P. Nausieda, and H.L. Klawans, *Geriatrics*, 35:65–70 (1980).
17. B.C. Szekely, K.N. Neiberg, and W. Sheppard, *Rehabil. Litl.*, 43:72–76 (1982).
18. W.J. Weiner and C. Singer, *J. Am. Geriatr. Soc.*, 37:359–363 (1989).
19. M. Schenkman and R.B. Butler, *Phys. Ther.*, 69:932–943 (1989).
20. M.P. Yekukutiel, A. Pinhasov, G. Shahar, and H. Sroka, *Clin. Rehabil.*, 5:207–214 (1991).
21. M. Schenlman, J. Donavan, J. Tsubota, M. Kluss, P. Stebbens, and R. Butler, *Phys. Phase*, 69:944–955 (1989).

22. A. Hurwitz, *J. Neurosci. Nursing*, 21:180–184 (1989).
23. W. Barnes, J. Seiz, D. Kiel, R.J. Elble, and B.V. Manyam, *Arch. Phys. Med. Rehabil.*, 72:796 (1991).
24. D.E. Herman, J. Seitz, D. Kiel, W. Barnes, R. Elble, and B.V. Manyam, *Phys. Ther.*, 00:000–000 (1993).
25. R.B. Harris, L.F. Hughes, R.J. Elble, and B.V. Manyam, Tenth International Symposium on Parkinson's Disease 145 (1991).
26. L. Cote and G. Reidel, *Exercises for the Parkinson Patient with Hints for Daily Living*, Parkinson's Disease Foundation, New York.
27. R. Wechmann, *Be Active! A Suggested Exercise Program for People with Parkinson's Disease*, The American Parkinson's Disease Association, New York (1990).
28. S. Grillner, *Physiol. Rev.*, 12:183 (1975).
29. M.I. Lipshits, K. Mauritz, and K.E. Popov, *Fiziol Cheloveka*, 7:411–419 (1982).
30. J. Massion, *Exp. Brain Res.*, 67:645–650 (1984).
31. J.E. Brown and J.S. Frank, *Exp. Brain Res.*, 67:645–650 (1987).
32. C.D. Marsden, Presented at the American Academy of Neurology Annual Meeting, Boston (1991).
33. S. Tse and D.M. Bailey, *Am. J. Occup. Ther.*, 46:295–300 (1991).
34. W.C. Koller, S. Glatt, B. Vetere-Overfield, and R. Hassanein, *Clin. Neuropharmacol.*, 12:98–105 (1989).
35. B. Flewitt, R. Capildeo, and F.C. Rose, *Research Progress in Parkinson's Disease* (F.C. Rose and R. Capildeo, eds.), Pitman Medical, Tunbridge Wells, pp. 404–413 (1981).
36. S. Franklyn, S. Kohout, I.J. Stern, and M. Dunning, *Research Progress in Parkinson's Disease* (F.C. Rose and R. Capildeo, eds.), Pitman Medical, Tunbridge Wells, pp. 397–400 (1981).
37. L. Gauthier, S. Dalziel, and S. Gautheir, *Am. J. Occup. Ther.*, 41:360–365 (1987).
38. D.P. Colvin, G.G. Bishop, T.W. Engel, A.L. Patra, and C.J. Lord, *Adv. Bioeng.*, 20:195–198 (1991).
39. T. Piller, R. Dickstein, and Z. Smolinski, *J. Rehab. Res.*, 28:47–52 (1991).
40. S.D. Dowd, *Parkinson Rep.*, 12:4–5 (1991).
41. M.B. Robinson, *Equipment and Suggestions to Help the Patient with Parkinson's Disease in the Activities of Daily Living*, The American Parkinson's Disease Association, New York (1989).
42. R.M. Dubinsky, C. Gray, D. Husted, K. Busenbark, B. Vetere-Overfield, D. Wiltfong, D. Parrish, and W.C. Koller, *Neurology*, 41:517–524 (1991).
43. P. Madeley, J.L. Hulley, H. Wildgust, and R.H.S. Mindham, *J. Neurol. Neurosurg. Psychiatry*, 53:580–582 (1990).
44. J. Atarashi and E. Uchida, *Recent Adv. Res. Nerv. Syst.*, 3:871–882 (1950).
45. J.A. Logemann and H.B. Fisher, *J. Speech Hearing Disord.*, 46:348–352 (1981).
46. M. Oxtoby, *Parkinson's Disease and Their Social Needs*, Parkinson's Disease Society, London (1982).
47. A.G. Mlcoch, *Handbook of Parkinson's Disease* (W.C. Koller, ed.), Marcel Dekker, New York, pp. 181–207 (1987).

48. E.M.R. Critchley, *J. Neurol. Neurosurg. Psychiatry*, 44:751–758 (1981).
49. E.H. Lenneberg, *The Biological Foundations of Language*, Wiley, New York (1967).
50. R. Luchsinger and G.E. Arnold, *Voice-Speech-Language*, Constable, London (1965).
51. F.L. Darley, A.E. Aronson, and J.R. Brown, *J. Speech Hearing Res.*, 12:246–269 (1969).
52. N. Biary, P.A. Pimental, and P.W. Langenberg, *Neurology*, 38:255–258 (1988).
53. A.W. Downie, *J. Neurol. Neurosurg. Psychiatry*, 44:852–853 (1981).
54. S. Scott and F. Caird, *J. Neurol. Neurosurg. Psychiatry*, 46:140–144 (1982).
55. American Parkinson's Disease Association, *Speech Problems and Swallowing Problems in Parkinson's Disease*, American Parkinson's Disease Association, New York (1989).
56. G.R. Paulson and R.H. Tafrate, *Neurology*, 20:14–17 (1970).
57. D.M. Calne, D.G. Shaw, A.S.D. Spiers, and G.M. Stern, *Br. J. Radiol.*, 43:456–457 (1970).
58. M. Bushmann, S.M. Dobmeyer, L. Leeker, and J.S. Perlmutter, *Neurology*, 39:1309–1314 (1989).
59. E. Brown, G.M. Brown, O. Kofman, and B. Quarrington, *Am. J. Psychiatry*, 135:1552–1555 (1978).
60. R.G. Brown, M. Jahanshahi, N. Quinn, and C.D. Marsden, *J. Neurol. Neurosurg. Psychiatry*, 53:480–486 (1989).
61. W.C. Koller, B. Vetere-Overfield, A. Williamson, K. Busenbark, J. Nash, and D. Parrish, *Clin. Neuropharmacol.*, 13:461–463 (1990).
62. R.J. Uitti, C.M. Tanner, A.H. Rajput, C.G. Goetz, H.L. Klawans, and B. Thiessen, *Clin. Neuropharmacol.*, 12:375–383 (1989).
63. P.J. Karstaedt and J.H. Pincus, *Arch. Neurol.*, 49:149–151 (1992).
64. J.K. Tsui, S. Ross, K. Poulin, J. Douglas, D. Postnikoff, S. Calne, W. Woodward, and D.B. Calne, *Neurology*, 39:549–556 (1989).
65. E.M. Berry, J.H. Growdon, J.J. Wurtman, B. Caballero, and R.J. Wurtman, *Neurology*, 41:1295–1297 (1991).
66. J.H. Pincus and K. Barry, *Arch. Neurol.*, 44:270–272 (1987).
67. R. Mayeux, Y. Stern, A. Herman, L. Greenbaum, and S. Fahn, *Ann. Neurol.*, 20:6:727–730 (1985).
68. B.V. Manyam, *Textbook of Clinical Neuropharmacology*, 2nd edition (H.L. Klawans, C. Gaetz, C. Tanner, eds.), Raven Press, New York, pp. 297–306 (1992).
69. P. Allard, J. Dansereau, P.S. Thiry, G. Geoffroy, J.V. Raso, and M. Duhaime, *Can. J. Neurol. Sci.*, 9:105–111 (1982).

24

Cerebral Palsy

Susan T. Iannaccone

*University of Texas Southwestern Medical Center
Dallas, Texas*

INTRODUCTION

"The pediatric patient is not just a small adult." Many clinicians are familiar with the frequently remarkable recovery of children after serious brain injury. Because it is a developing organism, the child's brain possesses biological plasticity or capacity for repair thought to be greater than that of adult brain. Brain plasticity is difficult to define but is often mentioned when considering transplantation of fetal tissue (considered to be very plastic) to adult brain or spinal cord (nonplastic) [1,2]. It is assumed that after the second trimester of human gestation, neurons are no longer capable of regeneration, because of their lowered plasticity, but the exact threshold for regeneration is not known [3,4].

We should avoid confusing "neuronal plasticity" with the morphological and physiological pluripotentiality of embryonic cells. Buchwald [5] has classified plasticity into four forms: developing brain, aging brain, traumatized brain, and learning brain. She defines plasticity as the ability to undergo "structural–functional changes." Such change is most easily attributed to developing brain, which undergoes rapid, gross, and easily recognizable structural modifications. However, recent work has shown that learning in the adult mammalian brain has been associated with conformational changes in the calcium channel of certain pathways [6]. Neuronal change that occurs with normal aging or with trauma is still poorly understood [4,7]. The plasticity of the young human brain must affect its pattern of recovery and ultimate outcome after injury.

Thus, goals for rehabilitation of the child are different from those of the adult patient in several ways. These goals will change with age because they must take into consideration the developmental potential appropriate for the child's chronological age. The assessment of outcome must include an acknowledgement that physiological recovery and normal developmental processes continue during rehabilitation.

Treatment goals should also allow for normal physical growth during the rehabilitation process. The child's nutritional needs may require feeding assessments with more aggressive intervention than in adult patients. For example, children normally gain height and weight continuously until age 16–18 years. Assessment and intervention would be indicated when the child stops gaining weight and before he or she ceases linear growth.

The stress of neurological injury and chronic disability will affect the whole family over many years, with both psychological and financial burdens. Recovery or outcome for the child has been shown to be maximal when the family participates actively in the treatment program and receives professional help in coping with management issues.

In this chapter, we discuss the rehabilitation aspects of the most common chronic neurological disorder of childhood: cerebral palsy. Rehabilitation of head injuries and neuromuscular disorders is discussed elsewhere in this book. Many principles necessary for the rehabilitation of children with chronic neurological disorders do not change with diagnosis. These principles will be discussed in this chapter.

INCIDENCE/PREVALENCE

Cerebral palsy (CP) can be defined as a fixed motor deficit caused by an injury of the brain early in life that may or may not be associated with a cognitive deficit. Both prenatal and perinatal causes are known [8]. In the United States, hypoxic/ischemic encephalopathy secondary to premature delivery is a common identifiable cause of CP [9]. The incidence of CP is 14.1:1000 live births [10] and 20.9:1000 neonatal survivors with a birth weight less than 2000 g. In 1991, there were an estimated 274,000 Americans with CP [11].

CLASSIFICATION

CP may be classified according to cause: anoxic/ischemic encephalopathy, neonatal sepsis, intraventricular hemorrhage, intrauterine viral infection, or associated type of epilepsy with or without cognitive deficit. Neuroimaging studies often reveal residual abnormalities related to the original insult (Figure 1). A practical rehabilitation classification of CP is often based on the

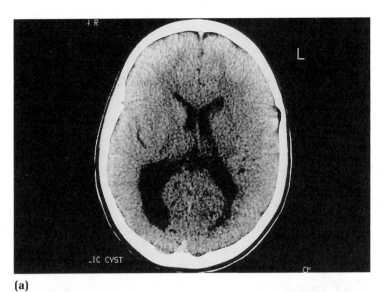

(a)

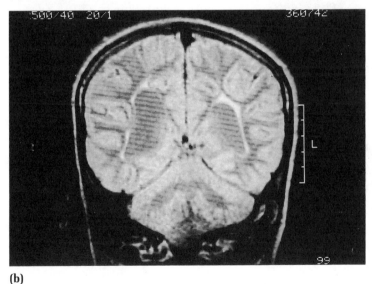

(b)

Figure 1 (a) Axial view of CT scan of the brain of a 9-year-old boy with static encephalopathy, spastic triparesis, and epilepsy. The lateral ventricles are asymmetrical and enlarged, suggesting cerebral atrophy. (b) Magnetic resonance imaging (T2-weighted) of the same brain in the coronal view indicates an abnormal signal in the periventricular white matter. These findings are consistent with periventricular leukomalacia secondary to premature delivery.

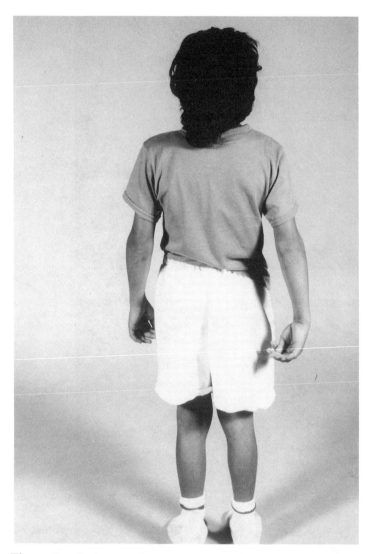

Figure 2   This boy was delivered at home in Mexico by a midwife. He experienced severe jaundice, according to his history but did not receive any specific treatment. He was developmentally delayed, had a sensory neural hearing loss, and decreased upward gaze. His father's main concern was the abnormal posturing on ambulation that affected all extremities, but especially the right upper. He also had variable muscle tone and pathologically brisk deep tendon reflexes. He was diagnosed as having kernicterus with dystonia.

type of motor deficit: which limbs are affected (hemiparesis, diparesis, triparesis, paraplegia); what type of muscle tone predominates (hypotonic, spastic); or whether there is an associated movement disorder (choreic, athetoid). Movement disorders may occur if the basal ganglia or lower brainstem nuclei were damaged, producing ataxia or chorea. Athetoid CP commonly occurred after hyperbilirubinemia. However, Rh incompatibility is now preventable, and this form of CP is rare (Figure 2).

ACUTE SEQUELAE

After the brain injury has occurred, the patient may suffer coma, cerebral edema, seizures, and pseudobulbar palsy. Decreased mental status in the presence of cerebral edema or seizure activity may be treatable and temporary. Such acute sequelae should be stabilized using standard medical therapy before embarking on a rehabilitation program, since the symptoms will interfere with the patient's attentiveness.

Pseudobulbar palsy may result in malnutrition as a result of decreased oral intake. Optimal nutritional status is critical to maximize the patient's ability to learn during therapy.

CHRONIC SEQUELAE

The chronic sequelae of cerebral palsy are lifelong and are the focus of the rehabilitation program. These include motor deficits, speech and swallowing disorders (usually secondary to pseudobulbar palsy), and the cognitive disorders that sometimes accompany CP. Children with CP are best served by a multidisciplinary group of professionals who are familiar with the complications of CP and their prevention/treatment.

Management of Motor Deficits

The motor deficit is the hallmark of CP. As noted above, the patient may be hypotonic, dystonic, rigid, or spastic. The character of muscle tone and the pattern of weakness reflect both the area of brain damage and the age of the patient. Many floppy infants with central hypotonia develop decorticate/decerebrate posture after infancy.

The upper motor neuron syndrome with increased muscle tone and abnormal stretch reflexes is the most visible impairment in most patients with CP. Depending on the severity, it may be the most stubborn neurological deficit to manage (Figure 3).

Physical Therapy

Physical therapy remains the most widely prescribed treatment for motor deficits. A commonly used method of physical therapy was derived from

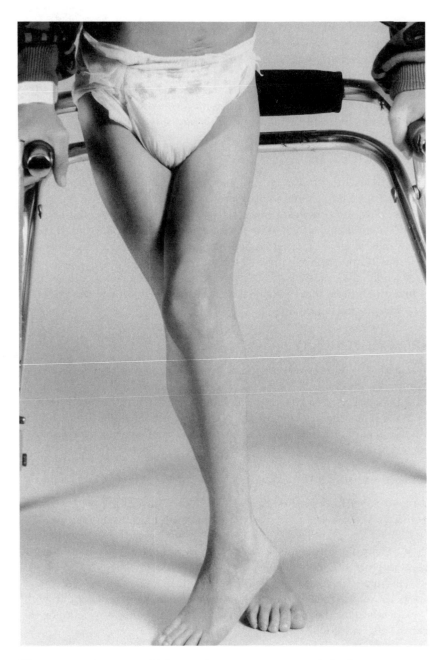

Figure 3 This 6-year-old boy with severe scissoring of the lower extremities requires a K walker to assist with ambulation.

Bobath and Bobath [12], whose theory was to increase stretch in antagonistic muscles so that spasticity is minimized and normal postural control can be achieved. The Bobath technique is now referred to as "neurodevelopmental therapy" (NDT). Position can also decrease extensor tone by inhibiting the tonic neck or other unopposed postural reflexes. Although many dollars, hours, and tears have been spent using this method, there are no *scientific* data to support its efficacy [13]. Almost no controlled trials have addressed whether certain subgroups of patients with CP may benefit more than others [14,15], and there are no data to indicate when or how much therapy is effective.

The Doman-Delacato method of therapy was developed based on a theory that the central nervous system must recapitulate the rostral–caudal phylogenic hierarchy of development before the goals of normal cognitive and motor skills can be achieved [16]. There is no scientific basis for this theory, nor is there any evidence that the stringent program of round-the-clock exercises is more effective than the more traditional range-of-motion protocols.

Despite controversies about the efficacy of various philosophies of therapy for cerebral palsy, there is excellent evidence that range-of-motion exercises and stretching can prevent and reverse some contractures. It is clear that stretching is useful only if done daily. If patients cannot do it themselves, someone with whom they live must do it. Therefore, parents should maintain primary responsibility for giving the child daily PT. The role of the therapist becomes that of monitor: Are the contractures improving? and are the parents using proper technique? Soon after a child has been enrolled in a physical therapy program, positive responses with increased socialization and rapid gain in developmental milestones are often noted. However, this response may be short-lived and could be the result of increased individual attention directed at the child [17,18].

Occupational Therapy

Early intervention programs (EIP), which are sometimes referred to as "infant stim programs," have become widespread in their application to the treatment of premature infants [19,20]. These programs are designed to encourage the social and language development of "high risk" infants (those who are premature, of low birth weight, or with neonatal asphyxia) by providing them early with a regular (weekly) developmental session. These sessions are usually conducted by occupational therapists, either in the home or in the therapist's office, and consist largely of directed play combined with NDT. The goals are to encourage social development while improving postural reflexes that are important for independent sitting and ambulation. A study of 134 infants discharged from a special care nursery (SCN) recently showed no advantage of weekly therapy [21]. In another study, low-birth-weight (LBW) infants who received neurodevelopmental therapy were no closer to normal control infants in function than LBW infants who did not receive therapy [22]. Russman [23] has reviewed the literature and concluded that the goals of EIP must be better defined before any judgment regarding its effectiveness can be made. There is a need for carefully controlled studies to compare infants who receive therapy with those who do not [24].

Medication

Several medications are available for the treatment of spasticity, the most widely used being diazepam and baclofen. Diazepam is probably safer for use in infants, but baclofen has been used for several years in older children without ill effects. Either drug requires close titration of response against adverse side effects, so the physician should begin treatment at a low dosage, with gradual increase while monitoring the degree of spasticity. As with physical therapy, a clear definition of the goals of treatment is necessary and an appropriate end point must be established. Treatment goals may include increased ease of diapering by elimination of scissoring, improved positioning during therapy sessions, or decreased frequency and severity of spasms. Many patients with CP are able to walk despite paraparesis because increased muscle tone allows them to bear weight on weak legs. Decrease in spasticity in these patients will lessen the ability to walk independently; thus, the use of medication should be conservative in ambulatory patients with CP.

In infants, diazepam 1 mg orally may be given every 12 hr and the frequency gradually increased to every 4–6 hr as needed. Diazepam frequently causes significant sedation and increases oral secretions, a potentially dangerous problem for children with pseudobulbar palsy. Baclofen should probably not be used in children under the age of 5 years and should be initiated orally at low dosages, such as 10 mg twice daily. Intrathecal baclofen seems safe and effective in adults and children with severe refractory spasticity in dosages of 25–100 μg [25].

Spinal Cord Stimulation

Waltz et al. [26] described their method of spinal cord stimulation in 1987, although the idea had been around since the discovery of electricity. Using a percutaneous technique developed in 1979, they introduced a multielectrode assembly through an epidural needle and threaded it to the C2 level [26]. This procedure was performed on 735 patients, of whom 212 had CP and ranged from 7 to 45 years of age. Seventy-three percent had "moderate to marked" improvement, but the authors' rating system and criteria for improvement were poorly documented and somewhat subjective. There is no systematic report of follow-up results, although in 5 patients described in the paper improvement persisted for 2, 3, 3, 5, and 7 years, respectively.

A double-blind study [27] of eight patients with CP failed to show any effect of spinal cord stimulation on spasticity. Waltz's method was used to implant electrodes in these patients between 11 and 18 years in age. Spasticity was evaluated before and after 4 consecutive months of continuous stimulation with a clinical rating system of functional and neurological status as well as neuropsychological testing. After 6 months' follow-up, 7 patients were no longer using the stimulator on a regular basis. None of the ratings improved after the spinal cord stimulation, in contrast to Waltz' conclusions that stimulation may improve all levels of functioning, including speech and frequency of seizures.

Cerebellar Stimulation

Chronic cerebellar stimulation (CCS) has fallen out of favor because of a lack of scientific evidence for its benefits. However, no controlled studies have been reported and it still has many proponents. A silicone-coated electrode mesh was applied over the surface of the anterior lobes of the cerebellum. Stimulation could be turned on or off by the patient or a parent, depending on the clinical state of the patient. The only "double-blind" studies to be published recently were single case reports [28] in which the patient was his or her own control. The patient was examined with and without the stimulator "on," while objective methods such as gait analysis were used to assess the effect of CCS. Now that computerized gait analysis is readily available, more controlled studies of CCS may be indicated.

Rhizotomy

Peacock and Staudt reviewed results of dorsal rhizotomy in 55 patients with CP and spasticity [29]. Their paper is an example of why this procedure has remained so controversial. The authors described their surgical methods and their goal: "to improve current functional performance," but they gave no measure of patients' function before or after surgery. Moreover, there were no control patients. It is difficult to separate the effect of surgery from that of the intensive physical therapy that usually followed postoperatively. We do know empirically that rhizotomy in ambulatory patients may result in such loss of tone that the patient loses the ability to stand [19]. Landau, in his editorial, reviewed the literature regarding this procedure, concluding that "to justify its use will require carefully controlled and persuasive objective evidence of its benefits" [30].

Assistive Devices and Orthoses

When appropriately utilized, assistive devices and orthoses may improve function for some patients. For a child with ataxia, crutches or a walker may improve balance. Upper or lower extremity orthoses may be used to inhibit tone or as a training device during certain stages of therapy. However, the limitations and disadvantages of orthoses must be understood. An orthosis will not stop a child from walking on his or her toes. The weight of orthoses will discourage some children from walking at all.

Mobility

Whenever possible, mobility for patients with CP should be consistent with the age-appropriate development of motor independence in able-bodied children. Methods to promote mobility include bracing to allow weight bearing, using a walker for added support, or using a wheelchair if needed. Standing frames may be helpful in preventing flexion contractures and promoting growth of long bones [31]. A properly fitting wheelchair should assist in maintaining good trunk and head alignment, preventing contractures (especially of the ankles), and improving function of the upper extremities [31–33]. Depending on the mental status of the patient, a motorized wheelchair may be introduced early so that the child develops independence of movement by the age of 2 years. Because of physical growth and motor maturation, it is important that mobility be reassessed on a regular basis. Wheelchair models should be adaptable to accommodate the growing child.

Orthopedic Surgery

Orthopedic surgery is not a treatment for CP or spasticity. It is a form of management for the complications of spasticity, such as joint contractures or limb deformities [34]. The neurologist should play an important role in helping define the goals of surgery and in determining the rationale for it. Since spasticity remains after surgery, any improvement that results may be temporary. Increased muscle tone may reproduce the deformity before the patient can achieve his or her goals. It is important for the patient and family not to have unrealistic expectations for reconstructive surgery.

Hip subluxation/dislocation is found in many children with CP, either early because of delayed ambulation or later because of spasticity and posturing. It is important to prevent subluxation to avoid intractable pain. This can be accomplished by soft tissue release, which will prevent dislocation. If there is not expectation for ambulation, frank dislocation generally does not require correction. However, older children frequently develop severe joint pain on motion or difficulty in positioning a dislocated hip. Surgical resection of the femoral head may be necessary to relieve this pain.

Scoliosis is a common deformity that occurs in CP, particularly if the patient has quadraparesis [35]. Unequal leg length during growth will tilt the pelvis and result in scoliosis in an ambulatory patient. Scoliosis is also common in patients with CP who are wheelchair dependent. When unchecked, progressive scoliosis will result in loss of pulmonary function and affect the patient's health and well-being. When scoliosis is not caused directly by spasticity, it is more amenable to surgical correction. Several types of spine instrumentation are used. Surgeons consider the degree of curve and rotation, underlying neurological disorder, and age and condition of the patient when choosing the type of instrumentation. Postoperative management is crucial for maintaining function; early weight bearing has been found to improve recovery times and to prevent loss of function secondary to muscle atrophy.

Management of Pseudobulbar Palsy

Pseudobulbar palsy occurs frequently in CP. It may be an early clue that the infant has suffered a cerebral insult. Early manifestations of pseudobulbar palsy include poor suck or uncoordinated suck, tongue thrusting, and dysphagia. The infant may require a long time to feed and appear disinterested, or he or she may choke and aspirate. When the mother attempts to breast feed first, the infant may present with failure to thrive because of poor weight gain secondary to inadequate nutrition.

Drooling

Drooling is particularly disturbing because it is socially distressful. Medications such as scopolamine [36] have been of some benefit. The patient is not producing an abnormal amount of saliva, but fails to swallow normally. Many patients are amenable to behavior modification, which should be stringent in order to succeed [37,38]. Some clinicians have used surgical divergence of the salivary duct, with variable results.

Dysphagia

A diagnosis of dysphagia may be documented by a modified barium video swallow, although this is not always necessary. The dysphagia usually improves as the infant grows, perhaps because of the increased mechanical advantage of a larger throat or because of maturation of central integration and control. Thus, temporary measures to improve oral feeding should be tried before more invasive methods such as gastrostomy. By increasing texture and seating and/or positioning the child correctly during and after the feeding, one can improve feedings significantly. Positioning is also helpful in preventing gastroesophageal (GE) reflux, a common problem among patients of all ages with CP [39].

Gastrostomy

Gastrostomy feedings should be instituted only if the above methods fail to maintain adequate nutrition or if the administration of drugs, particularly antiepileptic drugs (AEDs), has prevented good medical management [40,41]. The gastrostomy can now be performed with local anesthesia in a percutaneous procedure. The tube can be replaced with a "button" that keeps the gastrostomy closed but accessible at meal time for insertion of a tube. However, if a patient has GE reflux, the ostomy must be constructed with a Nissen procedure to prevent reflux. If the child develops oral control later, the gastrostomy may be removed.

Aspiration

Aspiration occurs frequently in patients with pseudobulbar palsy (Figure 4). A vigorous respiratory therapy program may be helpful in preventing pneumonia. Parents should undergo instruction in cardiopulmonary resuscitation and chest physiotherapy (CPT), and be instructed in the appropriate frequency of CPT, always avoiding treatments after feeding [42]. CPT just before a feeding may decrease the risk of aspiration by lessening secretions and preventing vomiting.

Dental Complications

Patients with pseudobulbar palsy may have serious dental complications as a result of not eating by mouth or secondary to bruxism [43]. A pedodontist with experience in treating patients with CP should be consulted to maintain oral hygiene and perform extractions when necessary.

Speech

Poor language development often accompanies pseudobulbar palsy and may be associated with oral apraxia. The speech pathologist can help to determine if the language delay is due to poor motor control or if there is an accompanying cognitive deficit. Speech therapy frequently begins in infancy with an attempt to develop oral sensation and motor control. As with physical therapy, controlled studies are difficult to perform because each patient's deficit may be unique. Most children seem to respond positively to speech therapy, which should be discontinued if the child does not enjoy the sessions. Older children who are unable to communicate verbally can learn to use communication boards or electronic devices [44]. Sign language may be introduced early as a means of learning the importance of symbols.

Cognitive Function

As stated above, EIPs may be helpful in encouraging social development in a child with CP who is at risk of becoming isolated because of language or motor deficit. Early socialization will help the child to make the transition to school, where he or she will be surrounded by other children and will face many challenges. Many schools will not accept children who are not toilet trained because of the increased requirement for personnel to maintain sanitation. Thus, one goal for the EIP or preschool may be to achieve independent

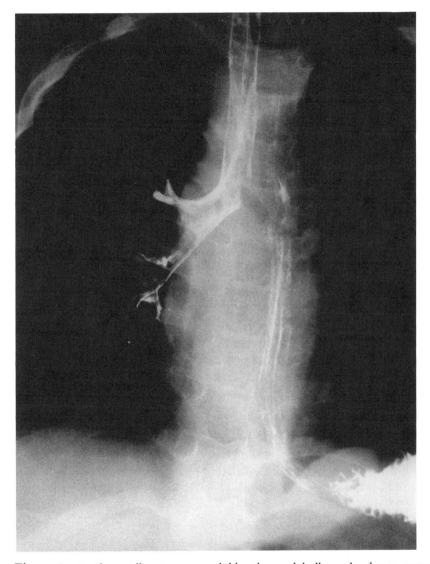

Figure 4 A video swallow in a young child with pseudobulbar palsy demonstrates aspiration of liquid barium into the bronchial tree.

toileting using behavior modification. This is probably a realistic goal for all except the most profoundly retarded persons.

School Placement

Psychometric testing should be obtained prior to school placement, usually around the age of 3–4 years. It should be done by a trained psychometrist under the guidance of a child psychologist and may indicate the need for more detailed neuropsychological testing. The latter is especially helpful if the child has exhibited a behavior disorder. Since the child's abilities and needs will change with age, the psychometrics should be repeated every 2 years throughout childhood.

Behavior

Several behavioral symptoms are common among children with CP secondary to ischemic/anoxic encephalopathy. These include aggressive/violent behavior, depression, attention deficit disorder (ADD), and sleep disorder. The child with encephalopathy is at higher risk for such problems both because of perinatal brain injury and because of psychosocial family stress associated with caring for and living with a child with chronic disability. Behavioral symptoms may be complicated by marital distress/divorce, codependency between mother and child, antiepileptic drug therapy, and economic stress. The evaluation of a patient with CP with a behavioral disorder is similar to that of any child with such symptoms. The behavior almost always will respond to a comprehensive program including parent education, behavior modification, counseling, and medication. It is important to recognize the adverse effects medication may have on behavior, and to consider discontinuing or changing medication if these interfere with the child's comprehensive therapeutic program.

Children with CP also exhibit normal childhood behavior. This occasionally takes parents by surprise and may be difficult to recognize if the patient has a language deficit. School phobia, fear of sleeping alone, and night terrors should be treated with behavior modification, as might be done in children without CP.

LONG-TERM PLANNING/GOALS

Most parents confronted with the "diagnosis" of CP will ask immediately, "What can we expect in the future?" The answer should not only be honest but also well-informed. The family should understand that CP is not a disease. This means that the child's neurological deficit will not worsen or progress, but may change with age, seizure frequency, or intercurrent illness. Some predictions can be offered, with the caveat that each child is an individual.

If the child is unable to sit independently by the age of 2.5–3 years, he or she is unlikely to become an independent ambulator (without assistive devices).

Although language development correlates well with intelligence, evaluation of cognition is necessary every 2 years throughout elementary school. Before the child finishes elementary school, a determination of long-range academic goals should be made so that planning can begin either for college or vocational school.

At the same time, an assessment of the child's possibility for attaining communication and life skills should be made. For instance, an attendant may be necessary for a patient who is quadriplegic and dependent for ADLs, although the patient may have the intellectual skills required for college.

Some discussion with parents regarding possible complications of CP should occur early after the diagnosis. Apparent worsening of the neurological deficit may be due to the development of epilepsy, or poor seizure control. Obesity may decrease a child's mobility by increasing load on a weak muscle. Poor compliance with an exercise program may increase flexion contractures or exacerbate posturing. Abdominal pain precipitating crying and abnormal posturing may occur after a Nissen procedure or indicate the presence of an ulcer.

Once the patient reaches high school, vocational counseling should begin. This can be done through vocational rehabilitation (VR) services that may be provided by the county or state [45]. There are also VR services available through the private sector. Such services include a comprehensive evaluation of the patient's/client's cognitive, neurological, social, and medical status. Recommendations are then made as to vocational training, placement in supported work environment, and residential arrangements. Success in the workplace and living independently seem to be more directly related to cognitive ability than to the motor deficit [11].

Although most persons with cerebral palsy have life-long disabilities, it is important for patients, parents, and professionals to understand that many persons with cerebral palsy enjoy productive and well-adjusted lives.

REFERENCES

1. G. Clowry, K. Sieradzan, and G. Vrbova, *Neuromusc. Disord.*, 1:87–92 (1991).
2. H. Hattori and C.G. Wasterlain, *Pediatr. Neurol.*, 6:219–228 (1990).
3. S.F. Farmer, L.M. Harrison, D.A. Ingram, and J.A. Stephens, *Neurology*, 41: 1505–1510 (1991).
4. R.L. Isaacson, *Clin. Perinatol.*, 17:67–75 (1990).
5. J.S. Buchwald, *Clin. Perinatol.*, 17:57–66 (1990).
6. D.N. Spinelli, *Clin. Perinatol.*, 17:77–82 (1990).

7. C.J. Woolf and E.T. Walters, *TINS*, *14*:74–78 (1991).
8. M.S. Scher, H. Belfar, J. Martin, and M.J. Painter, *Pediatrics*, *88*:898–906 (1991).
9. N. Paneth and J. Kiely, *The Epidemiology of the Cerebral Palsies* (F. Stanley and E. Alberman, eds.), Blackwell Scientific, Oxford, pp. 46–56 (1984).
10. E. Alberman, *The Epidemiology of the Cerebral Palsies* (F. Stanley and E. Alberman, eds.), Blackwell Scientific, Oxford, pp. 27–31 (1984).
11. *MMWR*, *40*:16–18 (1991).
12. K. Bobath and B. Bobath, *Management of the Motor Disorders of Children with Cerebral Palsy* (D. Scrutton, ed.), Blackwell Scientific, Oxford, pp. 6–18 (1984).
13. O. Goldkamp, *Arch. Phys. Med. Rehab.*, *65*:232–234 (1984).
14. F.B. Palmer, B.K. Shapiro, R.C. Wachtel, M.C. Allen, J.E. Hiller, S.E. Harryman, B.S. Mosher, C.L. Meinert, and A.J. Capute, *N. Engl. J. Med.*, *318*:803–808 (1988).
15. E. Tirosh and S. Rabino, *Am. J. Dis. Child.*, *143*:552–555 (1989).
16. D.J. Matthews, *Pediatr. Ann.*, *17*:762–764 (1988).
17. M.J. Craft, J.A. Lakin, R.A. Oppliger, G.M. Clancy, and D.W. Vanderlinden, *Dev. Med. Child Neurol.*, *32*:1049–1057 (1990).
18. S.V. Horton and D.C. Taylor, *Res. Dev. Disabil.*, *10*:363–375 (1989).
19. P.C. Ferry, *Arch. Neurol.*, *43*:281–282 (1986).
20. M. Rang and J. Wright, *Clin. Orthop. Rel. Res.*, *247*:55–60 (1989).
21. M.C. Piper, V.I. Kunos, D.M. Willis, B.L. Mazer, M. Ramsay, and K.M. Silver, *Pediatrics*, *78*:216–224 (1986).
22. M. Goodman, A.D. Rothberg, J.E. Houston-McMillan, P.A. Cooper, J.D. Cartwright, and M.A. VanDerVelde, *Lancet*, *1*:1327–1330 (1985).
23. B.S. Russman, *Arch. Neurol.*, *43*:282–283 (1986).
24. H.P. Parette and J.J. Hourcade, *Am. J. Occup. Ther.*, *38*:462–468 (1984).
25. A.L. Albright, A. Cervi, and J. Singletary, *JAMA*, *265*:1418–1422 (1991).
26. J.M. Waltz, W.H. Andreesen, and D.P. Hunt, *PACE*, *10*:180–204 (1987).
27. H. Hugenholtz, P. Humphreys, W.M.J. McIntyre, R.A. Spasoff, and K. Steel, *Neurosurgery*, *22*:707–714 (1988).
28. C. Hershler, A.R.M. Upton, H. Debruin, I. Burcea, R.N. King, and C. Zoghaib, *PACE*, *12*:861–869 (1989).
29. W.M. Landau and C.C. Hunt, *J. Child Neurol.*, *5*:174–178 (1990).
30. W.J. Peacock and L.A. Staudt, *J. Child. Neurol.*, *5*:179–185 (1990).
31. J. Noronha, A. Bundy, and J. Groll, *Am. J. Occup. Ther.*, *43*:507–512 (1989).
32. U. Myhr and L. VonWendt, *Dev. Med. Child. Neurol.*, *33*:246–256 (1991).
33. K. Katz, M. Liebertal, and E.H.W. Erken, *Dev. Med. Child. Neurol.*, *30*:222–226 (1988).
34. L.A. Koman, R.H. Gelberman, E.B. Toby, and G.G. Poehling, *Clin. Orthop. Rel. Res.*, *253*:62–74 (1990).
35. S.E. Koop, J.E. Lonstein, R.B. Winter, and F. Denis, *Dev. Med. Child. Neurol.*, *33*:19–20 (1991).
36. L.K. Siegel and M.A. Klingbeil, *Dev. Med. Child. Neurol.*, *33*:1013–1014 (1991).

37. R. Koheil, A.E. Sochaniwskyj, K. Bablich, D.J. Kenny, and M. Milner, *Dev. Med. Child. Neurol.*, *29*:19–26 (1987).
38. D. Reddihough, H. Johnson, M. Staples, I. Hudson, and H. Exarchos, *Dev. Med. Child. Neurol.*, *32*:985–989 (1990).
39. J.F. Bosma, *J. Neurol. Rehab.*, *4*:79–84 (1990).
40. K.D. Sanders, K. Cox, R. Cannon, D. Blanchard, J. Pitcher, P. Papathakis, L. Varella, and R. Maughan, *J. Parenter. Enteral Nutr.*, *14*:23–26 (1990).
41. G. Stringel, M. Delgado, L. Guertin, J.D. Cook, A. Maravilla, and H. Worthen, *J. Pediatr. Surg.*, *24*:1044–1048 (1989).
42. G.B. Mallory and P.C. Stillwell, *Arch. Phys. Med. Rehab.*, *72*:43–55 (1991).
43. P.L. Judd and D.J. Kenny, *J. Neurol. Rehab.*, *4*:85–96 (1990).
44. A. Arruabarrena, G. Buldain, L. Gardeazabal, E. Gomez, and J. Gonzalez, *J. Med. Eng. Technol.*, *13*:28–33 (1989).
45. P.H. Wehman, G. Revell, J. Kregel, J.S. Kreutzer, M. Callahan, and D. Banks, *Arch. Phys. Med. Rehab.*, *72*:101–105 (1991).

Index

About the Editors

David C. Good is an Associate Professor of Neurology and Director of Rehabilitation at the Bowman Gray School of Medicine of Wake Forest University, Winston-Salem, North Carolina. Formerly an Associate Professor of Medicine and Chief of the Neurorehabilitation Section at Southern Illinois University School of Medicine, Springfield, Illinois, Dr. Good is the author or coauthor of numerous professional papers, book chapters, and abstracts. He is a member of the American Academy of Neurology, the American Congress of Rehabilitation Medicine, and a certified member of the American Society of Neurorehabilitation, among others. Dr. Good received the B.S. degree (1970) in biochemistry and the M.D. degree (1974) from the University of Wisconsin—Madison.

James R. Couch, Jr., is a Professor in and Chairman of the Department of Neurology at the University of Oklahoma Health Sciences Center, Oklahoma City. The author or coauthor of numerous professional papers, Dr. Couch is a member of the American Neurologic Association and a Fellow of the American Academy of Neurology and the Stroke Council of the American Heart Association. He is a certified member of the American Society of Neurorehabilitation as well as a member of the American Association of University Professors of Neurology, among others. He has served on the boards of the American Academy of Neurology, the American Society of Neurorehabilitation, and the American Association of University Professors of Neurology. He received the B.S. degree (1961) in zoology from Texas A&M University, College Station, and the M.D. degree (1965) and the Ph.D. degree (1966) in physiology from Baylor University College of Medicine, Houston, Texas. Dr. Couch trained in neurology at Washington University School of Medicine, Saint Louis, Missouri, and was on the Faculty of Neurology at the University of Kansas School of Medicine, Kansas City, and Southern Illinois University School of Medicine, Springfield, prior to his present appointment.